VIROLOGY

Indianapolis, 27.3.1985

Gino

SECOND EDITION

VIROLOGY

EDITED BY

Wolfgang K. Joklik, D. Phil.

James B. Duke Distinguished Professor of Microbiology and Immunology
Chairman, Department of Microbiology and Immunology
Duke University Medical Center

ACC

APPLETON-CENTURY-CROFTS/ Norwalk, Connecticut

0-8385-9461-1

Notice: Our knowledge in the clinical sciences is constantly changing. As new information becomes available, changes in treatment and in the use of drugs become necessary. The author(s) and the publisher of this volume have taken care to make certain that the doses of drugs and schedules of treatment are correct and compatible with the standards generally accepted at the time of publication. The reader is advised to consult carefully the instruction and information material included in the package insert of each drug or therapeutic agent before administration. This advice is especially important when using new or infrequently used drugs.

85 86 87 88 89 90/10 9 8 7 6 5 4 3 2 1

Prentice-Hall International, Inc., London
Prentice-Hall of Australia, Pty. Ltd., Sydney
Prentice-Hall Canada, Inc.
Prentice-Hall of India Private Limited, New Delhi
Prentice-Hall of Japan, Inc., Tokyo
Prentice-Hall of Southeast Asia (Pte.) Ltd., Singapore
Whitehall Books Ltd., Wellington, New Zealand
Editora Prentice-Hall do Brasil Ltda., Rio de Janeiro
Prentice-Hall Hispanoamericana, S.A., Mexico

Library of Congress Cataloging in Publication Data
Main entry under title:

Virology.

Rev. ed. of: Principles of animal virology. c1980.
Includes bibliographies and index.
1. Virology. I. Joklik, Wolfgang K. II. Principles of animal virology. [DNLM: 1. Vertebrate Viruses. 2. Virus Diseases. QW 164 V189]
QR360.V512 1985 616'.0194 84-28299
ISBN 0-8385-9461-1

Cover Design: M. Chandler Martylewski

Cover photograph courtesy of Dr. Samuel Dales

PRINTED IN THE UNITED STATES OF AMERICA

Contributors

Wolfgang K. Joklik, D. Phil.
James B. Duke Distinguished Professor of Microbiology and Immunology
Chairman, Department of Microbiology and Immunology
Duke University Medical Center

David W. Barry, M.D.
Head, Department of Clinical Investigation and Virology
Burroughs-Wellcome Company
Associate Professor of Medicine
Duke University Medical Center

Cornelia L. Dekker, M.D.
Formerly Assistant Clinical Professor of Pediatrics
Duke University Medical Center
Presently Senior Clinical Research Scientist
Burroughs-Wellcome Company

Thomas E. Frothingham, M.D.
Professor of Pediatrics and Professor of Community Health Sciences
Duke University Medical Center

John D. Hamilton, M.D.
Associate Professor of Medicine
Duke University Medical Center

Samuel L. Katz, M.D.
Wilburt C. Davison Professor of Pediatrics
Chairman, Department of Pediatrics
Duke University Medical Center

Sandra N. Lehrman, M.D.
Formerly Clinical Assistant Professor of Pediatrics
Duke University Medical Center
Presently Senior Virologist
Burroughs-Wellcome Company

Catherine M. Wilfert, M.D.
Professor of Pediatrics and Professor of Clinical Virology
Duke University Medical Center

Contents

Preface

Virology occupies a unique position in contemporary biology. Many of the most important infectious agents that afflict humans, animals, and plants are viruses. Although viral infections cannot yet be cured—a rational system of antiviral chemotherapy, long a primary aim of virologists, is not yet at hand—conspicuous success has been achieved in preventing viral diseases by mobilizing the immune mechanism. The total elimination from the globe several years ago of the smallpox virus, for example, which has probably killed more human beings through the ages than any other infectious agent, represents one of the major triumphs of modern medicine. Interestingly, viruses that cause important human diseases are still being discovered. A case in point is provided by the various recently recognized human T cell leukemia virus (HTLV) species some of which are implicated in the pathogenesis of adult T cell leukemia (ATL), others in that of the acquired immune deficiency syndrome (AIDS).

The importance of viruses as infectious agents is matched by their importance as model systems for studies at the molecular level. The genomes of viruses are up to a million times smaller than the genomes of the cells in which they multiply; yet there is no doubt that the principles that govern the organization and expression of viral and cellular genetic information are the same. Indeed, studies of viruses as model systems have yielded a rich harvest of fascinating discoveries ranging from the demonstration of the existence of messenger RNA in 1959 to recently acquired, totally unexpected and surprising insight into the arrangement of genetic material and the nature of the promoters and enhancers that control gene expression during normal development and differentiation. Work with viruses has also led to the discovery of certain cellular genes, the oncogenes, inappropriate transcriptional activation of which appears to be the primary and fundamental cause of uncontrolled growth that, unless checked by the immune system, results in cancer.

Virology provides an important conceptual framework for biology students. This textbook, which represents the basic and clinical virology sections of the 18th edition of *Zinsser Microbiology*, is intended for advanced undergraduates who plan to proceed to graduate and medical school, graduate students in cell and molecular biology, and medical students. It comprises two sections: one discusses the biochemistry, molecular biology, and genetics of animal viruses (and also includes a chapter on the molecular virology of bacteriophages), and another describes the viruses that are pathogenic for man, the nature and symptoms of the diseases that they cause, and how to treat and prevent such diseases.

Regarding the bibliography, we have elected not to reference specific statements in the text, but have appended to each chapter a list of recent reviews and important original papers. The former will quickly guide readers to any specific aspect of virology they wish to pursue; the latter makes available the detailed considerations and circumstances that generated key discoveries. Many of the papers cited are now—or no doubt will soon become—"classics." This material should be of particular benefit to lecturers and instructors.

The list of individuals who helped produce this volume is long, and we are profoundly indebted to them. We would especially like to thank our many colleagues who permitted us to use illustrative material and who almost invariably supplied us with original photographs, and the many publishers who allowed us to reproduce previously published material. We would also like to thank the many artists who designed and drew the innumerable charts and graphs, and all the secretaries who cheerfully typed and retyped the manuscript. Finally, we wish to express our appreciation to the staff of Appleton-Century-Crofts for their very efficient cooperation in producing this book.

Wolfgang K. Joklik
David W. Barry
Cornelia L. Dekker
Thomas E. Frothingham
John D. Hamilton
Samuel L. Katz
Sandra N. Lehrman
Catherine M. Wilfert

SECTION I

BASIC VIROLOGY

CHAPTER 1

The Nature, Isolation, and Measurement of Animal Viruses

Many important infectious diseases that afflict mankind are caused by viruses. Some are important because they are often fatal; among such are rabies, smallpox, poliomyelitis, hepatitis, several hemorrhagic fevers, and some encephalitic diseases. Others are important because they are very contagious and cause acute discomfort; among such are influenza, the common cold, measles, mumps, and chickenpox, as well as respiratory–gastrointestinal disorders. Still other viruses, such as rubella and cytomegalovirus, can cause congenital abnormalities, and finally there are viruses that can cause tumors and cancer in animals and also in humans.

There is little that can be done to interfere with the growth of viruses, since they multiply within cells, using the cells' synthetic capabilities. Only a limited number of highly specialized reactions are under their own control. It is hoped that their selective inhibition will form the basis for a rational system of antiviral chemotherapy, thereby permitting virus diseases to be brought under effective control, just as antibiotics have brought most bacterial diseases under control.

In addition to their medical importance, viruses provide the simplest model systems for many basic problems in biology. The reason is that viruses are essentially small segments of genetic material encased in protective shells. Since the information encoded in viral genomes differs from that in host cell genomes, viruses afford unrivaled opportunities for the study of the mechanisms that control the replication and expression of genetic material. Knowledge of these mechanisms is fundamental to an understanding of the development and operation of differentiated functions in higher organisms and is, therefore, directly applicable to the practice of medicine and the improvement of human welfare.

Historical Background

There are three major classes of viruses: animal viruses, plant viruses, and bacterial viruses. Since knowledge concerning each of these classes has accumulated along distinctive lines, extensive specialization has developed. Bacterial viruses are, therefore, dealt with only briefly in this book, and plant viruses are not considered at all. Yet discoveries made concerning each of these classes of viruses have influenced profoundly our understanding of the nature of each of the others.

The existence of viruses became evident during the closing years of the 19th century when, as the result of newly acquired expertise in the handling of bacteria, the infectious agents of numerous diseases were being isolated. For some infectious diseases this proved to be an elusive task until it was realized that the agents causing them were smaller than bacteria. Iwanowski, in 1892, was probably the first to record the transmission of an infection (tobacco mosaic disease) by a suspension filtered through a bacteria-proof filter. This was followed in 1898 by similar experiments of Löffler and Frosch concerning foot-and-mouth disease of cattle. Beijerinck (1898) considered the infectious agents in bacteria-free filtrates to be living but fluid—that is, nonparticulate—and introduced the term "virus" (Latin, poison) to describe them. It quickly became clear, however, that viruses were particulate, and the term "virus" became the operational definition of infectious agents smaller than bacteria and unable to multiply outside living cells. In 1911 Rous discovered a virus that produced malignant tumors in chickens, and during World War I Twort and d'Herelle independently discovered the viruses that multiply in bacteria, the bacteriophages.

During the next 25 years the experimental approaches in the three areas of virology diverged. Plant viruses proved easy to obtain in large amounts, thus permitting extensive chemical and physical studies. This work first led to the demonstration that plant viruses consist only of nucleic acid and protein and culminated in the crystallization of tobacco mosaic virus by Stanley in 1935. This feat evoked great astonishment, since it cut across preconceived ideas concerning the attributes of living organisms and demonstrated that agents able to reproduce in living cells behaved under certain conditions as typical macromolecules.

Work with bacteriophages concentrated on their clinical application. It was hoped that bacteria could be destroyed inside the body by injecting appropriate bacteriophages. Their activity in vivo, however, never matched their activity in vitro, most probably because they are eliminated efficiently from the bloodstream.

Work with animal viruses concentrated on the pathogenesis of virus infections and on epidemiology. Throughout this period, fundamental studies on animal cell–virus interactions were severely hampered by the absence of rapid and efficient techniques for quantitating viruses. The only method then available was the expensive and time-consuming serial dilution end point method, using animals (p. 10).

Around the year 1940 came several breakthroughs. First, the advent of electron microscopy permitted visualization of viruses for the first time. As will become evident, not only is morphology an important criterion of virus classification, but the study of the morphology of viruses has also had a profound impact on our understanding of their behavior and function. Second, techniques for purifying certain animal viruses were being perfected, and a group of workers at the Rockefeller Institute headed by Rivers carried out some excellent chemical studies on vaccinia virus. Third, Hirst discovered that influenza virus agglutinates chicken red cells. This phenomenon, hemagglutination, was rapidly developed into an accurate method for quantitating myxoviruses, as a result of which this group of viruses became, in the 1940s, the most intensively investigated group of animal viruses. Finally, this period marked the beginning of the modern era of bacterial virology. Until then the interaction of bacteriophages with bacteria had been analyzed principally in terms of populations rather than at the level of a single virus particle interacting with a single cell. This conceptual block was removed by Ellis and Delbrück's study of the one-step growth cycle, as a result of which the bacteriophage–bacterium system became extraordinarily amenable to experimentation. Indeed, during the past three decades, many of the major advances in molecular biology have resulted from work in the bacteriophage field. Among these are the demonstration that initiation of virus infection involves the separation of viral nucleic acid and protein, the demonstration that the virus genome can become integrated into the genome of the host cell, the discovery of messenger RNA, and elucidation of the factors that control initiation and termination of both transcription and translation of genetic information.

In animal virology, rapid advances followed the development, in the late 1940s, of techniques for growing animal cells in vitro. Strains of many types of mammalian cells can now be grown in media of defined composition. As a result, animal cell–virus interactions can now be analyzed with the same techniques that have proved so powerful in the case of bacteriophages.

The Nature of Viruses

Viruses are a heterogeneous class of agents. They vary in size and morphology; they vary in chemical composition; they vary in host range and in the effect that they have on their hosts. There are certain characteristics, however, that are shared by all viruses:

1. Viruses consist of a genome, either RNA or DNA, that is surrounded by a protective protein shell. Frequently this shell is itself enclosed within an envelope that contains both protein and lipid.
2. Viruses multiply only inside cells. They are absolutely dependent on the host cells' synthetic and energy-yielding apparatus. They are parasites at the genetic level.

3. The multiplication of viruses involves as an initial step the separation of either their genomes or their nucleocapsids from their protective shells (see below).

In essence, therefore, viruses are nucleic acid molecules that can enter cells, replicate in them, and code for proteins capable of forming protective shells around them.

Given this definition of viruses, are they to be regarded as living organisms or as lifeless arrangements of molecules? The answer to this question depends on whether one is concerned with viruses as extracellular suspensions of particles or as infectious agents. Isolated virus particles are arrangements of nucleic and protein molecules with no metabolism of their own; they are no more active than isolated chromosomes. Within cells, however, virus particles are capable of reproducing their own kind manyfold by virtue of precisely regulated sequences of reactions. Considered in this light, viruses may indeed be said to possess at least some of the attributes of life. Such terms as "organism" and "living," however, are not really applicable to viruses. It is preferable to refer to viruses as being functionally active or inactive, rather than living or dead.

The Origin of Viruses

The question of the origin of viruses poses a fascinating problem. The two likeliest hypotheses are (1) viruses are the products of regressive evolution of free-living cells. An evolutionary pathway of this type has been suggested for mitochondria, which still retain vestiges of cellular organization as well as a mechanism for replicating, transcribing, and translating genetic information. The largest animal viruses, the poxviruses, are so complex that one could imagine them also to be derived from a cellular ancestor. (2) Viruses are derived from cellular genetic material that has acquired the capacity to exist and function independently. Nowadays the latter hypothesis is considered much more likely for all viruses with the possible exception of poxviruses.

The Characteristics of Cultured Animal Cells

The medical practitioner should understand not only how viruses affect the patient as a whole but also how viruses interact with cells. This understanding can be acquired far more readily by studying isolated infected cells than by examining infected cells in the intact organism. Animal virology provided the main impetus for the development of tissue culture—the technique of growing cells in vitro. Tissue culture is now used extensively in many fields of biologic and biomedical research. Since knowledge concerning the normal cell is crucial to an understanding of the virus–cell interaction, we will first examine briefly the characteristics of animal cells cultured in vitro.

The Establishment of Animal Cell Strains

Cells of many organs can be grown in vitro. As a rule, small pieces of the tissue in question are dissociated into single cells by treatment with a dilute solution of trypsin, and a suspension of the cells is then placed into a flask, bottle, or Petri dish. There the cells attach to the flat surface, and provided that they are supplied with a growth medium, they multiply. The essential constituents of a growth medium are physiologic amounts of 13 essential amino acids and 9 vitamins, salts, glucose, and a buffering system that generally consists of bicarbonate in equilibrium with an atmosphere containing about 5 percent carbon dioxide. This medium is supplemented to the extent of about 5 percent with serum, the source of which is not predicated by the species from which the cells were derived; calf and fetal calf serum are the two most commonly employed. Antibiotics, such as penicillin and streptomycin, are also usually added in order to minimize the growth of bacterial contaminants, and a dye, such as phenol red, is generally included as a pH indicator. This medium, or more complex versions of it, will permit most cell types to multiply with a division time of 24 to 48 hours.

When cells are brought into contact with a surface, they generally attach firmly and flatten so as to occupy the maximum surface area. The only time when they are not maximally extended is during mitosis, when they become round and are therefore easily dislodged from the substratum. Cells multiply until they occupy all available surface area—that is, until they are confluent—but no further. The reason for this is that cells cease dividing when they make contact with neighboring cells, a phenomenon known as "contact inhibition" (Chap. 8).

Animal cells can be cloned just like bacterial cells, although the efficiency of cloning is frequently less than 100 percent. Numerous genetically pure cell strains are now available. They fall into two morphologic categories, epithelial cells with a polygonal outline and fibroblasts with a narrow spindle-like shape (Fig. 1-1).

The first cultures after tissue dispersion are known as "primary cultures." When such cultures are confluent they are passaged by dislodgment from the surface by treatment with trypsin or the chelating agent ethylene diamine tetraacetate (EDTA) and reseeding into several new containers, in which they form secondary cultures. Passaging can be continued in this manner, provided that an adequate supply of growth medium is supplied at regular intervals.

The overall properties of cell strains are generally stable on continuous culturing. However, mutations occur constantly, so that one particular mutant, or variant, usually emerges as the dominant population component under

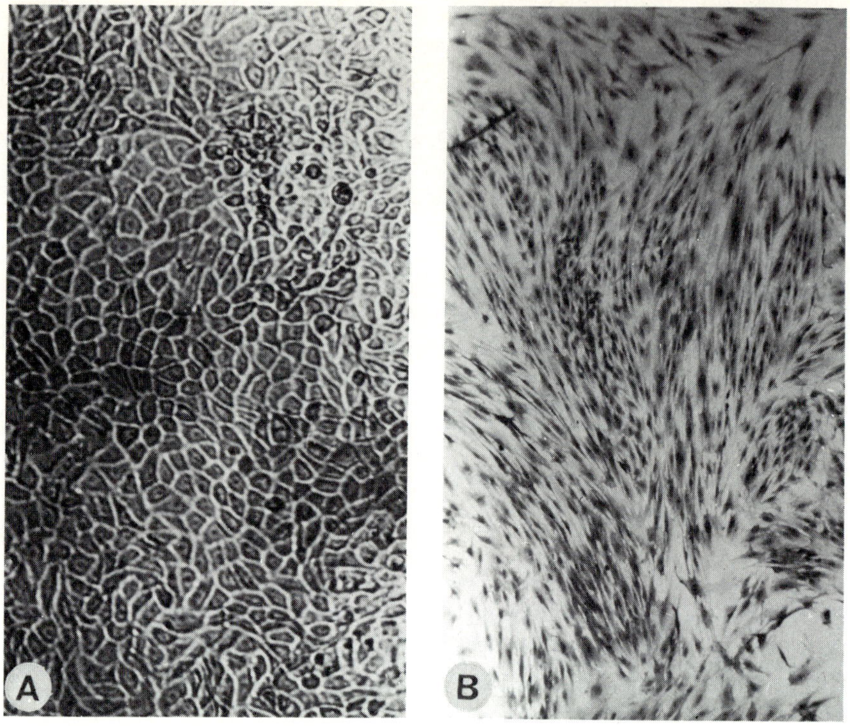

Figure 1-1. Cultured mammalian cells. **A.** Unstained monkey kidney cells, which exhibit a typical epithelioid morphology. **B.** Chick embryo fibroblasts (Giemsa stain). Note characteristic spindle shape and orderly alignment. (***A*** *from Eagle and Foley: Cancer Res 18: 1017, 1958;* ***B*** *courtesy of Dr. R.E. Smith.)*

any given set of conditions. As a result, the same cell strain cultured in two different laboratories may exhibit detectable phenotypic differences.

The Multiplication Cycle

The multiplication of each individual cell conforms to a regular pattern, which can be thought of as a cycle (Fig. 1-2). According to this scheme, the interval between successive mitoses is divided into three periods: the G1 period that precedes DNA replication, the S period during which DNA replicates, and the G2 period during which the cell prepares for the next mitosis. RNA and protein are not synthesized while mitosis proceeds—that is, during metaphase—but are otherwise synthesized throughout the multiplication cycle. Nongrowing cells are usually arrested in the G1 period; the resting state is often referred to as G0 (G zero).

Under conditions of normal growth, the individual cells of a growing culture pass through this multiplication cycle in an unsynchronized fashion, so that cells at all stages of the cycle are always present. It is, however, possible to synchronize cells so that they multiply in step for several generations. Synchronized cell cultures are useful in studies of the reactions that are essential for progression through the multiplication cycle.

The Aging of Cell Strains

Cells derived from normal tissues cannot be passaged indefinitely. Instead, after about 50 passages, which generally occupy about 1 year, their growth rate inevitably begins to slow. The amount of time that they spend in G0 following each mitosis gradually increases, fewer and fewer cells enter the S period, and the cells' karyotype (that is, their chromosomal complement) changes from the euploid (diploid) pattern characteristic of normal cells to an aneuploid one, characterized by the appearance of supernumerary chromosomes, chromosome fragments, and chromosomal aberrations (that is, changes in the structure of individual chromosomes). Finally, the cell strain dies out. Loss of cell strains in this manner is generally guarded against by growing large numbers of cells during the early passages and storing them at −196C, the boiling point of liquid nitrogen.

Continuous Cell Lines

While cells derived from normal tissues have the properties described thus far, malignant tissues give rise to aneuploid cell lines that have an infinite life span and are referred to as "established cell lines." Infrequently such

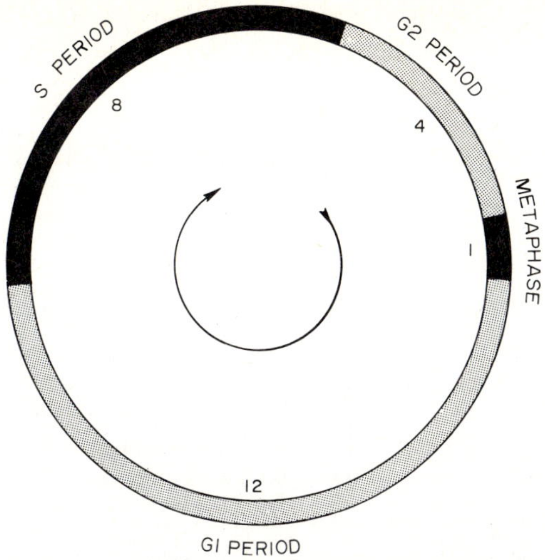

Figure 1-2. The multiplication cycle of mammalian cells. The duration of the cycle illustrated here is 25 hours; the average lengths (in hours) of the individual periods is indicated by the numbers inside the cycle.

cell lines seem to arise from euploid cell strains, but the possibility that malignant or premalignant cells were not present originally is difficult to rule out. In addition to being aneuploid and immortal, such cell lines usually have two other significant properties: they form tumors when transplanted into animals, and they can grow in suspension culture like bacteria. Cells growing in suspension are used extensively for studies of virus multiplication, since they are easier to handle experimentally than cells growing as monolayers.

Patterns of Macromolecular Biosynthesis

Since virus multiplication consists essentially of nucleic acid and protein synthesis, a brief description of the patterns of macromolecular synthesis in animal cells is relevant. The essential feature of the animal cell is its compartmentalization. The DNA of the animal cell is restricted to the nucleus at all stages of the cell cycle except during metaphase, when no nucleus exists. All RNA is synthesized in the nucleus. Most of it remains there, but messenger RNA and transfer RNA migrate to the cytoplasm. Ribosomal RNA is synthesized in the nucleolus; the two ribosomal subunits are assembled partly in the nucleolus and partly in the nucleus, and then they also migrate to the cytoplasm. All protein synthesis proceeds in the cytoplasm. The only exception to this brief summary concerns the mitochondria, which contain DNA-synthesizing, RNA-synthesizing, and protein-synthesizing systems of their own and which are located only in the cytoplasm.

The Detection of Animal Viruses

The presence of viruses is recognized by the manifestation of some abnormality in host organisms or host cells. In the organism, symptoms of virus infection vary widely, from inapparent infections (detectable only by the formation of antibody), the development of local lesions, or mild disease characterized by light febrile response to progressively more severe disease culminating in death. In cells, the symptoms of virus infection vary from changes in morphology and growth patterns to cytopathic effects, such as rounding, breakdown of cell organelles, the development of inclusion bodies, and general necrotic reactions, finally resulting in complete disintegration.

The Isolation of Animal Viruses

Many techniques have been developed for isolating viruses. The source of virus may be excreted or secreted material, the bloodstream, or some tissue. Samples are collected and, unless processed immediately, are sheltered from heat, preferably by storage at −70C, the temperature of dry ice. If necessary, a suspension is then prepared by grinding or sonicating in the presence of cold buffer solution, and this is then centrifuged in order to remove large debris and contaminating microorganisms.

This suspension is then tested for the presence of virus in several ways. First, it is injected back into the original host species in order to determine whether the first noted abnormality is produced. Second, the suspension is injected into other animals in order to establish whether there exist more susceptible hosts in which the disease develops more rapidly, more severely, or in a more easily recognizable manner. Newborn or suckling animals (often mice or hamsters) or developing chick embryos are hosts that permit many viruses to multiply more extensively than do adult animals and are accordingly widely used for virus isolation. Third, a search is conducted for a cultured animal cell strain or line in which the virus will multiply well, so that it may be isolated and characterized. Finally, cells are needed in which the virus rapidly elicits readily observable cytopathic effects and which can therefore be used to assay it.

The final stage of the isolation procedure is passage at limiting dilution in order to ensure that only a single unique virus is being isolated. This may be accomplished either by limiting serial dilution, when the virus suspension is diluted to such an extent that only one out of several aliquots inoculated gives a positive response, or by plaque isolation (p. 9). The latter is preferable, since plaques originate from single virus particles, just as bacterial colonies originate from single bacterial cells.

While virus isolation from severely diseased hosts may present no difficulty, it may be a formidable task if the original source is merely suspected of containing a small amount of virus. As a result, no symptoms may result when the initial virus suspension is inoculated into the various test systems. In such cases one generally resorts to so-called blind passaging, in the hope that gradual enrichment of virus will occur. In this procedure, cells are disrupted several days after inoculation even if they appear healthy and unaltered, and an extract of them is inoculated into fresh cells. This is repeated several times until symptoms appear. It is important that this procedure be adequately controlled by passaging extracts of uninfected cells under the same conditions, since animal cells are known to harbor latent viruses that may be induced to multiply and that may then be mistaken for the etiologic agent of whatever condition is under study.

Adaptation and Virulence

During the isolation of viruses, there may emerge variants capable of multiplying more efficiently in the host cells used for this purpose than the original wild-type virus. This phenomenon, which is known as "adaptation," has as its basis the selection of spontaneous mutants that constantly arise during virus multiplication. These mutants multiply more efficiently in the cells used for isolating the virus than in the cells of the original infected tissue. Such variants damage the original host less severely than the wild-type virus and are therefore said to be less "virulent." Viruses are often purposely adapted in order to alter growth and virulence characteristics. An example is provided by the attenuated vaccine virus strains, which are obtained by repeated passaging of virus virulent for one host in some different host, until virus strains with decreased virulence for the original host are selected.

The Measurement of Animal Viruses

Viruses are measured by several methods that can be divided into two categories. First, viruses may be measured as infectious units, that is, in terms of their ability to infect, multiply, and produce progeny. Second, viruses may be measured in terms of the total number of virus particles, irrespective of their function as infectious agents.

Measurement of Viruses as Infectious Units

Measurement of the amount of virus in terms of the number of infectious units per unit volume is known as titration. There are several ways of determining the titer of a virus suspension, all of them involving infection of host or target cells in such a way that each particle that causes productive infection elicits a recognizable response.

Plaque Formation

In this method a series of monolayers of susceptible cells are inoculated with small aliquots of serial dilutions of the virus suspension to be titrated. Wherever virus particles infect cells, progeny virus particles are produced and released and then immediately infect adjoining cells. This process is repeated until, after a period ranging from 2 to 12 days or more, there develop areas of infected cells that

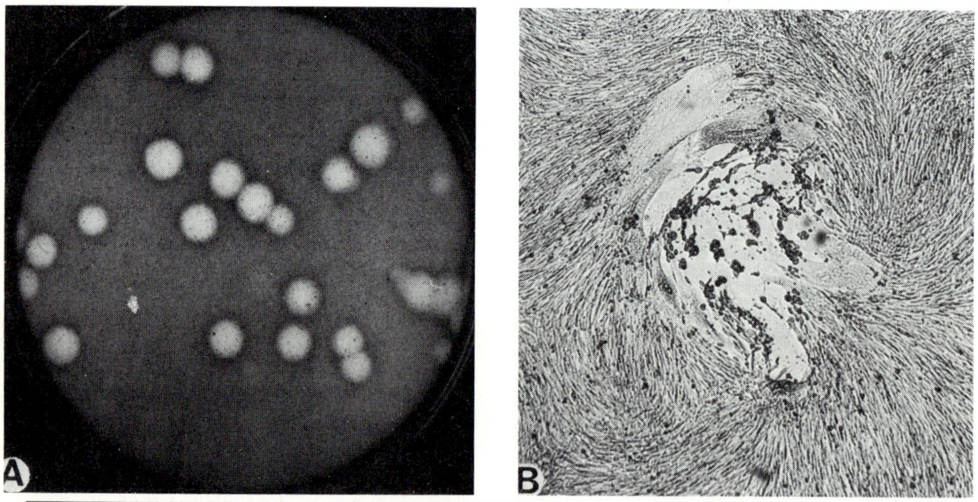

Figure 1-3. Virus plaques. **A.** Plaques of influenza virus on monolayers of chick embryo cells, 4 days after inoculation. The monolayers were stained with neutral red on day 3. **B.** Photograph showing the microanatomy of a herpesvirus plaque on BHK 21 cells. (***A*** *courtesy of Dr. G. Appleyard,* ***B*** *courtesy of Dr. S. Moira Brown.)*

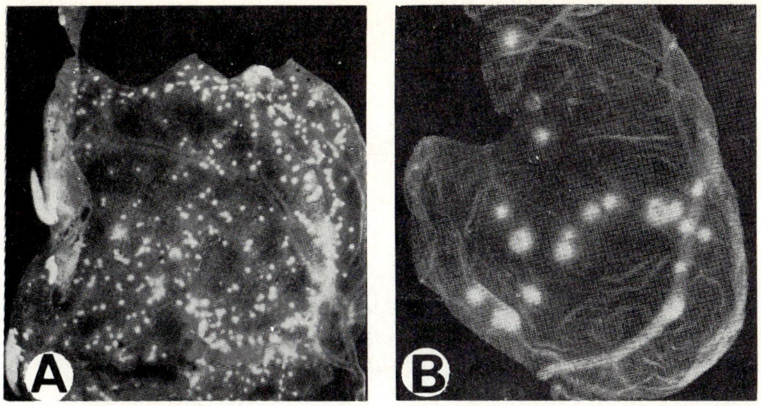

Figure 1-4. Pocks on the chorioallantoic membrane of the developing chick embryo. The membrane is cut out 2 or 3 days after inoculation, washed, and spread on a flat surface. **A.** Variola virus. **B.** Vaccinia virus. *(From Kempe: Fed Proc 14:468, 1955.)*

can be seen with the naked eye. These are called "plaques." In order to ensure that progeny virus particles liberated into the medium do not diffuse away and initiate separate (or secondary) plaques, agar is frequently incorporated into the medium.

The fundamental prerequisite for this method of enumerating infectious units is that the infected cells must differ in some way from noninfected cells; for example, they must either be completely destroyed, become detached from the surface on which they grow, or possess staining properties different from those of normal cells. In practice, the most common method of visualizing plaques is to apply the vital stain neutral red to infected cell monolayers after a certain number of days and to count the number of areas that do not stain (Fig. 1-3). Titers are expressed in terms of numbers of plaque-forming units (PFU) per milliliter.

There is a linear relationship between the amount of virus and the number of plaques produced; that is, the dose–response curve is linear. This indicates that each plaque is caused by a single virus particle. The virus progeny in each plaque therefore are clones, and virus stocks derived from single plaques are said to be "plaque purified." Plaque purification is an important technique for isolating genetically pure virus strains.

Plaque formation is often the most desirable method of titrating viruses. It is economical of cells and virus, as well as technically simple. However, not all viruses can be measured in this way, because there may be no cells that develop the desired cytopathic effects. For these viruses, alternative titration methods must be used.

Pock Formation

Many viruses cause macroscopically recognizable foci of infection or lesions on the choriollantoic membrane of the developing chick embryo. This membrane may be used in a manner similar to the cell monolayers employed for plaque assay. The main advantage is ready availability, wide virus susceptibility, and ease of handling. The main disadvantage is variation in virus susceptibility among different eggs of even the same hatch, so that a larger number of eggs than cultured cell monolayers is necessary to attain the same level of statistical significance. The lesions caused by viruses are known as pocks and are generally recognizable as opaque white or red areas caused by cell disintegration, migration, and proliferation, as well as edema and hemorrhage (in the case of red pocks) (Fig. 1-4). The actual titration is carried out as described for plaques, with enumeration of pocks taking the place of counting plaques.

Focus Formation

Many tumor viruses do not destroy the cells in which they multiply and, therefore, produce no plaques. However, they cause cells to change morphology and to multiply at a faster rate than uninfected cells. As a result, transformed cells develop into foci that gradually become large enough to be visible to the naked eye (Fig. 1-5). Assay by focus

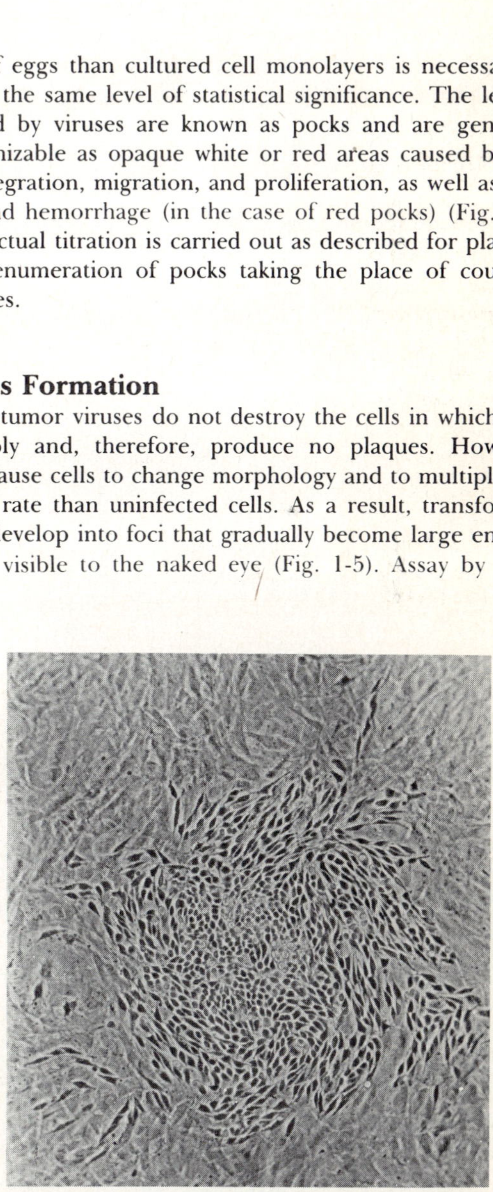

Figure 1-5. Focus of NRK (normal rat kidney) cells transformed by Kirsten murine sarcoma virus. × 200. *(Courtesy of Dr. S.A. Aaronson.)*

formation (counting the number of focus-forming units, or FFU) is analogous to assay by plaque and pock formation.

The Serial Dilution End Point Method

Although many viruses destroy cells, they do not produce the type of cytopathic effects necessary for visible plaque formation. Such viruses may be titrated by means of the serial dilution end point method. In this method serial dilutions of virus suspensions are inoculated into cell monolayers, which are then incubated until the cell sheet shows clear signs of cell destruction (Fig. 1-6). The end point is that dilution that gives a positive (cell-destroying) reaction, and the titer is calculated assuming that the last positive

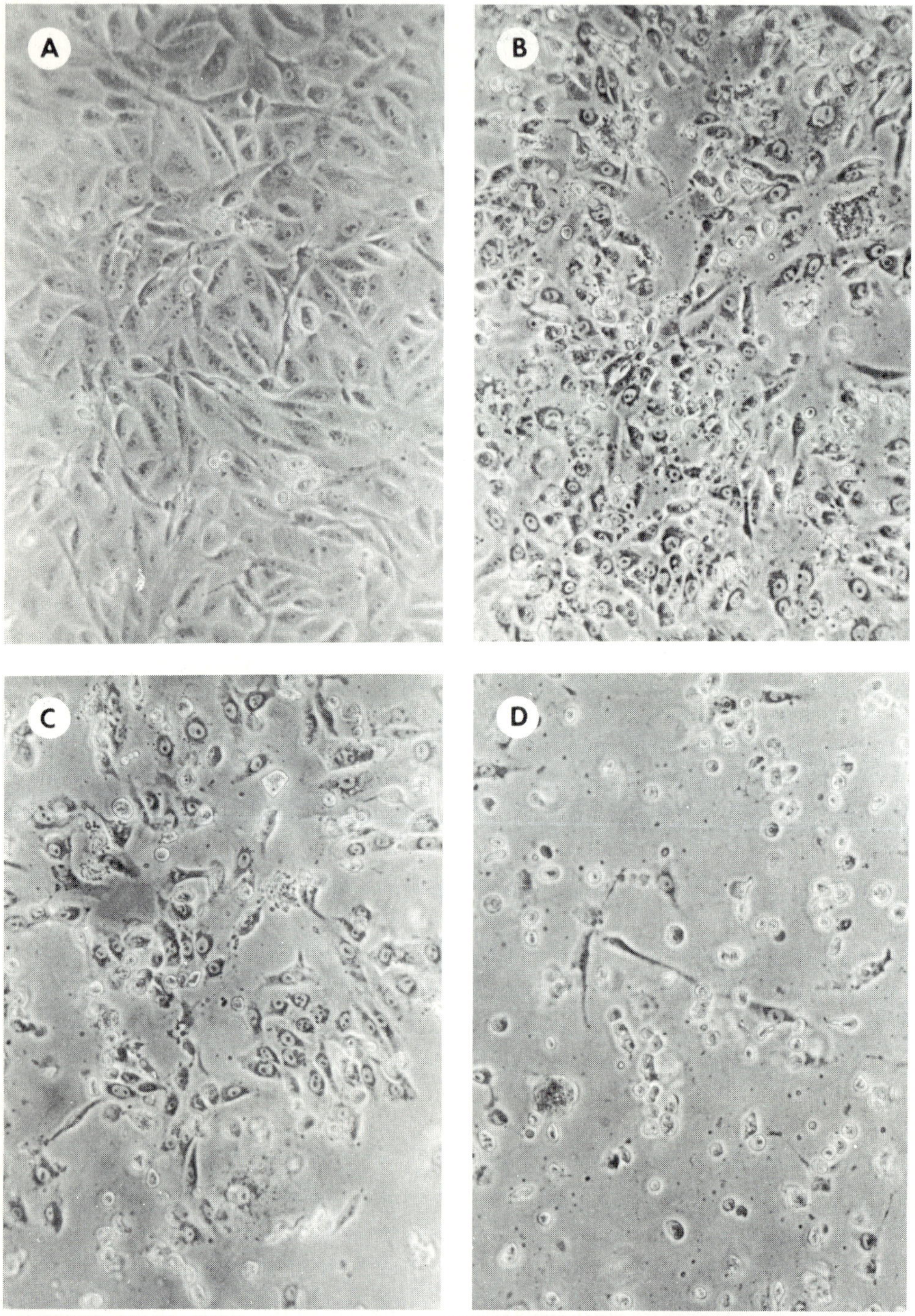

Figure 1-6. The cytopathic effects caused by reovirus serotype 3 in Vero monkey kidney cells. **A.** Normal cell sheet. **B.** Partial cell destruction at 20 hours after infection. **C.** 36 hours after infection. **D.** 48 hours after infection. × 125. *(Courtesy of Dr. E.C. Hayes.)*

dilution originally contained at least one infectious unit. Considerable accuracy can be attained by the use of statistical methods of treating results.

The dilution end point method is also employed when virus is titrated in laboratory animals. Examples are the titration of togaviruses (arboviruses) and Group A Coxsackie viruses in the brains of suckling mice, with death as the end point.

Enumeration of the Total Number of Virus Particles

It is universally true for animal viruses that even though one virus particle is capable of causing infection, not all particles in a population actually do so. The total number of virus particles in a given preparation can be determined by either direct or indirect methods.

Counting by Means of Electron Microscopy

Direct counting of virus particles by means of electron microscopic examination is carried out according to either of two methods. The first involves mixing virus preparations with suspensions of latex spheres of similar size and known concentration and spraying the mixture onto coated electron microscope grids. The number of virus particles and spheres in individual spray droplets is then counted; knowing the concentration of the spheres, the number of virus particles can be calculated (Fig. 1-7). The second method involves centrifuging virus preparations onto electron microscope grids and counting the virus particles; knowing what volume of the virus suspension was centrifuged, the virus concentration can be calculated.

Measurement of Optical Density

The concentration of highly purified virus preparations can be routinely determined by very simple methods once they have been standardized by electron microscopy. One of these methods is measurement of the optical density. For example, 1 ml of a suspension of reovirus particles that absorbs 90 percent of incident light at a wavelength of 260 nm (that is, 1 optical density unit or 1 $OD_{260\ nm}$) contains 2.1×10^{12} virus particles, and 1 $OD_{260\ nm}$ of vaccinia virus corresponds to 1.2×10^{10} virus particles.

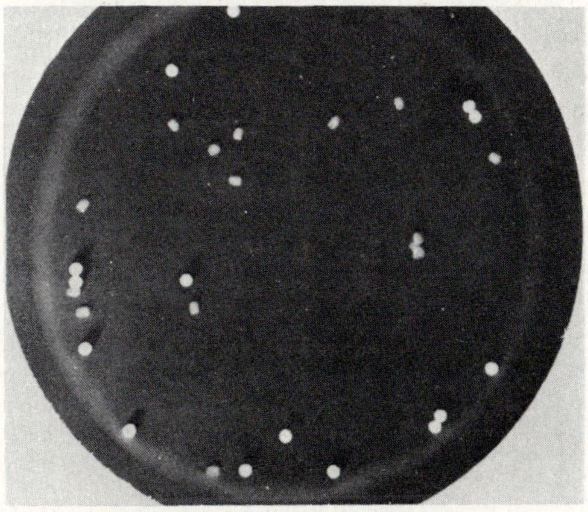

Figure 1-7. A spray droplet containing 15 latex particles (spheres) and 14 vaccinia virus particles (slightly smaller brick-shaped particles). × 6500. *(From Dumbell et al.: Virology 4:467, 1957.)*

The Hemagglutination Assay

The most common indirect method of measuring the number of virus particles is the hemagglutination assay. Many animal viruses adsorb to the red blood cells of various animal species. Each virus particle is multivalent in this regard; that is, it can adsorb to more than one cell at a time. In practice, the maximum number of cells with which any particular virus particle can combine is two, because red cells are far bigger than viruses. In a virus-cell mixture in which the number of cells exceeds the number of virus particles, the small number of cell dimers that may be formed is generally not detectable, but if the number of virus particles exceeds the number of cells, a lattice of cells is formed that settles out in a highly characteristic manner readily distinguishable from the settling pattern exhibited by unagglutinated cells.

The hemagglutination assay is performed by determining the virus dilution that will just hemagglutinate a given number of red cells (Fig. 1-8). Since the number of virus particles necessary for this is readily calculated, hemagglutination serves as a highly accurate and rapid method of quantitating virus particles. It was and still is particularly useful in studies with myxoviruses, particularly influenza virus, and many others.

The Significance of the Infectious Unit: Virus Particle Ratio

For all animal viruses the number of virus particles in any given preparation exceeds the number of demonstrably infectious units; usually the ratio of infectious units to particles is in the range of 1:10 to 1:1000 or even less. There are two possible explanations for this. The first is that virus preparations contain a majority of noninfectious particles. Although this may be so sometimes, it is unlikely to be the general rule. It is more likely that although all virus particles in a given preparation are capable of causing productive infection, only a small proportion of them are actually successful in doing so. Two lines of evidence support this view. The first is that the titer of a given virus preparation varies markedly, depending on the nature of the assay system. For example, the titer often differs with the route of inoculation if the virus is assayed in whole animals and with the type of cell if it is assayed in cultured cells. Second, before a virus particle can manifest itself (e.g. as a plaque, pock, or focus), it must initiate several productive infection cycles that require numerous reactions, many of which have a low probability of occurring (Chap. 4). Therefore, the number of infectious units can-

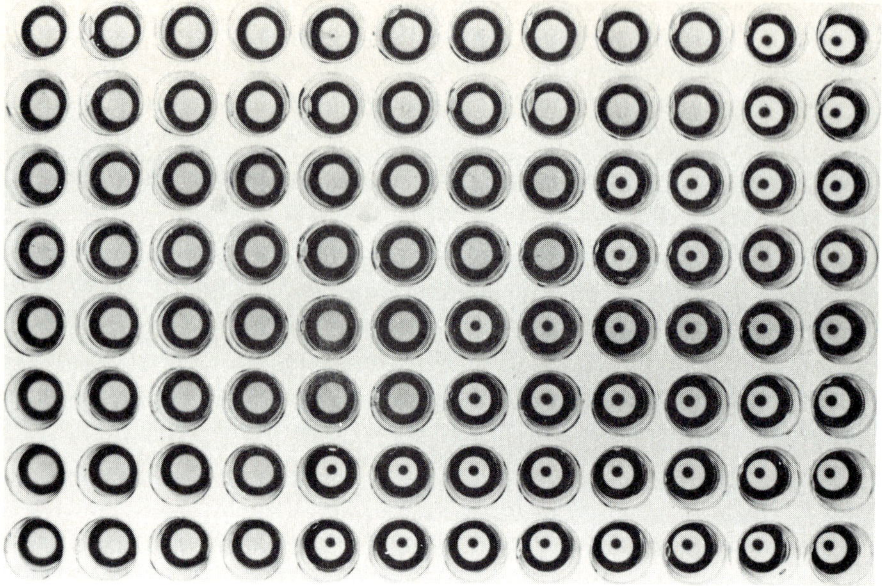

Figure 1-8. Hemagglutination titration of influenza virus. In the top two rows a sample of influenza virus was diluted in serial twofold steps from left to right; in the next two rows the amount of virus in the first well was the same as in the third well in the top row, and so on down. The same number of red blood cells was then added to all wells, and after mixing, the tray was placed at 4C for 2 hours. Unagglutinated cells form a dark button; where the virus has agglutinated cells, the resulting lattice has prevented button formation. The pattern developed in this tray attests to the reproducibility of the technique. *(Courtesy of Dr. E.C. Hayes.)*

not equal the total number of virus particles. The ratio of the number of infectious units to the total number of virus particles may generally be regarded as a measure of the probability with which virus particles achieve productive infection.

FURTHER READING

Books

VIRUSES

Andrews C, Pereira HG, Wildy P: Viruses of Vertebrates, 4th ed. London, Bailliere Tindall, 1978

Fenner FJ, McAuslan BR, Mims CA, et al.: Animal Viruses, 2nd ed. New York, Academic Press, 1974

Fenner FJ, White DO: Medical Virology, 2nd ed. New York, Academic Press, 1976

Fraenkel-Conrat H, Wagner RR (eds): Methods Used in the Study of Viruses, Comprehensive Virology. New York, Plenum, 1981, vol 17

Howard CR (ed): New Developments in Practical Virology. New York, Liss, 1982

Hughes SS: The Virus: A History of the Concept. New York, Neale Watson Academic Publication, 1977

Luria SE, Darnell JE Jr, Baltimore D, et al.: General Virology, 3rd ed. New York, Wiley, 1978

CELLS

Alberts B, Bray D, Lewis J, et al.: Molecular Biology of the Cell. New York, Garland Publishing, 1983

Barigozzi C (ed): Original and Natural History of Cell Lines. New York, Liss, 1978

Clarkson B, Marks PA, Till JE (eds): Differentiation of Normal and Neoplastic Hematopoietic Cells. New York, Cold Spring Harbor Laboratory, 1979

Crow R, Ozer H, Rifkin D (eds): Experiments with Normal and Transformed Cells. New York, Cold Spring Harbor Laboratory, 1979

Dingle JT, Gordon JL (eds): Cellular Interactions. Amsterdam/New York, Elsevier, 1981

Frederick JF (ed): Origins and Evolution of Eukaryotic Intracellular Organelles. New York, New York Academy of Sciences, 1980

Gall JG, Porter KR, Siekevitz P (eds): Discovery in Cell Biology. New York, Rockefeller University Press, 1981

Glick JL (ed): Fundamentals of Human Lymphoid Cell Culture. New York, Marcel Dekker, 1980

Goldstein L, Prescott DM (eds): The Structure and Replication of Genetic Material. Cell Biology. New York, Academic Press, 1979, vol 2

Hoffman JF, Giebisch GH, Bolis L (eds): Membranes in Growth and Development. New York, Liss, 1981

Jeter JR, Cameron IL, Padilla GM, et al. (eds): Cell Cycle Regulation. New York, Academic Press, 1978

Lerner RA, Bergsma D (eds): The Molecular Basis of Cell–Cell Interaction. New York, Liss, 1978

Lloyd CW, Rees DA (eds): Cellular Controls in Differentiation. New York, Academic Press, 1981

Lloyd D, Poole RK, Edwards SW (eds): The Cell Division Cycle. New York, Academic Press, 1982

Maul GG (ed): The Nuclear Envelope and the Nuclear Matrix. New York, Liss, 1981

Nicolini C (ed): Cell Growth. New York, Plenum, 1982

Pollack R (ed): Readings in Mammalian Cell Culture. New York, Cold Spring Harbor Laboratory, 1981

Poste G, Nicholson GL (eds): Cytoskeletal Elements and Plasma Membrane Organization. New York, Elsevier, 1981

Salmon SE (ed): Cloning of Human Tumor Stem Cells. New York, Liss, 1980

Sato G (ed): Functionally Differentiated Cell Lines. New York, Liss, 1981

Sato GH, Pardee AB, Sirbasku DA (eds): Growth of Cells in Hormonally Defined Media. New York, Cold Spring Harbor Laboratory, 1982

Whitson GL (ed): Nuclear–Cytoplasmic Interactions in the Cell Cycle. New York, Academic Press, 1980

Zimmerman AM, Forer A (eds): Mitosis/Cytokinesis. New York, Academic Press, 1982

Selected Reviews and Papers

Amsterdam A, Jamieson JT: Techniques for dissociating pancreatic exocrine cells. J Cell Biol 63:1037, 1974

Barnes D, Sato G: Serum-free culture. Cell 12:649, 1980

Branton D, Cohen CM, Tyler J: Interaction of cytoskeletal proteins on the human erythrocyte membrane. Cell 24:24, 1981

Conrad GW, Hart GW, Chen Y: Differences in vitro between fibroblast-like cells from cornea, heart and skin of embryonic chicks. J Cell Sci 26:119, 1977

Dustin P: Microtubules. Sci Am 243:66, 1980

Edelman GM: Cell adhesion molecules. Science 219:450, 1983

Mullinger AM, Johnson RT: Packing DNA into chromosomes. J Cell Sci 46:61, 1981

Osborn M, Weber K: Intermediate filaments: Cell-type-specific markers in differentiation and pathology. Cell 31:303, 1982

Pastan IH, Willingham MC: Journey to the center of the cell: Role of the receptosome. Science 214:504, 1981

Porter KR, Tucker JB: The ground substance of the living cell. Sci Am 244:56, 1981

Rothman JE: The Golgi apparatus. Science 213:1212, 1981

Smith JR, Hayflick L: Variation in the life span of clones derived from human diploid strains. J Cell Biol 62:48, 1974

Stack SN, Brown DB, Dewey WC: Visualization of interphase chromosomes. J Cell Sci 26:281, 1977

Watt FM, Harris H: Microtubule organizing centers in mammalian cells in culture. J Cell Sci 44:103, 1980

Wishnow RN, Steinfeld JL: The conquest of the major infectious diseases in the United States: A bicentennial retrospect. Ann Rev Microbiol 30:427, 1976

CHAPTER 2

The Structure, Components, and Classification of Viruses

The Morphology of Animal Viruses

Although animal viruses differ widely in shape and size, they are nevertheless constructed according to certain common principles. Basically, viruses consist of nucleic acid and protein. The nucleic acid is the genome that contains the information necessary for virus multiplication; the protein is arranged around the genome in the form of a layer or shell that is termed the capsid. The structure consisting of shell plus nucleic acid is the nucleocapsid. Many animal virus particles consist of naked nucleocapsids, whereas others possess an additional envelope that is usually acquired as the nucleocapsid buds from the host cell. The complete virus particle is known as the virion, a term that denotes both intactness of structure and the property of infectiousness.

Capsids

The essential feature of capsids is that they are composed of numerous repeating subunits—identical or belonging to only a few different species—arranged in precisely defined patterns. The simplest subunits are single protein molecules; more complex forms are morphologic subunits termed capsomers that can be seen with the electron microscope and that consist of several either identical or different protein molecules. The use of only a few types of subunits for capsid construction has two noteworthy consequences: (1) It minimizes the amount of genetic informa-

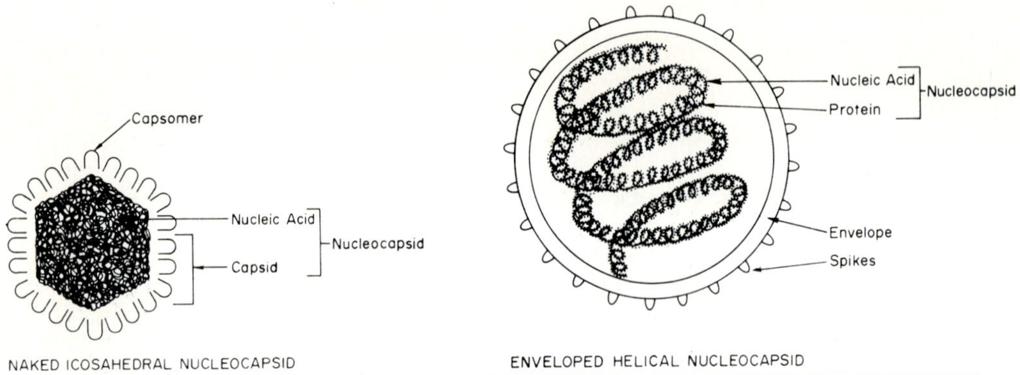

Figure 2-1. The two basic patterns of animal virus structure. **Left:** The condensed genome is enclosed by a shell of capsomers arranged so as to display 5:3:2 rotational symmetry. **Right:** The extended genome is enclosed by protein molecules arranged so as to display helical symmetry. The resultant structure, the nucleocapsid, is enclosed in an envelope to whose outer surface glycoprotein spikes are attached.

tion necessary to specify capsids, and (2) it assures that they will be assembled efficiently. Capsid proteins exhibit a strong tendency to bind to one another, and much of the information necessary for the morphogenesis of nucleocapsids is inherent in their amino acid sequence.

Capsids (and envelopes) have a dual function. The first is to protect viral genomes from potentially destructive agents in the extracellular environment, such as enzymes. All viral genomes are protected from nucleases by virtue of the capsids that enclose them. Animal viruses are generally resistant to attack by the proteases of higher animals, such as pepsin, trypsin, and chymotrypsin. Some, such as the enteroviruses, are completely resistant, whereas others, such as the poxviruses and reoviruses, possess susceptible outer shells but resistant cores. Glycoprotein spikes of enveloped viruses (see below) can generally be removed by treatment with proteolytic enzymes, and the resulting "bald" particles lack infectivity. Phospholipases usually inactivate enveloped viruses by hydrolyzing their phospholipids.

The second function of viral capsids is to introduce viral genomes into host cells. The need for this latter function stems from the fact that viral nucleic acids are often longer than cell diameters and cannot penetrate into cells by themselves. Capsids (and envelopes), on the other hand, adsorb readily to cell surfaces and can enter cells by several mechanisms (see Chap. 4).

Envelopes

Only six families of animal viruses exist as naked nucleocapsids. In all others the nucleocapsids are enclosed by membrane-containing envelopes that are acquired as the nucleocapsids bud through special patches of cell membrane—either in outer plasma cell membranes or in vacuolar membranes—on their way to the exterior of the cell. The membrane patches through which nucleocapsids bud are virus-modified; usually the cell-specified proteins in them are completely replaced by virus-specified proteins, and virus-specified glycoprotein spikes are attached to their outer surface. However, there are exceptions. The envelopes of herpesviruses and RNA tumor viruses probably still contain some host-coded proteins, and although herpesvirus envelopes contain glycoproteins, they do not possess obvious spikes.

Viral envelopes generally lack rigidity. As a consequence they usually appear heterogeneous in shape and size when fixed for electron microscopy, and enveloped

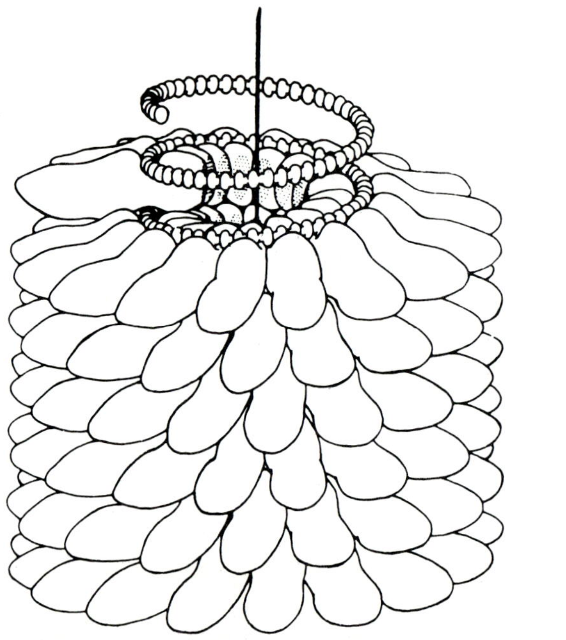

Figure 2-2. Schematic representation of tobacco mosaic virus. As can be seen in the cutaway section, the ribonucleic acid helix is associated with protein molecules in the ratio of three nucleotides per protein molecule. *(From Klug and Caspar: Adv Virus Res 7:225, 1960.)*

viruses are therefore often said to be pleomorphic. There is little doubt, however, that in their native state most enveloped viruses are spherical, enclosing either icosahedral nucleocapsids or spherically coiled helical nucleocapsids. However, two types of enveloped viruses are not spherical. These are the rhabdoviruses, which possess a highly characteristic bullet-like shape, rounded at one end and flat at the other, and certain strains of influenza virus, whose helical nucleocapsids become enveloped not in a coiled but in an extended configuration, which causes the enveloped virus particles also to be long and filamentous.

Nucleocapsids

Viral nucleocapsids are constructed according to a small number of basic patterns. Two of these have been studied in great detail at both the structural and the molecular level. In one, the nucleic acid is extended; in the other, it is condensed (Fig. 2-1). Superimposed on these two patterns are variations dictated both by the size of the genome and by the nature of the capsid proteins.

Nucleocapsids with Helical Symmetry. The prototype of nucleocapsids in which the nucleic acid occurs as an extended filament is a plant virus, tobacco mosaic virus (TMV), whose structure has been studied extensively by x-ray diffraction. In this virus, the extended nucleic acid molecule is surrounded by protein molecules arranged helically so as to yield a structure with a single rotational axis (Fig. 2-2). The ortho- and paramyxoviruses and rhabdoviruses possess nucleocapsids constructed in this manner, each with its own characteristic length, width, periodicity, flexibility, and stability (Fig. 2-3). It should be noted that these nucleocapsids are not the complete virus particles; the particles of these virus families consist of the nucleocapsids coiled more or less tightly inside envelopes (Figs. 2-4 and 2-5).

Nucleocapsids with Icosahedral Symmetry. In the second pattern of virus structure, the nucleic acid is condensed and forms the central portion of a quasispherical nucleocapsid. Here the capsid consists of a shell of protein molecules that are clustered into small groups called capsomers, with the bonds between molecules within capsomers being stronger than those between capsomers. Capsomers are morphologic units that can often be seen with the electron microscope; they vary in size and shape from virus to virus.

X-ray diffraction analysis indicates that in this type of nucleocapsid the capsomers are arranged very precisely ac-

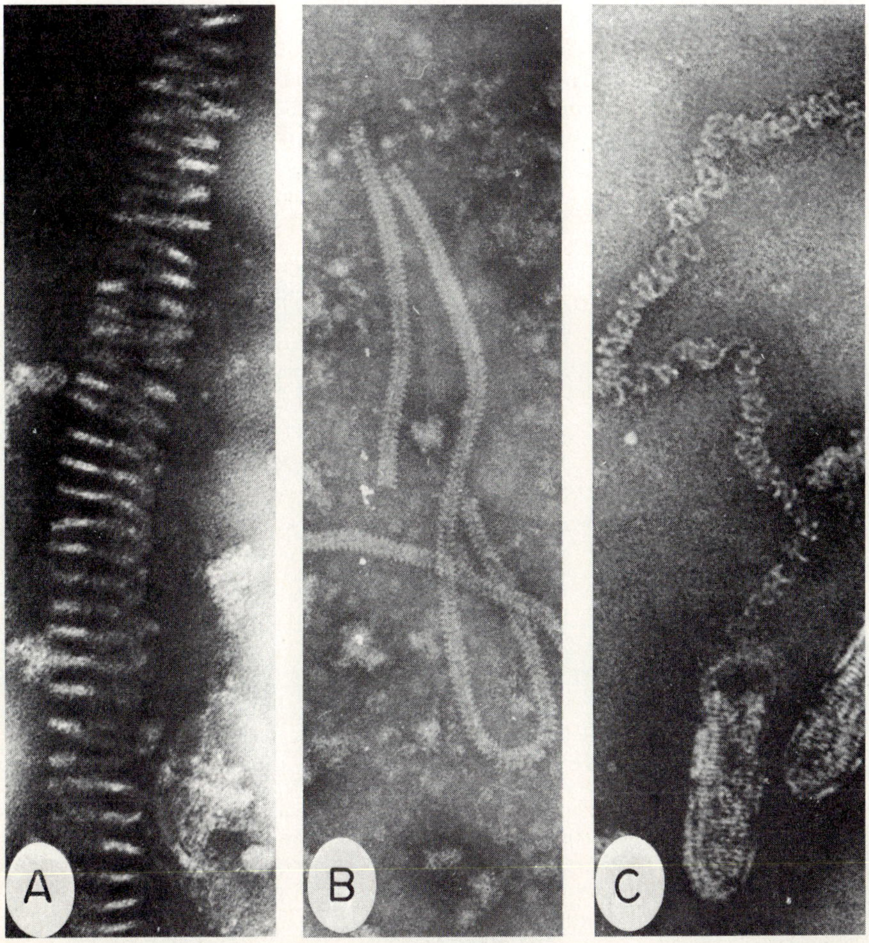

Figure 2-3. The nucleocapsids of (**A**) influenza virus strain PR8 (× 225,000); (**B**) measles virus (× 150,000); and (**C**) vesicular stomatitis virus (VSV) (× 160,000). The latter is emerging from a damaged virus particle. *(**A,** from Almeida and Waterson: In Barry and Mahy (eds): The Biology of Large RNA Viruses, 1970. New York, Academic Press; **B,** from Finch and Gibbs: J Gen Virol 6:144, 1970; **C,** from Simpson and Hauser: Virology 29:660, 1966.)*

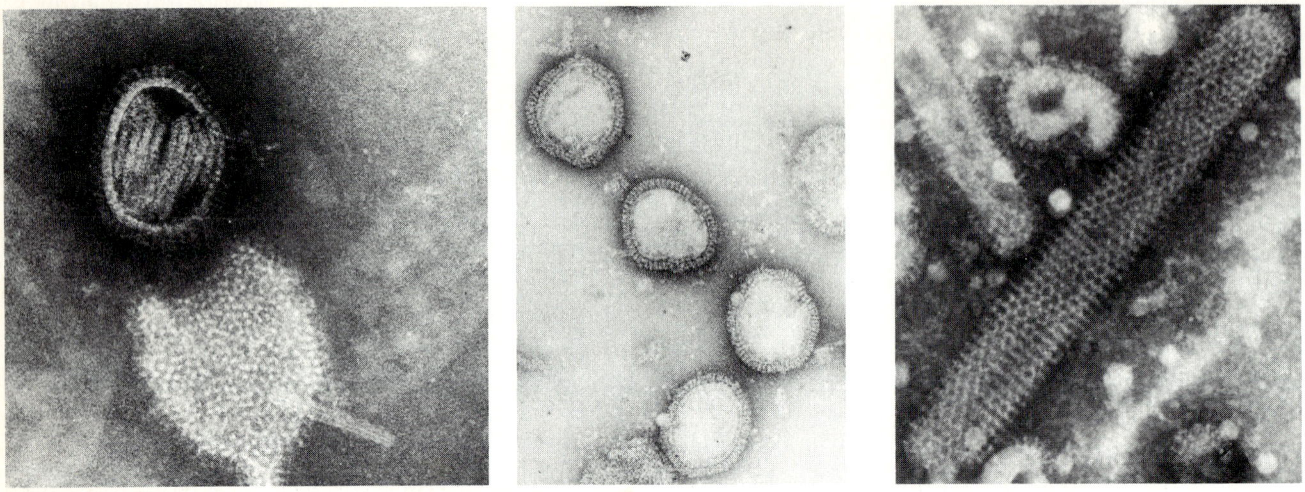

A B C

Figure 2-4. The structure of influenza virus. **A.** Influenza virus A_2, stained with phosphotungstate. One particle is penetrated by the stain, thereby revealing the arrangement of the internal nucleocapsid. × 155,000. *(Courtesy of Dr. M. V. Nermut.)* **B.** Influenza virus A_0/WSN, stained with phosphotungstate, revealing the characteristic arrangement of spikes on the particle surface. There are two types of spikes; hemagglutinin spikes are about six times more numerous than neuraminidase spikes. × 135,000. *(Courtesy of Dr. I. T. Schulze.)* **C.** A filamentous particle of an influenza C strain. Note the regular subunit surface pattern. × 115,000. *(From Apostolov and Flewett: J Gen Virol 4:366, 1969.)*

cording to icosahedral patterns characterized by 5:3:2-fold rotational symmetry (Fig. 2-6). Two such patterns are found among animal viruses. The first is exhibited most clearly by adenoviruses. The adenovirus capsid is constructed in the shape of an icosahedron with six capsomers along each edge and 252 capsomers altogether (Fig. 2-7). Of these, 240 are spherical and are situated along the edges and on the faces of the icosahedron; each has six nearest neighbors and is known as a hexon or hexamer. The remaining 12 are situated at the 12 vertices of the icosahedron and have five nearest neighbors; these are known as pentons or pentamers. They have a highly characteristic shape, consisting of a spherical base and a long fiber that may serve as the cell attachment organ.

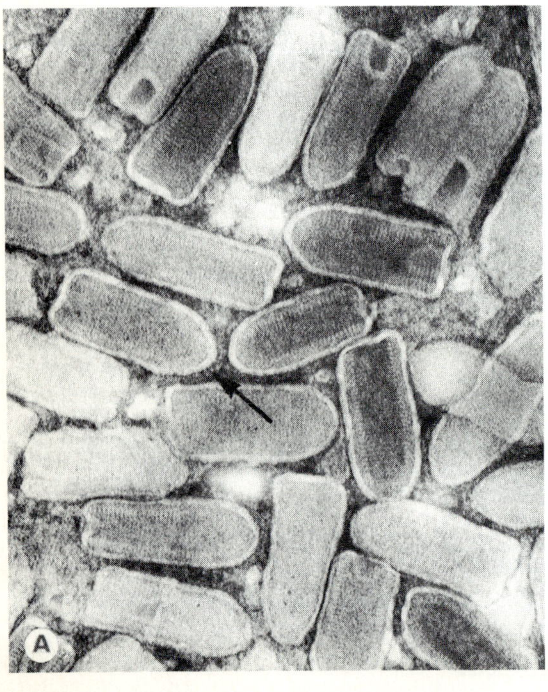

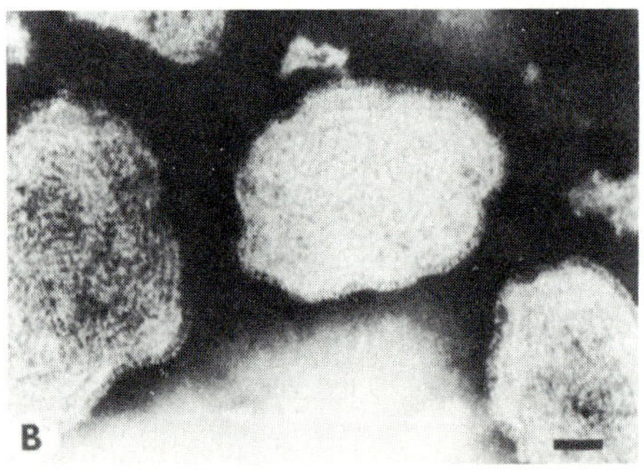

Figure 2-5. A. Highly characteristic bullet-shaped vesicular stomatitis virus (VSV) particles, some penetrated by stain, revealing the tightly coiled nucleocapsid. Note glycoprotein spikes (arrow). *(Courtesy of Dr. Erskine Palmer).* **B.** Sendai virus, a paramyxovirus. Note the tightly coiled nucleocapsid. × 73,500. *(From Maeno et al.: J Virol 6:492, 1970.)*

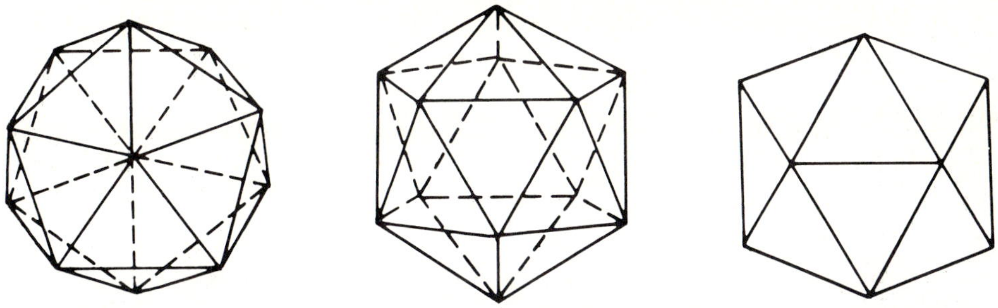

Figure 2-6. The icosahedron viewed normal to five-, three-, and two-fold rotational axes. Edges of the upper and lower surfaces are drawn in solid and broken lines respectively. The five-fold rotational axes pass through the vertices (**left**); the three-fold rotational axes pass through the centers of the triangular faces (**center**); and the two-fold rotational axes pass through the edges (**right**). In this view, the edges on the upper and lower surfaces coincide. Note that the icosahedron possesses 12 vertices, 20 triangular faces, and 30 edges.

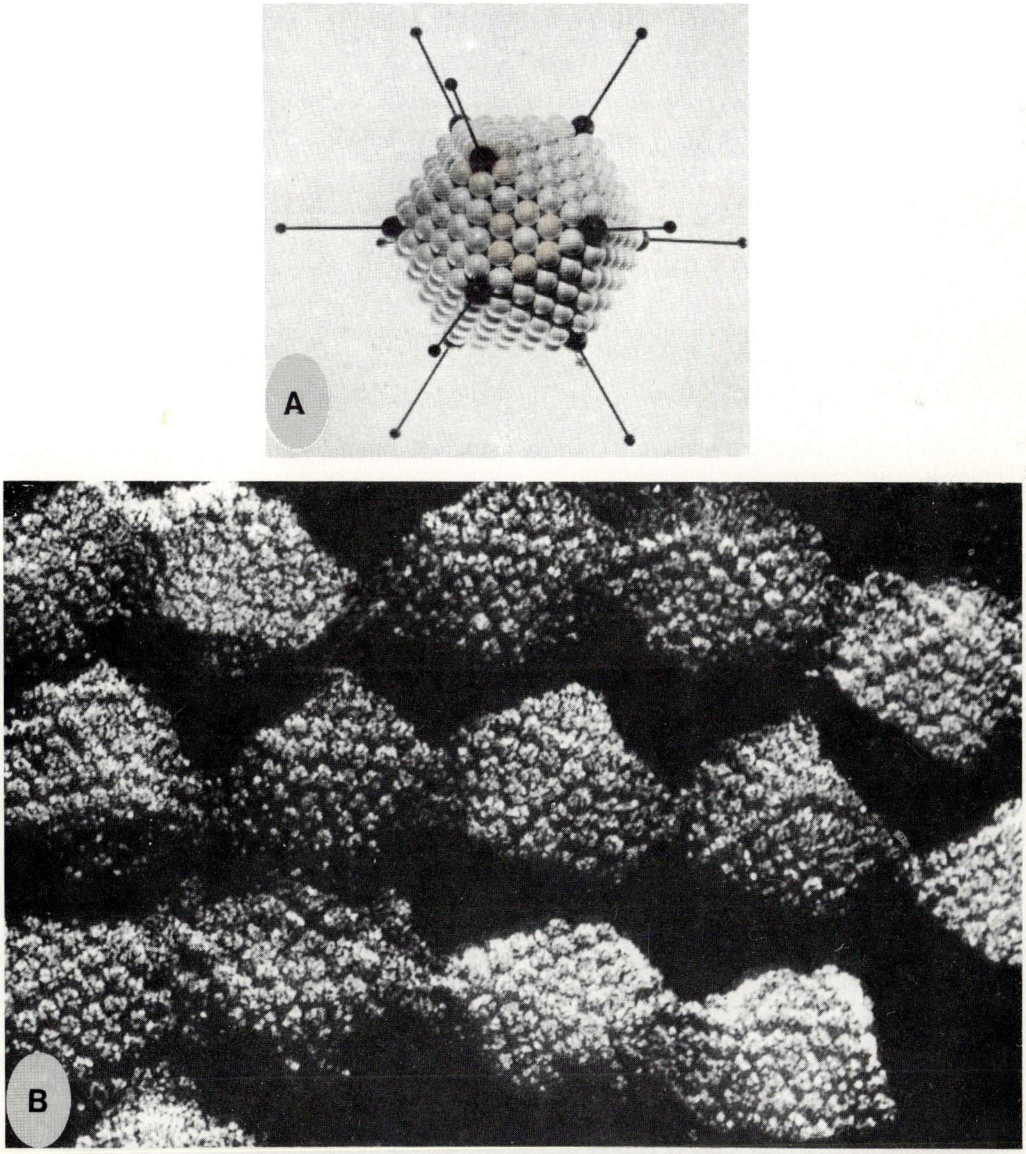

Figure 2-7. **A.** Model of the adenovirus particle constructed by R. C. Valentine. **B.** Adenovirus freeze-dried and shadowed with platinum. × 400,000. *(Courtesy of Dr. M.V. Nermut.)*

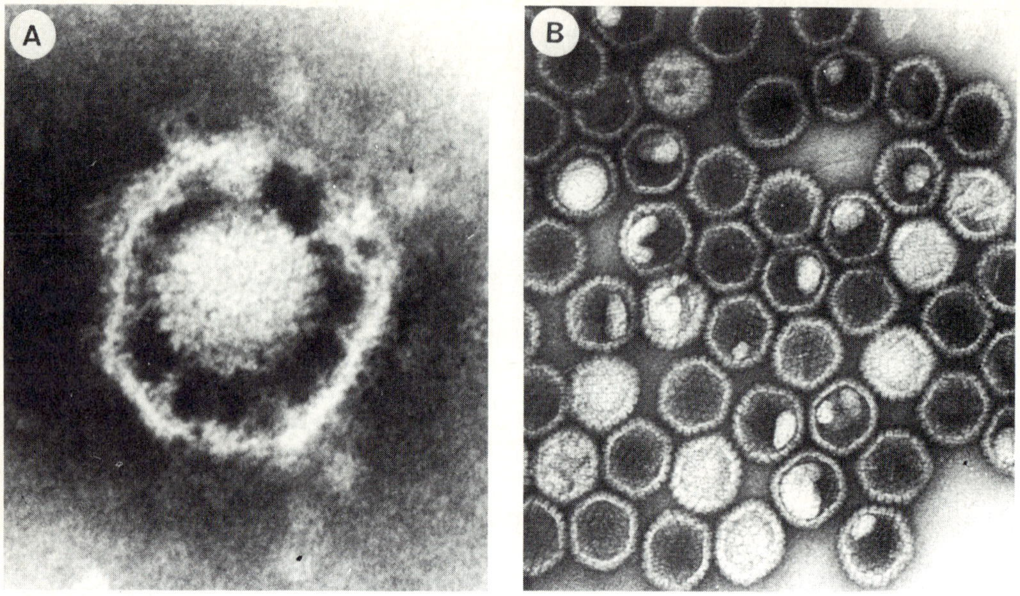

Figure 2-8. The morphology of herpesviruses. **A.** Enveloped equine abortion virus (EAV) particle. × 125,000. **B.** EAV particles from which the envelope has been removed by treatment with detergent. × 75,000. *(From Abodeely et al.: J Virol 5:513, 1970.)*

The capsids of four other virus families are constructed similarly. Iridovirus capsids possess 10 capsomers along each edge, and there are 1112 capsomers altogether—1100 hexons and 12 pentons; herpesvirus capsids possess five capsomers along each edge and 162 capsomer altogether—150 prism-shaped hexons and 12 pentons (Fig. 2-8); papovavirus capsids consist of 72 capsomers—60 hexons and 12 pentons (Fig. 2-9); and parvovirus capsids appear to be made up of 32 capsomers—20 hexons and 12 pentons (Fig. 2-9).

The second pattern is exhibited most clearly by picornaviruses. Here 60 identical capsomers, each composed of four different proteins, are situated equidistantly from a common center, which results in a spherical capsid (Fig. 2-10). However, instead of being bonded equally strongly to each other, these capsomers are bonded into groups of five, 12 of which make up the capsid. Reoviruses are unique in possessing two capsids shells (Fig. 2-11). Both possess icosahedral symmetry, but it has so far proved impossible to discern either the total number of capsomers or the precise manner in which they are arranged. The capsid shell of some members of this family,

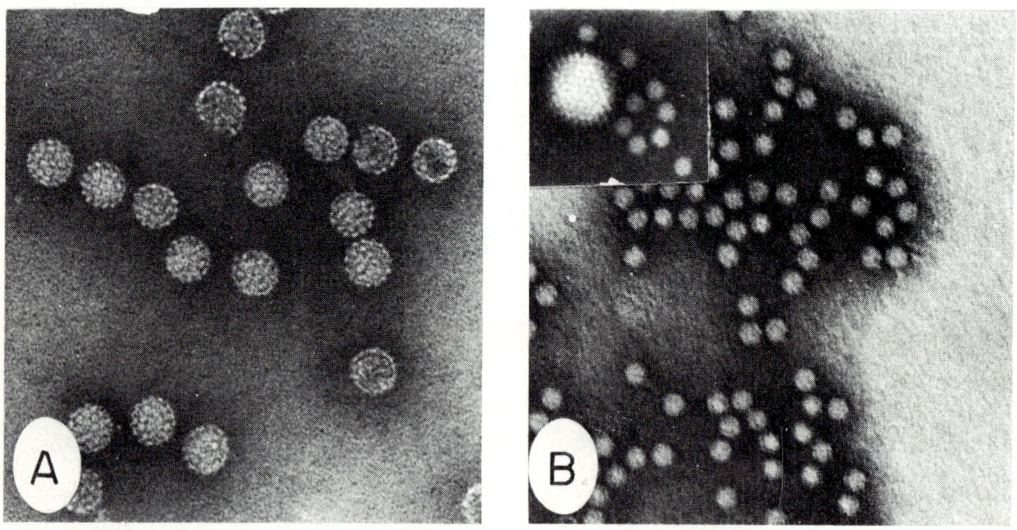

Figure 2-9. **A.** The papovavirus SV40 (× 160,000). **B.** The parvovirus adeno-associated virus (AAV) type 4 (× 150,000). **Insert:** A particle of the simian adenovirus SV15, which enabled the AAV to multiply (see Chap. 6). *(Courtesy of Dr. Heather Mayor.)*

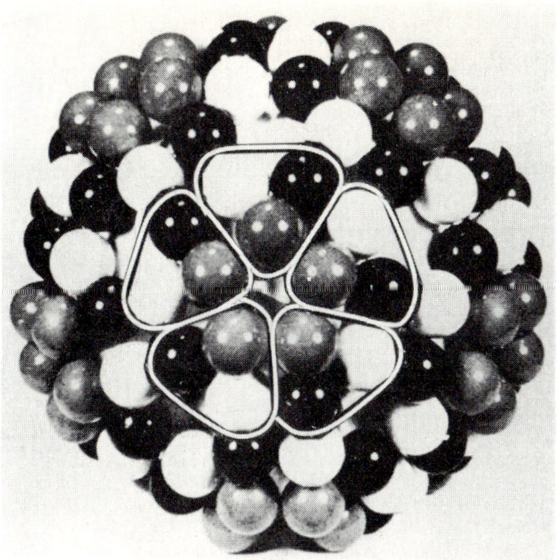

Figure 2-10. Model of the picornavirus capsid. There are 60 capsomers, each consisting of three protein molecules, represented here by white, gray, and black balls. (In fact, in the mature virion, one of these protein molecules is cleaved into a larger and a smaller fragment, both of which remain in position.) Groups of five capsomers (as outlined) form units that are intermediates during morphogenesis; the capsid is composed of 12 of these "groups of five." *(Adapted from Johnston and Martin: J Gen Virol 11:77, 1971.)*

such as the orbiviruses and the rotaviruses, appears to be composed of 32 large ring-shaped capsomers. It is more likely however that this type of capsid is composed of numerous small subunits arranged in ring-shaped (or hexagonal) patterns and that many of these subunits are shared by adjacent rings so that what is visible is 32 holes, rather than 32 capsomers. Reovirus capsids are probably structured similarly, although here the rings are much less prominent.

In the case of the picornaviruses, caliciviruses, adenoviruses, papovaviruses, parvoviruses, and reoviruses, the virus particles are the naked nucleocapsids. In the case of the herpesviruses and the sole iridovirus that is a mammalian virus, however, the naked nucleocapsids themselves are relatively noninfectious; here the virus particles consist of enveloped icosahedral nucleocapsids.

Structure of Togaviruses, Bunyaviruses, Arenaviruses, and Coronaviruses

These viruses are all enveloped particles to whose outer surface glycoprotein spikes are attached; the spikes are particularly prominent in coronaviruses (Fig. 2-12), where they are large and club-shaped and surround the virus particles like a corona (hence the name). The nucleocapsids of these viruses exhibit a variety of morphologic patterns. In the case of the togaviruses, the alphaviruses—which comprise the old group A arboviruses—contain condensed RNA molecules intimately associated with protein to form nucleocapsids that possess distinct icosahedral symmetry (Fig. 2-13); but the nucleocapsids of the slightly smaller flaviviruses—the old group B arboviruses, the name deriving from the prototype yellow fever virus—possess no obvious symmetry elements. The bunyaviruses have a diameter that is about twice that of togaviruses and possess three coiled circular nucleocapsids that possess helical symmetry (Fig. 2-14). The arenaviruses (Fig. 2-15)

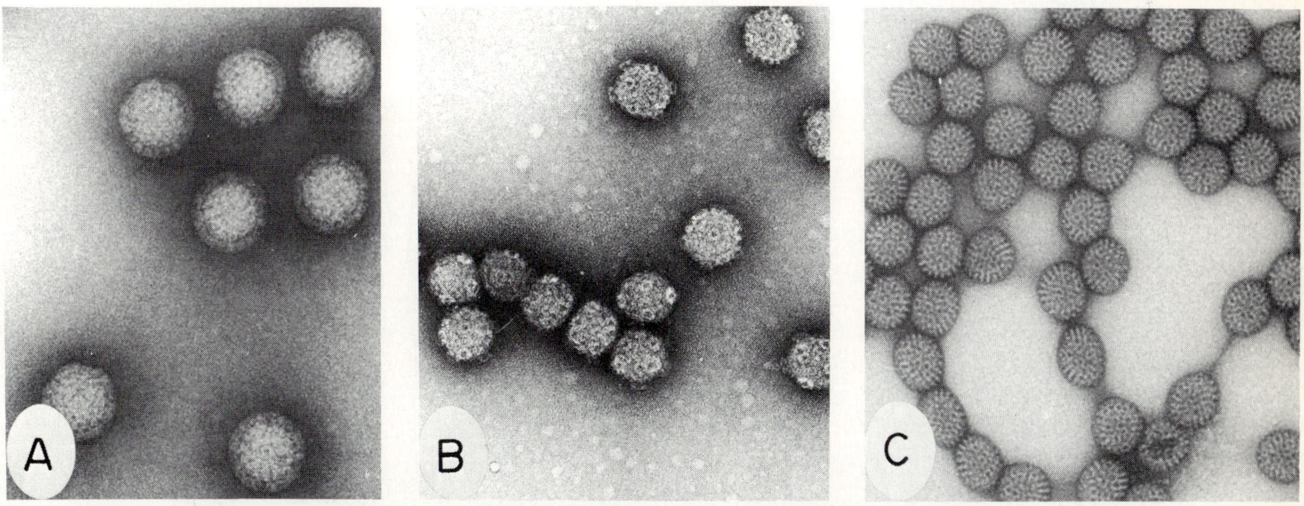

Figure 2-11. Morphology of reovirus and human rotavirus. **A.** Reovirus. Note double capsid shell. The arrangement of capsomers is clearly discernible at the periphery. × 120,000. **B.** Reovirus cores. Cores are derived from reovirus particles by digesting their outer capsid shell with chymotrypsin. Note the large spikes; there are 12, located as if situated on the 12 vertices of an icosahedron. **C.** Human rotavirus. Its structure is similar to, but not identical with, that of orbiviruses. × 136,000. ***(A, B,** courtesy of Drs. R.B. Luftig and W.K. Joklik; **C,** courtesy of Dr. Erskine Palmer, Centers for Disease Control, Atlanta.)*

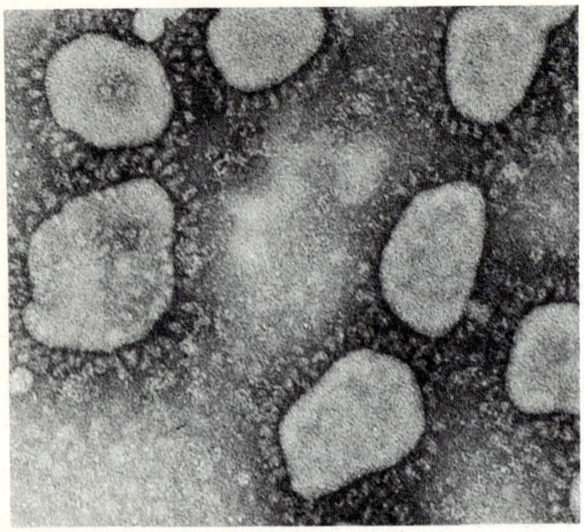

Figure 2-12. Coronavirus particles. Note pleomorphic envelopes studded with characteristic widely spaced club- or pear-shaped surface projections. × 144,000. *(From Kapikian: In Lennette and Schmidt (eds): Diagnostic Procedures for Viral and Rickettsial Infections, 4th ed, 1969. New York, American Public Health Assoc.)*

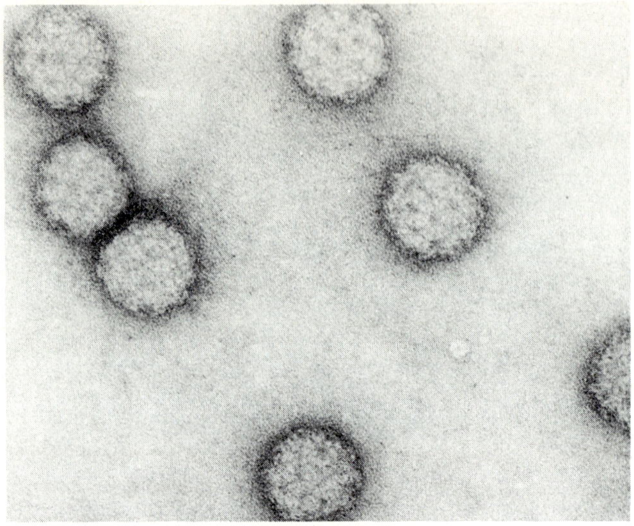

Figure 2-13. The togavirus Sindbis virus, stained with uranyl acetate. × 240,000. *(Courtesy of Dr. P.J. Enzmann.)*

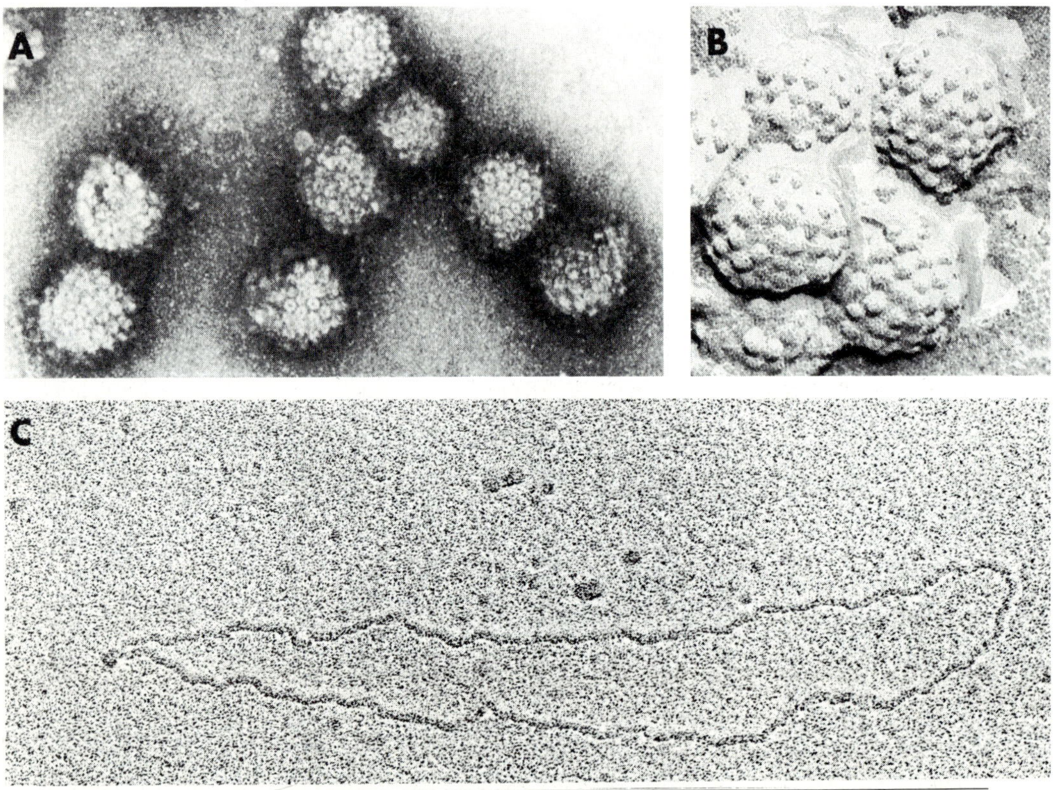

Figure 2-14. The structure of Uukuniemi virus, a bunyavirus. **A.** Virus particles fixed with glutaraldehyde and negatively stained with uranyl acetate. × 100,000. **B.** Freeze-etched, glutaraldehyde-fixed virus particles: a group of particles showing the icosahedral arrangement of the surface projections. × 180,000. **C.** Circular nucleocapsid of this virus, shadowed with platinum. Nucleocapsids are released from virus particles by treatment with the nonionic detergent Triton X-100. × 60,000. *(From von Bonsdorff: J Virol 16:1296, 1975.)*

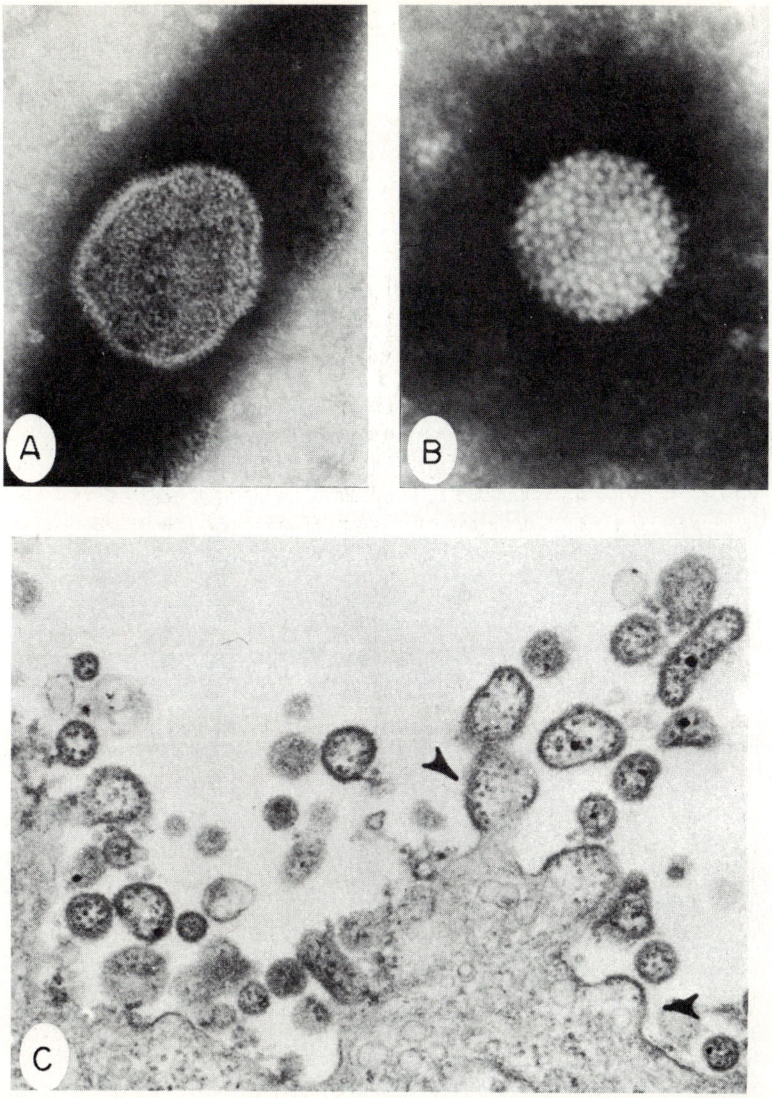

Figure 2-15. Tacaribe virus, an arenavirus. **A, B.** Two virus particles, one of which has been partially penetrated by negative contrast medium, showing the glycoprotein spikes that cover their surface. × 135,000 and × 235,000, respectively. **C.** Thin section of Paraña virus particles budding from the plasma membrane of Vero African green monkey kidney cells. Note the characteristic dense granules, which are ribosomes. × 45,000. *(From Murphy et al.: J Virol 6:507, 1970.)*

are slightly larger than bunyaviruses and contain two circular coiled nucleocapsids; they also contain several highly characteristic granules (Latin *arenosus,* sandy) that have been shown to be ribosomes (which, however, are not required for virus multiplication). Finally, the coronaviruses (Fig. 2-12), which are about the same size as bunyaviruses, possess linear helical nucleocapsids that resemble those of myxoviruses.

Structure of RNA Tumor Viruses, Poxviruses, and Some Miscellaneous Viruses

RNA tumor viruses have a more complex structure; they consist of a concentrically coiled nucleocapsid that possesses icosahedral symmetry and is closely associated with an "inner coat" that is itself bounded by a membrane bearing more or less prominent glycoprotein spikes (Fig. 2-16) (see Chap. 8).

Poxviruses are the largest and most complex of all animal viruses. Morphologically, there are two classes of poxviruses. Most poxvirus particles are prolate ellipsoids that are often brick-shaped when fixed for electron microscopy. They are covered on their outer surface with tubules or filaments arranged in a characteristic whorled or mulberry pattern (Fig. 2-17). Within this outer layer there is a protein coat that contains two lateral bodies of unknown composition and function, and a DNA-containing nucleoid or core bounded by a layer of well-defined protein subunits.

Parapoxviruses are somewhat smaller, ovoid rather than brick-shaped, and covered on their outer surface by tubules or filaments similar to those that cover the poxvirus particles just described, except that they are arranged

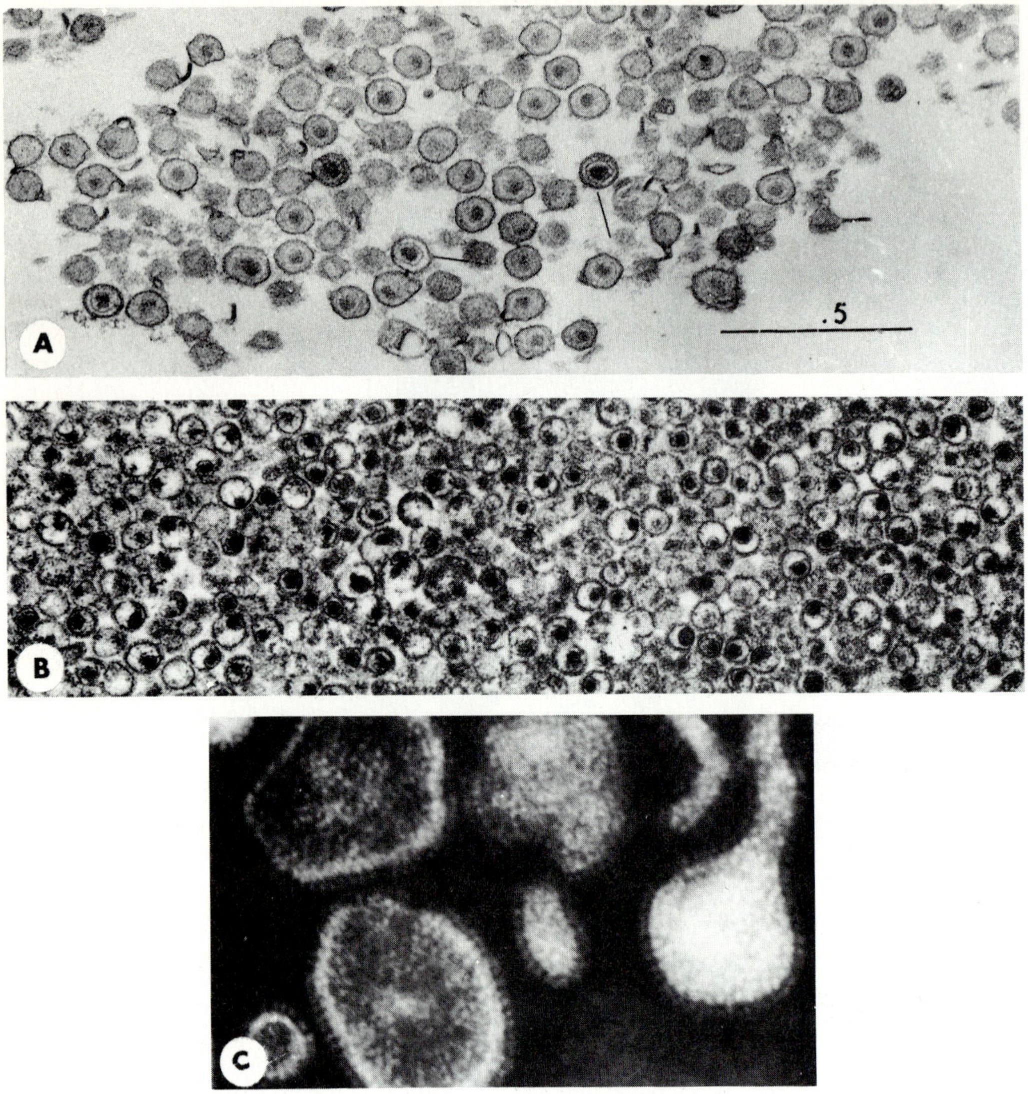

Figure 2-16. The structure of RNA tumor viruses. **A.** Thin section of Rous sarcoma virus, a C-type virus. Outer and inner membranes as well as nucleoids are clearly visible (arrows); note the central location of the nucleoid. × 52,000. **B.** Thin section of mouse mammary tumor virus, a B-type virus. Note the eccentric location of the nucleoid. **C.** Mouse mammary tumor virus stained with phosphotungstate. Note the prominent glycoprotein spikes. *(**A,** from Courington and Vogt: J Virol 1:400, 1967; **B, C,** courtesy of Dr. D. Moore.)*

in a highly regular, crisscross pattern, which is probably caused by one continuous filament wound round each particle in 12 to 15 left-handed turns (Fig. 2-18). The internal components of parapoxvirus particles are similar to those of the poxvirus particles described above.

Finally, there are several viruses that have not yet been assigned to any virus family. Among these are hepatitis B virus (serum hepatitis virus), which has a diameter of 42 nm (Dane particles, see Chaps. 8 and 22); and the chronic infectious neuropathic agents.

The relative sizes of some important animal viruses are illustrated in Fig. 2-19. Their morphology is summarized in Table 2-1.

The Nature of the Components of Animal Viruses

Purification of Viruses

Little serious work on the properties, composition, and molecular biology of viruses is possible unless pure virus is available. The starting material for virus purification may be any material that contains a sufficiently large amount of virus. This may be cellular material such as infected organs or cultured cells, or it may be extracellular material such as plasma, allantoic fluid, or cell culture medium. If the virus concentration in such material is not high

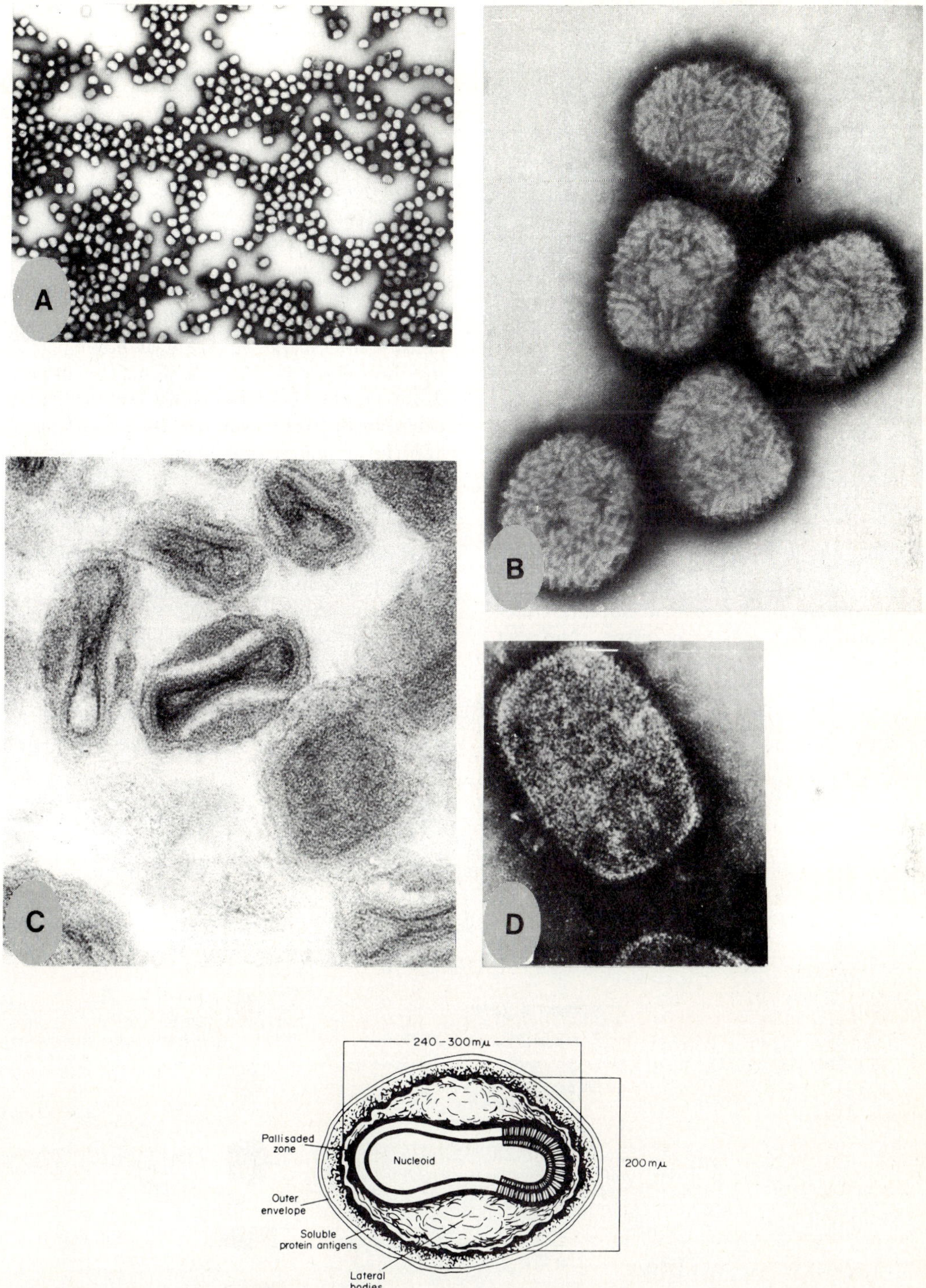

E

Figure 2-17. The structure of vaccinia virus. **A.** A purified virus preparation. Note characteristic brick shape. × 6,000. **B.** Vaccinia virus particles stained with phosphotungstate to reveal surface structure. Note the characteristic arrangement of rodlets or tubules. × 60,000. **C.** Cross-section of vaccinia virus particle. × 70,000. **D.** An isolated core, showing regular surface elements. × 90,000. **E.** A model of the vaccinia virus particle. *(**A, B, C,** courtesy of Dr. Samuel Dales; **D,** from Easterbrook: J Ultrastr Res 14:484, 1966; **E,** adapted from Westwood et al.: J Gen Microbiol 34: 67, 1964.)*

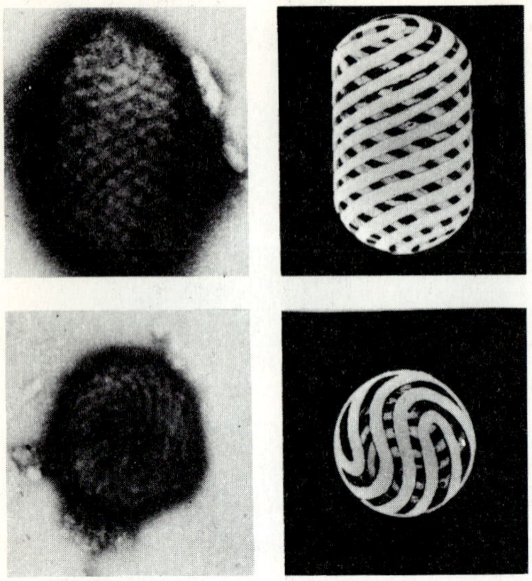

Figure 2-18. Parapoxvirus particles. These are particles of contagious pustular dermatitis virus (ORF), negatively stained so as to reveal the crisscross arrangement of surface strands or tubules. × 90,000. *(From Buttner et al.: Arch Ges Virusforsch 14: 657, 1964.)*

enough, an initial concentration step that employs either precipitation or centrifugation may be necessary. The next step is then generally designed to achieve a preliminary purification by removing the bulk of nonviral material. This may be achieved by treatment with detergents or emulsification with organic solvents followed by centrifugation or by adsorption to and elution from red blood cells (in the case of myxoviruses), or by pasage through columns that contain materials capable of separating viral and cellular components. For the final purification step, fractionation by means of density gradient centrifugation is almost always used. There are two modes of employing this technique (Fig. 2-20). In velocity density gradient or rate zonal centrifugation, the virus suspension is layered onto a density gradient; that is, a solution of either sucrose or glycerol or some salt of gradually increasing density, the maximum density being such that virus particles would migrate to the bottom of the tube if centrifuged long enough. If centrifuged for shorter periods, particles with the same sedimentation coefficient, which depends on size, density, and shape, sediment as homogeneous bands that may be collected. This step eliminates all impurities except those with the same sedimentation coefficient as virus particles. In order to eliminate the remaining impurities, the particles in the virus-containing band recovered from the first density gradient are then centrifuged to equilibrium in a second density gradient composed of solutions of higher density. Here particles form bands where the density of the medium is identical to their own buoyant density. Because contaminants with both the same sedimentation coefficient and the same density as virus particles are rare, virus purified by two such density gradient centrifugation steps is generally considered to be essentially pure (that is, at least 97 to 99 percent free of nonviral material).

The purification of icosahedral viruses generally presents no difficulties. Some enveloped viruses, however, are

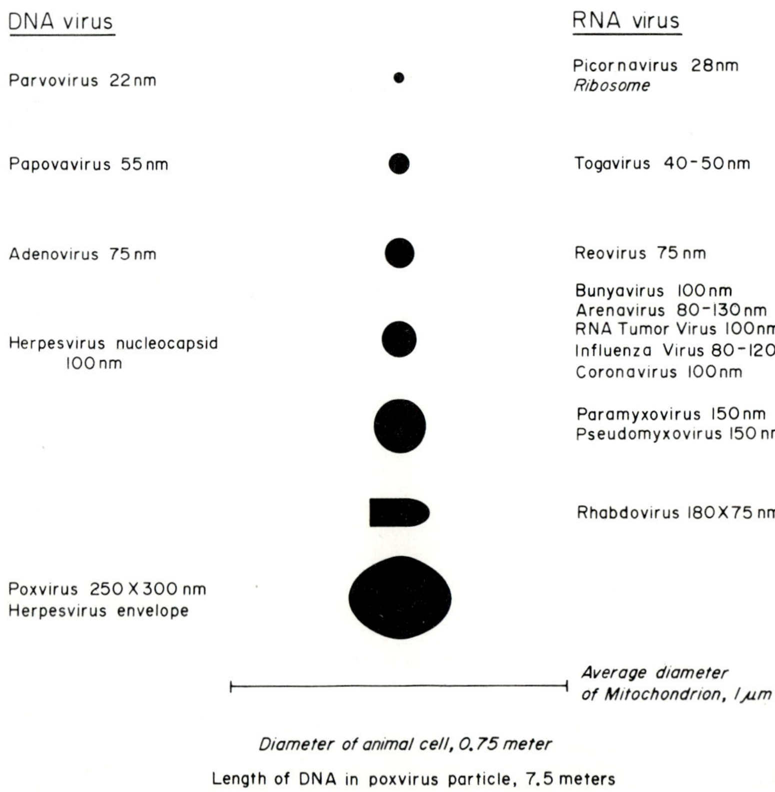

Figure 2-19. The relative sizes of the principal families of animal viruses. Unless otherwise indicated, the scale is the same for all.

TABLE 2-1. THE MORPHOLOGY OF ANIMAL VIRUSES

Virus	Morphology
DNA Virus	
Poxvirus	Complex
Iridovirus	Enveloped icosahedral nucleocapsid
Herpesvirus	Enveloped icosahedral nucleocapsid
Adenovirus	Naked icosahedral nucleocapsid
Papovavirus	Naked icosahedral nucleocapsid
Parvovirus	Naked icosahedral nucleocapsid
RNA Viruses	
Picornavirus	Naked icosahedral nucleocapsid
Togavirus	Enveloped icosahedral nucleocapsid
Bunyavirus	Enveloped helical circular nucleocapsids
Reovirus	Naked double-shelled icosahedral nucleocapsid
Orthomyxovirus	Enveloped helical nucleocapsid
Paramyxovirus	Enveloped helical nucleocapsid
Rhabdovirus	Enveloped helical nucleocapsid
RNA tumor virus	Enveloped icosahedral nucleocapsid
Arenavirus	Enveloped helical nucleocapsid
Coronavirus	Enveloped helical nucleocapsid

not easily purified because the amount of envelope per virus particle may be variable, which causes them to be heterogeneous with respect to both size and density.

It is almost impossible to establish absolute criteria of purity for viruses, mainly because small amounts of cellular constituents tend to absorb to them. Absence of particulate impurities is best assessed by electron microscopic examination.

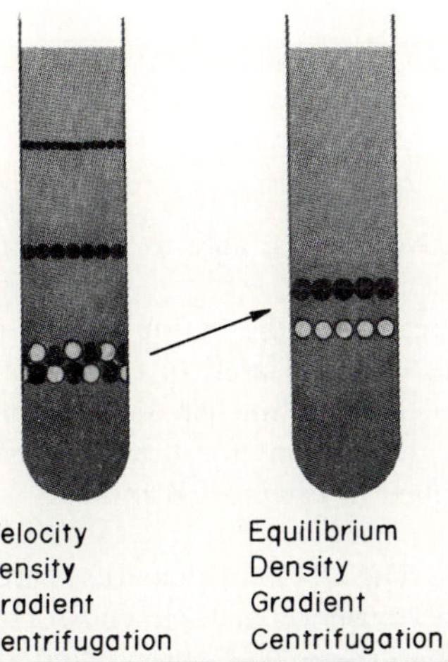

Figure 2-20. Application of the technique of density gradient centrifugation to virus purification. A partially purified virus preparation is layered onto the left-hand density gradient, which is centrifuged so that particles with the same sedimentation coefficient form distinct bands. Three such bands are shown, one of which contains virus (open spheres). This band is then centrifuged to equilibrium in the right-hand density gradient, in which particles are separated according to their buoyant density. See text for further details.

Viral Nucleic Acids

The nucleic acids of animal viruses are astonishingly diverse. Some are DNA, others RNA; some are double-stranded, others single-stranded; some are linear, others circular; some have plus polarity, others minus polarity. Information concerning these and other properties of viral nucleic acids is essential for an understanding of the key reactions during virus multiplication cycles.

Size of Viral Nucleic Acids

The nucleic acid content of animal viruses varies within wide limits. At the lower end of the scale, only about 2 percent of influenza virus particles are RNA, and only about 5 percent of poxvirus particles are DNA; at the upper end, about 25 percent of picornavirus particles are RNA. However, the proportion of nucleic acid in virus particles is not as significant as its absolute amount, which is the factor that determines the amount of genetic information that it contains. The smallest animal virus genomes are those of the picornaviruses and parvoviruses, whose molecular weights range from 1.5 to 3×10^6. Because the coding ratio (the ratio of the molecular weight of single-stranded nucleic acid to the molecular weight of the protein for which it can code) is about nine, these viral genomes can code for protein with a total molecular weight of from 150,000 to 300,000, which is equivalent to four to eight average-sized proteins. The largest animal virus genomes, those of the poxviruses and herpesviruses, are about 100 times larger; their molecular weights range from 100 to almost 200×10^6 (Fig. 2-21). The molecular weights of viral genomes are listed in Table 2-2.

Structure of Viral Nucleic Acids

Strandedness. Both double-stranded and single-stranded DNA as well as RNA can act as the genome of animal viruses (Table 2-2).

Terminal Redundancy. The nucleic acids of several animal viruses are terminally redundant or repetitious, that is, their base composition may be represented as A, B, C. . . . X, Y, Z, A, where A, B, C, and so on are nucleotide sequences. This is most readily demonstrated, in the case of double-stranded DNAs, by treating them briefly with bacteriophage λ exonuclease, which digests DNA strands from their 5′-phosphate-containing termini. In this way, one end of one strand and the other end of the other strand are digested. On melting and reannealing, DNA digested in this manner circularizes, indicating that the two single-stranded regions at the two ends are complementary, hence that their sequences must be repetitious (Fig. 2-22). In the case of herpesvirus DNA, the length of the repeated sequences is about 400 nucleotide base pairs, which is about 0.25 percent of its total length. Terminal redundancy of this type is also exhibited by the RNA of RNA tumor viruses.

Figure 2-21. Electron micrograph of an intact herpesvirus DNA molecule. It is about 44-μm long. The small circular molecules are intact DNA molecules of the bacteriophage ϕX 174 (see Chap. 9), which were added to provide a size marker. *(Courtesy of Dr. Edward K. Wagner.)*

Adenovirus, parvovirus, and poxvirus DNAs, as well as rhabdovirus, bunyavirus, arenavirus RNA, are also terminally redundant, but here the repeated sequences are the inverted or reversed complements of each other; that is, their structure is of the form 5′-GATCAT. . . . ATGATC-3′. This is demonstrated by the fact that here single-stranded DNA circles form upon melting and reannealing, without first having to be digested with nuclease (Fig. 2-23). The length of the repeated sequence in adenovirus DNA is about 100 base pairs (0.3 percent of its length); for adeno-associated virus and poxvirus DNAs, the corresponding figures are 145 bases (about 3 percent) and 10,000 base pairs (about 5 percent), respectively. For rhabdovirus RNA the repeated inverted complementary sequence is about 20 residues long. Bunyavirus and arenavirus RNA exist in circular form in the native state, but not following denaturation. The reason for this appears to be the presence of inverted complementary base sequences some 10 to 30 nucleotides long at their ends, which causes them to be sticky or cohesive, that is, able to hybridize and therefore circularize.

The significance of the various forms of terminal redundancy is no doubt related to the mode of replication and expression of these nucleic acids. Examples of situations in which the reasons for terminal redundancy seem clear are described in Chapters 8 and 9.

Crosslinking. The DNAs of poxviruses are unique in being crosslinked covalently at their ends. This is shown by the fact that when these DNAs are melted and reannealed, single-stranded circles are generated whose circumference is twice the length of the linear double-stranded poxvirus DNA molecules. The structure of the ends of vaccinia virus DNA is shown in Fig. 2-24.

Covalent Linkage With Protein. Several viral nucleic acids are linked covalently to protein molecules. Thus the RNAs of picornaviruses like poliovirus are liked at their 5′-

TABLE 2-2. CHARACTERISTICS OF VIRAL NUCLEIC ACIDS

Virus	Nature of Nucleic Acid	Mol Wt ($\times 10^6$)	Strandedness	Structure	Number of Segments	Polarity	Infectivity of Naked Nucleic Acid
Poxvirus	DNA	125–185	Double	Linear crosslinked	1		
Herpesvirus	DNA	100, 150*	Double	Linear	1		+
Adenovirus	DNA	23	Double	Linear	1		+
Papovavirus	DNA	3, 5†	Double	Supercoiled circular	1		+
Parvovirus	DNA	2	Single	Linear	1	+ and − or −§	+ −
Hepatitis B virus	DNA	2	Partially double	Linear, cohesive ends	1		−
Picornavirus	RNA	2–3	Single	Linear	1	+	+
Calicivirus	RNA	2–3	Single	Linear	1	+	+
Togavirus	RNA	4.5	Single	Linear	1	+	+
Bunyavirus	RNA	5	Single	Linear, cohesive ends	3	−	−
Reovirus	RNA	15	Double	Linear	10, 11‖		−
Orthomyxovirus	RNA	4	Single	Linear	8	−	−
Paramyxovirus	RNA	6	Single	Linear	1	−	−
Rhabdovirus	RNA	3–4	Single	Linear	1	−	−
RNA tumor virus	RNA	5–8	Single	Linear	2‡	+	−
Arenavirus	RNA	5	Single	Linear, cohesive ends	2	−	−
Coronavirus	RNA	5.5	Single	Linear	1	+	+

*100×10^6 for α- and γ-herpesviruses; 150×10^6 for β-herpesviruses.
†5×10^6 for papilloma viruses; 3×10^6 for all others.
‡The genome is not really segmented; the two molecules are identical.
§Adeno-associated viruses, + and −; most others, −.
‖ Orthoreoviruses and orbiviruses, 10 segments; rotaviruses, 11 segments.

termini to a 22 amino acid-long protein (through a tyrosine residue), and each 5′-terminus of the double-stranded DNA of adenoviruses is linked to a protein with a molecular weight of about 55,000. The 5′-terminus of calicivirus RNA and of the minus strand of hepatitis B virus DNA is also linked to a protein. These proteins probably function as primers in the replication of these nucleic acids.

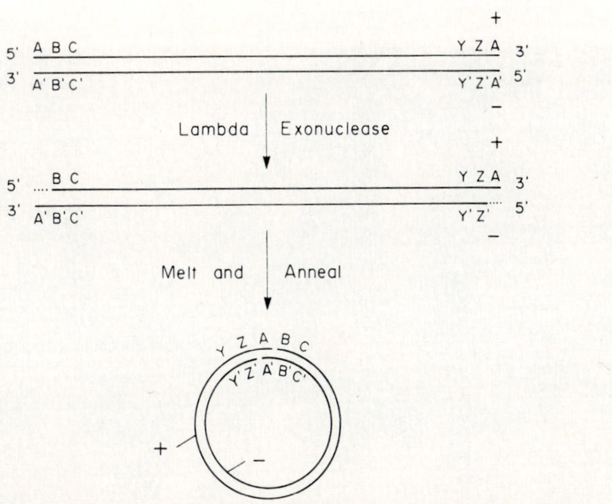

Figure 2-22. Demonstration of terminal redundancy in double-stranded DNA. Note that the A-A′ sequences that are paired in the circularized molecule were originally located at opposite ends of the linear molecule.

Circularity and Supercoiling. Most viral nucleic acids are linear, but papovavirus DNA exists in the form of double-stranded circles, circles that are supercoiled. The reason why papovavirus DNA circles are supercoiled is as follows. Papovavirus DNAs, like SV40 DNA, exist in virus particles in the form of minichromosomes, that is, chains of beads or nucleosomes (Fig. 2-25) that resemble in structure the chromatin of eucaryotic cells. Nucleosomes consist of pairs of the four histones H3, H4, H2A, and H2B, around which the viral DNA is wound. There are about 24 nucleosomes per SV40 DNA molecule. Because it is about 5200 base pairs long, there are about 220 base

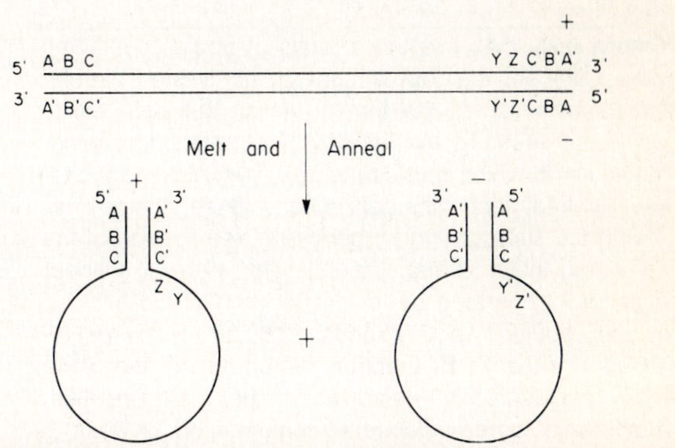

Figure 2-23. Demonstration of the presence of inverted terminally redundant sequences in double-stranded DNA.

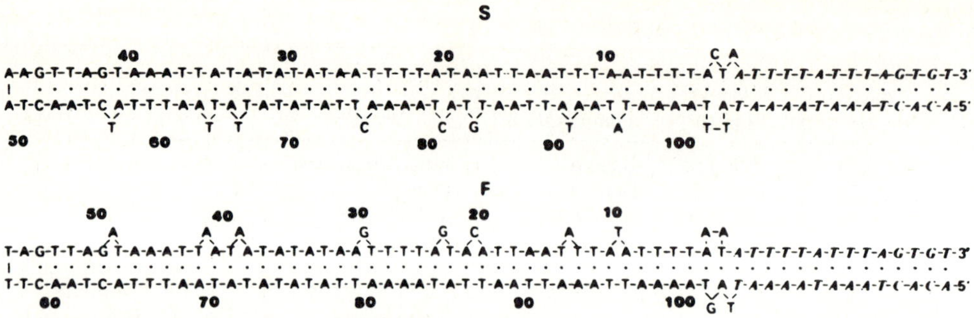

Figure 2-24. The structure of the ends of the DNA of vaccinia virus strain WR. Its plus and minus strands are crosslinked by normal phosphodiester bonds. Note the slight deviations from perfect double-strandedness near the crosslinks, which means that the DNA can assume a variety of configurations. Two of the most highly base-paired configurations are illustrated. The sequences of the two strands are identical from base pair 105 on into the interior of the molecule, which is toward the right. Because vaccinia virus DNA possess inverted terminal repeats (see text), its two ends are identical. *(From Baroudy et al.: Cell 28:315, 1982; Pickup et al.: Virology 124:215, 1983.)*

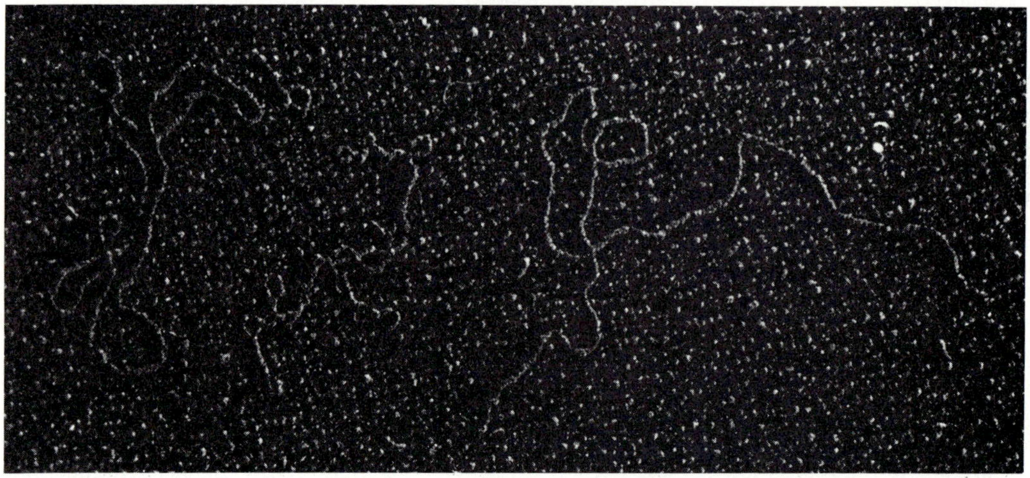

A

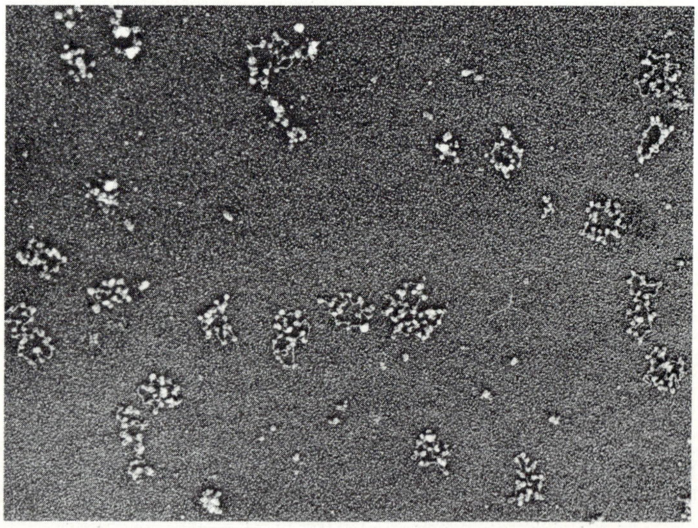

B

Figure 2-25. A. The three forms of bovine papilloma virus DNA. At the top, a supercoiled twisted circular molecule, which is the form in which the DNA exists within the virus. To the left of it is a "relaxed" circular molecule, in which one strand has been nicked, or broken, by treatment with deoxyribonuclease, thereby relieving the supercoiling by permitting free rotation of the remaining intact strand. On the right, there is a linear molecule, generated by the introduction of nicks close to one another in both strands. × 66,000. *(Courtesy of Dr. H. J. Bujard.)* **B.** Electron micrograph of the SV40 DNA nucleoprotein complex in the chromatin-like, beads-on-a-string nucleosome conformation. × 50,000. *(From Keller and Mueller: Science 201:406, 1978.)*

pairs per nucleosome, 180 of which are initimately associated with each nucleosome, whereas 40 are present in the space between adjacent nucleosomes. Coiling the circular DNA molecule around each nucleosome requires a reduction in the number of superhelix turns if the resulting structure is to be devoid of strain. Therefore, when the nucleosomes are removed and the naked DNA is examined in pure form, it is supercoiled, the supercoiling having been caused by the deficiency in superhelical turns. For the SV40 DNA molecule, the deficiency is about 24 superhelical turns. The negative supercoils are introduced into the DNA by the enzyme DNA gyrase, which is a topoisomerase, a class of enzymes that catalyze adenosine triphosphate-dependent changes in the linking number of circular DNA; that is, they coil the DNA helix axis itself by permitting DNA strands to move or pass "through" DNA strands by transiently breaking such strands. Supercoiling is relieved by the action of widespread untwisting enzymes, which are also topoisomerases (DNA gyrase being the only topoisomerase that introduces supercoils), or by nicking one strand with a nuclease, or by the intercalation of substances such as ethidium bromide (Fig. 2-26).

The significance of circularity is not known. It is not essential for infectivity, as the DNA in poxviruses, herpesviruses, and adenoviruses is linear. Conceivably, circularity is a prerequisite for integration into the host genome (see Chap. 8), and the DNAs of adenoviruses and herpesviruses, which, like papovaviruses, can transform cells (see Chap. 8), circularize before being integrated.

Circular Permutation. As discussed in Chapter 9, bacteriophage DNAs are frequently circularly permuted. The DNAs of mammalian animal viruses are generally not circularly permuted. However recent evidence indicates that the DNA of a vertebrate iridovirus is circularly permuted and terminally redundant, and that the genome of the porcine herpesvirus pseudorabies virus possesses features that can best be explained on the basis of circular permutation of some of its sequences.

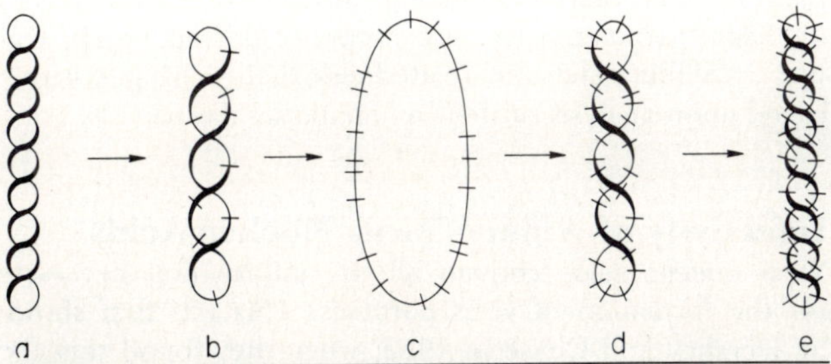

Figure 2-26. Diagrammatic representation of the removal and reversal of supercoiling turns by intercalation of ethidium bromide. The Watson–Crick helix is here represented as a single continuous line. The number of supercoiling turns in the original molecule (**a**) decreases as ethidium bromide molecules (represented by bars perpendicular to the helix axis) bind to the DNA and intercalate between base pairs (**b**). At equivalence, the accumulated untwisting due to the number of intercalated drug molecules balances the initial number of supercoiling turns (**c**). Intercalation of further drug molecules (**d**) leads to the introduction of supercoiling turns in the opposite sense (**e**). *(From Crawford and Waring: J Gen Virol 1:387, 1967.)*

Segmentation. For a long time it was assumed that viral genomes consist of unbroken strands of nucleic acid. However, this is not always so. The genomes of reoviruses and rotaviruses consist of 10 and 11 segments of double-stranded RNA, respectively (Fig. 2-27); the genomes of influenza viruses, bunyaviruses, and arenaviruses consist of eight, three, and two single-stranded RNA molecules, respectively; and the genome of RNA tumor viruses consists

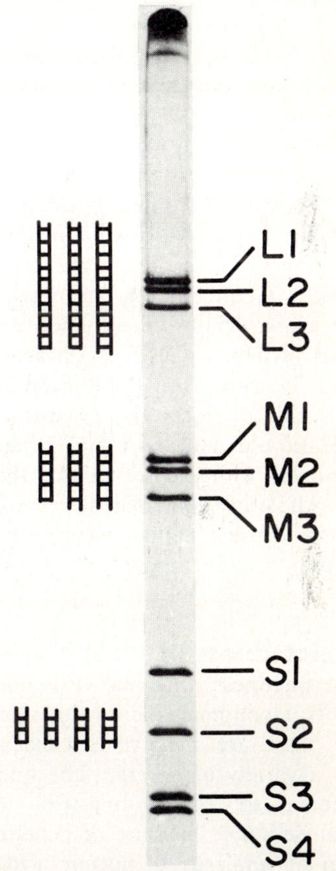

Figure 2-27. The structure of the reovirus genome. RNA extracted from reovirus particles by treatment with the detergent sodium dodecyl sulfate (SDS) was subjected to electrophoresis in a polyacrylamide gel. In such gels, molecules of various sizes migrate as discrete bands, with the smallest ones moving fastest. The direction of migration in the gel shown here was from top to bottom. Bands of RNA were visualized by autoradiography. Each band corresponds to a reovirus gene. The reovirus genome is seen to consist of 10 molecular species that fall into three size classes, designated L, M, and S. Because the rate of migration is inversely proportional to the square of the molecular weight, estimates of relative molecular weights can be made by measuring the distances traveled by the various bands. The relative sizes of the 10 reovirus genes are indicated at the left of the gel.

of two single-stranded RNA molecules that are identical (so that the genome is not really segmented [see Chap. 8]). One of the consequences of segmentation is highly efficient genetic recombination caused by random reassortment of segments in multiply infected cells (see Chap. 6).

Polarity of Viral Nucleic Acids

The single-stranded RNA molecules present in picornavirus, calicivirus, togavirus, coronavirus, and RNA tumor virus particles can be translated by ribosomes and serve as messenger RNA. All the genetic information necessary for the formation of progeny virus is translated directly from them. This is not the case for the RNA molecules present in ortho- and paramyxovirus, rhabdovirus, bunyavirus, and arenavirus particles. These RNAs must first be transcribed into RNA strands of opposite polarity, and it is these transcripts that are then translated by ribosomes. Because the polarity of messenger RNA is generally designated as plus, the polarity of the RNA in the former group of viruses is plus, and that of the RNA in the latter group is minus.

The adeno-associated satellite viruses, which belong to the parvovirus family and contain single-stranded DNA, present a unique situation. There are two kinds of these virus particles; one contains plus strands, the other minus strands. These two kinds of particles are produced in equal amounts. When the DNA is extracted from them it hybridizes rapidly, thus giving the illusion that it is double-stranded. It is only when the DNA is extracted under conditions where the plus and the minus strands are prevented from hyridizing with each other that the true situation is revealed. All other parvoviruses (except the insect Densonucleosis viruses) contain single-stranded DNA of one polarity only, namely minus.

Genetic Relatedness of Viral Nucleic Acids

The genetic relatedness of animal virus nucleic acids is of interest for its taxonomic and evolutionary significance. For example, there are many viruses that are poxviruses, according to a variety of criteria. The question naturally arises as to how closely related they are.

The most definitive measure of genetic relatedness is determination of similarity of nucleic acid-base sequence by direct sequence analysis. Very efficient techniques for sequencing both RNA and DNA have been perfected, and the genomes of many animal viruses have been sequenced either completely or in part.

Another, less laborious, way to assess genetic relatedness, which is still sensitive enough to be useful taxonomically, is measurement of how extensively nucleic acids can hybridize with each other. If the nucleic acids under investigation are double-stranded, the two molecules whose relatedness is to be determined are denatured to the single-stranded state, mixed, and allowed to reanneal. Single strands derived from the two genomes are thus presented with the opportunity of pairing with each other, and conditions are readily arranged so that such pairing can be quantitated. If the two genomes are very closely related, pairing will occur extensively; if there is no relatedness, no pairing will occur. For example, the genomes of highly oncogenic adenoviruses hybridize with each other to the extent of 80 percent or more; in other words, they share over 80 percent of their base sequences. However, they share only about 25 percent of base sequences with the genomes of the nononcogenic adenoviruses, which, on the other hand, share over 80 percent of base sequences among themselves. Another example is provided by strains of the three serotypes of reovirus. The RNAs of strains of serotypes 1 and 3 hybridize with each other to the extent of about 70 percent, but both hybridize only to the extent of about 10 percent with the RNAs of reovirus strains of serotype 2.

If the viruses that are to be compared possess single-stranded nucleic acid, the strategy is to hybridize the viral nucleic acid in question to the double-stranded, or replicative form (see Chap. 4) of the nucleic acid of the virus strain whose genetic relatedness is to be assessed.

Another interesting application of this methodology is heteroduplex analysis, in which the hybrid molecules are examined in the electron microscope. Regions of genomes that are identical or nearly identical, that is, homologous, are then seen to be double-stranded, whereas regions that are so dissimilar that they will not base-pair with each other, or regions that are present in only one genome and not in the other (either insertions or deletions) appear as single-stranded regions. An example of heteroduplex analysis is shown in Figure 4-12.

Another measure of genetic relatedness employs comparison of proteins rather than of nucleic acids. Similarity of nucleic acid-base sequences signifies similarity of the amino acid sequences of the proteins encoded by them. This in turn implies antigenic similarity; that is, ability of proteins to react with each other's antibodies. Ability of nucleic acids to hybridize, and of the proteins coded by them to cross-react immunologically, are thus measures of the same parameter. As an example of this approach, Figure 2-28 illustrates the relatedness of five herpesviruses, based upon analysis of their antigenic similarity.

Infectivity of Animal Virus Nucleic Acids

Viral nucleic acids contain all the information necessary for the formation of virus particles. This was first shown by Hershey and Chase in 1952, when they found that the injection of bacteriophage DNA into the host cell causes the formation of progeny virus particles. Later, in 1956, Gierer and Schramm showed that the same was true for RNA when they found that RNA extracted from tobacco mosaic virus particles was infectious.

The nucleic acids of several groups of animal viruses, such as that of the picornaviruses, caliciviruses, togaviruses, coronaviruses, papovaviruses, adenoviruses, and herpesviruses, are also infectious (see Table 2-2). These are all nucleic acids that either can act as messenger RNA themselves or that are transcribed into messenger RNA by host-coded RNA polymerases. Viral nucleic acids that are transcribed into messenger RNA by virus-coded polymer-

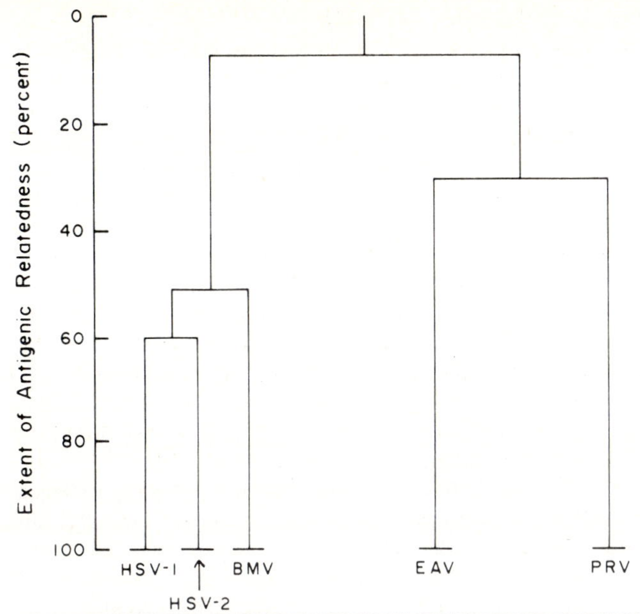

Figure 2-28. Dendrogram illustrating the serologic relatedness of five herpesviruses, herpes simplex virus type 1 (HSV-1), herpes simplex virus type 2 (HSV-2), bovine mammillitis virus (BMV), equine abortion virus (EAV), and pseudorabies virus (PRV). The extent of antigenic relatedness was assessed by counting the number of precipitin bands formed in agar gel immunodiffusion reactions, using antisera to the various herpesviruses and the virus-coded proteins in extracts of cells infected with homologous and heterologous herpesviruses. *(Adapted from Honess and Watson: J Gen Virol 37:15, 1977.)*

ases, such as the minus-stranded RNAs of ortho- and paramyxoviruses, rhabdoviruses, bunyaviruses, and arenaviruses; the double-stranded RNA of reovirus; and the double-stranded DNA of poxviruses, are not infectious, as they cannot express themselves in the cell.

In all cases, the naked nucleic acids are less infectious by factors ranging from 10^3 to 10^6 than the virus particles from which they were extracted. There are two principal reasons for this. First, naked viral nucleic acids are quickly degraded by nucleases, which are generally present in extracellular fluids, as well as on outer cell membranes; second, naked nucleic acids are taken up very poorly by cells. Uptake can be increased significantly by (1) treating cells briefly with concentrated salt solutions, which promotes pinocytosis, thereby facilitating nucleic acid entry; or (2) complexing the naked nucleic acids with polycations such as protamine of DEAE-dextran; or (3) adsorbing them to precipitated calcium phosphate, which is taken up well by cells. The inefficiency with which naked viral nucleic acids penetrate into cells emphasizes the role of the viral capsid in this vital function.

The host range of naked viral nucleic acids is very much broader than that of the respective virus particles. This stems from the fact that the host range of a virus particle is restricted by the specificity of the interaction between the capsid and cell surface receptors (see Chap. 4). This is not the case for naked viral nucleic acids. For example, whereas poliovirus can infect and therefore multiply only in cells of human or primate origin, poliovirus RNA can also infect chick cells and mouse cells.

Infectious viral nucleic acid can be extracted not only from infectious virus particles but from all virus particles that contain undamaged nucleic acid. Among such are virus particles inactivated by heat, proteolytic enzymes, and detergents.

Presence of Host Cell Nucleic Acids in Virus Particles

As a rule, capsids enclose viral nucleic acids. However, sometimes segments of host nucleic acid become encapsidated instead. For example, particles exist that contain, within a papovavirus capsid, a linear piece of host DNA roughly the same size as papovavirus DNA. Each such particle, known as a pseudovirion, contains a different segment of host DNA. Pseudovirions usually make up only a small fraction of the yield, but in some cell lines the majority of the particles formed as a result of infection with polyoma virus are pseudovirions. Another example is provided by virus particles that are formed when papovaviruses are passaged repeatedly at high multiplicity; that is, in cells infected with many virus particles. These virus particles contain DNA molecules that consist partly of viral and partly of host cell sequences. They are formed when the viral genomes, which become integrated into host cell DNA prior to replication (see Chaps. 8 and 9), are imperfectly excised (cut out of the host genome).

Viral Proteins

The principal constituent of all animal viruses is protein. Proteins are the sole component of capsids, the major component of envelopes, and are also intimately associated with the nucleic acids of many icosahedral viruses as internal or core proteins. All these proteins are referred to as structural proteins, as their primary function is to serve as virus particle building blocks. They are almost always encoded by the viral genome.

Viral proteins vary widely in size, from less than 10,000 to more than 150,000 daltons. They also vary in number, with some virus particles containing as few as three species, and others containing more than 50. Viral proteins are characterized most conveniently by dissociating highly purified virus preparations with detergent and subjecting the resulting protein mixtures to electrophoresis in polyacrylamide gels. The most commonly used detergent is sodium dodecyl sulfate (SDS), which not only destroys the secondary structure of proteins but also forms complexes with them. These complexes carry numerous strong negative charges, so that upon electrophoresis in polyacrylamide gels they migrate strictly according to size. As a result, SDS-polyacrylamide gel electrophoresis provides a very convenient method for determining not only the number of different protein species that make up virus particles, but also their sizes. The polyacrylamide gel electrophoresis profile of vaccinia virus proteins is shown in Figure 2-29.

All members of the same virus family display the same or almost the same highly characteristic electrophoretic protein patterns. The patterns of reovirus, rhinovirus, murine encephalomyelitis (ME) virus, and Sendai virus (a paramyxovirus) proteins are illustrated in Figure 2-30.

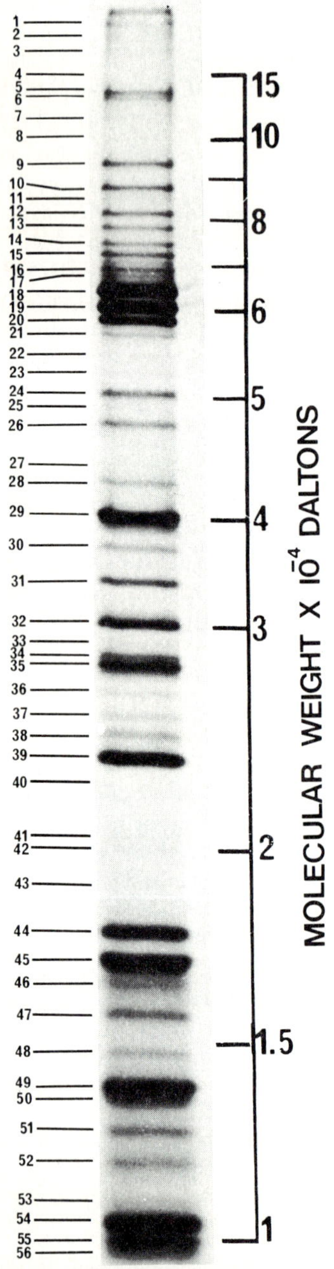

Figure 2-29. Polyacrylamide gel of vaccinia virus structural proteins. Vaccinia virus labeled with ^{35}S-methionine was dissolved in a buffer containing sodium dodecyl sulfate, and the resulting solution was electrophoresed in an 11 percent polyacrylamide gel. An autoradiogram was then prepared from it by exposing x-ray film to it. The direction of electrophoresis was from top to bottom. Over 50 proteins are clearly visible. There is evidence that the vaccinia virus particle may comprise as many as 100 different species of proteins. *(From Dales: Virology 95:355, 1979.)*

Glycoproteins

Viral envelopes often contain glycoproteins in the form of spikes or projections. Their carbohydrate moieties consist of oligosaccharides comprising 10 to 15 monosaccharide units, which are linked to the polypeptide backbone through N- and O-glycosidic bonds involving asparagine and serine or threonine, respectively. Their principal components are generally galactose and galactosamine, glucose and glucosamine, fucose, mannose, and neuraminic acid, which always occupies a terminal position.

It was long thought that the structure of the oligosaccharides of viral glycoproteins is specified solely by the nature and relative abundance of the various host cell glycosyl transferases that assemble them from their monosaccharide components. This is certainly a very important factor, but it now appears that the nature of the protein that is being glycosylated also influences oligosaccharide structure, particularly near the chain termini. As a result, the oligosaccharides of viral glycoproteins probably differ from those of cells. Further, the oligosaccharides of glycoproteins of different viruses grown in the same cell are probably not identical, and the oligosaccharides of the glycoproteins of the same virus grown in different cells, although closely related, are probably different. The structure of the oligosaccharide of the spike glycoprotein of vesicular stomatitis virus is shown in Figure 2-31.

Viral Proteins with Specialized Functions

Some viral proteins have specialized properties and functions. Among them are the following:

Hemagglutinins. Many animal viruses, both naked and enveloped (such as picornaviruses, togaviruses, reoviruses, ortho- and paramyxoviruses, adenoviruses, and papovaviruses), agglutinate the red blood cells of certain animal species. This property, which is called hemagglutination, reflects the fact that these red blood cells possess recep-

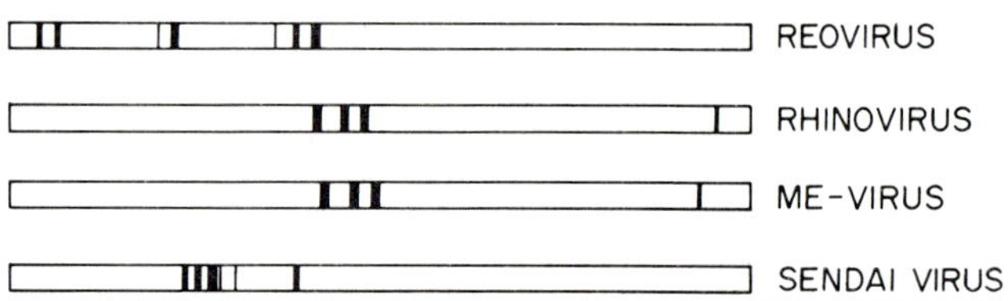

Figure 2-30. Drawings of polyacrylamide gel patterns of the proteins of reovirus, rhinovirus, murine encephalomyelitis (ME) virus, and Sendai virus. Highly purified preparations of these viruses were dissolved in buffer containing sodium dodecyl sulfate (SDS); the illustration shows gels in which the SDS complexes of the proteins of these four viruses had been electrophoresed from left to right. The location of each band is a measure of its molecular weight; thus the largest protein shown is the left-most protein of reovirus (mol wt 150,000), and the smallest is the right-most protein of rhinovirus (mol wt about 8000). The relative amount of each protein is indicated by the thickness of the band representing it. It is clear from the gel patterns shown that the protein complements of rhinovirus and ME virus, both picornaviruses, are very similar, and that they are quite different from those of reovirus and Sendai virus.

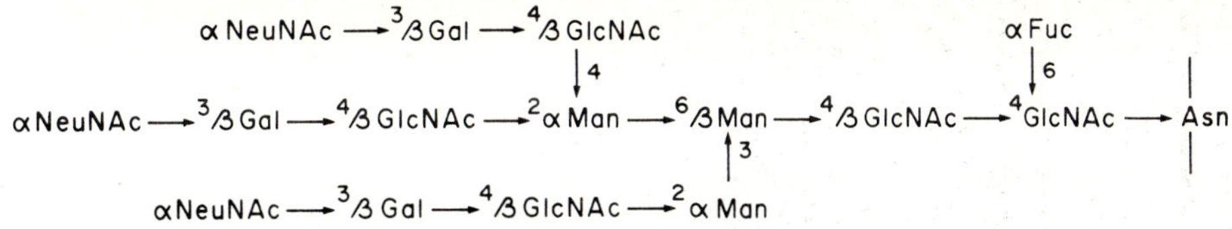

Figure 2-31. The structure of the oligosaccharide unit of the vesicular stomatitis virus spike glycoprotein. There are two of these units per protein molecule. Asn, asparagine; GlcNAc, N-acetylglucosamine; Man, manose; Gal, galactose; NeuNAc, N-acetyl-neuraminic acid; Fuc, fucose. *(From Reading, et al.: J Biol Chem 253:5600, 1978.)*

tors for certain surface components of virus particles. In the case of ortho- and paramyxoviruses, these viral surface components, called hemagglutinins, are glycoprotein spikes present on the virus particle surface (see Fig. 2-4). The ability to hemagglutinate can be used to quantitate virus (see Chap. 1).

Enzymes. Virus particles often contain enzymes (Table 2-3). Among them are the following:

1. Orthomyxovirus and paramyxovirus particles contain an enzyme, neuraminidase, that hydrolyzes the galactose-N-acetylneuraminic acid bond at the ends of the oligosaccharide chains of glycoproteins and glycolipids, thereby liberating N-acetylneuraminic acid. Like the hemagglutinin, this enzyme is located on glycoprotein spikes. Orthomyxoviruses possess two types of spikes, one with hemagglutinin and the other with neuraminidase activity (See Fig. 2-4), whereas paramyxoviruses also possess two types of spikes, on one of which both activities are located. The primary function of neuraminidase appears to be to release virus particles from the cells in which they were formed. The reason why the release of these viruses requires a special enzyme is that their hemagglutinins possess strong affinity for the galactose-N-acetylneuraminic acid (sialic acid) residues at the ends of oligosaccharide chains of glycoproteins. By hydrolyzing them, the enzyme permits the liberation of virus particles that would otherwise not be released or that would readsorb immediately after being liberated.
2. Many virus particles contain RNA polymerases. The necessity for such enzymes stems from the fact that the nucleic acid present in virus particles must be able to express itself once it has gained access to the interior of the host cell. If this nucleic acid itself can act as messenger RNA, like picornavirus or togavirus RNA, there is no problem. If it cannot, either because it is double-stranded or because it is RNA with minus polarity, RNA with plus polarity must first be synthesized. There are two possible sources for the enzymes necessary for this purpose. The first is enzymes existing in the host cell. Herpesvirus, adenovirus, and papovavirus DNAs are transcribed into messenger RNA by DNA-dependent RNA polymerases specified by the host cell. The alternative is that the virus particle itself contains the enzyme. Examples of this type are the poxviruses that possess a DNA-dependent RNA polymerase in their cores, reoviruses that possess an RNA-dependent RNA polymerase in their cores, and negative RNA-stranded viruses that contain RNA polymerases that synthesize plus RNA strands from the minus RNA strands present within them. These enzymes are usually not active

TABLE 2-3. ENZYMES IN ANIMAL VIRUSES

Virus	Enzyme
DNA Viruses	
Poxvirus	DNA-dependent RNA polymerase
	Messenger RNA capping enzymes
	Poly (A) polymerase
	Nucleases (nicking enzymes)
	DNA-dependent nucleotide phosphohydrolase
	Topoisomerase
	Protein kinase
Herpesvirus	None
Adenovirus	Protein kinase
Papovavirus	None
Parvovirus	DNA polymerase
Hepatitis virus	DNA polymerase
RNA Viruses	
Picornavirus	None
Calicivirus	None
Togavirus	None
Bunyavirus	RNA polymerase
Reovirus	RNA-dependent RNA polymerase
	Nucleotide phosphohydrolase
	Messenger RNA capping enzymes
Orthomyxovirus	Neuraminidase
	RNA polymerase
Paramyxovirus	Neuraminidase
	RNA polymerase
	Messenger RNA capping enzymes
	Poly (A) polymerase
Rhabdovirus	RNA polymerase
	Messenger RNA capping enzymes
	Poly (A) polymerase
	Protein kinase
RNA tumor virus	RNA-dependent DNA polymerase (reverse transcriptase)
	Ribonuclease H
	Protein-cleaving enzyme
	Protein kinase
Arenavirus	RNA polymerase
	Poly (A) polymerase
Coronavirus	None

in intact virus particles but are activated when the envelope or capsid is partially degraded, which generally occurs very soon after infection.

3. RNA tumor viruses possess a DNA polymerase, the so-called reverse transcriptase, which transcribes their single-stranded RNA into double-stranded DNA, which is then integrated into the genome of the host cell (see Chap. 8). Furthermore, hepatitis B virus contains a DNA polymerase that appears to be able to transcribe both DNA and RNA into DNA (see Chap. 8).

All these enzymes are virus-specified. The evidence for this conclusion is provided by the existence of virus strains that contain variant enzymes and the fact that the enzymes in question often simply do not exist in uninfected cells.

Viruses also often contain other enzymes. Among them are the enzymes that modify both ends of the messenger RNA molecules synthesized by these polymerases, notably the capping enzymes (that is, the enzyme that guanylylates their 5′-termini and the methylases that methylate both the terminal G as well as the ribose residue that was N-terminal in the uncapped molecule), and poly (A) polymerases that polyadenylate the 3′-termini of messenger RNA molecules. Protein kinases, the function of which is unknown, are also often present, and the very complex poxviruses also contain deoxyribonucleases, DNA-dependent phosphohydrolases, and topoisomerases that may function in DNA replication.

Viral Lipids

Viral envelopes contain complex mixtures of neutral lipids, phospholipids, and glycolipids. As a rule, the composition of these mixtures resembles that of the membranes of the host cells in which the virus multiplied. As the lipid composition of membranes varies markedly from one cell strain to another and even for the same cell strain depending on the composition of the medium, this means that the same virus grown in different cell strains may have widely differing neutral lipid, phospholipid, and glycolipid complements, even though its biologic properties, including infectivity, are identical.

The nature and extent of the differences in composition that are encountered are best illustrated by the example of the paramyxovirus SV5. On the average, this virus contains about 20 percent total lipid, of which roughly 25 percent and 5 percent are cholesterol and triglyceride, respectively; 55 percent are phospholipid; and 15 percent are glycolipid. If grown in cells the membranes of which have a molar ratio of cholesterol to phospholipid of 0.81, the ratio for the viral envelope is 0.89; if the cellular ratio is 0.51, that for the viral envelope is 0.60. The same holds for the relative amounts of several phospholipids. If the ratio of phosphatidylcholine to phosphatidylethanolamine in host cell membranes is 3.55, the ratio in the viral envelope is 2.55; if the ratio in host cell membranes is 0.8, the ratio in the viral envelope is 0.6. However, for one cell the ratio is 1.6, whereas that in the viral envelope derived from it is 0.6, which suggests that a limited degree of lipid selection is possible.

The Classification of Animal Viruses

Attempts to devise a system of classification for animal viruses began almost as soon as their importance as pathogens became apparent. However, the criteria on which to base such a system have changed with advances in our knowledge of their nature and properties. For example, host range cannot be such a criterion; not only is each animal species subject to infection by a wide variety of viral agents, but also numerous viruses infect several different animal species. Similarly, the pattern of pathogenesis of the disease that is caused is an unreliable foundation on which to base a system of classification.

It has become more and more apparent that a system of classification must be based on the physical and chemical properties of the virus particles themselves.

Criteria for Classification

Morphology

The primary criterion for classification is morphology. It is easy to apply because it does not require purified virus. Virus particles can be examined either within cells, that is, in thin sections of infected tissue, or in their extracellular state. Morphologic detail is usually brought out by shadowing with thin films of some heavy metal, such as uranium or tungsten; by staining with osmic acid or uranyl acetate; or by negative staining with phosphotungstic acid.

Physical and Chemical Nature of Viral Components

Morphologic similarity correlates closely with similarity of viral components. For example, all viruses with the morphology of adenoviruses contain double-stranded DNA genomes with a molecular weight of about 23 million; all papovaviruses contain circular supercoiled DNA genomes with molecular weights of 3 to 5 million, and all reoviruses contain segmented double-stranded RNA genomes. In fact, a system of virus classification based on the structure and size of viral genomes yields the same grouping as one based on morphology. Similarly, viruses with similar morphology are composed of similar populations of proteins; and a classification system based on polyacrylamide gel patterns, such as illustrated in Figures 2-29 and 2-30, again yields the same grouping.

Genetic Relatedness

Although the members of the major virus families presumably derived from a common ancestor, genetic relationships among them are often no longer discernible. For example, several groups of mammalian poxviruses exist (Table 2-4) whose members are unrelated genetically as

TABLE 2-4. THE MAJOR FAMILIES OF ANIMAL VIRUSES

DNA-containing Viruses

Classification	*Description*
I. POXVIRIDAE	All genera except *Parapoxvirus*: Brick-shaped complex particles, whorled surface filament pattern Dimensions: 225 × 300 nm *Parapoxvirus*: Ovoid complex particles, regular surface filament pattern Dimensions: 150 × 200 nm

Strains pathogenic for many animal species exist. There are seven genera; the members of each are closely related antigenically but share only one antigen with members of the others. Poxviruses multiply in the cytoplasm.

Subfamily	*Host*	*Symptoms in humans*
Chordopoxvirinae (poxviruses of vertebrates)		
A. Genus *Orthopoxvirus*		
Variola major	Humans	Smallpox
Variola minor	Humans	Alastrim
Monkeypox	Monkey, humans	Smallpox-like disease
Vaccinia	Cattle	—
Cowpox	Cattle, humans	Vesicular eruption of the skin
Buffalopox	Buffalo	—
Rabbitpox	Rabbit	—
Ectromelia (mousepox)	Mouse	—
B. Genus *Leporipoxvirus*		
Myxoma	Rabbit	—
Fibroma	Rabbit	—
C. Genus *Avipoxvirus*		
Fowlpox	Chicken	—
Other birdpox viruses	Various birds	—
D. Genus *Capripoxvirus*		
Sheeppox	Sheep	—
Goatpox	Goat	—
E. Genus *Suipoxvirus*		
Swinepox	Pig	—
F. Genus *Parapoxvirus*		
Orf (contagious postular dermatitis [CPD])	Sheep, goats, humans	Nodules on hands
Pseudocowpox (milker's nodule virus)	Cattle, humans	Nodules on hands
Bovine papular stomatitis	Cattle	—
G. Ungrouped		
Molluscum contagiosum	Humans	Benign epidermal tumors
Yaba monkey tumor virus	Monkeys, humans	Benign subcutaneous tumors
Tanapoxvirus	Monkeys, humans	Benign subcutaneous tumors
Entomopoxvirinae (poxviruses of insects)		
Various strains	Coleoptera, lepidoptera, diptera	—

Classification

II. IRIDOVIRIDAE

These are the icosahedral cytoplasmic deoxyviruses. Many iridoviruses are insect viruses and nonenveloped. The sole mammalian iridovirus is enveloped. The size of its DNA is about 150×10^6.

	Host	*Symptoms in humans*
African swine fever virus	Swine	—
Frog virus 2	Amphibia	—
Frog virus 3		
Lymphocystis virus of fish	Fish	—
Tipula iridescent viruses	Insects	—
Iridescent viruses of	Molluscs, annelids, protozoa	—

(continued)

TABLE 2-4. (cont.)

DNA-containing Viruses

Classification	*Description*
III. HERPESVIRIDAE	Enveloped icosahedral nucleocapsids Diameter of enveloped virions: 180–250 nm Diameter of naked nucleocapsids: 100 nm

The most logical classification of herpesviruses is based on a combination of biologic properties and genome structure. α-Herpesviruses have a variable host range (from very wide to very narrow); most, but not all, have a relatively short replication cycle; most, but not all, are highly cytopathic in cultured cells; they frequently establish latent infections in sensory ganglia; and their DNA has a molecular weight of about 100×10^6. β-Herpesviruses have a narrow host range and a relatively long replication cycle; are less cytopathic; frequently establish latent infections in the salivary gland and in other tissues; and their DNA has a molecular weight of about 150×10^6. γ-Herpesviruses have a narrow host range; a predilection for lymphoblastoid cells which they can transform (that is, they can cause tumors); and their DNA has a molecular weight of about 100×10^6. Few herpesviruses are closely related to each other as judged by DNA–DNA hybridization, but most show some relatedness (2 to 10 percent cross-hybridization). Almost all herpesviruses possess some common antigenic determinants. Herpesviruses cause type A nuclear inclusions (single large acidophilic inclusion bodies separated from basophilic marginated chromatin by a nonstaining halo).

	Host	*Symptoms in humans*
A. *α-Herpesviruses*		
Herpes simplex virus type 1 (human (α-)herpesvirus 1)	Humans	Stomatitis, upper respiratory infections, generalized systemic disease, severe and generally fatal encephalitis
Herpes simplex virus type 2 (human (α-)herpesvirus 2)	Humans	Genital infections
Varicella-zoster (human (α-)herpesvirus 3)	Humans	Chickenpox, herpes zoster
B virus	Monkey, humans	Fatal encephalitis in humans
Equine abortion virus (EAV) (equine herpesvirus 1)	Horse	—
LK virus (equine herpesvirus 2)	Horse	—
Coital exanthema virus (equine herpesvirus 3)	Horse	—
Pseudorabies virus (suid herpesvirus)	Pig	—
Infectious bovine rhinotracheitis (IBR)	Cattle	—
Infectious bovine keratoconjunctivitis (IBKC)	Cattle	—
Feline rhinotracheitis virus	Cat	—
Infectious laryngotracheitis virus (ILT)	Chicken	—
B. *β-Herpesviruses*		
Human cytomegalovirus (human (β-)herpesvirus 5)	Humans	Jaundice, hepatosplenomegaly, brain damage, death
Other Cytomegaloviruses	Monkey	—
	Rodents	—
	Swine	—
C. *γ-Herpesviruses*—All these viruses either cause, or are strongly suspected of causing, tumors		
Epstein–Barr virus (human (γ-)herpesvirus 4)	Humans	Burkitt lymphoma Nasopharyngeal carcinoma Infectious mononucleosis
Marek's disease virus	Chicken	—
Herpesvirus saimiri	Squirrel monkey	—
Herpesvirus ateles	Spider monkey	—
Herpesvirus sylvilagus	Rabbit	—
Guinea pig herpesvirus	Guinea pig	—
Lucké tumor virus	Frog	—

(continued)

TABLE 2-4. (cont.)

DNA-containing Viruses

Classification	*Description*
IV. ADENOVIRIDAE	Naked icosahedral nucleocapsids Diameter: 70 nm

Adenoviruses have been isolated from many species of animals; their host range is generally rather narrow. Adenoviruses share common group-specific complement-fixing antigenic determinants (on hexons) and, in addition, possess type-specific determinants (on pentons and fibers). Host-specific adenoviruses are often represented by numerous serotypes. For example, there are 35 human adenovirus serotypes that can be grouped into subgroups on the basis of antigenic cross-reactivity, DNA hybridization characteristics, ability to transform cells of various animal species, and ability to agglutinate rhesus monkey and rat erythrocytes. More specifically, viruses of subgroup A possess 48 percent (G + C) and regularly cause tumors in newborn hamsters (high tumorigenicity); those in subgroup B possess 51 percent (G + C) and sometimes cause tumors in newborn hamsters (low tumorigenicity); and members of subgroups C, D, and E possess 58 percent (G + C) and do not cause tumors, but still transform cultured cells. Members of subgroup A exhibit about 60 percent homology with each other. For members of the other subgroups, this value is 90 to 100 percent. The extent of homology between subgroups is 10 to 20 percent. Recombination occurs only within, not among, subgroups. Members of the various subgroups exhibit different pathogenicities. Adenoviruses produce intranuclear type B inclusions (basophilic masses sometimes connected to the nuclear periphery by strands of chromatin).

	Host	*Symptoms in humans*
A. Genus *Mastadenovirus*		
Human adenoviruses 35 serotypes	Humans	
Subgroup A Serotypes 12,18,31		No known pathogenicity; regularly isolated from feces of apparently healthy individuals; high incidence of antibodies
Subgroup B Serotypes 3,7,11,14,16,21,34		Acute respiratory disease (7, also 3,14, and 21); pharyngitis (3,7); acute hemorrhagic cystitis in children (11,21); low incidence of antibodies
Subgroup C Serotypes 1,2,5,6		Mild infections of the respiratory tract, especially in infants and children; latent infections in lymphoid tissue
Subgroup D Serotypes 8,9,10,13,15,17,19,20,22–30,32,33		Epidemic keratoconjunctivitis (8, also 19); no known pathogenicity for others; low incidence of antibodies
Subgroup E Serotype 4		Acute respiratory disease
Ungrouped Serotypes 31,35		
Simian adenoviruses 23 serotypes	Monkey	—
Canine adenoviruses (infectious canine hepatitis [ICH])	Dog	—
Adenoviruses of	Cattle, pigs, sheep, frogs, and many other species	—
B. Genus *Aviadenovirus*		
Avian adenoviruses (CELO, chicken-embryo-lethal-orphan; GAL, gallus-adeno-like)	Chicken, quail, other birds	—
C. Noncultivatable adenoviruses (Enteric adenoviruses [EA])	Humans	Enteritis-associated enteric infections

(continued)

TABLE 2-4. (cont.)

DNA-containing Viruses

Classification	*Description*
V. PAPOVAVIRIDAE	Naked icosahedral nucleocapsids Diameter: 55 nm (papilloma viruses) 45 nm (all other papovaviruses)

Papovaviruses (papilloma-polyoma-simian vacuolating agent) fall into two distinct groups on the basis of size; members of the genus papillomavirus possess both larger capsids and larger genomes than members of the genus polyomavirus. All except K virus produce tumors in animals; all produce latent and chronic infections in their natural hosts. Most adults possess antibodies against BK virus and JC virus. Polyomaviruses agglutinate erythrocytes of certain animal species.

	Host	*Symptoms in humans*
A. Genus *Papillomavirus*		
Human papilloma viruses (HPV) 1–15	Humans	
HPV 1 and 4		Plantar warts
HPV 2		Common warts (verruca vulgaris)
HPV 3,5,8,9,10,12,14, and 15		Flat warts (verruca plana) and/or epidermodysplasia verruciformis (EV)
HPV 6 and 11		Anogenital warts (condylomata acuminata), otolaryngeal warts
HPV 7		Meat-handlers' warts
HPV 13		Oral focal hyperplasia
Bovine papilloma viruses 1–5	Cattle	—
Shope rabbit papilloma virus	Rabbit	—
Various viruses pathogenic for other animal species		—
B. Genus *Polyomavirus*		
Polyoma virus	Mouse	—
Simian vacuolating agent (SV-40)	Monkey, humans(?)	—
Rabbit vacuolating agent (RKV)	Rabbit	—
K virus	Mouse	—
BK virus	Humans	Isolated from the urine of renal transplant patients
JC virus	Humans	Isolated from brains of patients with progressive multifocal leucoencephalopathy (PML)
Other primate polyomaviruses [Lymphotrophic papovavirus (LPV)]	African green monkey	Multiplies only in monkey or human B lymphoblasts. About 30 percent of humans have antibody against it

Classification	*Description*
VI. PARVOVIRIDAE	Naked icosahedral nucleocapsids Diameter: 22 nm

These viruses are grouped together on the basis of morphology and nucleic acid structure (single-stranded DNA). All multiply in the nucleus. Most are antigenically unrelated. Adeno-associated viruses (AAVs) multiply only in cells simultaneously infected with adenoviruses (Chap. 6); rat virus (RV) multiplies only in cells that are themselves multiplying actively. Aleutian mink diseases virus causes a slow disease characterized by hypergammaglobulinemia, systemic proliferation of plasma cells, glomerulonephritis, and hepatitis, and is invariably fatal. The disease condition is caused by activation of the immune response; it is exacerbated by administration of inactivated virus or passive antibody. Although it causes a slow disease, Aleutian mink disease virus replicates as rapidly in cultured cells as viruses that cause acute disease.

	Host	*Symptoms in humans*
A. Genus *Adeno-associated virus*		
Human AAV 4 serotypes	Humans	No known symptoms
Other AAVs	Cattle, dog, chicken	

(continued)

TABLE 2-4. (cont.)

DNA-containing Viruses		
	Host	*Symptoms in humans*
B. Genus *Parvovirus*		
Rat virus (Kilham)	Rat	Latent viruses isolated from various hosts including human tumors; none is oncogenic or capable of transforming cultured cells. They produce a mongoloid osteolytic deformity in newborn hamsters
Hamster osteolytic viruses (H-1, H-3, X-14, etc.)		
Minute virus of mice (MVM)	Mouse	—
Other parvoviruses (porcine parvovirus, feline panleukopenia virus, bovine parvovirus, canine parvovirus, etc.)	Pig, cattle, cat, dog	—
Aleutian mink disease virus	Mink	—
C. Genus *Densovirus*		
Densonucleosis viruses	Insects	—

RNA-containing Viruses		
Classification	*Description*	
I. PICORNAVIRIDAE	Naked icosahedral nucleocapsids Diameter: 25–30 nm	

Picornaviruses comprise a large number of virus strains pathogenic for many animal species. They are subdivided into four genera: *Enterovirus* and *Cardiovirus,* whose members are acid-stable, and *Rhinovirus* and *Aphthovirus,* whose members are acid-labile.

	Host	*Symptoms in humans*
A. Genus *Enterovirus*		
Human enteroviruses		
Poliovirus 3 serotypes	Humans, monkey	Poliomyelitis
Coxsackie virus A 23 serotypes	Humans, mouse	Differentiated from Group B Coxsackie viruses primarily on the basis of selective tissue damage: Group A, primarily general striated muscle damage; Group B, primarily fatty tissue and central nervous tissue damage. Group A viruses are associated with herpangina, aseptic meningitis, paralysis, and the common cold syndrome
Coxsackie virus B 6 serotypes	Humans, mouse	Pleurodynia (Bornholm disease), aseptic meningitis, paralysis, severe systemic illness of newborns
ECHO viruses (enteric cytopathogenic human orphan) 32 serotypes	Humans	Paralysis, diarrhea, aseptic meningitis
Human enterovirus 72 (hepatitis A virus)	Humans	Infectious hepatitis, jaundice
Simian enteroviruses 18 serotypes	Monkey	—

(continued)

TABLE 2-4. (cont.)

RNA-containing Viruses

	Host	Symptoms in humans
Murine encephalomyelitis (ME) viruses	Mouse	—
Poliovirus muris		
(Theiler's virus)		
GDVII strain and others		
Bovine enteroviruses	Cattle	—
7 serotypes		
Porcine enteroviruses	Swine	—
8 serotypes		
B. Genus *Cardiovirus*		
Encephalomyocarditis virus (EMC)	Various species including humans	Mild febrile illness
Mengovirus	Mouse	—
ME virus	Mouse	—
C. Genus *Rhinovirus*		
Human rhinoviruses	Humans	Common cold, bronchitis, croup, bronchopneumonia
113 serotypes		
Other rhinoviruses	Strains pathogenic for horses, cattle	—
D. Genus *Aphthovirus*		
Foot-and-mouth disease virus (FMDV)	Cattle, swine, sheep, goats	—
7 serotypes		

Classification	*Description*
II. CALICIVIRIDAE	Naked icosahedral nucleocapsids Diameter: 35–40 nm

Caliciviruses differ significantly from picornaviruses in size and structure, but the primary reason they have been constituted a separate family is that the strategy of genome expression during the multiplication cycles of picornaviruses and caliciviruses is quite different. Vesicular exanthema (VE) virus and San Miguel sealion virus (SMSV) are very closely related; feline picornaviruses are related to them to the extent of about 10 percent as judged by RNA hybridization analysis.

	Host	*Symptoms in humans*
VE of swine virus	Swine	—
SMSV	Seals	—
Feline picornaviruses	Cat	—
Probable calicivirus	Humans	Gastroenteritis
Norwalk virus		

Classification	*Description*
III. TOGAVIRIDAE	Enveloped icosahedral nucleocapsids Diameter: 60–70 nm (alphaviruses and rubiviruses) 45–55 nm (flaviviruses and pestiviruses)

Togaviruses include many of the viruses previously known as arboviruses (arthropodborne). They multiply in bloodsucking insects as well as in vertebrates; in their natural environment they alternate between an insect vector (usually a mosquito or tick) and a vertebrate reservoir, rarely producing disease in either. Many cause subclinical infections in humans, particularly in the tropics, but several are among the most virulent and lethal of all viruses. They are commonly named for the geographic site where they were isolated. They are divided into four genera, primarily on the basis of antigenic relationships (neutralization, complement fixation and hemagglutination inhibition). The alphaviruses and flaviviruses are the old arbovirus groups A and B.

	Reservoir	*Symptoms in humans*
A. Genus *Alphavirus* (mosquito-borne)		
Eastern equine encephalitis (EEE)	Birds	Encephalitis: frequently fatal
Semliki forest virus	Monkey	Undifferentiated febrile illness
Sindbis	Monkey	None
Chikungunya	Monkey	Myositis-arthritis
O'Nyong-Nyong	?	Fever, arthralgia, rash

(continued)

TABLE 2-4. (cont.)

RNA-containing Viruses		
	Reservoir	*Symptoms in humans*
Ross river virus	Mammals	Fever, rash, arthralgia
Venezuelan equine encephalitis (VEE)	Rodents	Encephalitis
Western equine encephalitis (WEE)	Birds	Encephalitis
B. Genus *Flavivirus*		
1. Mosquito-borne		
Yellow fever	Monkey	Hemorrhagic fever, hepatitis, nephritis, often fatal
Dengue (4 serotypes)	Humans	Fever, arthralgia, rash
Japanese encephalitis	Birds	Encephalitis: frequently fatal
St. Louis encephalitis	Birds	Encephalitis
Murray Valley encephalitis	Birds	Encephalitis
West Nile	Birds	Fever, arthralgia, rash
Kunjin	Birds	—
2. Tickborne		
Central European tickborne encephalitis (biphasic meningoencephalitis)	Rodents, hedgehog	Encephalitis
Far Eastern tickborne encephalitis [Russian spring–summer encephalitis (RSSE)]	Rodents	Encephalitis
Kyasanur forest	Rodents	Hemorrhagic fever
Louping Ill	Sheep	Encephalitis
Powassan	Rodents	Encephalitis
Omsk hemorrhagic fever	Mammals	Hemorrhagic fever
C. Genus *Rubivirus*		
Rubella virus	Humans	Severe deformities of fetuses in first trimester of pregnancy
D. Genus *Pestivirus*		
Mucosal disease virus (bovine virus diarrhea virus)	Cattle	—
Hog cholera virus (European swine fever)	Pig	—
Border disease virus	Sheep	—
E. Also included among the togaviruses are several as yet unclassified viruses. Among them are:		
Riley's lactic dehydrogenase elevating virus (LDHV)	Mouse	Produces lifelong chronic viremia in mice; elevates lactic dehydrogenase levels by decreasing the rate of enzyme clearance
Equine arteritis virus	Horse	—
Simian hemorrhagic fever	Monkey	—

Classification	*Description*	
IV. BUNYAVIRIDAE	Enveloped nucleocapsids Diameter: about 100 nm	
Bunyaviruses include all former arbovirus group C viruses, as well as previously ungrouped arboviruses.		
	Host	*Symptoms in humans*
A. Genus *Bunyavirus*		
Bunyamwera and related viruses	Mammals	—
California encephalitis group including La Crosse, Lumbo, and Snowshoe hare virus	Mammals	Encephalitis
B. Genus *Phlebovirus*		
Sandfly fever Sicilian virus	Sandfly, mammals	Facial erythema
Rift Valley fever virus	Humans, sheep, cattle	Fever, arthralgia, retinitis
C. Genus *Nairovirus*		
Crimean–Congo hemorrhagic fever (CCHF) (2 serotypes)	Mammals	Hemorrhagic fever

(continued)

TABLE 2-4. (cont.)

RNA-containing Viruses

	Host	*Symptoms in humans*
Five other serotypes including Nairobi sheep disease virus	Mammals	
D. Genus *Uukuvirus*		
Uukuniemi and related viruses	Birds, mammals	—

Classification	*Description*
V. REOVIRIDAE	Naked nucleocapsids possessing two capsid shells (except cytoplasmic polyhedrosis virus), each with icosahedral symmetry Diameter: 75 nm

The name is an acronym based on respiratory-enteric-orphan (because of lack of association with any disease in humans). The primary criterion for inclusion in this family is possession of a genome consisting of 10, 11, or 12 segments of double-stranded RNA. There are six genera with widely differing host ranges and somewhat differing morphologies. The vertebrate reoviruses possess two clearly defined capsid shells; the orbiviruses (many of which are transmitted by arthropods and are functionally arboviruses) possess a structurally featureless outer shell and an inner shell composed of 32 large ring-shaped capsomers (hence the name, Latin *orbis,* ring; however, see p. 17). The cytoplasmic polyhedrosis viruses possess only one capsid shell with clearly defined icosahedral symmetry. Phytoreoviruses closely resemble the vertebrate reoviruses, while Fijiviruses possess a structure more reminiscent of cytoplasmic polyhedrosis viruses. Rotaviruses present a wheel-like appearance (see Fig. 2-11), hence the name. The members of the six genera are not related antigenically.

	Host	*Symptoms in humans*
A. Genus *Orthoreovirus*		
Mammalian reoviruses 3 serotypes	Humans, other mammals	Pathogenicity not established
Avian reoviruses 5 serotypes	Chicken, duck	—
B. Genus *Orbivirus*		
Bluetongue virus	Culicoides, sheep	—
Eugenangee virus	Mosquitoes	—
Kemerovo	Ticks	—
African horse sickness virus	Culicoides, horse	—
Colorado tick fever virus	Ticks, humans	Encephalitis
C. Genus *Cypovirus*		
Cytoplasmic polyhedrosis virus Numerous strains	*Bombyx mori* (silkworm) and other Lepidoptera, Diptera, and Hymenoptera	—
D. Genus *Phytoreovirus*		
Wound tumor virus	Plants, leaf hoppers	—
Rice dwarf virus	Plants, leaf hoppers	—
E. Genus *Fijivirus*		
Maize rough dwarf virus	Plants, leaf hoppers	—
Fiji disease virus	Plants, leaf hoppers	—
F. Genus *Rotavirus*		
Human rotavirus	Humans	Diarrhea in infants
Calf rotavirus (Nebraska calf diarrhea virus)	Calf	—
Murine rotavirus (Epizootic diarrhea of infant mice [EDIM])	Mouse	—
Simian rotavirus (SA11)	Monkey	—
Bovine or ovine rotavirus ("O" agent)	Cattle or sheep	—
Numerous other rotaviruses	Guinea pig, goat, horse, deer, antelope, rabbit, dog, duck	—

Classification	*Description*
VI. ORTHOMYXOVIRIDAE	Enveloped helical nucleocapsids Diameter: 80–120 nm

(continued)

TABLE 2-4. (cont.)

RNA-containing Viruses

The term myxovirus was coined to denote the unique affinity of influenza viruses for glycoproteins. Nowadays, members of this family are characterized by possession of nucleocapsids with helical symmetry that reside within envelopes, to whose outer surface are attached glycoprotein spikes of two types: One is the hemagglutinin, the other the neuraminidase. Influenza virus strains of type C differ from those of type A and type B in that (1) their buoyant density is lower, (2) the receptors for their hemagglutinins do not appear to contain sialic acid, and (3) their receptor-destroying enzyme seems to cleave some bond other than the -gal-neuraminic acid bond.

	Host	*Symptoms in humans*
A. Genus *Influenza virus*		
Influenza virus type A		
Human subtypes	Human	Acute respiratory disease
A_0 1933–1947*		Acute respiratory disease
A_1 1947–1957		Acute respiratory disease
A_2 1957–1964 (Asian)		Acute respiratory disease
A_2 1968 (Hong Kong)		Acute respiratory disease
Swine influenza virus	Swine	Acute respiratory disease
Avian subtypes		
Fowl plague virus and numerous other strains	Chicken, duck, turkey and others	—
Equine subtypes	Horse	—
Influenza virus type B		
Human subtypes		
B_0 1940–1945	Human	Acute respiratory disease
B_1 1945–1955		Acute respiratory disease
B_2 1962–1964		Acute respiratory disease
B_3 1962 (Taiwan)		Acute respiratory disease
Influenza virus type C (possible separate genus)	Humans	Acute respiratory disease

Classification	*Description*
VII. PARAMYXOVIRIDAE	Enveloped helical nucleocapsids Diameter: about 150 nm

Members of this family were until recently grouped with the orthomyxoviruses in the family Myxoviridae. They have been placed in a separate family because they differ from orthomyxoviruses in that their genomes are not segmented and their hemagglutinin and neuraminidase are located on the same glycoprotein spike. The other type of spike is responsible for the cell-fusing and hemolyzing activities (genus *Paramyxovirus*). Members of the *Morbillivirus* and *Pneumovirus* genera possess no neuraminidase, and members of the genus *Pneumovirus* possess no hemagglutinin either.

	Host	*Symptoms in humans*
A. Genus *Paramyxovirus*		
Parainfluenza virus type 1		
Sendai virus (hemagglutinating virus of Japan [HVJ])	Human, pig, mouse	Croup, common cold syndrome
HA-2 (hemadsorption virus)	Human	Mild respiratory disease
Parainfluenza viruses types 2 to 5		
Numerous strains including HA-1, SV5	Human and other animals	Respiratory tract infections
Newcastle disease virus (NDV)	Chicken	—
Mumps	Human	Parotitis, orchitis, meningoencephalitis
B. Genus *Morbillivirus*		
Measles	Human	Measles
Subacute sclerosing panencephalitis (SSPE)	Human	Chronic degeneration of the central nervous system
Distemper	Dog	—
Rinderpest	Cattle	—

(continued)

TABLE 2-4. (cont.)

RNA-containing Viruses

	Host	*Symptoms in humans*
C. Genus *Pneumovirus*		
Respiratory syncytial virus (RSV)	Human	Pneumonia and bronchiolitis in infants and children, common cold syndrome
Bovine respiratory syncytial virus	Cattle	—
Pneumonia virus of mice (PVM)	Mouse	—

Classification	*Description*
VIII. RHABDOVIRIDAE	Bullet-shaped, enveloped helical nucleocapsids Dimensions: 180 × 75 nm

This group comprises all viruses with the unique bullet-shaped morphology, as well as some that are bacilliform (rounded at both ends). It includes vesicular stomatis virus (VSV), rabies, and some viruses isolated from insects that do not appear to cause disease in vertebrates, but antibodies to them are found in birds and mammals, including humans. Some members of this family multiply in arthropods as well as in vertebrates.

	Host	*Symptoms in humans*
A. Genus *Vesiculovirus*		
VSV	Cattle, horse, swine	—
Chandipura virus	Isolated from humans	—
Flanders-Hart Park virus	Mosquitoes, birds	—
Kern Canyon virus	Bats	—
B. Genus *Lyssavirus*		
Rabies	All warm-blooded animals	Encephalitis, almost invariably fatal
C. Fish Rhabdoviruses (Two genera)	Fish	—
D. Other Rhabdoviruses		
Drosophila sigmavirus	Drosophila	—
Lettuce necrotic yellow virus	Plants	—
Other plant rhabdoviruses		—
E. Possible Rhabdoviruses		
Marburg virus	Monkey	Hemorrhagic fever, frequently fatal
Ebola hemorrhagic fever	?	Acute hemorrhagic fever, almost 90 percent case mortality

Classification	*Description*
IX. RETROVIRIDAE (RNA tumor viruses)	Enveloped particles containing a coiled nucleocapsid with an icosahedral core shell Diameter: about 100 nm

The RNA tumor virus family comprises a large group of viruses characterized by possession of an RNA genome that comprises two identical molecules, a common morphology, and reverse transcriptase. There are three subfamilies. The first, the Oncovirinae, comprises the C-, B-, and D-type RNA tumor viruses. The second subfamily, the Lentivirinae, comprises the Visna group of viruses. They resemble the Oncovirinae with respect to morphology, nature of the genome, possession of a DNA polymerase, and ability to transform cultured cells in vitro, but have not yet been shown to possess oncogenic potential. The third subfamily, the Spumavirinae, comprises the foamy viruses, which are found in spontaneously degenerating kidney (and other) cell cultures, causing the formation of multinucleated vacuolated giant cells that have a highly characteristic appearance. Spumavirinae resemble Oncovirinae in morphology and in certain key characteristics of their mode of replication.

Subfamily	*Host*	*Symptoms in humans*
Oncovirinae		
A. Genus *Oncornavirus C*		
Subgenus Oncornavirus C avian		
Endogenous leukemia/leukosis viruses (RAV-0, RAV-1, RAV-2, etc.)	Chicken	—

(continued)

TABLE 2-4. (cont.)

RNA-containing Viruses		
Subfamily	*Host*	*Symptoms in humans*
Avian sarcoma viruses (ASV), Nondefective	Chicken	—
Rous Sarcoma virus (RSV)		
Sarcoma/acute leukemia viruses, defective	Chicken and other birds	—
Fujinami sarcoma virus (FSV)		
Y73 Sarcoma virus and		
Esh sarcoma virus		
UR-2 virus		
Avian myeloblastosis virus (AMV)		
Avian erythroblastosis virus (AEV)		
Avian myelocytomatosis virus (MC29)		
Reticuloendotheliosis virus (REV)	Duck, chicken	—
Lymphoproliferative disease virus of turkeys (LPDV)	Turkey	—
Subgenus Oncornavirus C mammalian		
Endogenous leukemia viruses, numerous strains	Mammals	—
Sarcoma/acute leukemia viruses, defective	Rodents	
Abelson murine leukemia virus		
Murine sarcoma viruses (Harvey, Kirsten, Moloney, Rasheed)		
Feline sarcoma viruses (Snyder–Theilen, Gardner–Arnstein, McDonough)	Cats	—
Simian sarcoma virus	Woolly monkey	—
Subgenus Oncornavirus C Reptilian	Reptiles	—
Reptilian Type C retroviruses		
B. Genus *Oncornavirus B*		
Mouse mammary tumor virus (Bittner virus (milk factor))	Mouse	—
Viruses of guinea pigs, baboons and other mammals	Mammals	—
C. Genus *Oncornavirus D*		
Mason–Pfizer monkey virus (MPMV)	Rhesus monkey	—
Viruses from primates	Primates	?
Guinea pig virus	Guinea pig	—
Lentivirinae		
Visna	Sheep	—
Maedi	Sheep	—
Progressive pneumonia virus	Mice	—
Spumavirinae		
Human foamy virus	Human cells	—
Simian foamy viruses (9 serotypes)	Monkey kidney cells	—
Canine foamy virus	Dog kidney cells	—
Bovine syncytial virus	Bovine kidney cells	—
Feline syncytial virus	Feline cells	—
Hamster syncytial virus	Hamster cells	—
Probable Retrovirus		
Equine infectious anemia virus	Horse	—

Classification	*Description*
X. ARENAVIRIDAE	Enveloped coiled nucleocapsids Diameter: 80–130 nm

This family comprises viruses characterized by well-defined envelopes that bear closely spaced projections and enclose an unstructured interior containing a variable number of characteristic electron-dense granules about 25 nm in diameter that have been shown to be ribosomes. They share a group-specific antigen, but antisera do not cross-neutralize.

(continued)

TABLE 2-4. (cont.)

RNA-containing Viruses	Host	Symptoms in humans
Lymphocytic choriomeningitis virus (LCM)	Mouse	Latent infection in mice, may produce fatal meningitis in many other species, including humans
Tacaribe virus complex		
Several viruses including Argentinian (Junin) and Bolivian (Machupo) hemorrhagic fever	Isolated from insects and rodents	Hemorrhagic fever, Machupo frequently fatal
Lassa virus	?	Hemorrhagic fever, frequently fatal

Classification	*Description*
XI. CORONAVIRIDAE	Enveloped helical nucleocapsids Diameter: about 100 nm

Nucleocapsids helical, characteristic large club-shaped projections (spikes). There is some antigenic relationship between certain human and murine strains.

	Host	*Symptoms in humans*
Infectious bronchitis virus (IBV)		
Avian strains	Chicken	—
Human strains	Human	Acute upper respiratory disease
Mouse hepatitis virus	Mouse	—
Probable coronaviruses		
Human enteric coronavirus	Humans	Intestinal disorders
Feline infectious peritonitis (feline coronavirus)	Cats	—

XII. MISCELLANEOUS VIRUSES

Several viruses do not fit into any of the families listed so far. The most important are:

A. Hepatitis B Virus. Clinically, two types of viral hepatitis are distinguished. One is characterized by a short incubation period (infectious hepatitis, or epidemic jaundice); the other is characterized by a long incubation period and usually requires parenteral transmission (serum hepatitis). The etiologic agent of the former, hepatitis virus A, is a picornavirus. The etiologic agent of the latter, hepatitis B virus (HBV), appears to infect only humans in nature, and experimental infection has only been achieved in a few additional primates. Its infectious form appears to be a particle about 40 nm in diameter, the Dane particle, that contains a partially double-stranded circular DNA molecule consisting of a complete minus strand and a plus strand that is about two thirds as long. Evidence is accumulating that HBV is implicated in the etiology of hepatomas. Recently, several viruses have been discovered that closely resemble HBV, namely the woodchuck hepatitis virus, the ground squirrel hepatitis virus, and the Pekin duck hepatitis virus. These viruses are used as models for studies on HBV.

B. Chronic infectious neuropathic agents (CHINA viruses). These agents have a preclinical period lasting months to several years, succeeded by a slowly progressing, usually fatal disease. Most of them affect the central nervous system. Degenerative diseases of other organs and tissues may be caused by similar agents. They include the agents that cause Kuru and Creutzfeldt–Jakob disease in humans, scrapie in sheep, and transmissible mink encephalopathy in mink. All are slow degenerative disorders of the central nervous system, marked by ataxia and wasting, and end in death. The etiologic agents have been transmitted, but not yet isolated or even visualized.

*In 1971 a WHO Study Group adopted a new nomenclature for influenza type A viruses. In this system virus strains are described in terms of both the hemagglutinin (HA) and neuraminidase (NA) antigens. A_0 strains are now designated as HON1, A_1 strains as H1N1, the Asian type A_2 of 1957 as H2N2, and the Hong Kong type A_2 of 1968 as H3N2.

judged by nucleic acid hybridization, immunologic cross-reactivity, or ability to recombine (see Chap. 6). The same applies to members of the herpesvirus family; the human, simian, canine, and avian adenoviruses; and so on. These groups form the basis for subdividing the viruses within families into genera.

Major Families of Animal Viruses

Table 2-4 presents a summary of the distinguishing characteristics of the major families of animal viruses, together with a list of the most important animal and human pathogens in each. It is based in large part on recommendations made by the International Committee on Taxonomy of Viruses.

FURTHER READING

Books and Reviews

Bishop DHL: Virion polymerases. In Fraenkel-Conrat H, Wagner RR (eds): Comprehensive Virology. New York, Plenum, 1977, vol 10, p 117

Caspar DLD, Klug A: Physical principles in the construction of regular viruses. Cold Spring Harbor Symp Quant Biol 27:1, 1962

Compans RW, Klenk H: Viral membranes. In Fraenkel-Conrat H, Wagner RR (eds): Comprehensive Virology. New York, Plenum, 1979, vol 13, p 293

Diener TO: Viroids and their interactions with host cells. Ann Rev Microbiol 36:239, 1982

Tooze J (ed): DNA tumor viruses. New York, Cold Spring Harbor Laboratory, 1980

Wimmer E: Genome-linked proteins of viruses. Cell 29:199, 1982

POXVIRUSES

Baxby D: Jenner's Smallpox Vaccine: The Riddle of Vaccinia Virus and Its Origin. London, Heineman, 1981

HERPESVIRUSES

Roizman B: The structure and isomerization of herpes simplex virus genomes. Cell 16:481, 1979

Roizman B (ed): The Herpesviruses. New York, Plenum, 1982

ADENOVIRUSES

Nermut MV: The architecture of adenoviruses: Recent views and problems. Arch Virol 64:175, 1980

PARVOVIRUSES

Berns KI, Hauswirth WW: Adeno-associated viruses. Adv Virus Res 25:407, 1980

PICORNAVIRUSES

Perez-Bercoff R (ed): The Molecular Biology of Picornaviruses. New York, Plenum, 1978

Putnak JR, Phillips BA: Picornaviral structure and assembly. Microbiol Rev 45:287, 1981

TOGAVIRUSES

Schlesinger RW (ed): The Togaviruses. New York, Academic Press, 1980

BUNYAVIRUSES

Calisher CH, Thompson WH (eds): California Serogroup Viruses. New York, Alan R. Liss, 1983

REOVIRUSES

Joklik WK (ed): The Reoviridae. New York, Plenum, 1983

RHABDOVIRUSES

Bishop DHL (ed): Rhabdoviruses. Boca Raton, Fla, CRC Press, 1979

RETROVIRUSES

Weiss R, Teich N, Varmus H, et al. (eds): RNA Tumor Viruses. New York, Cold Spring Harbor Laboratory, 1982

ARENAVIRUSES

Howard CR, Simpson DIH: The biology of the Arenaviruses. J Gen Virol 51:1, 1981

CORONAVIRUSES

MacNaughton MR, Davies, HA: Human enteric Coronaviruses. Arch Virol 70:301, 1981

Selected Papers

POXVIRUSES

Baroudy BM, Venkatesan S, Moss B: Incompletely base-paired flip-flop terminal loops link the two DNA strands of the vaccinia virus genome into one uninterrupted polynucleotide chain. Cell 28:315, 1982

Essani K, Dales S: Biogenesis of vaccinia: Evidence for more than 100 polypeptides in the virion. Virology 95:385, 1979

Geshelin P, Berns KI: Characterization and localization of the naturally occurring cross-links in vaccinia virus DNA. J Mol Biol 88:785, 1974

Kates JR, McAuslan BR: Messenger RNA synthesis by a "coated" viral genome. Proc Natl Acad Sci USA 57:314, 1967

Nevins JR, Joklik WK: Isolation and properties of the vaccinia virus DNA-dependent RNA polymerase. J Biol Chem 252:6930, 1977

Oie M, Ichihashi Y: Characterization of vaccinia polypeptides. Virology 113:263, 1981

Pickup DJ, Bastia D, Stone HO, et al.: Sequence of terminal regions of cowpoxvirus DNA: arrangement of repeated and unique sequence elements. Proc Natl Acad Sci USA 79:7112, 1982

Preston VG, Davison AJ, Garon CF, et al.: Visualization of an inverted terminal repetition in vaccinia virus DNA. Proc Natl Acad Sci USA 75:4863, 1978

Sarov I, Joklik WK: Studies on the nature and location of the capsid polypeptides of vaccinia virions. Virology 50:579, 1972

IRIDOVIRUSES

Lee MH, Willis DB: Restriction endonuclease mapping of the frog virus 3 genome. Virology 126:317, 1983

HERPESVIRUSES

Graham FL, Veldjuisen G, Wilkie NM: Infectious herpesvirus DNA. Nature [New Biol] 245:265, 1973

Heine JW, Honess RW, Cassai E, et al.: Proteins specified by herpes simplex virus. XII. The virion polypeptides of type 1 strains. J Virol 14:640, 1974

Palmer EL, Martin ML, Gary GW: The ultrastructure of disrupted herpesvirus nucleocapsids. Virology 65:260, 1975

ADENOVIRUSES

Brown DP, Westphal M, Burlingham BT, et al.: Structure and composition of the adenovirus type 2 core. J Virol 16:366, 1975

Everitt E, Lutter L, Philipson L: Structural proteins of adenoviruses. Virology 67:197, 1975

Nermut MV: Fine structure of adenovirus type 5. I. Virus capsid. Virology 65:480, 1975

Rekosh DMK, Russell WC, Bellett AJD: Identification of a protein linked to the ends of adenovirus DNA. Cell 11:283, 1977

Roberts RJ, Arrand JR, Keller W: The length of the terminal repetition in adenovirus-2 DNA. Proc Natl Acad Sci USA 71:3829, 1974

PAPOVAVIRUSES

Fiers W, Conteras R, Haegeman G, et al.: Complete nucleotide sequence of SV40 DNA. Nature 273:113, 1978

Finch JT: The surface structure of polyoma virus. J Gen Virol 24:359, 1974

Gibson W: Polyoma virus proteins: A description of the structural proteins of the virion based on polyacrylamide gel electrophoresis and peptide analysis. Virology 62:319, 1974

Müller U, Zentgraf H, Eicken I, et al.: Higher order structure of simian virus 40 chromatin. Science 201:406, 1978

Reddy VB, Dhar R, Weissman SM: Nucleotide sequence of the genes for the simian virus 40 proteins VP2 and VP3. J Biol Chem 253:621, 1978

Reddy VB, Thimmappaya B, Dhar R, et al.: The genome of simian virus 40. Science 200:494, 1978

PARVOVIRUSES

Berns KI, Kelley TJ: Visualization of the inverted terminal repetition of adeno-associated DNA. J Mol Biol 82:267, 1974

Chesebro B, Bloom M, Hadlow W, et al.: Purification and ultrastructure of Aleutian disease virus of mink. Nature 254:456, 1975

McPherson RA, Rose JA: Structural proteins of adenovirus-associated virus: Subspecies and their relatedness. J Virol 46:523, 1983

Mayor HD, Torikai K, Melnick JL: Plus and minus single-stranded DNA separately encapsidated in adeno-associated satellite virions. Science 166:1280, 1969

Spear IS, Fife KH, Hauswirth WW, et al.: Evidence for two nucleotide sequence orientations within the terminal repetition of adeno-associated virus DNA. J Virol 24:627, 1977

Türler H: Interactions of polyoma and mouse DNAs. III. Mechanism of polyoma pseudovirion formation. J Virol 15:1158, 1975

PICORNAVIRUSES

Ambros V, Baltimore D: Protein is linked to the 5′ end of poliovirus RNA by a phosphodiester linkage to tyrosine. J Biol Chem 253:5263, 1978

Coulepis AG, Locarnini SA, Westaway EG, et al.: Biophysical and biochemical characterization of hepatitis A virus. Intervirology 18:107, 1982

Golini F, Nomoto A, Wimmer E: The genome-linked protein of picornaviruses. Virology 89:112, 1978

Lund GA, Ziola BR, Salmi A, et al.: Structure of the mengo virion. V. Distribution of the capsid polypeptides with respect to the surface of the virus particle. Virology 78:35, 1977

Medappa KC, McLean C, Rueckert RR: On the structure of rhinovirus 1A. Virology 44:259, 1971

CALICIVIRUSES

Black DN, Brown F: A major difference in the strategy of the calici- and picornaviruses and its significance in classification. Intervirology 6:57, 1975/1976

Burroughs JN, Doel TR, Smale CJ, et al.: A model for vesicular exanthema virus, the prototype of the calicivirus group. J Gen Virol 40:161, 1978

TOGAVIRUSES

Aliperti G, Schlesinger MJ: Evidence for an autoprotease activity of Sindbis virus capsid protein. Virology 90:366, 1978

Bell JR, Bond MW, Hunkapillar MW, et al.: Structural proteins of western equine encephalitis virus: Amino acid compositions and N-terminal sequences. J Virol 45:708, 1983

Burke D, Keegstra K: Carbohydrate structure of Sindbis virus glycoprotein E2 from virus grown in hamster and chicken cells. J Virol 29:546, 1979

Enzmann PJ, Weiland F: Studies on the morphology of the alphaviruses. Virology 95:501, 1979

de Madrid AT, Porterfield JS: The flaviviruses (group B arboviruses): A cross-neutralization study. J Gen Virol 23:91, 1974

Pedersen CE, Eddy GA: Separation, isolation, and immunological studies of the structural proteins of Venezuelan equine encephalomyelitis virus. J Virol 14:740, 1974

von Bonsdorff CH, Harrison SC: Hexagonal glycoprotein arrays from Sindbis virus membranes. J Virol 28:578, 1978

BUNYAVIRUSES

Dahlberg JE, Obijeski JS, Korb J: Electron microscopy of the segmented RNA genome of La Crosse virus: Absence of circular molecules. J Virol 22:203, 1977

Hewlett MJ, Petterson RF, Baltimore D: Circular forms of Uukuniemi virion RNA: An electron microscopic study. J Virol 21:1085, 1977

Murphy FA, Harrison AK, Whitefield SG: Bunyaviridae: Morphologic and morphogenetic similarities of Bunyamwera serologic supergroup viruses and several other arthropod-borne viruses. Intervirology 1:297, 1973

Petterson RF, von Bornsdorff CH: Ribonucleoproteins of Uukuniemi virus are circular. J Virol 15:386, 1975

Smith JF, Pifat DY: Morphogenesis of Sandfly fever viruses (Bunyaviridae family). Virology 121:61, 1982

REOVIRUSES

Esparza J, Gil F: A study on the ultrastructure of human rotavirus. Virology 91:141, 1978

Luftig RB, Kilham SS, Hay AJ, et al.: An ultrastructural study of virions and cores of reovirus type 3. Virology 48:170, 1972

Nicolas JC, Cohen J, Fortier B, et al.: Isolation of a human pararotavirus. Virology 124:181, 1983

Palmer EL, Martin ML: The fine structure of the capsid of reovirus type 3. Virology 76:109, 1977

Palmer E, Martin ML: Further observations on the ultrastructure of human rotavirus. J Gen Virol 62:105, 1982

Shatkin AJ, Sipe JD, Loh P: Separation of ten reovirus genome segments by polyacrylamide gel electrophoresis. J Virol 2:986, 1968

Smith RE, Zweerink HJ, Joklik WK: Polypeptide components of virions, top component and cores of reovirus type 3. Virology 39:791, 1969

Urasawa S, Urasawa T, Taniguchi K: Three human rotavirus serotypes demonstrated by plaque neutralization of isolated strains. Infect Immun 38:781, 1982

ORTHOMYXOVIRUSES

Desselberger U, Palese P: Molecular weights of RNA segments on influenza A and B viruses. Virology 88:394, 1978

Inglis SC, McGeoch DJ, Mahy BWJ: Polypeptides specified by the influenza virus genome. II. Assignment of protein coding functions to individual genome segments by in vitro translation. Virology 78:522, 1977

Murti KG, Bean WJ Jr, Webster RG: Helical ribonucleoproteins of influenza virus: An electron microscopic analysis. Virology 104:227, 1980

Racaniello VR, Palese P: Influenza B virus genome: Assignment of viral polypeptides to RNA segments. J Virol 29:361, 1979

Schwartz RT, Klenk H: Carbohydrates of influenza virus. IV. Strain-dependent variations. Virology 113:584, 1981

PARAMYXOVIRUSES

Orvell C: Structural polypeptides of mumps virus. J Gen Virol 41:527, 1978

Scheid A, Choppin PW: Identification of biological activities of paramyxovirus glycoproteins. Activation of cell fusion, hemolysis, and infectivity by proteolytic cleavage of an inactive precursor protein of Sendai virus. Virology 57:475, 1974

Shimizu K, Shimizu YK, Kohama T, et al.: Isolation and characterization of two distinct types of HVJ (Sendai virus) spikes. Virology 62:90, 1974

RHABDOVIRUSES

Emerson SU, Wagner RR: L protein requirement for in vitro

RNA synthesis by vesicular stomatitis virus. J Virol 12:1325, 1973

Reading CL, Penhoet EE, Ballou CE: Carbohydrate structure of vesicular stomatitis virus glycoprotein. J Biol Chem 253:5600, 1978

Tabas I, Schlesinger S, Kornfeld S: Processing of high mannose oligosaccharides to form complex type oligosaccharides on the newly synthesized polypeptides of the vesicular stomatitis virus G protein and the IgG heavy chain. J Biol Chem 253:716, 1978

Wagner RR, Prevec L, Brown F, et al.: Classification of rhabdovirus proteins: A proposal. J Virol 10: 1228, 1972

ARENAVIRUSES

Palmer EL, Obijeski JF, Webb PA, et al.: The circular, segmented nucleocapsid of an arenavirus—Tacaribe virus. J Gen Virol 36:541, 1977

Young PR, Howard CR: Fine structure analysis of Pichinde virus nucleocapsids. J Gen Virol 64:833, 1983

CORONAVIRUSES

Guy JS, Brian DA: Bovine coronavirus genome. J Virol 29:293, 1979

King B, Brian BA: Bovine coronavirus structural proteins. J Virol 42:700, 1982

MacNaughton MR, Davies HA, Nermut MV: Ribonucleoprotein-like structures from coronavirus particles. J Gen Virol 39:545, 1978

MacNaughton MR, Madge MH: The genome of human coronavirus strain 229 E. J Gen Virol 39:497, 1978

HEPATITIS B VIRUS

Barker LF, Almeida JD, Hoofnagle JG, et al.: Hepatitis B core antigen: Immunology and electron microscopy. J Virol 14:1552, 1974

Krugman S, Gregg MB, Kabat EA, et al.: Nomenclature of antigens associated with viral hepatitis B. Intervirol 2:134, 1974

Robinson WS, Greenman RL: DNA polymerase in the core of human hepatitis B virus. J Virol 13:1231, 1974

VIROIDS

Dickson E, Diener TO, Robertson HD: Potato spindle tuber and citrus exocortis viroids undergo no major sequence changes during replication in two different hosts. Proc Natl Acad Sci USA 75:951, 1978

Owens RA, Erbe E, Hadidi A, et al.: Separation and infectivity of circular and linear forms of potato spindle tuber viroids. Proc Natl Acad Sci USA 74:3859, 1977

CHAPTER 3

Viruses and Viral Proteins as Antigens

Many proteins coded by viruses are good antigens. This is of vital significance both medically and scientifically. Although great strides have been made during the past two decades in defining the biochemistry and molecular biology of the multiplication cycles of animal viruses, the chemotherapeutic control of viral diseases is not yet practical. In fact, with very few exceptions, there is no way in which virus infections can be controlled; in almost all cases one relies on the natural ability of the host to form antibody to the invading virus. When the spread of virus infection to essential organs is too rapid, or when for some reason antibody formation does not take place early enough, the patient may succumb. Gammaglobulin from hyperimmune sera is sometimes administered as a last resort; even then, one must rely on antibodies, not on drugs. By the same token, the only presently practical form of antiviral prophylaxis is provided by antibodies produced in response to vaccines (Chap. 7).

Structural viral proteins stimulate the formation of antibodies not only as components of virus particles, but also as components of virus particle subunits, such as capsomers or nucleocapsids, and also in the free state. The principal antigenic determinants are often the same in all three forms, but extra antigenic sites are sometimes generated as individual proteins become part of more complex structures. For example, adenovirus hexons exhibit antigenic determinants not expressed by free hexon proteins, and the capsids of picornaviruses possess antigenic specificities that are not exhibited by their component structural proteins.

The range of antiviral antibodies formed under conditions when viruses can and cannot multiply differs greatly. If a virus cannot multiply, either because it has been inactivated or because the host is not susceptible, only antibodies to surface components of the virus particle are usually formed. However, if the virus can multiply, not only is far more antibody formed because progeny virus will also act as antigen, but also the range of antibodies produced is much wider. This is because antibodies are then also formed to the unassembled and partially assembled viral components that are synthesized as a result of virus multiplication, as well as to nonstructural virus-coded proteins. For example, antisera to inactivated vaccinia virus contain only a few species of antibody directed against its surface components; but antisera from animals in which vaccinia virus has multiplied contain antibodies against at least 30 different viral proteins in readily detectable amounts.

The antigenic determinants of virus-coded proteins are of great importance for virus classification. Viruses that belong to the same genus or major group share common determinants, or group-specific antigens, that are generally located on internal virus components. The most specific, or individual, viral antigenic determinants are usually located on surface components of virus particles, which are the type-specific antigens that identify individual virus strains.

Possession of group- and type-specific antigenic determinants provides an important tool for epidemiology. Newly isolated virus strains are usually characterized on the basis of their reaction with antisera of known specificity, which reveals the nature of their group- and type-specific antigens. Furthermore, it is possible to determine whether a given human or animal population has been exposed to a particular virus strain by testing serum samples for the presence of antiviral antibody.

The interaction of viruses and viral proteins with antibodies can be recognized and measured in several ways. The four most important ways are described below.

Interaction of Virus with Neutralizing Antibody

Antibodies to viral surface components neutralize infectivity; these are the neutralizing antibodies that protect against disease. They usually persist in the body for many years, and even when their level drops, a secondary or anamnestic response to virus generally boosts their titers to very high levels, so that no second cycle of infection ensues. This explains the fact that animals generally contract any particular virus disease only once. Exceptions, such as the common cold and influenza, are due to special circumstances. The reason for the frequent recurrence of the common cold syndrome is that it is elicited by a large group of viruses, among which are rhinoviruses, enteroviruses, adenoviruses, ortho- and paramyxoviruses, and coronaviruses. The reason for recurrent epidemics caused by influenza virus is that new antigenic variants arise readily, and are readily selected in humans (Chap. 6).

The reaction between neutralizing antibody and virus follows first-order kinetics, which indicates that one antibody molecule can inactivate one virus particle. It does so by interfering with the initial events of the virus multiplication cycle. There are two likely mechanisms. The first is steric hindrance—virus particles combined with antibody molecules are unlikely to be able to react with their receptors on cell surfaces. The second mechanism involves interference with uncoating. Under conditions of normal infection, viral genomes are liberated into the interior of the cell, ready to start multiplication (see below); but virus–antibody complexes are apparently engulfed by and inactivated in phagocytic vacuoles, so that no intact viral genomes are able to reach the interior of the cell (Chap. 4).

Complement-fixing Antigen and Antibody

The virus–antibody interaction can also be measured by taking advantage of the fact that complexes of viral protein and antibody often fix complement. As sensitive methods for titrating complement are available, this provides a convenient and accurate method of measuring either the amount of viral antigens (complement-fixing antigens or CFA), or of antibody to such antigens. The chief advantage of this method of detecting viral antigens is that any virus-coded protein may be a complement-fixing antigen; both structural and nonstructural virus-coded proteins, as well as viral subunits and virus particles themselves, may form complexes with antibody that fix complement. This method of quantitating viral proteins is particularly useful for detecting abortive virus infections when only part of the genetic information present in the viral genome is expressed and no virus particles are produced (Chap 5). It is also of great importance in epidemiology, as it is often far easier to identify newly isolated virus strains by determining whether extracts of cells infected with them fix complement with antisera of known specificity than by measuring the ability of such antisera to neutralize infectivity.

Hemagglutination Inhibition

As described in Chapter 1, many viruses can agglutinate red blood cells. Virus particles coated with antibody molecules cannot do so, and antisera that contain virus-specific antibodies therefore inhibit hemagglutination. The antigens that are involved here are viral surface components, which, as pointed out above, possess the most type-specific antigenic determinants; hemagglutination-inhibition therefore provides a highly specific characterization of viruses. Because it is also very easy to perform, this technique is very useful in virus identification and epidemiology.

Gel Immunodiffusion and Immunoelectrophoresis

Under appropriate conditions of antigen–antibody equivalence, antigen–antibody complexes are insoluble. This property is used in gel immunodiffusion and gel immunoelectrophoresis, techniques that are widely employed for resolving mixtures of viral antigens such as occur in extracts of infected cells.

The most widely used version of gel immunodiffusion is the Ouchterlony method, which employs Petri plates containing agar into which are cut a number of wells, one being situated centrally and the others equidistantly from it and from each other. Antiserum or antibody is placed into the center well, antigen is placed into the outer ones, and diffusion is then allowed to proceed. Where the concentration of antigen–antibody complexes exceeds their solubility product, precipitin lines form, the location of which depends on the relative diffusion rates, and therefore on the relative sizes, of antigen and antibody. Identity of antigens is revealed by the familiar fusion of precipitin lines (Fig. 3-1).

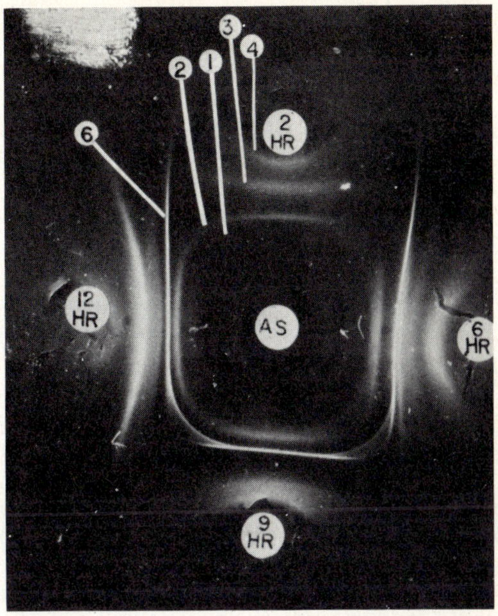

Figure 3-1. The use of gel diffusion analysis to detect virus-specified proteins in extracts of infected cells. Antiserum to vaccinia virus was placed into the center well (AS) of a Petri dish containing a layer of agar. Extracts of HeLa cells infected for 2, 6, 9, and 12 hours, respectively, with vaccinia virus were placed into the other four wells, and the antibodies and antigens were allowed to diffuse toward each other. Precipitin lines, formed as described in the text, were then stained with Poinceau S. The pattern becomes increasingly complex with increasing time after infection, as more virus-specified proteins are synthesized. The advantage of this method is that virus-specified proteins are revealed without the necessity for purification. *(From Salzman and Sebring: J Virol 1:16, 1967.)*

In the gel immunoelectrophoresis technique, antigens are not separated by free diffusion but by electrophoresis in agar slabs, after which antiserum is applied in a trough cut parallel to the direction of electrophoresis. After diffusion, precipitin lines form as above (Fig. 3-2). The concentrations of antibody and antigen used in both these techniques are generally adjusted so that the precipitin lines are very thin, thus permitting great resolution.

A modification of this technique is rocket immunoelectrophoresis, in which proteins are electrophoresed into agarose gels that contain antibodies to them. If the pH of such gels is adjusted so that antibody molecules remain stationary (about pH 8.6), rocket-shaped zones of precipitation result that are demonstrable with protein stains and the area of which is proportional to the quantity of antigen that is applied. This technique is very versatile because it permits not only the quantitation of single antigens in complex mixtures, provided that the appropriate monospecific antibody is available, but is also applicable to mixtures of antigens. The technique is then known as crossed immunoelectrophoresis, and the antigens are first separated by electrophoresis in a standard agarose gel before being electrophoresed at right angles into the gel that contains the appropriate mixture of antibodies. An example of this technique is to use extracts of infected cells as the source of virus-coded antigens, and antiserum from an infected rabbit as the source of the gamut of antibodies to all these antigens. This combination yields a profile which permits the simultaneous quantitation of numerous virus-coded proteins.

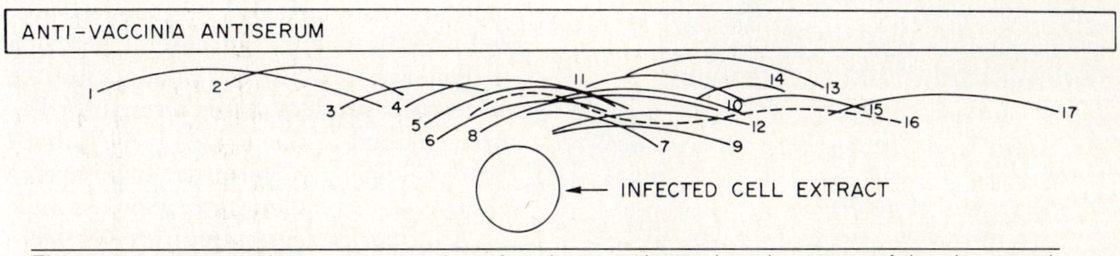

Figure 3-2. Diagrammatic representation of an immunoelectrophoretic pattern of the virus-specified proteins present in an extract of chick cells infected with vaccinia virus. In this technique, the cell extract is placed into a circular well cut into an agar slab and an electric field is applied, causing antigens to migrate at rates governed by their charge and size. After electrophoresis, antiserum to vaccinia virus is placed into a trough cut parallel to the direction of electrophoresis and allowed to diffuse toward the separated cell extract components. Virus-specified proteins able to react with antibodies in the antiserum form precipitin lines. Seventeen such proteins can be detected in the extract shown here. *(From Rodriguez-Burgos et al.: Virol 30:569, 1966.)*

Visualization of Viral Antigens Using Tagged Antibody

There are many occasions when direct visual localization of viral antigens is desired. This can be achieved by using antibody that is tagged, conjugated, or labeled with some material that can be visualized with either the light microscope or the electron microscope.

Antibody labeled with the dye fluorescein fluoresces brightly when viewed with a microscope equipped with a source of ultraviolet light (Fig. 3-3). Such antibody is a sensitive research tool in viral pathogenesis—that is, in studies of the route of infection and the spread of virus within the organism—because it can reveal a small number of infected cells. It is also useful for measuring the proportion of infected cells in a variety of experimental situations, and it can serve as a rapid diagnostic tool, as minute amounts of infected biopsy material can be treated with fluorescein-labeled antibodies to several suspected viruses, one of which will cause the infected cells to fluoresce. Finally, as fluorescein-labeled antibody can also reveal the pattern of viral antigen distribution within infected cells, and because this pattern is often highly characteristic (nuclear or cytoplasmic, diffuse or highly localized), it can also serve as a useful adjunct to virus identification.

Antibody molecules can also be tagged with large molecules or particles that can be seen with the electron microscope. Among these are ferritin, a large iron-containing protein, bacteriophage or virus particles with characteristic shapes, and latex spheres. Use of such antibody permits exquisitely detailed observation of the distribution of viral antigens in infected cells. It is therefore invaluable in studies aimed at establishing the exact location of the sites of synthesis, accumulation, and assembly of viral protein components (Fig. 3-4).

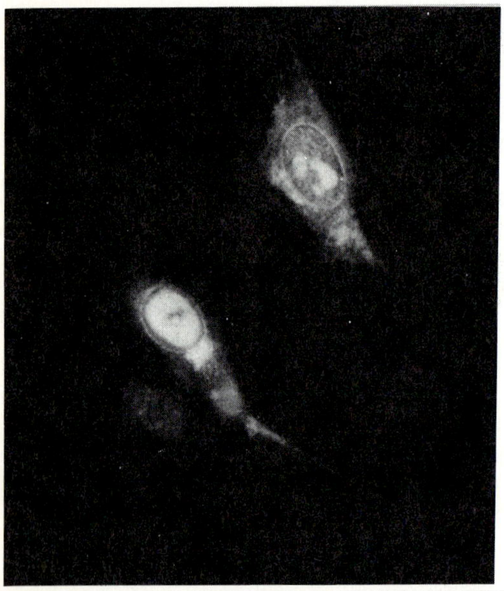

Figure 3-3. Visualization of viral antigens by means of immunofluorescence. Cells infected with herpes simplex virus were washed, fixed in acetone, and allowed to react either with herpesvirus antibody conjugated with fluorescein isothiocyanate (direct immunofluorescence), or with herpesvirus antibody prepared in rabbits, followed by antirabbit globulin conjugated with fluorescein isothiocyanate (indirect immunofluorescence). Cells were then examined under ultraviolet light. The cells shown here were stained by the indirect method. The top cell shows fluorescent nuclear patches as well as fluorescence at the nuclear membrane and some diffuse cytoplasmic fluorescence. The other cell shows bright fluorescence of practically the whole nucleus, as well as cytoplasmic fluorescence. × 550. *(From Ross et al.: J Gen Virol 2:115, 1968.)*

Detection of Minute Amounts of Viral Antigens and Antibodies

Appropriate patient management frequently depends on early detection of virus infections or on the recognition of persistent virus infections. In both situations, diagnosis requires the correct and rapid identification of minute amounts of viral antigens and antibodies, and in recent years great strides have been made in the development of extremely sensitive techniques for this purpose. Two such techniques are as follows. The first is radioimmunoassay. Not only is this technique capable of detecting extremely small amounts of virus-coded proteins, but it is also very useful for assessing serologic relatedness, as one can measure the efficiency with which unknown antigens can prevent antibody from precipitating the standard labeled test antigen—the closer the serologic relationship, the more efficient the competition.

The second technique is the enzyme-linked immunosorbent assay (ELISA), in which antigen is immobilized on some surface, such as the wells of a plastic microtiter plate (see Fig. 1-8), and specific antiserum coupled with alkaline phosphatase or peroxidase is then added. Following extensive washing, substrate is added, and the reaction product that is formed by the antibody-linked enzyme bound to the antigen is measured colorimetrically. This technique can be made to be over 100 times more sensitive than complement fixation assays.

A further dimension has recently been added to these techniques by the use of the "protein A" that is present in the cell walls of certain strains of *Staphylococcus,* which possesses high affinity for the Fc portion of most mammalian IgGs. Cells of such strains, or isolated A protein coupled to inert particles such as agarose, can be used to adsorb minute amounts of antigen–antibody complexes from complex mixtures, and the antigens in them can then be analyzed.

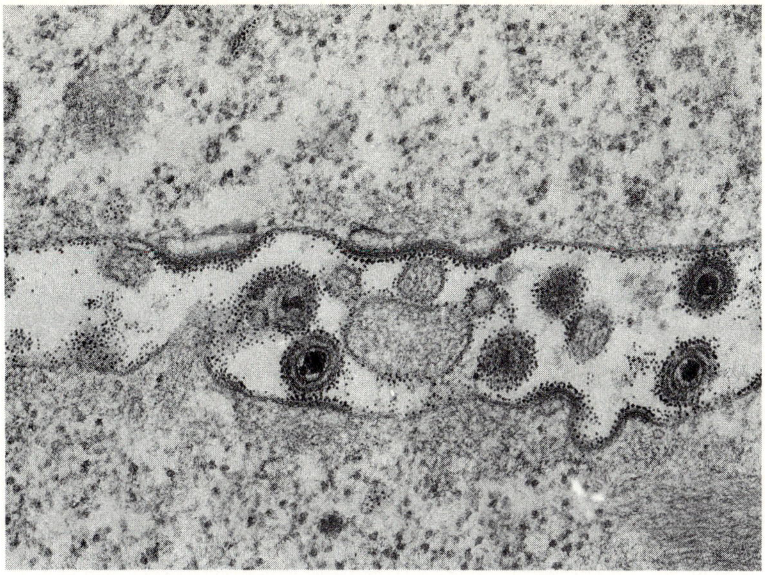

Figure 3-4. Visualization of viral antigens by means of ferritin-conjugated antibody. This electron micrograph reveals the localization of virus-specified proteins on the surfaces of cells infected with herpes simplex virus. Infected cells were allowed to react with herpesvirus antibody conjugated with ferritin; the cells were then washed, fixed, embedded, and sectioned. The surfaces of two adjacent cells are seen, both with intensely labeled patches. Budding virus particles and detached cytoplasmic fragments are also labeled. × 48,000. *(From Nii et al.: J Virol 2: 1172, 1968.)*

Virus-coded Cell Surface Antigens

As described in Chapters 4 and 5, new antigenic determinants frequently appear on the surfaces (outer plasma membranes) of infected cells. These new determinants are on virus-coded proteins. In the case of enveloped viruses, these proteins become, in due course, part of the viral envelope. In the case of nonenveloped viruses, they are nonstructural proteins that are synthesized early during the infection cycle. In either case, virus-coded cell surface proteins provide a clear signal to the immune mechanism that cells are infected; antibodies are formed against them and destroy the cells.

Immune Response to Virus Infection

During virus infection, antibodies are formed against all classes of virus-coded antigens. Those that are most important for eliminating virus from the body are those directed against virus particle components and against virus-coded cell surface antigens. The former include the neutralizing and complement-fixing antibodies that eliminate virus particles as infectious units (p. 54). As for the latter, their combination with virus-coded antigens on cell surfaces renders the cells subject to destruction by at least two mechanisms: combination with complement followed by lysis, and attack by cytolytic T lymphocytes. In either case, the infected cell is eliminated as a source of progeny virus.

Usually the mechanisms for destroying infectious virus and infected cells are beneficial to the host. However, it is now recognized that sometimes these mechanisms may be harmful. Let us consider first the destruction of infected cells. As a rule, the number of cells that are destroyed is not large enough to cause serious problems for the host organism, but there are exceptions. An example is provided by lymphocytic choriomeningitis virus (LCM), which causes encephalitis in mice and also in humans. LCM, an enveloped virus, is not a very "lytic" virus; cells infected with it are not severely damaged and may survive for long periods of time. In mice, LCM produces no overt disease if the immune mechanism is not operative (in tolerant or immunosuppressed animals). However, in immunologically competent mice, LCM causes a fatal meningitis within a week, that is, as soon as antibody begins to be formed, death being due to the destruction of infected cells by activated macrophages. Thus the disease is not caused by the destruction of the host's cells by the virus, but by the destruction of infected cells by the host's immune mechanism. A similar interaction between immune lymphocytes and virus-coded cell surface antigens may account for the symptoms associated with some viral diseases of humans, such as hepatitis.

The same is true for the second mechanism for destroying infected cells—namely, combination with antibody and complement, which will destroy infected cells long before cells break down as a direct result of virus infection. This mechanism also, though no doubt generally very valuable as a defense against infection, may sometimes cause severe damage to the host. For example, it appears that the sometimes fatal hemorrhagic shock syndrome associated with dengue fever is caused by sudden increases in vascular permeability that may be triggered by the interaction of immune complexes with the complement and clotting systems.

Although virus–antibody complexes are usually eliminated from the body without difficulty either before or after combination with complement, they may cause diseases quite unrelated to those caused by viruses alone. This realization has come from studies of several virus infections in animals, particularly LCM and lactic dehydrogenase elevating virus (LDHV). Infection with both these viruses results in the presence in the bloodstream of large amounts of virus–antibody complexes; it is also characterized by the development of glomerulonephritis and the presence in kidney capillaries of large amounts of virus–antibody–complement complexes. Similar observations have been made with respect to Aleutian mink disease and equine infectious anemia, in which the inflammatory changes are not confined to the kidneys but also involve the blood vessels (with the development of arteritis) and other parts of the body. Some forms of human glomerulonephritis may also be caused by virus–antibody complexes.

Finally, it is now suspected that autoimmune diseases, such as rheumatoid arthritis and lupus erythematosus, are also caused by the interaction of viruses with the immune system.

FURTHER READING

Books and Reviews

Cooper NR: Humoral immunity to viruses. In Fraenkel-Conrat H, Wagner RR (eds): Comprehensive Virology. New York, Plenum, 1979, vol 15, p 123

Della-Porta AJ, Westaway EG: A multi-hit model for the neutralization of animal viruses. J Gen Virol 38:1, 1977

Haller O (ed): Natural resistance to tumors and viruses. Curr Top Microbiol Immunol 92, 1981

Mandel B: Interaction of viruses with neutralizing antibodies. In Fraenkel-Conrat H, Wagner RR (eds): Comprehensive Virology. New York, Plenum, 1979, vol 15, p 37

Mogensen SC: Role of macrophages in natural resistance to virus infections. Microbiol Rev 43:1, 1979

Norrild B: Immunochemistry of herpes simplex virus glycoproteins. Curr Top Microbiol Immunol 90:67, 1980

Notkins A (ed): Viral Immunology and Immunopathology. New York, Academic Press, 1976

Oldstone MBA: Virus neutralization and virus-induced immune complex disease. Prog Med Virol 19:85, 1975

Oldstone MBA: Immune responses, immune tolerance, and viruses. In Fraenkel-Conrat H, Wagner RR (eds): Comprehensive Virology. New York, Plenum, 1979, vol 15, p 1

Oldstone MBA, Fujinami RS, Lampert PW: Membrane and cytoplasmic changes in virus-infected cells induced by interactions of antiviral antibody with surface viral antigen. Prog Med Virol 26:45, 1980

Sissons JGP, Oldstone MBA: Killing of virus-infected cells: The role of antiviral antibody and complement in limiting virus infection. J Infect Dis 142:442, 1980

Selected Papers

Babiuk LA, Acres SD, Rouse BT: Solid-phase radioimmunoassay for detecting bovine (neonatal calf diarrhea) rotavirus antibody. J Clin Microbiol 6:10, 1977

Ghose LH, Schnagl RD, Holmes IH: Comparison of an enzyme-linked immunosorbent assay for quantitation of rotavirus antibodies with complement fixation in an epidemiological survey. J Clin Microbiol 8:268, 1978

Halstead SB, O'Rourke EJ: Antibody enhanced dengue virus infection in primate leukocytes. Nature 265:739, 1977

Harmon SA, Summers DF: Characterization of monospecific antisera against all five vesicular stomatitis virus-specific proteins: Anti-L and anti-NS inhibit transcription in vitro. Virology 120:194, 1982

Icenogele J, Gilbert SF, Grieves J, et al.: A neutralizing monoclonal antibody against poliovirus and its reaction with related antigens. Virology 115:211, 1981

Minor PD, Schild GC, Bootman J, et al.: Location and primary structure of a major antigenic site for poliovirus neutralization. Nature 301:674, 1983

Oldstone MBA: Immune complexes in cancer: Demonstration of complexes in mice bearing neuroblastomas. J Natl Cancer Inst 54:223, 1975

Stollar V: Immune lysis of Sindbis virus. Virology 66:620, 1975

Zinkernagel RM, Oldstone MBA: Cells that express viral antigens but lack H-2 determinants are not lysed by immune thymus-derived lymphocytes but are lysed by other antiviral immune attack mechanisms. Proc Natl Acad Sci USA 72:3666, 1976

CHAPTER 4

The Virus Multiplication Cycle

Virus particles represent the static or inert form of viruses. The very existence of viruses is recognizable only in terms of their interaction with cells, which is the central theme of virology.

The interaction of virus and cell generates a novel entity, the virus–cell complex, the fate of which varies widely, as it depends both on the nature of the cell and on the nature of the virus. The two most commonly observed virus–cell interactions are: (1) the lytic interaction, which results in virus multiplication and lysis of the host cell; and (2) the transforming interaction, which results in the integration of the viral genome into the host genome and the permanent transformation or alteration of the host cell with respect to morphology, growth habit, and the manner in which it interacts with other cells with which it comes into contact.

In studying the virus–host interaction, one can focus primarily either on the fate and functioning of the invading virus particle and on the production of virus progeny, or on the reaction of the host cell to virus infection. Both approaches are of fundamental importance to the medical practitioner. The former is particularly relevant to the development of a rational approach to antiviral chemotherapy; the latter to an understanding of chronic virus infection and cancer. This chapter focuses on the invading virus particle; the next chapter focuses on the response of the cell.

Lytic Virus–Cell Interaction

The lytic virus–cell interaction is best thought of in terms of a cycle—the infection or multiplication cycle—during which the virus enters cells, multiplies, and is released. This cycle is repeated many times when a virus particle infects an organism, until, for one reason or another, further multiplication is arrested, or the host dies.

One of the principal goals of virology is to define in molecular terms all the various reactions that proceed during the virus multiplication cycle. As an example, when a poliovirus particle infects a cell, one RNA molecule and about 200 protein molecules are introduced into it. How does this RNA molecule replicate? What are the proteins for which it codes, and what are their functions? How are mature virus particles assembled? What is the fate of the 200 parental protein molecules? What effect do they have on the host cell? What are the reactions that cause the host cell to die?

It is impossible to answer these and many other questions by studies in the intact organism. Instead, simple experimental systems that can be manipulated at will are required. Such systems are provided by cloned strains of cultured animal cells that grow in vitro and can be infected under any desired set of conditions with pure (plaque-purified) strains of virus. Among their many advantages is that they permit focusing on one multiplication cycle, rather than on many repeated cycles, which is achieved by infecting all cells at the same time. In fact, one of the major conceptual breakthroughs in virology occurred about 40 years ago when Ellis and Delbrück demonstrated how very much simpler the analysis of the one-step growth cycle is than that of numerous successive unsynchronized cycles. In populations of cultured cells infected at high multiplicity—that is, with many virus particles per cell—so as to ensure that infection commences at the same time in all cells, the various reactions that together comprise virus multiplication proceed synchronously according to a regulated progressive pattern that is amenable to study by the techniques of biochemistry, biophysics, and cellular and molecular biology.

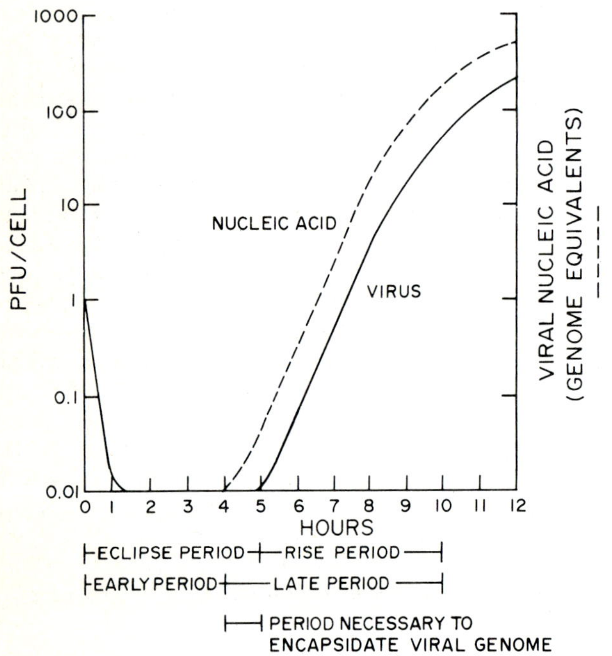

Figure 4-1. The one-step growth cycle. Its essential features are: Following adsorption, infectivity is abolished or "eclipsed"; this is caused by uncoating of the infecting virus particles. During the eclipse or early period, which can last from a few minutes to many hours, the stage is set for viral nucleic acid replication. The appearance of the first progeny genome marks the beginning of the late period, and the appearance of the first mature progeny virus particle marks the beginning of the rise period. It should be noted that the interval between the beginning of the late and rise periods represents the average time necessary for virus maturation; that is, the incorporation of a free nucleic acid molecule into a mature virus particle. The lengths of all periods, as well as the extent of virus multiplication, vary greatly for different viruses and cells.

One-Step Growth Cycle: General Aspects

The virus multiplication cycle can be divided into several periods, using events of critical importance as markers (Fig. 4-1). As discussed below, infectivity of virus particles is destroyed or eclipsed when they adsorb; the initial period of the cycle is therefore often referred to as the eclipse period. This period ends with the formation of the first mature progeny virus particle, which marks the beginning of the rise period. Alternatively, the synthesis of the first progeny genome is often regarded as dividing the multiplication cycle into the early and late periods. The eclipse and early periods and the rise and late periods overlap substantially, with the interval between the beginning of the late and rise periods representing the time necessary for the incorporation of a viral genome into a mature virus particle.

Eclipse Period

Adsorption

The first step of the virus–cell interaction is adsorption, which can itself be separated into several stages. The first of these is ionic attraction. Both cells and virus particles are negatively charged at pH 7, and positive ions are therefore required as counter-ions. As a rule this requirement is met most efficiently by magnesium ions. The second stage involves the interaction of virus particles with specific receptor molecules. Indirect evidence for the existence of such specific virus receptor molecules has been available for some time. For example, poliovirus adsorbs only to cells of human or primate origin. In fact, in the body, poliovirus adsorbs only to cells of the central nervous system and to cells lining the intestinal tract; other human and primate cells develop the ability to adsorb poliovirus only after being cultured in vitro, which causes unmasking of receptors (the gene for which is located on human chromosome 19). Recently, techniques have been devised for isolating such specific receptor molecules in the form of virus–receptor complexes. The fact that attachment of human rhinovirus type 2 and of poliovirus type 2 to human cells is inhibited by concanavalin A, a lectin that reacts with α-D-mannose residues, suggests that some of these receptors are glycoproteins.

The time course of virus adsorption follows first order kinetics. The rate of adsorption is independent of temperature if suitable corrections are made for changes in the viscosity of the medium, but the rate is directly proportional to the amount of surface to which virus can adsorb, that is, to the cell concentration. The kinetics of adsorption are described by the relation

$$\frac{V_t}{V_o} = e^{-Ktc},$$

where V_o and V_t are the concentrations of free virus at time 0 and after t minutes, respectively; c is the cell concentration; t is time in minutes; and K is the adsorption rate constant.

The number of virus particles or infectious units adsorbed per cell is referred to as the multiplicity of infection (moi). Animal cells are generally capable of adsorbing very large amounts of virus. It has been shown, for example, that cells contain about 100,000 receptor sites for Sindbis virus (Fig. 4-2).

Penetration and Uncoating

The second stage of the virus multiplication cycle involves penetration and uncoating, which are considered together because, although they are separated both temporally and spatially for some viruses, they occur simultaneously for others. Penetration, sometimes referred to as viropexis, concerns the entry into the cytoplasm of either the whole virus particle or that part of it that contains the genome. It may be observed directly by means of the electron microscope or indirectly by measuring the loss of ability of antiviral antiserum to arrest initiation of virus multiplication. The reason for this is that as long as virus particles remain outside the cell, combination with antibody significantly decreases their ability to cause productive infection; but once the particles are within the cell, they are no longer accessible to antibody.

Uncoating signifies the physical separation of viral nucleic acid from viral protein or, in the case of negative-stranded RNA viruses, the disruption of virus particles with resultant liberation of nucleocapsids. Double-stranded RNA-containing viruses also are not uncoated completely, but only to subviral particles (see below). Uncoating is of taxonomic significance because viruses are the only intracellular infectious agents or parasites for which this is an obligatory step of the multiplication cycle.

Uncoating is best assessed by measuring physical and chemical changes in the adsorbed virus particles. Among these changes are progressive labilization of the capsid structure as judged by loss of its ability to shield the viral genome from hydrolysis by nucleases, development of susceptibility to reagents such as urea to which intact virus particles are resistant, loss of antigenic determinants, and progressive loss of capsid protein. The total time from adsorption to final uncoating ranges from several minutes to several hours.

The actual pathways of penetration and uncoating of the various types of virus particles differ markedly—a fact not surprising in view of their diversity. The essential features of this process are as follows. Virus particles usually bind to the surface of microvilli, elongated projections extending from the cell surface. They then move down the microvillus shaft toward the body of the cell, where they encounter coated pits. These are specialized regions of the cell membrane that are formed continually and that are coated on their cytoplasmic, or inner, side by clathrin, a large protein. These coated pits, with the virus particles attached to them, then fold inward, pinch off, and move into the interior of the cell as coated vesicles, or phagocytic vacuoles. After the clathrin, which is now on their outer surface, is removed, they fuse with lysosomes. It is within the resulting vesicles, which now contain the lysomal proteolytic enzymes, that virus particles are uncoated or that the uncoating process begins. In the case of adenoviruses, the fibers and pentons are removed and partially uncoated virus particles are released into the interior of the cell (Fig. 4-3). In the case of reoviruses, the outer capsid shell is partially digested and subviral particles, consisting of the inner capsid shell or core to which about one half of the components of the outer capsid shell are still attached, are released into the cytoplasm, where they remain throughout the multiplication cycle, free reovirus RNA never being liberated (see p. 81). In the case of poxviruses, the outer regions of the virus particles are removed and viral cores are liberated into the cytoplasm. The degradation of these cores, which results in the uncoating of the viral DNA, requires the synthesis of a special virus-encoded uncoating

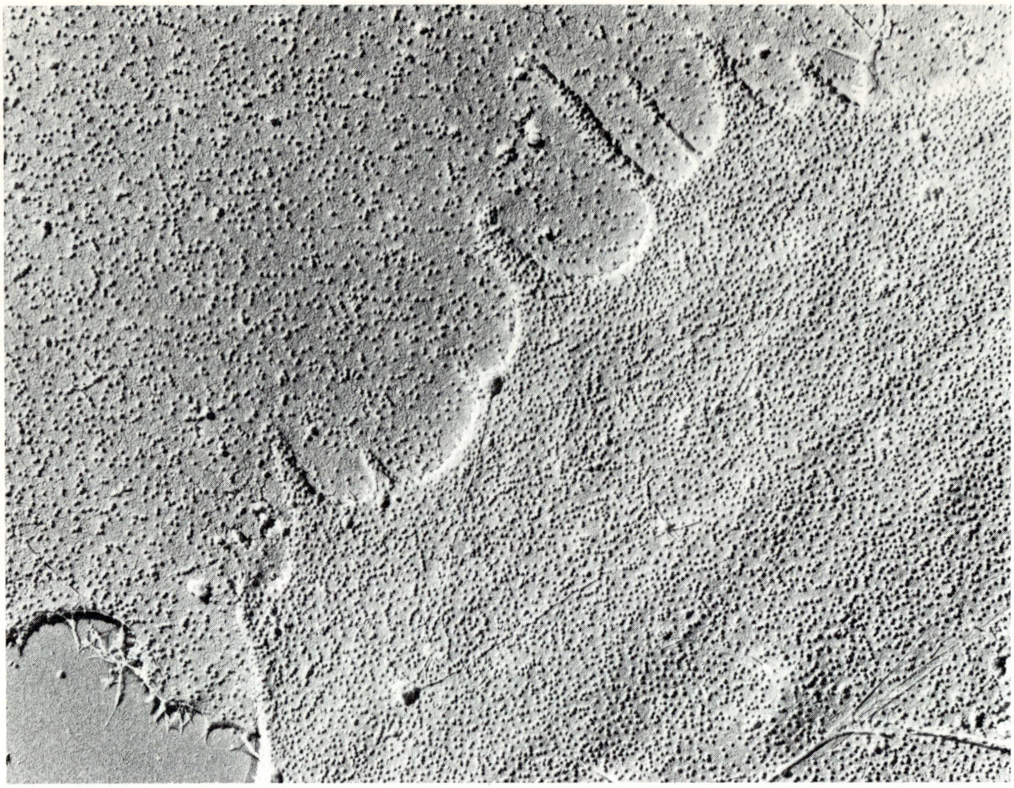

Figure 4-2. Surface replica of Sindbis virus adsorbed to the surface of two chick cells. × 9,300. *(From Birdwell and Strauss: J Virol 14:672, 1974.)*

protein (Fig. 4-4). In the case of most enveloped viruses except paramyxoviruses, the very acidic vesicle milieu causes the viral envelope to fuse with the vesicle membrane, thereby liberating the helical nucleocapsid into the interior of the cell.

The only viruses that are not taken up and uncoated by this mechanism are the paramyxoviruses. Here the viral envelope—probably through the mediation of the glycoprotein F spikes, which possess powerful cell-fusing activity—fuses directly with the plasma cell membrane, thereby liberating the nucleocapsid directly into the cytoplasm. There are several lines of evidence for this pathway, including direct morphologic evidence and the fact that cells infected with such viruses are killed by antiviral antibody plus complement (because fusion of the viral envelope with the host cell membrane causes viral antigens to be incorporated into it).

Eclipse

Adsorption, penetration, and uncoating result in loss of infectivity, which is referred to as eclipse. The only residual infectivity is that due to the viral nucleic acid itself (or to the nucleocapsid, as the case may be), which, however, is never more than a small fraction of that of the virus particles themselves.

The first three stages of infection are usually inefficient processes. Virus particles often adsorb to portions of the cell surface at which penetration will not proceed; viral genomes may be damaged by ribonuclease, which is frequently associated with outer (or plasma) cell membranes; and virus particles may fail to be released from the phagocytic vacuoles in which they have become engulfed. All these inefficiencies account in large part for the fact that the ratio of infectious to total animal virus particles is almost always far less than 1 (Chap. 1).

Synthetic Phase of the Virus Multiplication Cycle

Once the viral genome is uncoated, the synthetic phase of the virus growth cycle commences. In essence, this encompasses, in a precisely regulated program, the replication of the viral genome, the synthesis of viral proteins, and the formation of progeny virus particles.

The location of viral genome replication is characteristic for each virus (Table 4-1). There is no correlation between this location and any other property, such as chemical nature or size of genome. Viral protein is always synthesized in the cytoplasm on polyribosomes composed of viral messenger RNA, host cell ribosomes, and host cell

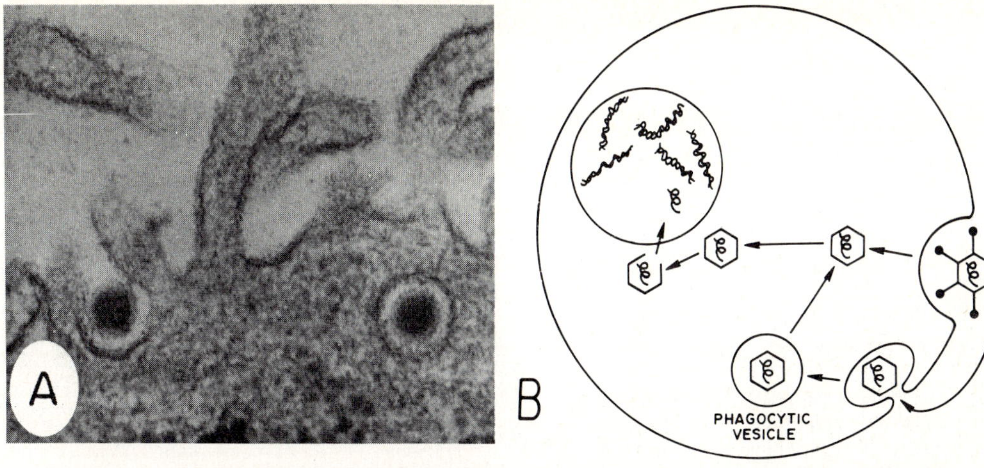

Figure 4-3. The penetration and uncoating of adenovirus. **A.** One virus particle about to be engulfed in a coated pit; another inside a coated vesicle. Virus particles that have lost their fibers and pentons are liberated from such vesicles. These particles are then transported to the nucleus, where uncoating is completed near the nuclear pore complex; only viral DNA enters the nucleus. *(From Chardonnet and Dales: Virology 40:462, 1970.)* **B.** Diagrammatic representation of the uptake and uncoating of adenovirus particles.

transfer RNA. In the case of RNA-containing viruses most, if not all, their genetic information is expressed soon after uncoating. In the case of the double-stranded DNA-containing viruses, however, the multiplication cycle can be divided into clearly defined early and late periods, with the onset of viral DNA replication marking the beginning of the late period (see Fig. 4-1).

Early Period

The early period of the synthetic phase is devoted primarily to the activation of reactions that are prerequisites for the initiation of viral genome replication. This activation proceeds as the result of viruses exercising certain early functions. Among them are: (1) inhibition of host DNA, RNA, and protein synthesis—which may involve the syn-

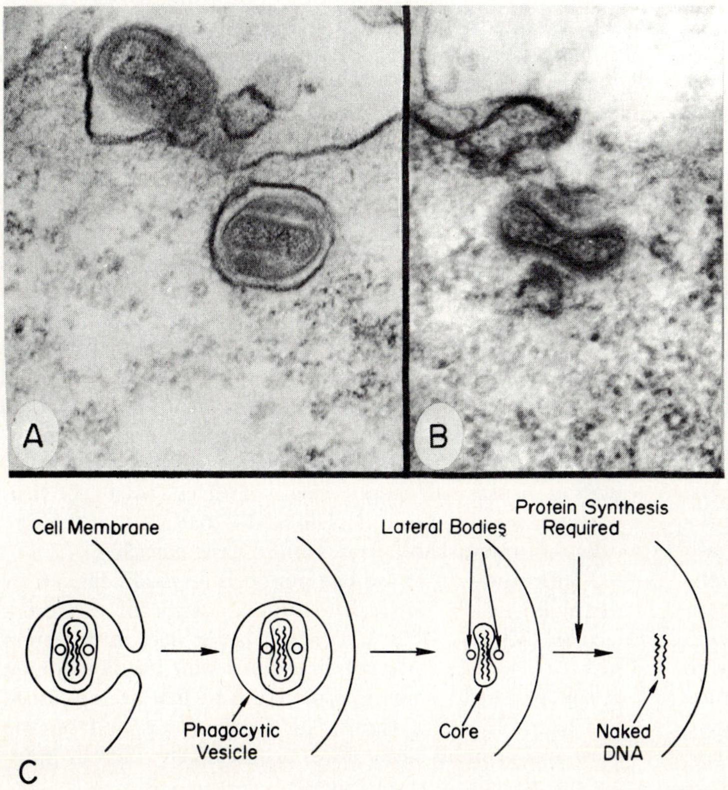

Figure 4-4. The penetration and uncoating of vaccinia virus. Three stages are shown. **A.** One of the two virus particles is in a coated pit; the other is already in the cytoplasm within a coated vesicle. **B.** The vesicle has broken down, as has the virus particle's outer protein coat. The core is now free, and the two laterial bodies have moved some distance away. The final stage of uncoating is the breakdown of the core, which results in the liberation of the DNA. This step is not achieved if protein synthesis is inhibited. This indicates that the synthesis of a special uncoating protein is required. Poxviruses are the only viruses that require the synthesis of a special protein for uncoating. The whole process is depicted diagrammatically in **C. A** and **B,** × 80,000. *(**A, B,** from Dales: J Cell Biol 18: 63, 1963; **C,** modified from Joklik: J Mol Biol 8:277, 1964.)*

TABLE 4-1. UNCOATING, VIRAL GENOME REPLICATION, AND VIRUS MATURATION

Virus	Uncoated to	Genome Replication	Virion Maturation
Poxviruses	Free DNA	Cytoplasm	Cytoplasm
Herpesviruses	Free DNA	Nucleus	At nuclear membrane
Adenoviruses	Free DNA	Nucleus	Nucleus
Papovaviruses	Free DNA	Nucleus	Nucleus
Picarnaviruses	Free RNA	Cytoplasm	Cytoplasm
Togaviruses	Free RNA	Cytoplasm	At membranes
Bunyaviruses	Nucleocapsid	Cytoplasm	At membranes
Reoviruses	Subviral particle	Cytoplasm	Cytoplasm
Orthomyxoviruses	Nucleocapsid	Nucleus	At membranes
Paramyxoviruses	Nucleocapsid	Cytoplasm	At membranes
Rhabdoviruses	Nucleocapsid	Cytoplasm	At membranes
RNA tumor viruses	Free RNA	Nucleus	At membranes
Arenaviruses	?	Cytoplasm	At membranes
Coronaviruses	Free RNA	Cytoplasm	At membranes

thesis of virus-coded proteins that either inhibit or alter the specificities of the DNA-replicating, RNA-transcribing, and protein-synthesizing systems—so that viral rather than host cell genetic information is processed; (2) synthesis of proteins that form the matrix of inclusions, either in the nucleus or in the cytoplasm, within which viral nucleic acids replicate and viral morphogenesis proceeds; and (3) synthesis of enzymes that synthesize viral DNA and RNA.

The extent to which early functions are expressed varies greatly from virus to virus. Some viruses possess so little genetic information that only very few early functions are expressed; others possess so much that they may express from 30 to 50 early functions. Early functions are expressed through (early) virus-coded proteins that are transcribed from early viral messenger RNA species. Viral genomes that are plus-stranded RNA serve directly as messenger RNA. For all other viruses, plus-stranded messenger RNA must first be transcribed from infecting parental genomes by means of polymerases either associated with them or preexisting in the host cell.

Late Period

During the late period, the late viral functions are expressed. The late viral proteins are primarily virus particle components and enzymes and other nonstructural proteins that function during viral morphogenesis; they are encoded by late viral messenger RNA molecules that are transcribed from different regions of the viral genome than early ones. Furthermore, late messenger RNA molecules are transcribed from progeny genomes; and because there are always more progeny than parental genomes, many more late messenger RNA molecules are always formed than early ones. Therefore, the amount of late proteins that is synthesized always greatly exceeds that of early ones. Activation of the regions of the viral genome that code for late functions may or may not be accompanied by deactivation of the regions that code for early functions. In either case, a mechanism exists that specifies that one set of genes (the early set) is transcribed from parental genomes, whereas another set (the late set) is transcribed only from progeny genomes. The basis for this mechanism lies in the specificity of the enzyme(s) that transcribes DNA. Indeed, work with certain bacteriophages has indicated that the host-specified DNA-dependent RNA polymerase is modified early during infection to a form that can transcribe those sites on the phage genome that code for early functions, and that at the beginning of the late period its specificity is altered again so as to enable it to respond to those signals that specify late functions (Chap. 9). Similar mechanisms may also operate in the case of animal viruses.

During the late period, the newly formed virus genomes and capsid proteins are assembled into progeny virus particles, a process that is known as morphogenesis. This is a spontaneously occurring process, as most of the information for virus assembly resides in the amino acid sequences of the capsid proteins. Nucleic acid performs no essential function during morphogenesis, a fact demonstrated by the occurrence among the yield of most icosahedral viruses of empty virus particles—that is, virus particles containing no nucleic acid—that are morphologically indistinguishable from mature virus particles.

The duration of the late period is generally limited by the ability of the host cell to supply energy for macromolecular synthesis. This is a critical factor because infection with lytic viruses invariably interferes with the functioning of the host cell by multiple mechanisms that are discussed in Chapter 5. As a result, the synthesis of viral nucleic acids and proteins slows down progressively, thereby limiting the amount of viral progeny.

Release of Progeny Virus

The final step of the infection cycle is the release of progeny virus. There is no special mechanism for the release of unenveloped viruses and poxviruses; infected cells simply disintegrate more or less rapidly, liberating the viral progeny that has accumulated within them. The amount of cell-associated virus therefore exceeds the amount of released virus until the very last phase of the multiplication cycle (Fig. 4-5). A special mechanism does, however, exist for the enveloped viruses, for which release is the final stage of morphogenesis. Here virus-coded envelope proteins are incorporated into certain areas of host cell membranes while nucleocapsids are being synthesized. The nucleocapsids then bud through the modified membrane patches and become enveloped by them (p. 86). Budding occurs both at the outer plasma cell membrane and at the membranes lining intracytoplasmic vacuoles, which then transport the virus to the exterior of the cell. These viruses do not exist in mature infectious form within cells, and the amount of extracellular virus, therefore, greatly exceeds the amount of cell-associated virus at all stages of the multiplication cycle (Fig. 4-5).

The duration of the phases of the virus multiplication cycle varies greatly, depending on the nature of the virus and on the nature of the host cell. Table 4-2 lists the minimum lengths of the eclipse periods and of the complete multiplication cycles of some well-studied viruses.

Multiplication Cycles of Several Important Viruses

Of the many facets of virus multiplication, the two that are central are: (1) the nature of the information encoded in viral genomes; and (2) the manner in which this information is expressed. Not only does description of a virus in this manner define it in its most fundamental terms, but it also provides the framework of knowledge essential for a rational approach to antiviral chemotherapy. A discussion of the strategy used by several important and intensively studied viruses to encode and express their information content follows.

Multiplication Cycles of Double-stranded DNA-containing Viruses

Knowledge concerning the multiplication of double-stranded DNA-containing viruses has expanded greatly in recent years owing to the advent of techniques for mapping their genomes by the use of bacterial restriction endonucleases. These enzymes, which are components of the restriction-modification systems in bacteria, cleave DNA at palindromic sequences that are highly specific for each enzyme. These sequences, which possess two-fold rotational symmetry, may be as simple as

↓
5′ . . . GGCC . . .
. . . CCGG . . . 5′,
↑

or as complex as

↓
5′ . . GCCNNNNNGGC . . .
. . . CGGNNNNNCCG . . . 5′.
↑

Clearly, the simpler the recognition site, the more often it will occur and the more often the DNA will be cut. The fragments that result may be ordered or mapped by

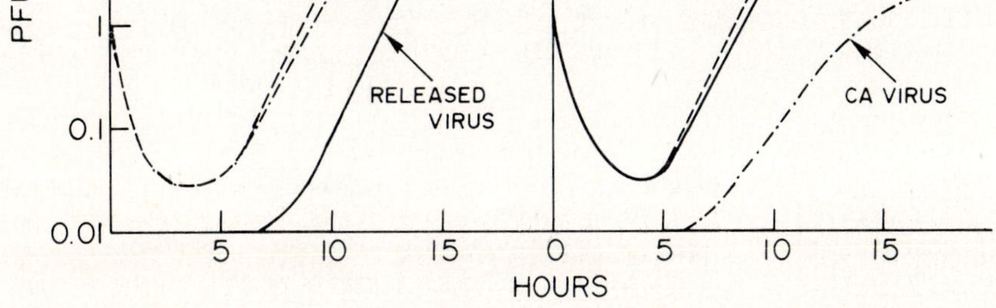

Figure 4-5. The relationship between virus multiplication and release. **A.** This graph refers to viruses with icosahedral nucleocapsids. Such viruses are not released readily from cells. Viral progeny accumulates within cells, so that for much of the rise period the amount of cell-associated (CA) virus greatly exceeds the amount of released virus. Release of virus occurs only when cells break down at the end of the rise period. **B.** This graph refers to all enveloped viruses. Such viruses mature only in the process of being released, as it is only then that they acquire their envelope. The amount of liberated virus therefore always greatly exceeds the amount of cell-associated virus. The only cell-associated virus particles are those in the process of budding from the plasma membrane and those that bud into intracytoplasmic vacuoles.

TABLE 4-2. APPROXIMATE DURATION OF ECLIPSE PERIOD AND OF ENTIRE MULTIPLICATION CYCLE

Virus	Eclipse Period (hours)	Total Multiplication Cycle (hours)
Poxvirus: vaccinia virus	4	24
Herpesvirus: herpes simplex virus	3–5	24–36
Adenovirus	8–10	48
Papovavirus: polyoma virus	12–14	48
Poliovirus	1–2	6–8
Togavirus: Sindbis virus	2	10
Reovirus	4	15
Orthomyxovirus: influenza virus	3–5	18–36
Rhabdovirus: vesicular stomatitis virus	2	8–10

digesting DNA under conditions when it is only partially cleaved, and analyzing the incompletely hydrolyzed pieces for neighboring fragments. Figure 4-6 shows the 6 *Hind* III restriction endonuclease fragments of SV40 DNA, and Figure 4-7 shows the order in which they are arranged, that is, the *Hind*III map. Several other restriction endonuclease maps of SV40 DNA are also shown. Given such maps—and almost 100 restriction endonucleases are now available—this type of analysis is capable of defining precisely the position in the viral genome of even short DNA sequences. It also permits one to determine to which endonuclease fragment the messenger RNA molecules that are transcribed at any time during the multiplication cycle will hybridize, which can provide information concerning when and how frequently each portion of the viral genome is transcribed during the multiplication cycle. This technique is known as physical mapping because here the viral DNA is treated as a sequence of nucleic acid bases. Physical maps can be correlated with genetic maps if they are available. In that case it becomes possible to determine the order of the various genes that comprise the viral genome and the extent to which they are expressed. The ultimate aim of this type of analysis is to define exactly where each gene is located in the viral genome, when it is transcribed during the virus multiplication cycle, how frequently it is

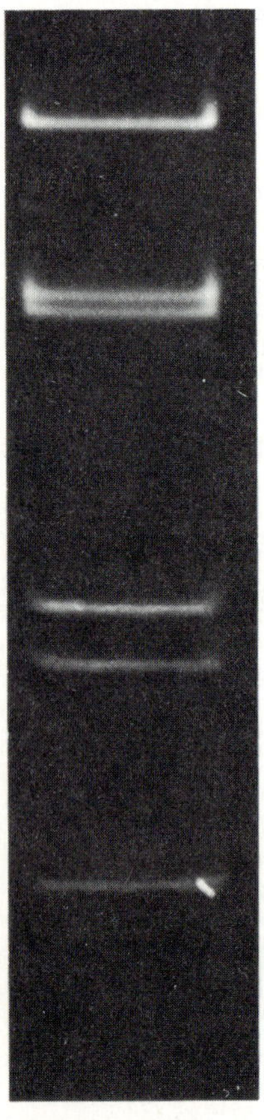

Figure 4-6. Autoradiogram of a polyacrylamide gel in which the six fragments were electrophoresed that result when circular ^{32}P-labeled SV40 DNA is digested with restriction endonuclease *Hind* III. *(Courtesy of Drs. J.K. Li and C. Huang.)*

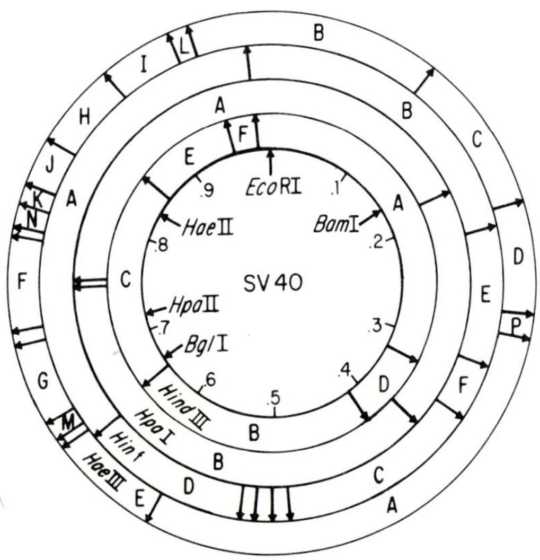

Figure 4-7. Restriction endonuclease cleavage maps of SV40 DNA, using *Hind*III, *Hpa*I, *Hin*f and *Hae*III. *Eco*RI, *Bam*I, *Bgl* I, *Hpa*II and *Hae*II cleave only once. The origin of DNA replication is at a palindromic sequence, part of which forms the recognition sequence for *Bgl*I.

transcribed, and, finally, what controls or regulates the transcription program.

Papovaviruses

Papovaviruses are the smallest double-stranded DNA-containing viruses. Although practically nothing is known of the multiplication cycles of papillomaviruses (because they do not grow in cultured cells), a great deal is known about how polyoma virus and SV40 multiply. It should be noted that two human viruses, namely BK virus and JC virus (see Chap. 8), are more or less closely related to SV40.

When these viruses infect certain cells of their natural hosts, viral DNA replicates, viral proteins are made, progeny virus particles are formed, and the cells lyse; in other words, they initiate productive infection. These host cells are known as permissive cells. In contract, many other types of cells are more or less nonpermissive—that is, they do not support efficient multiplication. Instead, the viral DNA becomes integrated into that of the host cells, thereby creating new, genetically different cells, namely, virus-transformed cells. Such cells form tumors in animals. The transforming papovavirus–host cell interaction is discussed in Chapter 8. The present chapter considers the nature of their lytic multiplication cycles.

The basic feature of the multiplication cycle of polyoma virus and SV40, like that of all double-stranded DNA-containing viruses, is that it can be divided into well-defined early and late phases (see Fig. 4-1). During each phase, different portions of the viral genome are transcribed into messenger RNAs, which are then processed and translated into proteins by the cellular protein-synthesizing system.

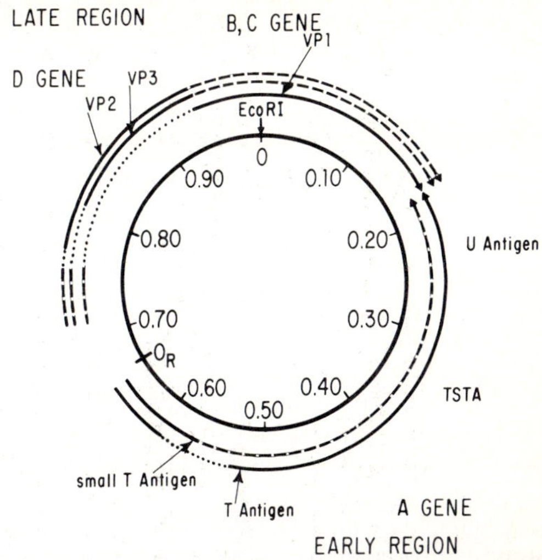

Figure 4-8. The genetic and transcription map of SV40 DNA. It is located so that the restriction endonuclease *Eco*RI cleavage site is at the 12 o'clock position. O_R is the origin of replication of SV40 DNA. The coding sequences of messenger RNAs are indicated by solid lines, noncoding sequences by dashed ones. Sequences spliced out during the processing of transcripts to messenger RNAs are indicated by dotted lines.

Early Period

The multiplication cycle of SV40 is best understood by reference to the genetic and transcription maps of its genome, a circular molecule of 5226 nucleotide base pairs that has been completely sequenced (Fig. 4-8). During the early phase, which lasts a surprisingly long time (14 to 18 hours), about 50 percent of the viral DNA, namely the region that extends from map position 0.65 (relative to the *Eco*RI restriction endonuclease cleavage site) to map position 0.17, is transcribed into RNA. This region comprises a single gene, known as the A gene; however the transcripts of the region are processed into not one, but two species of messenger RNA. The first is about 2230-nucleotides long and is composed of two parts, about 330- and 1900-nucleotides long, that map from map position 0.65 to 0.60 and from 0.54 to 0.17, respectively. RNA corresponding to the DNA between map position 0.60 and 0.54 is not present in this messenger RNA; this region is spliced out of the original transcript by a mechanism that is not yet clear. Splicing-out of regions of RNA transcripts is a common phenomenon even among the transcripts of cellular genes; numerous cellular messenger RNAs are now known to comprise sequences from widely separated regions of DNA. A well-known example is the messenger RNA of the β-globin gene of the mouse. This messenger RNA is derived from the transcript of a DNA sequence that is about 1700-base pairs long, which is processed so that two sequences of 780 and 125 nucleotides, respectively, are spliced out. Thus the β-globin messenger RNA consists of three sequences of about 480, 205, and 155 nucleotides, respectively, that are covalently joined but were originally separated. Regions that are spliced out are known as introns (inserted sequences); regions that are not spliced out are known as exons. Splicing-out is a very widespread feature of the mechanism by which RNA transcripts of eucaryotic DNA are processed to messenger RNAs; other features of this mechanism are capping of their 5′-termini and polyadenylation of their 3′-termini.

The second species of early SV40 messenger RNA is 2500-nucleotides long and is also composed of two exons, 630- and 1900-nucleotides long, respectively, that map from map position 0.65 to 0.55 and from 0.54 to 0.17, respectively.

The two messenger RNAs code for two proteins. First, the 2230-nucleotide long messenger RNA codes for the T antigen, a protein with a molecular weight of about 95,000 that is located in the nucleus, binds to SV40 DNA near the origin of replication (see below) and may function in initiating or facilitating the initiation of its replication. The T antigen may also be responsible for inducing the synthesis of substantial amounts of cellular DNA (generally it replicates at least once) and of several enzymes involved in DNA synthesis during the initial stages of the multiplication cycle. These must be cellular enzymes because SV40 DNA is too small to code for them. Finally, the T antigen is also responsible for the maintenance of the transformed state when SV40 transforms cells (see Chap. 8).

The second species of early messenger RNA, that which is 2500-nucleotides long, encodes a protein that is known as the small t antigen, whose molecular weight is about 17,000 and which is essential for initiating the transformed cell state. Whereas the T antigen is encoded by the sequences that extend from map position 0.65 to 0.60 and from 0.54 to 0.17, small t antigen is encoded by the sequence from 0.65 to 0.55. T antigen and small t antigen therefore share amino acid sequences and they cross-react immunologically. The reason small t antigen is so short is that there are several termination codons near map position 0.55. These condons are spliced out of the messenger RNA species that codes for T antigen.

In polyoma virus-infected cells there is yet a third protein, middle T antigen (mol wt 55,000), which shares antigenic determinants with both the T and the small t antigens. Its amino-terminal portion is the same as that of the T and small t antigens, but its carboxyl-terminal end is different, as it is encoded by the portion of the messenger RNA that follows the splice junction; that is, by the second exon, but in a different reading frame from that used for the T antigen. Like T antigen and small t antigen, middle t antigen plays an essential role in transformation, but cannot transform cells completely by itself.

Cells infected with SV40 also contain a protein, the U antigen (mol wt 28,000), which corresponds to the carboxyl-terminal portion of the T antigen. Its existence was first detected in cells infected with virus particles that are SV40-adenovirus hybrids (Ad2^{+}ND$_1$) (see Chap. 6) and that only contain SV40 DNA corresponding to map positions 0.28 to 0.11.

The SV40 72-bp Repeat. A very interesting feature of the early SV40 transcription unit is that about 150-base pairs (bp) upstream from the transcription start site two identical 72-bp sequences are located directly adjacent to each other. This 72-bp repeat acts as a powerful promoter element. It potentiates, activates, or enhances transcription by eucaryotic RNA polymerase II, even if it is thousands of base pairs away in either direction. It appears to act as a bidirectional super entry site for RNA polymerase II. This element has been positioned near a variety of genes by genetic engineering techniques, and always greatly enhances transcription. Its action is similar to that of the long terminal repeat (LTR) of retroviruses (see Chap. 8). The recognition and characterization of such transcriptional super promoters, which no doubt also exist in eucaryotic genomes including the human genome, are extremely important "fall-out" by-products of molecular virology.

Late Period

During the late period, the A gene continues to be transcribed, and in addition, the remainder of the SV40 genome is also transcribed. This region contains three genes —known as the B, C, and D genes—which overlap, as shown in Fig. 4-8; it is transcribed in the opposite direction, that is, from the opposite strand, as the A gene. Its transcripts are processed into three messenger RNAs that correspond to map positions 0.76 to 0.17, 0.83 to 0.17, and 0.95 to 0.17, respectively. In addition, all three messenger RNAs possess leader sequences that are about 120-nucleotides long and that are transcribed from the region between map positions 0.72 to 0.76. (The region that is spliced out in the first messenger RNA species is very short, and except for it, this messenger RNA species is a transcript of the entire late region of the SV40 genome.) These messenger RNAs are translated into three proteins. The map position 0.95 to 0.17 RNA species, which is the most abundant, is transcribed into VP1, a 46,000-dalton protein that is the major component of the SV40 capsid. The map position 0.83 to 0.17 messenger RNA species is translated only for part of its length—namely, the portion that corresponds to the region from map position 0.83 to about 0.97. This portion yields VP3, a 25,000 dalton protein that is a minor capsid component. Finally, the map position 0.76 to 0.17 RNA species also is translated only for part of its length—namely, the portion that corresponds to the region between map positions 0.76 and 0.97 —and its translation product is VP2, a 35,000-dalton protein that is also a minor capsid component. The fascinating feature of this mode of gene expression is that the gene for VP3 lies entirely within the gene for VP2; their messenger RNAs are read in the same phase, and translation of both is terminated by the same termination codon, which is a long way from the 3′-terminus of their messenger RNAs. Furthermore, the initiation signal for VP1 lies about 120 nucleotides within the genes for VP2 and VP3, and VP1 is read in a different phase from VP2 and VP3.

Replication of SV40 DNA

The replication of SV40 DNA starts at map position 0.67, the origin of replication, where there is a remarkable palindromic sequence 27-base pairs long. Replication proceeds bidirectionally until the two forks meet again, with one DNA strand being synthesized in a continuous manner, and the other in the form of Okazaki fragments that are then joined. Newly replicated SV40 DNA does not exist in free form within infected cells, but is complexed with histones into a chromatin-like structure. This structure differs from that of the minichromosomes present in SV40 particles (see Chap. 2) in being more condensed. The reason for this is that the intracellular SV40 chromatin also contains histone H1 (in addition to histones H3, H4, H2A, and H2B), which causes the intranucleosomal distance to be reduced. Upon removal of histone H1 by the addition of salt, this structure unfolds into the beads-on-a-string conformation. SV40 DNA cannot be transcribed while in the compact chromatin configuration, but can be transcribed in the beads-on-a-string conformation.

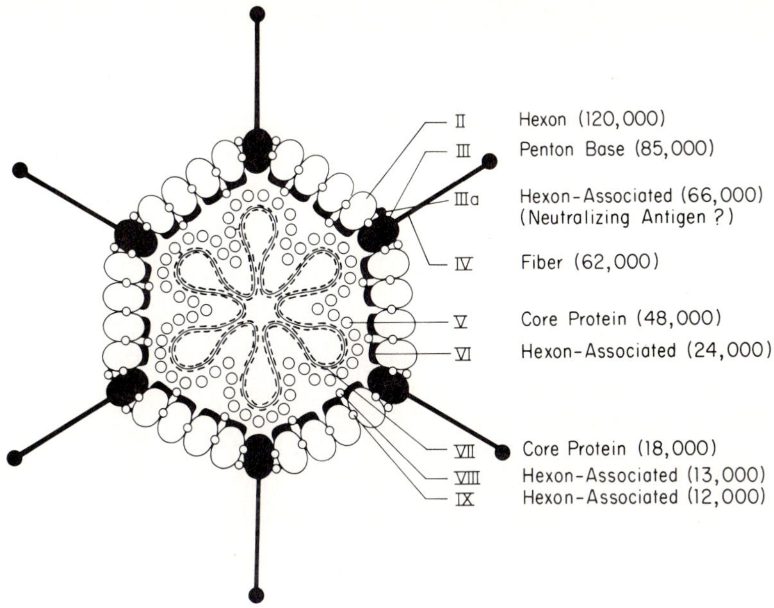

Figure 4-9. Model of adenovirus showing the inner DNA protein core and the outer icosahedral capsid, as well as the location and sizes of the various structural proteins. The fiber is the viral cell attachment organ, as well as the hemagglutinin. Proteins VI, VII, and VIII are synthesized in the form of precursors that are cleaved to the actual virus particle components. *(Adapted from Brown et al.: J Virol 16:366, 1975.)*

General Observations on the Strategy of Papovavirus Gene Expression

The preceding discussion of the multiplication cycle of SV40 and polyoma virus highlights the remarkable strategy according to which these viruses express the information encoded in their genomes. Most astonishing is that many of their coding sequences are used twice, and even three times. One obvious advantage of this strategy is that it minimizes the amount of DNA necessary to encode their proteins. It is also noteworthy that the functions of the early and late proteins are quite different. All early proteins have regulatory functions, and at least one, the T antigen, appears to act in a pleiotropic manner—that is, it seems to be multifunctional. In contrast, the late proteins are the structural virus particle components. Finally, it is remarkable that the DNA of these viruses exists in the form of a complex that has many of the properties of cellular chromatin, and that it uses cellular histones for this purpose.

Adenoviruses

The multiplication cycle of adenoviruses (Fig. 4-9, Table 4-3), whose genome (mol wt 23×10^6; 36,500 base pairs) is six to seven times the size of SV40 or polyoma virus, lasts about 36 to 48 hours. It can be divided into an early period of about 8 hours, during which about 30 percent of the viral genome is transcribed, and a late period during which the remainder of the information that it encodes is expressed. Viral DNA replication begins at 6 to 8 hours. Host macromolecular biosynthesis (synthesis of

TABLE 4-3. STRUCTURAL PROTEINS OF ADENOVIRUS (SEROTYPE 2)

Protein	Designation	Number per Virus Particle	Size (Mol Wt)
Hexon	II	720 (3 per hexon)	120,000
Penton	III	60 (5 per penton)	85,000
Fiber	IV	36 (3 per fiber)	62,000
Major core protein	VII	1000	18,000
Minor core protein	V	200	48,000
Hexon-associated	VI	450	24,000
Hexon-associated	VIII	?	13,000
Hexon-associated (peripentonal)	IIIa	?	66,000
Hexon-associated	IX	?	12,000

Additional structural proteins IVa1, IVa2, X, XI, and XII (mol wt 60,000, 56,000, 6500, 6000, and 5000, respectively) have been described, but not studied in detail.

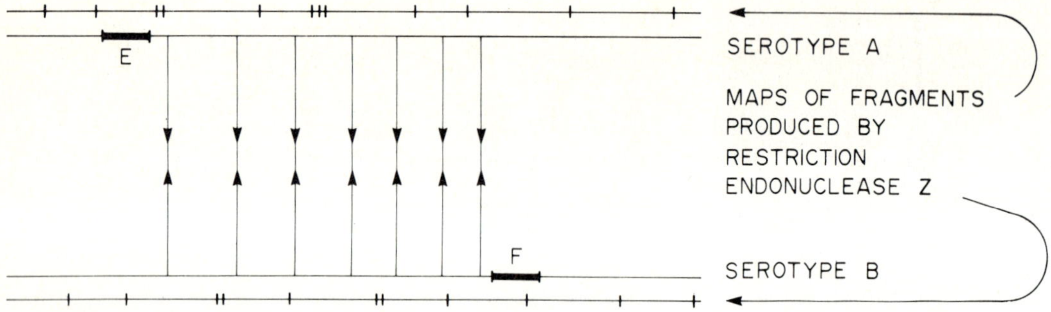

Figure 4-10. Mapping of genes by restriction endonuclease analysis of recombinant DNA. Two temperature-sensitive mutants (see Chap. 6) are taken, one in gene E of serotype A, the other in gene F of serotype B. (Note that there are 35 serotypes of human adenvovirus; see Table 2-4.) Wild-type recombinants (that is, recombinants able to grow at the normal temperature) are then isolated and their restriction endonuclease cleavage pattern profiles compared with those of the two mutants. Restriction endonuclease Z is used here as an example. Note that all recombination events must occur in the sequence between genes E and F. Clearly the DNAs of recombinants will have profiles partially characteristic of one parent and partially of the other. Fixing the distance between the two genes is thus a matter of defining the limits of the DNA segment between them; the more recombinants that are examined, and the more restriction endonucleases that are used, the more accurately can this distance be determined.

host protein, RNA, and DNA) is not shut off until the late period has commenced. Late proteins are often synthesized in very large amounts, greatly in excess over what is assembled into progeny virus particles; much of this protein may be deposited in infected cells in the form of quasicrystalline arrays (see below). Usually about 20 virus-coded proteins can be detected in infected cells, about half of which are structural components of adenovirus particles. But this is no more than about one half of the total number of adenovirus-coded proteins, because at least 45 virus-specific messenger RNA species have been identified.

Adenovirus Genetic Map

The location of many adenovirus genes has been determined by a variety of techniques, all of which take advantage of the fact that completely ordered, detailed restriction endonuclease cleavage maps are available for the DNAs of adenovirus strains of several serotypes. In one such method, the mixture of virus-specific messenger RNAs from infected cells is hybridized to individual restriction endonuclease fragments. The messenger RNA species that hybridize with each fragment, and are therefore transcribed from it, are then dissociated from the DNA and translated in cell-free protein-synthesizing systems, and the proteins that are formed are identified by reference to authentic samples of adenovirus-coded proteins. As the position on the viral genome of each restriction endonuclease cleavage fragment is known, the location of the genes coding for the proteins that are translated is also known. In a variation of this technique, known as the hybridization-arrested translation method, the nature of the proteins that can be translated in vitro from the messenger RNAs isolated from infected cells is compared with the proteins that are translated from such messenger RNA mixtures after they have been hybridized to individual restriction endonuclease fragments. Such hybridization prevents individual species of messenger RNA from being translated, which results in the absence of specific proteins in the mixtures of translated proteins. Another method involves analysis of wild-type recombinants between mutants of viruses of different serotypes. The use of mutants permits the selection of recombinants; because the DNAs of viruses that differ in serotype have different restriction endonuclease patterns, it is possible to map the position of the crossover points on the viral genome (Fig. 4-10); and because some of the proteins encoded by the different serotypes differ detectably in size (as determined by electrophoresis in sodium dodecyl sulfate-containing polyacrylamide gels), it is possible to assign their genes to specific regions on the adenovirus genetic and physical maps.

The location of several genes on the adenovirus genome is shown in Figure 4-11. Interestingly, not all sequences of the adenovirus genome are essential for infectivity. For example, a deletion mutant that lacks the sequences between map positions 79 to 85, which include the gene that codes for the 21K glycoprotein that is present on the surface of infected cells, grows well; these sequences are therefore not necessary for growth.

Nature of Adenovirus Transcripts and Messenger RNAs

Just as in the case of SV40 described above, the primary adenovirus genome transcripts are not messenger RNAs; rather they must be processed to messenger RNAs. Processing involves three major modifications. First, the 5′-termini of transcripts must be capped (which involves

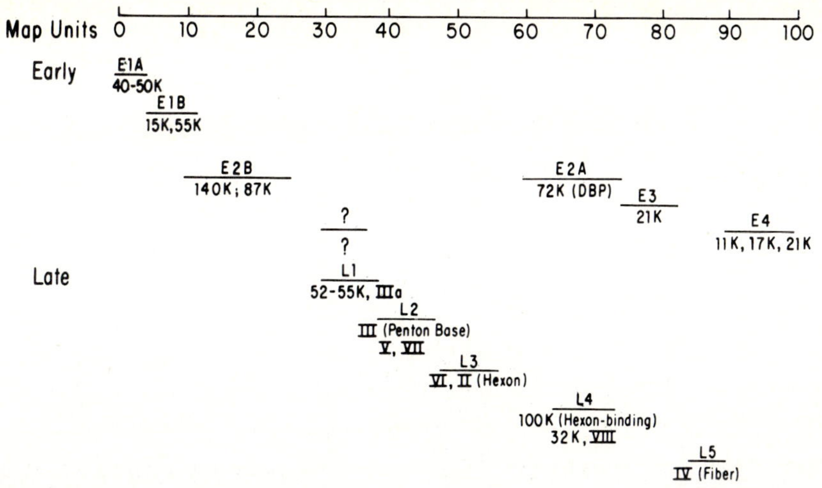

Figure 4-11. Location of the genes for various adenovirus proteins. The 55K protein (region E1B) is probably the adenovirus T antigen; the 140K protein and the 87K protein (region E2B) are, respectively, the adenovirus-coded DNA polymerase and the precursor of the 55K terminal protein that is covalently linked to the 5′-termini of adenovirus DNA; the 72K protein (region E2A) is a DNA-binding protein; the 100K protein (region L4) binds strongly to hexon protein and functions during morphogenesis; and the 21K protein (region E3) is a glycoprotein that is present on the surface of infected cells. Other adenovirus-specific proteins have been detected in infected cells. Some may be cleavage products of other adenovirus-specified proteins.

guanylylation and methylation); second, the 3′-termini of transcripts must be polyadenylated; and third, the transcripts must be spliced. The purpose of capping is most probably to provide strong ribosome binding sites to ensure efficient translation (although some messenger RNAs are known that are translated very efficiently, yet are not capped; and vice versa). The purpose of polyadenylation is not known; again, some messenger RNAs are known that are translated very efficiently, yet are not polyadenylated. As for splicing, the discovery of spliced adenovirus RNAs in the spring of 1977, and the demonstration shortly thereafter that splicing is a general phenomenon that applies not only to viral but also to most eucaryotic cellular messenger RNAs, was one of the major discoveries in biology in recent times—one that changed fundamentally our ideas and concepts concerning the nature and arrangement of eucaryotic genetic material.

The basic discovery was that a single messenger RNA species hybridizes to (and therefore is transcribed from) several widely separated regions of the adenovirus genome. One of the techniques for showing this was the so-called R-loop technique in which adenovirus DNA and RNA transcripts are mixed and partially melted; the DNA–DNA strands dissociate and more stable RNA–DNA hybrids are formed instead. When these hybrids are examined with the electron microscope, the regions where RNA and DNA have hybridized are seen as loops (R-loops), one arm of which is seen to be single stranded (a DNA strand), and the other double stranded (the RNA–DNA hybrid) (Fig. 4-12). This technique is extremely powerful for defining the precise locations of transcribed regions, as not only the length of R-loops, but also their distance from the ends of DNA molecules can be measured very precisely. Using this technique it was shown that most late adenovirus messenger RNA molecules begin with a leader sequence that is derived from three locations at map positions 16.7, 19.7, and 26.7, the combined length of which is about 200 nucleotides (Fig. 4-13). Presumably the original transcripts encompass not only the leader sequences and the coding sequences, but also the intervening sequences, the introns, that are then spliced out as part of the processing mechanism.

Adenovirus Transcription Program

Two transcription programs control the expression of adenovirus genes, one during the early period, and the other during the late period. During the early period, four widely separated regions of the genome are transcribed (Fig. 4-14). The first of these, region E1A and E1B at the left-hand end of the adenovirus genome, controls the earliest events in the multiplication cycle and the functions involved in cell transformation. The second region, which controls primarily DNA replication, consists of region E2A, which is transcribed into four messenger RNAs, all from different promoters; and region E2B, which gives rise to three messenger RNAs that use a promoter near map position 76. Finally, there is region E3, which is nonessential for virus growth, and region E4, the function of which is not known. Less than half the proteins coded by these early messenger RNA species have been identified.

Adenovirus late proteins are translated from about 20 messenger RNAs that are all processed from a transcript that covers the entire region between map positions 30 and 100. This was documented by measuring their relative

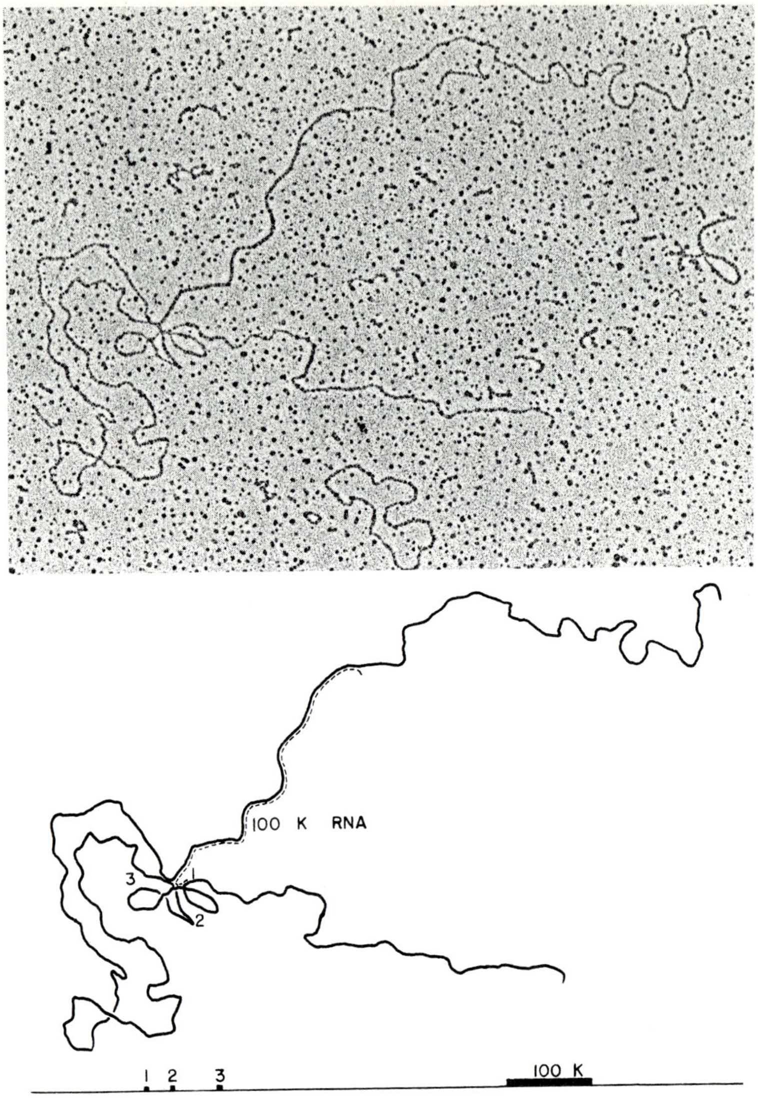

Figure 4-12. R-loops. An electron micrograph of a heteroduplex of human adenovirus serotype 2 (Ad2) RNA and single-stranded Ad2 DNA. The RNA was extracted from HeLa cells at a late time after infection. The DNA is constrained into a series of deletion loops corresponding to the intervening sequences removed from the spliced RNA. The first, second, and third leader segments and the main coding body of the messenger RNA are clearly visible. *(From Chow and Broker: Cell 15:497, 1978.)*

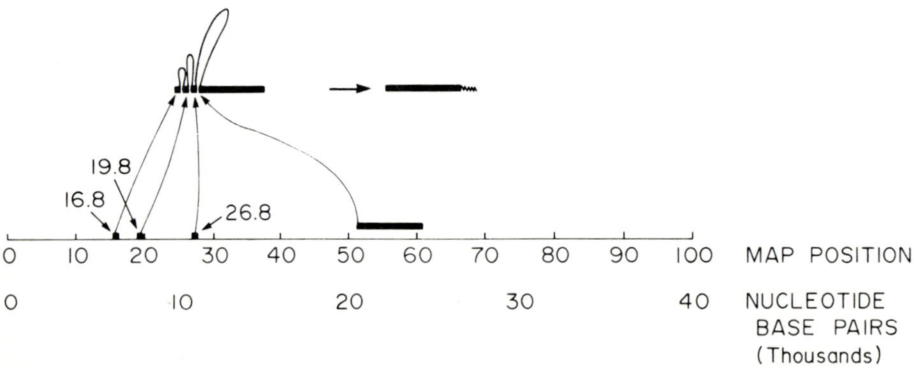

Figure 4-13. Structure of the adenovirus hexon messenger RNA. It consists of five portions: (1) a leader sequence about 50-nucleotides long, transcribed at map position 16.7; (2) a leader sequence about 80-nucleotides long, transcribed at map position 19.7; (3) a leader sequence about 75-nucleotides long, transcribed at map position 26.7; (4) a coding sequence about 3800-nucleotides long, transcribed from a genome sequence beginning at map position 51.7; and (5) a poly (A) sequence about 200-nucleotides long. The intervening sequences between map position 16.7 and 19.7, 19.7 and 26.7, and 26.7 and 51.7, which are present in the primary transcript, are spliced out.

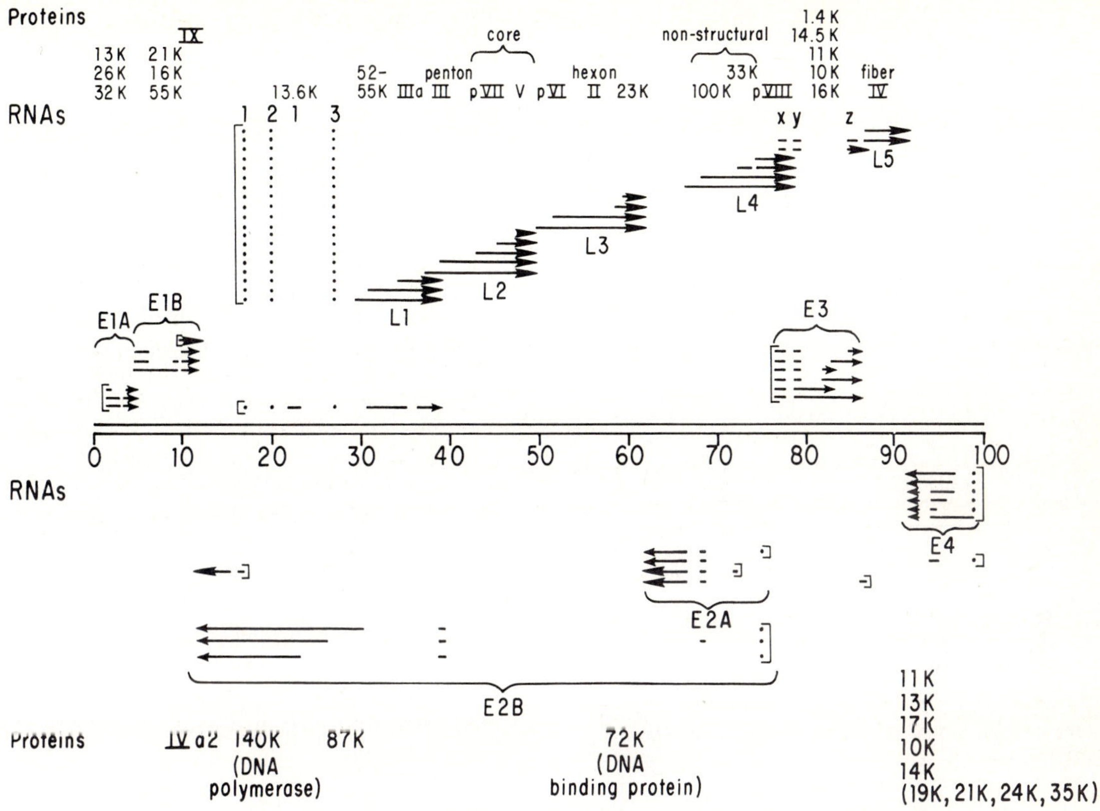

Figure 4-14. The adenovirus transcription map. Some transcripts are transcribed from one strand, others from the other. For each messenger RNA the following are indicated: the transcription region; the location of the promoters ([or]) and of the exons; and the proteins encoded by various messenger RNAs.

resistance to ultraviolet irradiation. Cells infected with adenovirus were irradiated with increasing doses of ultraviolet light, and the amount of each messenger RNA that accumulated was measured. It was found that the sensitivity to ultraviolet irradiation of each transcript of the four early regions was proportional to its physical size; but that the sensitivity of accumulation of each late messenger RNA species was proportional to the distance of the sequence from which it was transcribed from map position 30 (see Fig. 4-14). This indicated the existence of several discrete early region transcription units, but of only one late transcription unit. This late transcript is about 25,000-nucleotides long and is processed into the individual late messenger RNA species, all of which possess the same tripartite leader transcribed from the short sequences at map positions 16, 19, and 27, and falling into five groups that share common 3′-termini (which are polyadenylated) at map positions 39, 49, 61, 78, or 91. Their coding sequences vary, as shown in Figure 4-14. Neither the signals for splicing, nor the signals for polyadenylation, are known. Presumably, the nature of the cleavage/polyadenylation signals controls how many messenger RNA molecules of each type are made. (Clearly, many of some and few of other species are required, depending on how many of the corresponding protein molecules are needed.)

Whereas the preceding describes the overall features of the adenovirus transcription program, there are exceptions. For example, protein IX, a small hexon-associated protein (see Fig. 4-9) is a late protein, but is transcribed from a region around map unit 10, which is in early region E1B. Another messenger RNA uses the late messenger RNA promoter, possesses the late tripartite leader sequence, and maps in late region L1, yet is transcribed early. Clearly, the transcription program is fine-tuned by additional subtle features that remain to be defined.

In summary, the adenovirus transcription program provides an extremely sophisticated system for regulating both when each gene is transcribed and the extent to which it is transcribed (Fig. 4-15). The controlling features of this system are the existence of promoters where transcription is initiated, and the transcript processing mechanism that provides the means, through splicing and cleaving/polyadenylation, for specifying both the untranslated and the translated regions of messenger RNAs. This system permits any given region of DNA to be used over and over again, given the fact that there are three reading frames and that there is flexibility as to where coding regions start and finish. In other words, many adenovirus genes overlap, both on the same strand and on the complementary strand.

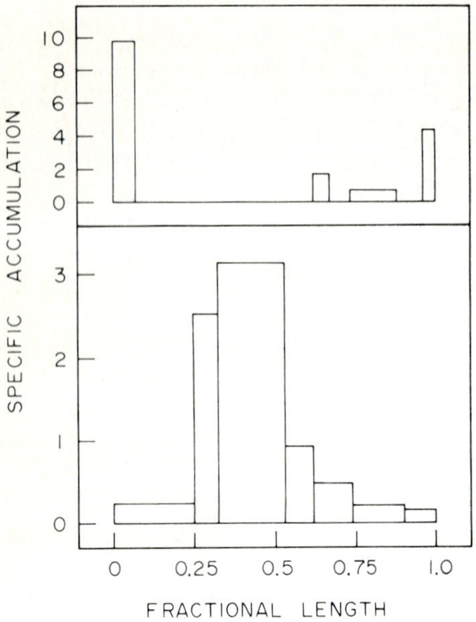

Figure 4-15. Frequency of accumulation of messenger RNAs transcribed from various regions of the adenovirus genome during the early and late periods of the multiplication cycle. Upper panel, early RNA (5.5 to 7.5 hours after infection); lower panel, late RNA (24 to 26 hours after infection). *(From Smiley and Mak: J Virol 28:227, 1978.)*

Adenovirus DNA Replication

Adenovirus DNA replication commences 6 to 8 hours after infection and reaches its peak rate 6 to 10 hours later. Adenovirus codes for a new DNA polymerase, but host cell DNA polymerase α may also function in adenovirus DNA replication. Replication begins at each end of the DNA molecule (Fig. 4-16) and proceeds in the 5′ to 3′ direction by displacement and complementary strand synthesis, the products being two double-stranded and two single-stranded molecules. The latter then probably cyclize by virtue of their inverted terminally repeated sequences, which would again permit complementary strand synthesis by 5′ to 3′ displacement, the products being two more double-stranded DNA molecules. This replication mechanism, parts of which are known to occur while others still lack rigorous proof, is unique because it does not involve the formation of Okazaki fragments and because the transcription of the two parental strands does not proceed simultaneously, but sequentially. Presumably, the two 5′-terminally linked protein molecules play some critical role in adenovirus DNA replication, possibly as primers.

There is some evidence that adenovirus DNA is integrated into host DNA during the lytic multiplication cycle. The significance of this phenomenon is not yet clear. It would seem that such integration is not essential for productive infection.

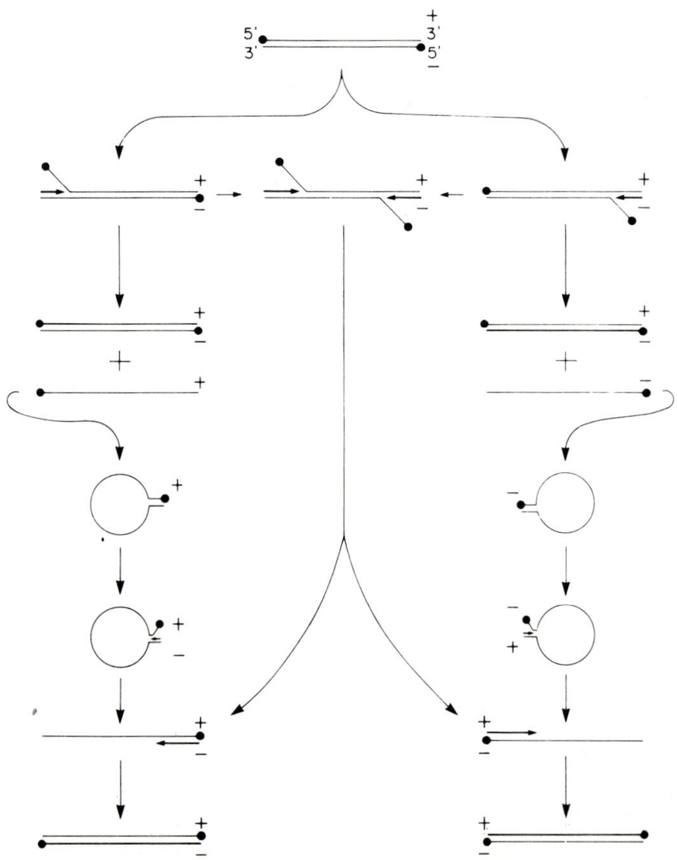

Figure 4-16. Proposed model for adenovirus DNA replication. Replication commences at either end and causes the displacement of either the plus or the minus strand. The resulting single strands then cyclize via their inverted terminally repeated sequences (see Chap. 2) and are transcribed again, yielding double-stranded molecules. Occasionally replication starts simultaneously at both ends, which yields replication intermediates of the type indicated. ●, the protein (mol wt 55,000) that is linked covalently to the 5′-termini of both DNA strands. *(Adapted from Lechner and Kelly: Cell 12:1007, 1977.)*

Adenovirus Morphogenesis

The morphogenesis of adenovirus, like that of papovaviruses and herpesviruses, proceeds in the nucleus, where paracrystalline arrays of mature virus particles, of incomplete empty particles, and even of the structural proteins that are often synthesized in great excess (see below) may be formed (Fig. 4-17).

Herpesviruses

The Herpesvirus Particle

Herpesvirus particles possess four distinct morphologic elements: (1) an electron-opaque core; (2) an icosahedral capsid that surrounds the core; (3) electron-dense amorphous material called the tegument, which surrounds the capsid; and (4) an envelope whose outer surface is studded with small glycoprotein spikes. The tegument, which has a fibrous structure, is unique to herpesviruses. Its amount varies greatly from strain to strain, and even from virus particle to virus particle.

Herpesvirus particles contain many (probably at least 30) proteins; the exact number is difficult to determine, as herpesviruses are not easily purified because the amount of tegument and envelope material per virus particle is not constant, and because many proteins are present in small amounts only. At least six proteins are present in the nucleocapsid, including the major component, the hexon (mol wt 155,000); and at least five glycoproteins are located on the outer surface of the envelope. Little is known concerning the protein composition of the tegument.

The DNA of herpesvirus (mol wt 96×10^6; 160,000 base pairs) is 30 times larger than that of SV40 and polyoma virus, and four times larger than that of adenovirus; the DNA of cytomegalovirus is 50 percent larger still. It consists of two regions, L and S, which comprise 82 and 18 percent of the viral DNA, respectively. Each component consists of largely unique sequences, U_L and U_S, bracketed by inverted repeated sequences (Fig. 4-18). Herpesvirus DNA extracted from virus particles consists of four isomers in which the orientations of the L and S components are inverted relative to each other; the herpesvirus ge-

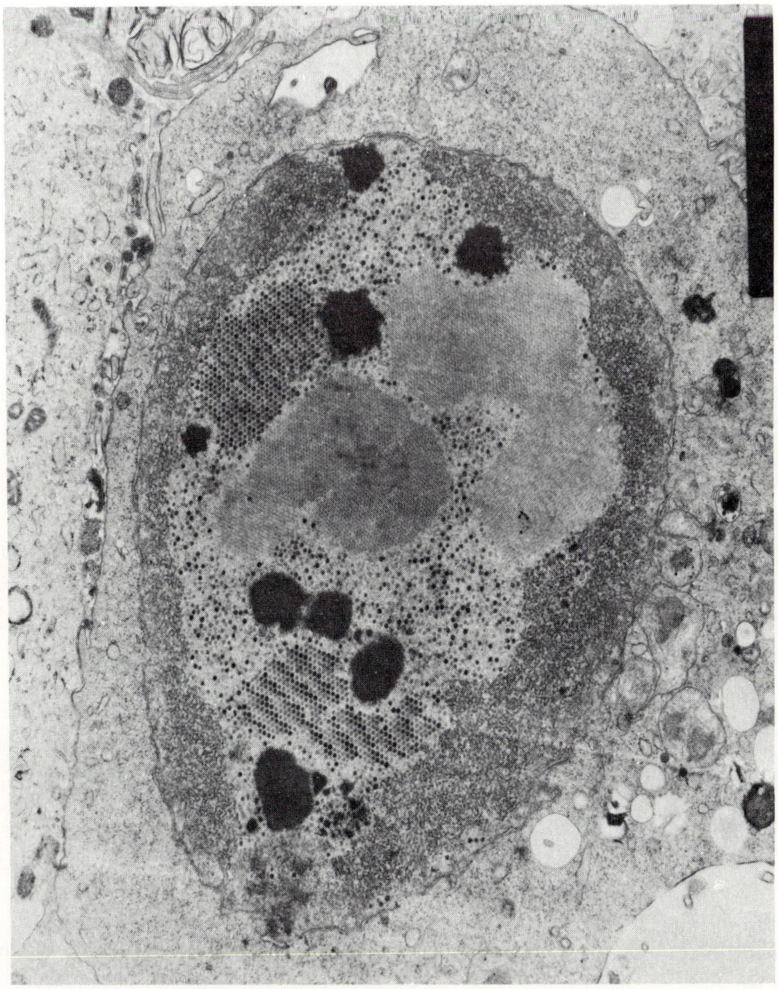

Figure 4-17. The nucleus of a Vero African green monkey kidney cell, 70 hours after infection with adenovirus type 2. Paracrystalline arrays of virus particles, crystals of vertex or core proteins, and intranuclear inclusions (the densely staining masses) are visible. × 10,000. *(From Henry et al.: Virology 44:215, 1972).*

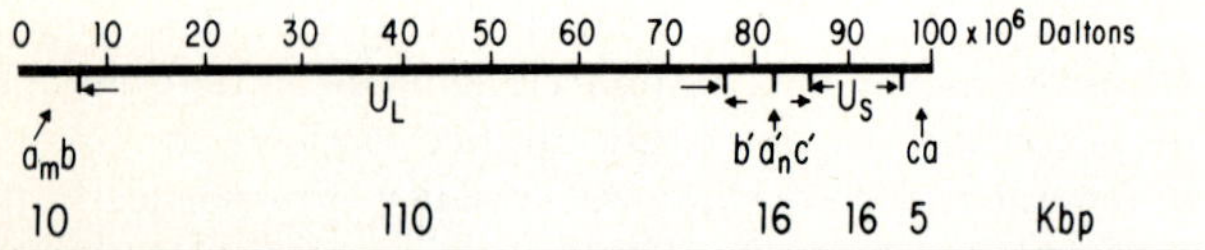

Figure 4-18. The sequence arrangement in herpes simplex virus DNA. U_L and U_S are unique regions flanked by inverted repeats. Regions *a, a'*, etc., are inverted forms of the same sequence. U_L is flanked by *b* sequences (about 8000 base pairs) and a variable number of *a* sequences (about 400 base pairs); U_S is flanked by *c* sequences (about 5000 base pairs) and *a* sequences. The *a* sequence is itself composed of five smaller sequence elements (from 12- to 64-base pairs long), two of which are unique, with the others present in 2, 2 to 3, and 19 to 22 copies, respectively. Note that the *a* sequence is present in the same orientation at the ends of the molecule and in the inverted orientation at the L–S junction. During the course of infection, the L and S components invert relative to each other such that the progeny DNA consists of equimolar amounts of four isomers that differ from each other solely in the relative orientation of the two components. The signal that directs the inversion of L and S components relative to each other is contained solely in the *a* sequence; in fact, insertion of *a* sequences into the U_L region causes additional inversions to occur. As a rule, the segment that inverts is flanked by *a'* sequences; segments that are flanked by *a* sequences do not invert. The inversion itself results from intramolecular recombination between terminal and inverted *a* sequences.

nome therefore exists in four configurations. The mechanism that causes this state of affairs is intramolecular recombination within a small region of the DNA (see Fig. 4-18). The significance of the extraordinary sequence anatomy of herpes simplex virus DNA is not clear, especially because it is modified or absent in other herpesviruses. Thus, in the genome of pseudorabies virus, a porcine herpesvirus, only the S segment is flanked by inverted repeated sequences and only the S segment inverts relative to the L segment, so that there are only two sequence isomers; and the genome of Epstein–Barr virus exists in only one configuration (see Chap. 8). Also, herpes simplex virus containing DNA that has been modified by recombinant DNA technology so that it can exist in only one configuration is infectious.

Herpesvirus Multiplication Cycle

The manner in which herpesvirus particles penetrate into cells is still a matter for debate; the evidence favors fusion of the viral membrane with the plasma cell membrane and liberation of naked nucleocapsids into the cytoplasm. Certainly, the herpesvirus envelope, most probably through the activity of one or more of the glycoproteins on its surface, causes cell membranes to fuse very readily, resulting in the formation of giant syncytia (see Chap. 5).

Once the parental DNA is uncoated, it moves to the nucleus where it begins to replicate after about 4 hours. The peak rate of herpesvirus DNA replication occurs at 6 to 8 hours, but the DNA continues to replicate at a gradually decreasing rate until the end of the multiplication cycle at about 36 hours. Herpesvirus DNA replication is mediated by a virus-coded DNA polymerase, which is an early protein, and probably proceeds via a rolling circle mechanism.

Substantial progress has recently been made in defining the herpesvirus genetic map. Using the techniques described above for adenovirus, more than 50 genes have so far been mapped on the herpesvirus physical map.

Herpesvirus Transcription Program

The herpesvirus transcription program has been intensively investigated by the techniques described above for SV40 and adenovirus. Like the transcription programs of these viruses, it can be divided into an early and a late period. The early period can be divided into two stages. During the first stage, which proceeds in the absence of de novo protein synthesis, about one third of the viral genome is transcribed by the host cell DNA-dependent RNA polymerase II into a series of apparently large, extensively processed transcripts; only about one third of their sequences reaches the cytoplasm in the form of messenger RNA molecules. The nature of the processing is not known; some herpesvirus messenger RNAs are spliced, but the majority appear to be unspliced. Only 4 of the 10 to 20 proteins that could be translated from these messenger RNA molecules have been detected and mapped on the herpesvirus genome; the others are probably formed in small amounts only. The proteins that are formed during this period are known as the immediate early or α proteins. Their rate of formation reaches a peak between 2 and 4 hours after infection and declines rapidly thereafter.

The second stage of the early period proceeds only when the α proteins have been synthesized. This stage is termed the β or true early stage. During this stage, which, like the α stage, proceeds even if herpesvirus DNA replication is inhibited, about 40 percent of the viral genome is transcribed, and the messenger RNAs that are translated in the cytoplasm correspond to about a quarter of the information encoded in herpesvirus DNA. Presumably, transcription is now initiated at new promoters, which are recognized by a new DNA-dependent RNA polymerase, perhaps the host cell RNA polymerase II modified by an α protein.

Once viral DNA replication has commenced, the transcription program changes again. The late period of the herpesvirus multiplication cycle can also be divided into two stages, the $\beta\gamma$, or leaky, late stage, and the γ late stage; $\beta\gamma$ genes are those that are transcribed marginally before DNA replication, and more strongly thereafter. During the late period more than one half of the viral DNA is transcribed.

The α, β, and γ herpesvirus proteins are rapidly being characterized (Fig. 4-19). Four α proteins are known; they seem to be phosphoproteins, and presumably are all regulatory proteins. About 10 β proteins have been identified, among them a DNA polymerase, a deoxypyrimidine kinase, and a DNA-binding protein. A deoxyribonuclease,

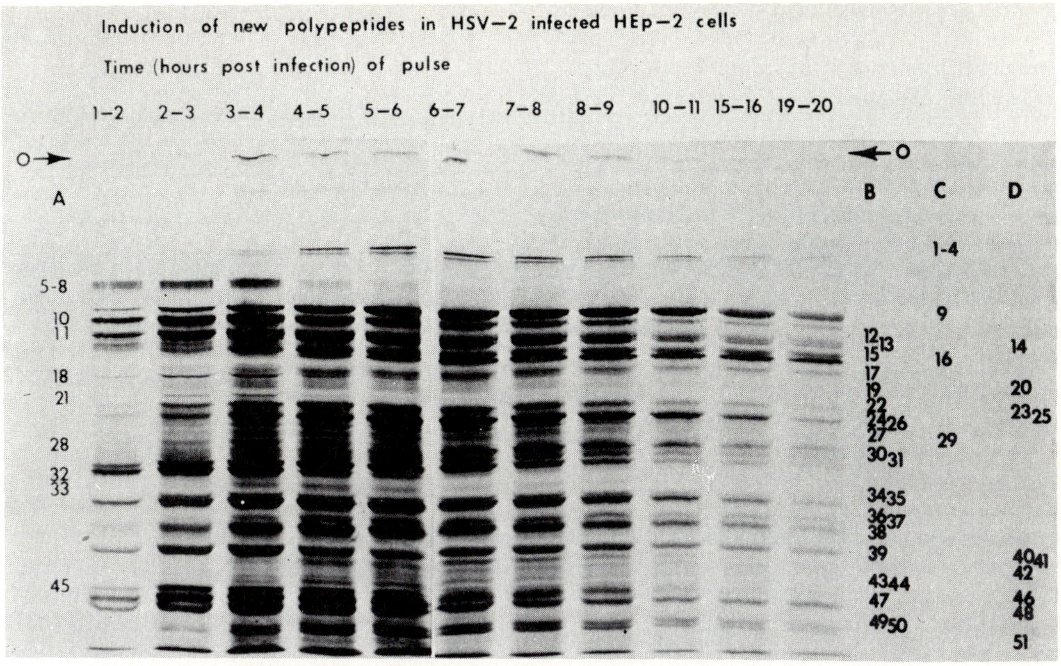

Figure 4-19. Autoradiogram of a polyacrylamide gel in which the proteins synthesized at various stages of the herpesvirus infection cycle (1 to 2 hours, 2 to 3 hours, 3 to 4 hours, and so on) had been electrophoresed. The direction of electrophoresis was from O (origin) downward. A, B, C, and D refer to kinetic groups to which the individual numbered proteins can be assigned, and which correspond roughly to the products of the α, β, and γ genes. *(Courtesy of Dr. Richard J. Courtney.)*

a ribonucleotide reductase, and a deoxycytidylic acid deaminase also appear to be early proteins. Another interesting early herpesvirus protein is an Fc receptor that begins to appear on the surface of infected cells at about this time. These virus-induced Fc receptors have affinity for normal immunoglobulin Gs and appear to be operationally equivalent to the Fc receptors expressed on certain cells of the immune system. The herpesvirus Fc receptor activity is associated with glycoprotein E, which also appears to be present in the envelopes of herpesvirus particles. The role of Fc-binding receptors in herpesvirus replication and biology is not understood. It is conceivable that the Fc-binding activity is fortuitous and that the receptor serves some entirely different function; but it has also been suggested that the binding of normal immunoglobulin or antiviral immunoglobulin to the Fc receptors can somehow interfere with cytotoxic immune reactions, thus sparing the infected cells and perhaps favoring the establishment of latency. Aggregated immunoglobulin G can in fact protect herpesvirus-infected cells from immune cytolysis in vitro. The binding of immunoglobulin to the Fc receptor may also repress the expression of viral functions in the cell, again favoring the establishment of latency. The other side of the coin, of course, is that cells infected with herpesvirus may be lysed nonspecifically by Fc receptor-positive killer cells; this has actually been observed.

As for the late proteins, they are predominantly structural components of virus particles.

Herpesvirus Morphogenesis and Release

Little is known concerning these processes except that assembly of herpesvirus nucleocapsids takes place in the nucleus, the capsid being formed first, followed by insertion of the viral DNA, and that the major site of envelopment is the inner nuclear membrane. Thus the envelopment of herpesvirus nucleocapsids differs sharply from the two important processes by which RNA-containing nucleocapsids are enveloped (budding through the plasma membrane or budding into vacuoles, see below). Instead, enveloped herpesvirus particles are transported through the cytoplasm by an as yet unidentified mechanism and are released from the plasma cell membrane without acquiring significant extra material in the process.

Poxviruses

Poxviruses are unique among animal viruses in that they require a newly synthesized protein for uncoating. Vaccinia virus particles are taken up into cells via phagocytic vacuoles (coated vesicles, see above) from which they are liberated into the cytoplasm in the form of cores. In the presence of inhibitors of protein synthesis, these cores are not uncoated; they do not liberate the DNA that they contain. Instead, uncoating of cores requires a protein that is encoded by the DNA that they contain and that is transcribed by the DNA-dependent RNA polymerase that is present within them. In fact, this uncoating protein gene is not the only gene that is expressed by cores. About one third of the vaccinia virus DNA is transcribed into capped and polyadenylated messenger RNA—the immediate early messenger RNAs—while it is still present within cores, that is, before it is uncoated.

Once vaccinia virus DNA is fully uncoated, it initiates the formation of inclusions, or factories, in the cytoplasm, within which it is transcribed further, replicates, and is encapsidated into progeny virions. The inclusions, which are easily visible with light microscopy, are composed of fibrillar material and may be located anywhere in the cytoplasm. Their number per cell is proportional to the multiplicity of infection, which suggests that each infecting virus particle initiates its own factory (Fig. 4-20).

During the early period of the multiplication cycle, almost one half of the vaccinia virus genome is transcribed into messenger RNA. Among the early proteins are several enzymes, such as a thymidine kinase and a DNA polymerase, as well as several structural proteins.

Vaccinia virus DNA replication commences at about 1.5 hours after infection and is complete by about 5 hours (Fig. 4-21). Its onset heralds the commencement of the late period of the multiplication cycle, which is characterized by new patterns of viral gene expression. Synthesis of at least some of the early structural proteins continues into the late period, but synthesis of the early enzymes ceases. Cessation of their synthesis is due to the so-called switch-off phenomenon (Fig. 4-22), which is of interest because it provides one of the few well-documented examples of

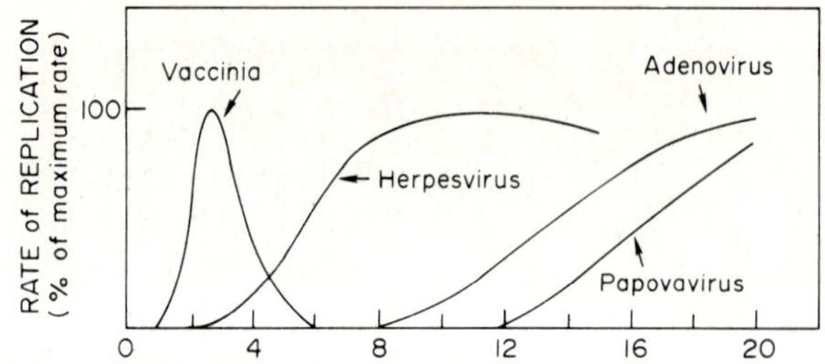

Figure 4-21. The replication of vaccinia virus, herpesvirus, adenovirus, and papovavirus DNA. Vaccinia virus DNA is atypical in replicating only during a brief period early in the multiplication cycle. Progeny DNA molecules form a pool from which individual molecules are selected at random for incorporation into progeny virus particles.

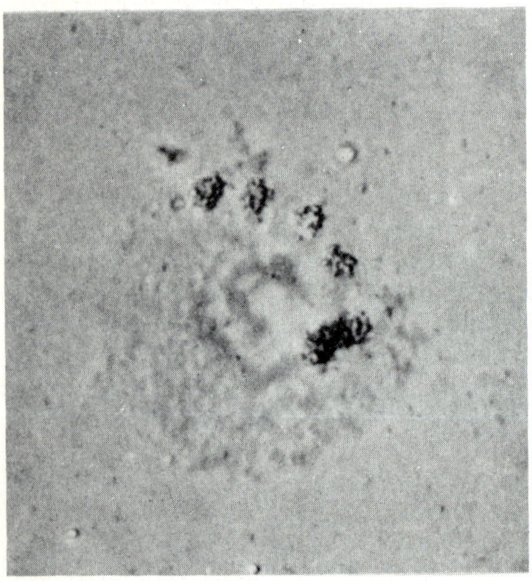

Figure 4-20. Vaccinia virus factories in the cytoplasm of HeLa cell. Cells growing on a cover slip were infected at a multiplicity of 6 plaque forming units (PFU) per cell. At 6 hours after infection tritiated thymidine was added, and at 7 hours the cells were fixed. Autoradiographic stripping film was then applied, and the slide stored for 2 weeks. On developing, the picture shown here was obtained. There are no grains (indicative of thymidine incorporation and, therefore, DNA replication) over the nucleus, but there are five labeled areas or factories in the cytoplasm (one actually composed of two coalesced areas)—this is where viral DNA is being synthesized. This cell had been stained with antibody to vaccinia virus coupled to fluorescein before autoradiography, and it was thereby demonstrated that the only areas in the cell that contained appreciable amounts of vaccinia virus antigens were the factories. Both viral DNA replication and viral morphogenesis therefore proceed within the factories. *(From Cairns: Virology 11:603, 1960.)*

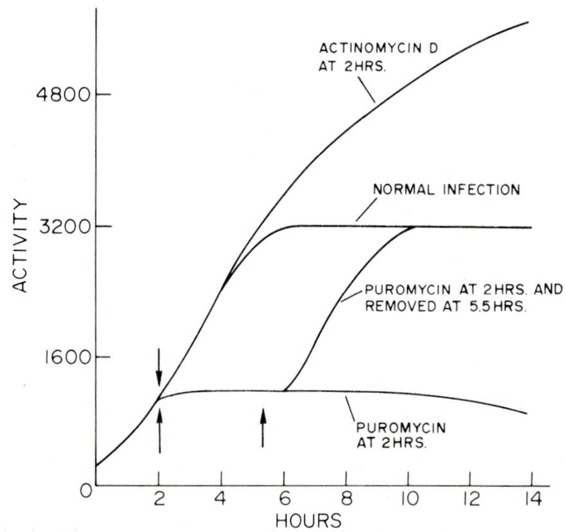

Figure 4-22. The switch-off phenomenon. This graph depicts the synthesis of early enzymes, such as thymidine kinase and DNA polymerase, during vaccinia virus infection. Under normal conditions these enzymes begin to be formed soon after infection, and their synthesis is "switched-off" at about 4 hours. If actinomycin D, which inhibits messenger RNA formation, is added at 2 hours, switch-off does not occur. This demonstrates (1) that the messenger RNAs from which these enzymes are translated are very stable, and (2) that switch-off itself requires the synthesis of some other messenger RNA. If protein synthesis is inhibited with puromycin at 2 hours, enzyme synthesis immediately ceases; if puromycin is removed at 5.5 hours, enzyme synthesis resumes and is again switched off after a time interval equivalent to that between the addition of puromycin and the onset of normal switch-off. This indicates that switch-off is due to the accumulation of a certain amount of some specific protein. *(Modified from McAuslan: Virology 21:383, 1963.)*

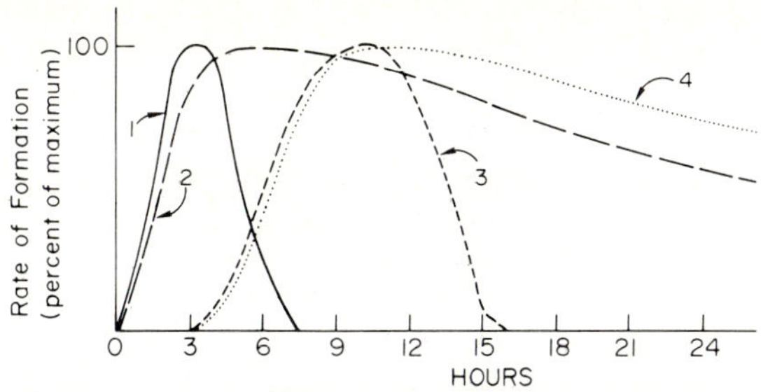

Figure 4-23. The synthesis of four classes of vaccinia-specified proteins. First, there are some early proteins whose synthesis is switched off when DNA replication commences. Early enzymes and several structural vaccinia virus proteins belong to this class. Second, there are those early proteins whose synthesis continues throughout the multiplication cycle. One of the major components of immature virus particles belongs to this class. Third, there are late proteins that are synthesized for some time following the onset of DNA replication and that are then switched off; finally, there are late proteins that are synthesized throughout the entire late period of the multiplication cycle. Most structural vaccinia virus proteins belong to this class. *(Modified from Holowczak, and Joklik: Virology 33:726, 1967.)*

regulation of gene expression at the level of translation. In essence, cessation of the synthesis of early enzymes is not due to inhibition of the transcription of their genes, to instability of their messenger RNA species, or to instability of the enzymes themselves. Rather it is due to a suddenly developing inability of the messenger RNA species that code for early enzymes to be translated. If viral DNA replication and protein synthesis are inhibited, this inability does not develop. It is thought, therefore, that one of the first late proteins to be synthesized specifically prevents the translation of the messenger RNA molecules that code for early enzymes. This mechanism of controlling protein synthesis is obviously highly selective, as many other viral messenger RNA molecules—for example, those that code for structural proteins—continue to be translated. It is of potential significance for antiviral chemotherapy because it implies the existence of a chemical difference between those messenger RNA molecules that continue to be translated and those that are switched off. In may prove possible to expoit this difference (see Chap. 7).

Another class of vaccinia proteins whose synthesis is switched off comprises certain late proteins that are formed for only several hours. Together with the early and late proteins whose synthesis is never switched off, there are thus at least four different vaccinia virus protein translation patterns, and there may be many more (Fig. 4-23).

Somewhat more than one half of vaccinia virus DNA codes for late proteins. By far the quantitatively most important of these are the structural viral proteins, most of which, like DNA, are usually formed in great excess. The vaccinia virus-coded proteins that are synthesized as the multiplication cycle progresses are shown in Figure 4-24; it is readily seen that different proteins are synthesized at

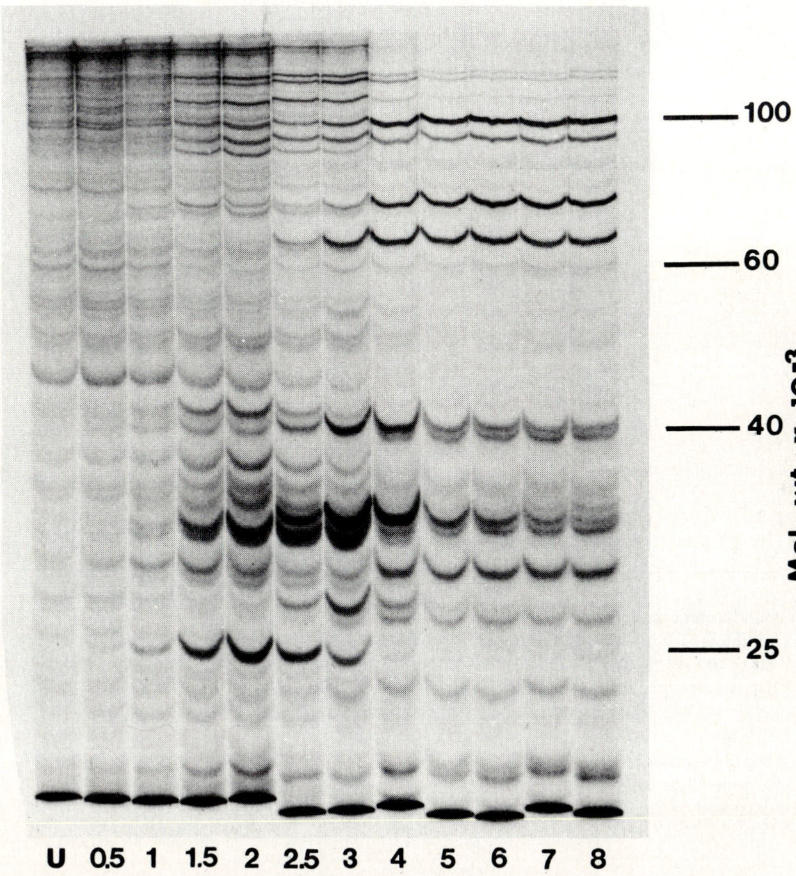

Figure 4-24. Autoradiogram of a 9 percent polyacrylamide slab gel in which the proteins synthesized at various stages of the vaccinia virus multiplication cycle had been electrophoresed. At the times indicated (hours after infection) the cells were labeled for 15 minutes with [^{14}C]-protein hydrolysate. At the right is a molecular weight scale as determined by electrophoresing proteins of known size under identical conditions. *(Courtesy of Dr. T.H. Pennington.)*

different times. It should be noted that very few host-coded proteins are formed even at the earliest times; like herpesvirus, vaccinia virus shuts down host–cell protein synthesis very efficiently (see Chap. 5).

Another way of analyzing the vaccinia virus transcription program is to hybridize early and late vaccinia messenger RNA populations to a series of mapped restriction endonuclease fragments of vaccinia virus DNA, and to translate the messenger RNAs that hybridize to each in an in vitro cell-free protein-synthesizing system. The results of such an analysis are summarized in Table 4-4. Clearly, numerous proteins are translated during both periods of the multiplication cycle, and some portions of the vaccinia virus genome are transcribed predominantly in the early period, others in the late period.

Progeny genomes of DNA-containing viruses generally replicate faster than they are incorporated into virus particles. They therefore accumulate to form pools from which individual genomes are withdrawn at random for encapsidation. Whereas some DNA molecules are withdrawn very soon after they are formed, others may remain naked for long periods of time. This is true particularly in the case of the vaccinia virus multiplication cycle, where DNA replication ceases at about 5 hours after infection, whereas viri-

TABLE 4-4. TRANSLATION MAP OF THE VACCINIA VIRUS GENOME*

Hind III Fragment		C		N+M+K	F	E	O+I	G	L+J	H	D	A	B	Total
Size (mol wt × 10^{-6})	5.9	4.4	3.8	5.3	8.9	9.9	5.3	6.0	5.8	5.6	10.3	30	19	120
Early Proteins (mol wt × 10^{-3})	42	60	38	54	68	95	80	54	41	40	86	58	42	
	19	21	32	53	62	67	79		21	39	84	45	35	
	8	19	21	46	59	64	33		17	14	79	41	35	
		13	15	40	54	62	32			11	52	40	31	
		6	14	30	45	55	25				34	39	27	
			12	23	39	36					28	37	19	
				20	35	34					27	35	8	
				16	33	32					24	31		
				11	27	30					17	27		
				9	17	26					14	24		
					16	22					12	23		
					16	17						20		
					10	15						18		
												16		
Medium–Early Proteins			23					33	110					
								30						
Late Proteins	—	22	40	—	52	12	46	65	44	55	70	96		
					40		35	44	37	46	35	84		
					15		11	33	36	36	17	45		
								30	33	30	14	22		
								14	30	28				
								12	28	18				
								9	28	17				
									19	16				
									19	13				
									18					
									14					

Adapted from Isle et al.: Virology 112:306, 1981.

*Extracts were prepared of HeLa cells infected with vaccinia virus under three sets of conditions: (1) In the presence of cycloheximide, an inhibitor of protein synthesis, when vaccinia virus cores are not uncoated and only early messenger RNA is made; (2) in the presence of cytosine arabinoside, an inhibitor of DNA replication, when both early and medium–early messenger RNAs are made; and (3) during the late period of the multiplication cycle, when some early and medium–early, but also all late messenger RNAs are made. The viral messenger RNAs in these extracts were hybridized to cloned *Hind* III restriction endonuclease fragments of vaccinia virus DNA, and those that hybridized were translated in a cell-free protein synthesizing system prepared from reticulocytes in order to determine which proteins they encoded. The *Hind* III C fragment was further divided into its *Eco*RI fragments, A, B, C, and D; because they are small, C and D are combined in this map. For the same reason, *Hind* III fragments N, M, and K, O and I, and L and J are also combined. *Hind* III fragments A and B are too large to be cloned readily and were used in uncloned form. Note the sizes of the proteins that were obtained, which range from over 100,000 to less than 10,000; and the fact that the early and late proteins are clustered on the vaccinia virus genome, late proteins being encoded primarily in the regions defined by *Hind* III fragments G, L, J, and H.

on morphogenesis continues for about 25 hours. The time necessary for a complete virus particle to be assembled around a vaccinia DNA molecule is about 1 hour.

Vaccinia Virus Morphogenesis. The morphogenesis of vaccinia virus proceeds in the cytoplasm, where mature virus particles accumulate (Fig. 4-25). Most virus particles are released only when infected cells disintegrate. However, mature vaccinia virus particles can also migrate to the

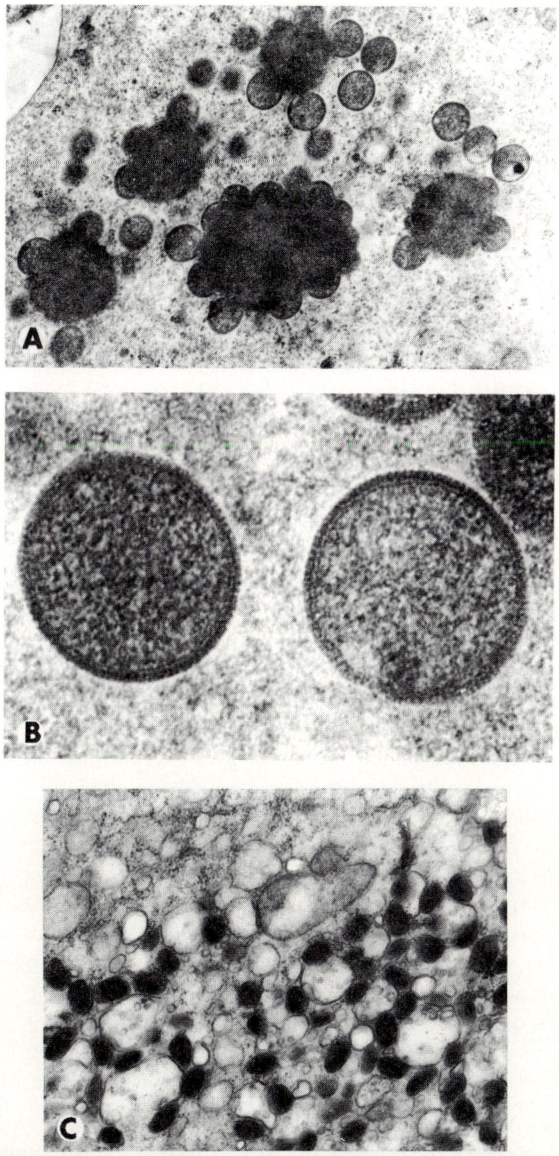

Figure 4-25. Vaccinia virus particles in the cytoplasm of infected cells. **A.** Immature virus particles developing from intracytoplasmic inclusions 1 hour after reversal of vaccinia virus morphogenesis arrest by rifampicin (see Chap. 7). × 9,000. **B.** Characteristic structure of immature vaccinia virus particles. × 48,000. **C.** Mature vaccinia virus particles in the cytoplasm of infected cells. × 12,000. *(**A, B,** courtesy of Dr. T.H. Pennington; **C,** from Dales and Siminovitch: J Biochem Biophys Cytol 10:475, 1961.)*

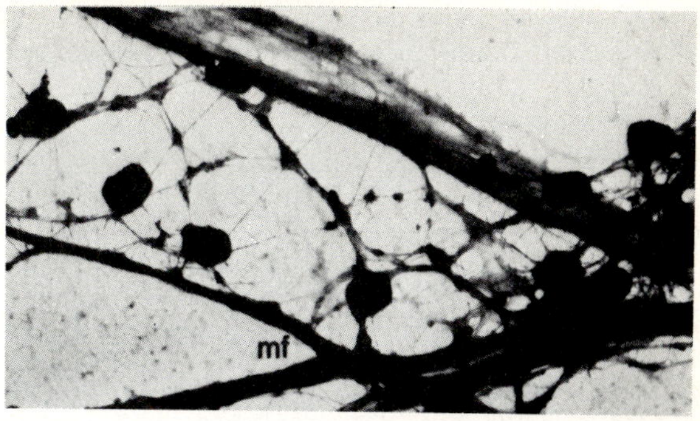

Figure 4-26. Vaccinia virus particles associated with elements of the cytoskeleton. Infected cells, extracted with 0.5 percent triton X-100. Uranyl acetate staining. Magnification, × 30,000. For details see text. *(From Hiller et al.: Virology 98:142, 1979.)*

plasma cell membrane in association with the actin-containing microfilaments of the cytoskeleton (Fig. 4-26). Late in infection, numerous specialized microvilli that contain predominantly F-actin and F-actin–binding proteins (α-actinin, filamin, and fimbrin) are formed on the surface of infected cells, and these microvilli usually contain a vaccinia virus particle at their tip. They may provide a second mechanism for vaccinia virus release and dissemination.

Multiplication Cycle of Double-stranded RNA-containing Viruses

When reovirus infects cells, its outer capsid shell is partially degraded to form an entity known as a subviral particle (SVP) (Fig. 4-27). This process activates an RNA polymerase (known as the transcriptase) within them that transcribes all 10 reovirus genes into capped, but unspliced and not polyadenylated, messenger RNA molecules. The parental double-stranded RNA never escapes from the SVP, which persists in infected cells throughout the multiplication cycle.

The messenger RNA molecules are translated for several hours and then begin to associate with viral proteins to form complexes within which they are transcribed once —and once only—into minus strands with which they remain associated, thereby giving rise to double-stranded RNA molecules, the progeny genes. These immature progeny virus particles then transcribe more messenger RNA molecules, which are translated into more proteins, and so on. At the same time, immature virus particles associate with the proteins of the outer capsid shell to form mature virus particles. It should be noted that the stages of the multiplication cycle when the plus and minus strands of progeny double-stranded RNA are synthesized are separated by an interval of several hours. Double-stranded RNA is thus synthesized by a mechanism that is quite different from that by which double-stranded DNA is formed.

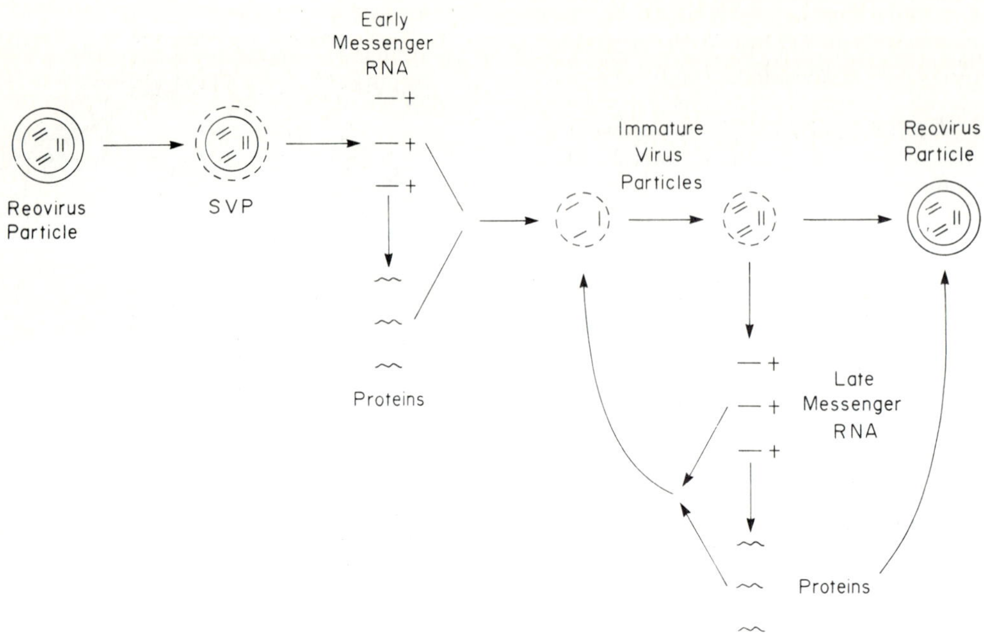

Figure 4-27. The reovirus multiplication cycle. For details, see text. Note that here early and late messenger RNA and protein molecules are identical. Because many immature virus particles are formed from each parental subviral particle, most viral messenger RNA molecules are transcribed from progeny templates.

Multiplication Cycles of Single-stranded RNA-containing Viruses

The principles involved in the multiplication of single-stranded RNA-containing viruses differ in several aspects from those described for the double-stranded DNA-containing viruses. Most importantly, their multiplication cycles cannot be divided into clearly defined early and late periods, as can those of the double-stranded DNA-containing viruses. A brief description of the multiplication cycles of several families of single-stranded RNA-containing viruses follows.

Multiplication Cycles of Plus-stranded RNA-containing Viruses

Picornaviruses

The multiplication cycle of poliovirus is considered here, as it has been investigated in most detail. The strategy of the poliovirus multiplication cycle is summarized schematically in Fig. 4-28.

After uncoating, the poliovirus RNA, a 7441-nucleotide long molecule that has been completely sequenced, is translated into one very large protein with a molecular weight of about 240,000. This protein, the polyprotein, is then cleaved in a precisely defined sequence of reactions into about 20 smaller proteins, among which are the four structural proteins, the RNA-linked protein VPg, an RNA polymerase, and a protease that carries out this cleavage program (Fig. 4-29). Little is known concerning the nature of the intermediate cleavage products or whether any of them exercise a specific function during the poliovirus multiplication cycle. They clearly possess the potential for doing so, and if they did, this would be another example of the multiple use of viral genetic information. In this respect, it is of interest that posttranslational cleavage of viral proteins occurs frequently; there are numerous examples of vaccinia virus, adenovirus, myxovirus, togavirus, retrovirus, and other viral capsid proteins being synthesized in the form of precursors larger than themselves. The reason in most cases is not expansion of the pool of genetic information, but rather one of the following:

1. Viral capsid proteins may be too insoluble to be transported from the site where they are synthesized to the site of morphogenesis unless their solubility is increased by the presence of removable amino acid sequences.
2. Precursors may be the forms in which capsid proteins must exist prior to assembly to enable them to interact correctly with other capsid proteins.
3. Cleavage of precursors to capsid proteins may provide at least part of the energy for morphogenesis.

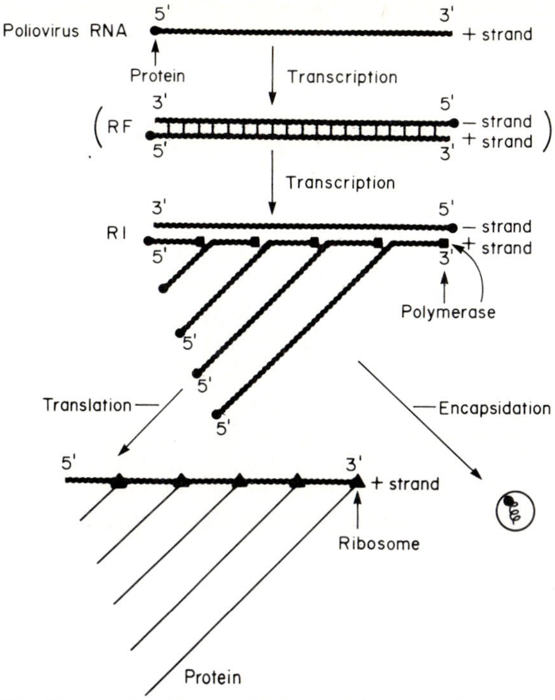

Figure 4-28. Replication and functioning of poliovirus RNA. Parental RNA strands are translated into the polyprotein, and the polymerase derived from the polyprotein then transcribes them into strands of minus polarity, to yield double-stranded replicative forms (RF), which probably have a very short half-life. Progeny plus strands are then transcribed repeatedly from the minus-strand templates by a peeling-off type mechanism. The structure consisting of minus-stranded template and several plus-stranded transcripts at various stages of completion is known as the replicative intermediate (RI). Early during the infection cycle, the number of RFs, and therefore of RIs, increases, so that the rate of formation of progeny plus strands first increases and then becomes constant. Progeny plus strands are either translated or encapsidated.

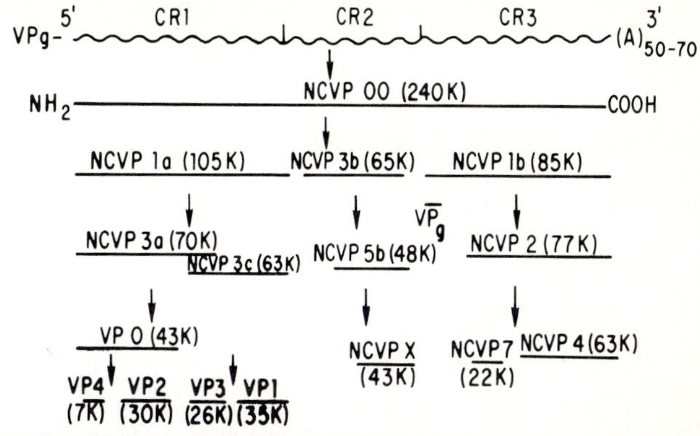

Figure 4-29. Synthesis and processing of the poliovirus precursor polyprotein NCVP 00 (noncapsid viral protein 00). Poliovirus RNA can be subdivided into three coding regions; CR1, which encodes the structural proteins; CR2, which encodes the protease, and CR3, which encodes the RNA polymerase. Some precursor proteins can be cleaved at more than one location. The small 5'-terminal genome-linked protein VPg has been mapped to a location at or near the amino terminus of the replicase precursor protein NCVP 1b. Cleavages that occur before the putative proteases, NCVP X and NCVP 7, have been formed probably occur autocatalytically.

The enzyme that cleaves the precursors is not known with certainty but appears to be either NCVP X, NCVP 7, or both. All cleavages occur between glutamine and glycine residues. The only exception is the cleavage of VP 0 to VP 4 and VP 2, which occurs only during morphogenesis. Proteins of other viruses with protease function are capsid protein C of togaviruses and p15 of retroviruses (see Chap. 8).

Poliovirus RNA replication, which starts within an hour of infection and appears to be catalyzed by the poliovirus polymerase NCVP 4 in concert with a cellular protein, takes place in two stages: First, the parental plus strand is transcribed into a minus strand; and then, the minus strand serves as the template for repeated transcription into progeny plus strands. Some progeny plus strands are then again transcribed into minus strands, but this is not a common occurrence. The total number of minus strands in the infected cell probably does not exceed 1000, whereas up to a million plus strands may be formed. RNA strands of both plus and minus polarity are covalently linked at their 5'-termini to a tyrosine residue of VPg, a protein with 22 amino acids that probably serves as a primer for transcription. This protein is also present on the RNA that is present in virus particles, but is not present on poliovirus RNA molecules that serve as messenger RNA. Thus, progeny RNA molecules that are encapsidated have never served as messenger RNAs, and poliovirus RNA molecules that serve as messengers do not become encapsidated.

Whereas translation of the poliovirus genome into a single precursor protein has many advantages, there are also potential disadvantages. In particular, it implies that all portions of the viral genome are expressed with equal frequency. This is very wasteful, as many more capsid protein molecules are required than, for example, polymerase molecules. In practice, the various processed poliovirus-specified proteins are not formed in equimolar amounts, especially during the later stages of the multiplication cycle when most of the proteins that are formed are indeed capsid components. The mechanism by which such translational control is achieved is probably as follows. It is known that the capsid proteins are encoded in the 5'-terminal region of the poliovirus RNA molecule. This means that in the event of premature termination of translation, which is not unlikely for a long messenger RNA such as poliovirus RNA, the formation of capsid proteins would be favored over those like the polymerase that are encoded by sequences in its 3'-terminal half.

As is the case for other icosahedral viruses, poliovirus progeny often accumulates in the form of large, intracytoplasmic, paracrystalline arrays (Fig. 4-30).

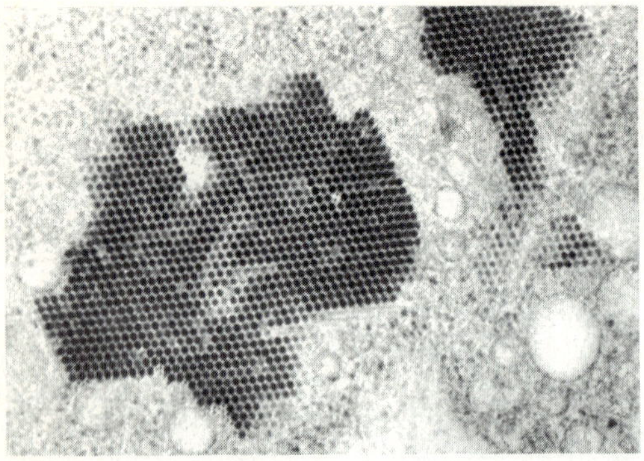

Figure 4-30. A large crystal of poliovirus in the cytoplasm of a HeLa cell infected for 7 hours. × 50,000. *(From Dales et al.: Virology 26:379, 1965.)*

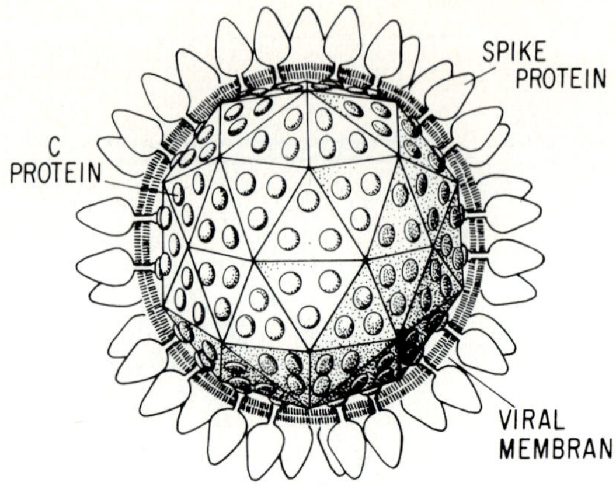

Figure 4-31. Structure of the alphavirus Semliki Forest virus. One hundred eighty molecules of the C protein (mol wt 30,000) form the icosahedral nucleocapsid; and 180 spikes are inserted into the lipid bilayer of the envelope. *(Adapted from Simons et al.: Sci Am 246:58, 1982.)*

Togaviruses

Togavirus particles, as exemplified by the alphavirus Semliki Forest virus, consist of an icosahedral nucleocapsid made up of 180 molecules of a single protein, the C protein, surrounded by an envelope that consists of a lipid bilayer into which 180 spikes are inserted (Fig. 4-31). Each spike consists of three glycoproteins, E1, E2, and E3, two of which span the lipid bilayer, and is associated with a C protein molecule (Fig. 4-32). Interestingly, proteins E1 and E2 are not only glycosylated, but also acylated; that is, several molecules of fatty acid are linked to them covalently via ester bonds, presumably in the regions that are most intimately associated with the lipid bilayer.

The RNA of alphaviruses, which form one of the togavirus genera, is a plus stranded RNA molecule about 12,700-nucleotides long (mol wt 4.3×10^6), with a sedimentation coefficient of 42S. The strategy of the alphavirus multiplication cycle (Fig. 4-33) is quite different from that of picornaviruses. When the alphavirus genome is uncoated, about two thirds of it, starting from the 5′-terminus, is translated into one large protein that is cleaved into four nonstructural proteins. They are, from the amino terminus, ns70-ns26-ns78-ns60 (the numbers being their molecular weights), and two of them form the RNA polymerase. This enzyme transcribes the parental plus strands into minus strands, which then act as templates for plus strand synthesis. The crucial point is that two types of plus strands are transcribed: (1) full-length 42S plus strands that, like the progeny plus strands of poliovirus RNA, can function either as messenger RNA, act as templates for the synthesis of additional minus strand synthesis, or be encapsidated into progeny virus particles; and (2) strands that are only about one third as long and possess a sedimentation coefficient of 26S (mol wt 1.6×10^6, about 4800-nucleotides long). These RNA molecules represent the 3′-terminal one third of the 42S RNA molecules, and they code for the four structural alphavirus proteins that are translated from them in the form of a 130,000-dalton precursor (Fig. 4-34).

In essence, then, the alphavirus genome expresses itself via two messenger RNAs instead of via only one. The special 26S messenger RNA is transcribed about three times as frequently as the 42S RNA, which acts as the messenger RNA only for the nonstructural protein precursor. These relative transcription frequencies are controlled by at least two proteins: one of the nonstructural proteins described above, which promotes transcription of 26S RNA; and the C protein, which represses it.

The morphogenesis of alphaviruses involves the formation of cores or nucleocapsids that consist of 42S plus-stranded RNA and C protein, and the budding of these

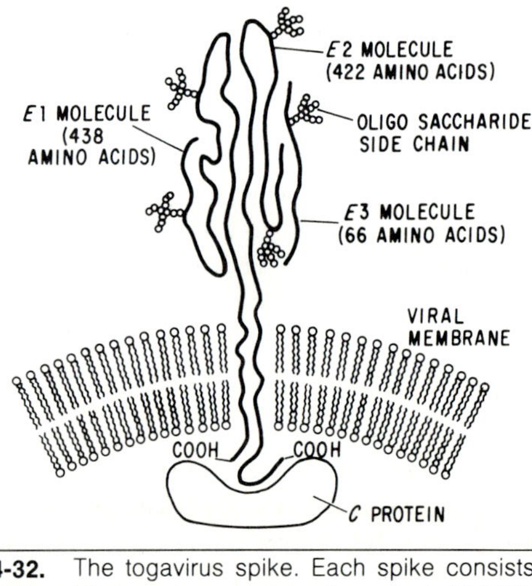

Figure 4-32. The togavirus spike. Each spike consists of three glycoproteins, E1 (envelope protein 1) (mol wt 48,000), E2 (mol wt 46,000), and E3 (mol wt 7,000). E1 and E2 possess two carbohydrate chains; E3 possesses only 1. The two large glycoproteins are anchored in the lipid bilayer by spanning it; thirty-one amino acids of E2 and two amino acids of E1 penetrate through it into the interior of the particle where they make contact with C protein molecules. *(Adapted from Simons et al.: Sci Am 246:58, 1982.)*

cores through patches of plasma cell membrane into which the glycosylated envelope proteins have been inserted. This process is discussed in more detail below.

Members of the *Flavivirus* genus, which are considerably smaller than alphaviruses (50 nm in diameter, rather than 60 to 65 nm), use a different strategy of genome expression and maturation. Here the viral RNA itself serves as messenger RNA for all virus-coded proteins. There is good evidence that this RNA—which, in contrast to that of alphaviruses, is not polyadenylated—possesses multiple internal protein synthesis initiation sites, a unique property for eucaryotic messenger RNAs. Furthermore, flaviviruses tend to mature in association with cytoplasmic membranes, bud into cytoplasmic vacuoles, and are liberated by exocytosis and cell lysis, instead of by budding through plasma cell membranes (see below).

Multiplication Cycles of Negative-stranded RNA-containing Viruses

Rhabdoviruses

One of the most intensively investigated negative-stranded RNA-containing viruses is the rhabdovirus vesicular stomatitis virus (VSV). The VSV particle consists of a helical nucleocapsid composed of a minus-stranded RNA molecule about 11,300-nucleotides long, and 2300 molecules of N protein (mol wt 52,000), 230 molecules of NS protein (mol wt 32,000), and 60 molecules of L protein (mol wt 175,000). The latter two proteins constitute the RNA polymerase. This nucleocapsid is surrounded by an envelope that consists of a layer of M protein (mol wt 25,000; 4700 molecules) and a lipid bilayer, to which about 700 spikes consisting of trimers of the G protein (mol wt 67,000; 2100 molecules) are attached. The G protein is a transmembrane protein; about 30 amino acids at its carboxyl-terminal end penetrate through the lipid bilayer into the interior of the particle, where they contact not only M protein molecules, but also the nucleocapsid.

These five structural proteins are the only proteins encoded by VSV RNA. The order of their genes, from the 3′-end of the RNA in virus particles, is N-NS-M-G-L. They are separated by short 13-residue long sequences of almost identical structure.

VSV enters the cell via invagination into coated vesicles in which its envelope is removed, and from which the nucleocapsid is liberated into the cytoplasm. Removal of the envelope activates the RNA polymerase in the nucleocapsid, which then transcribes the minus-stranded RNA within it into plus-stranded RNA of two types, using two quite different mechanisms. The first consists of the faithful transcription of the minus-strands into plus-strands, which in turn serve as templates for the synthesis of numerous progeny minus-strands. This is the process of minus-strand replication. The second mechanism involves the transcription of the minus-stranded RNA into plus-stranded RNA molecules that can serve as the messenger RNA through which the VSV genome expresses itself. For this purpose a different type of transcript is synthesized. In its simplest terms, this type of transcription process can be visualized as follows. The first gene to be transcribed is

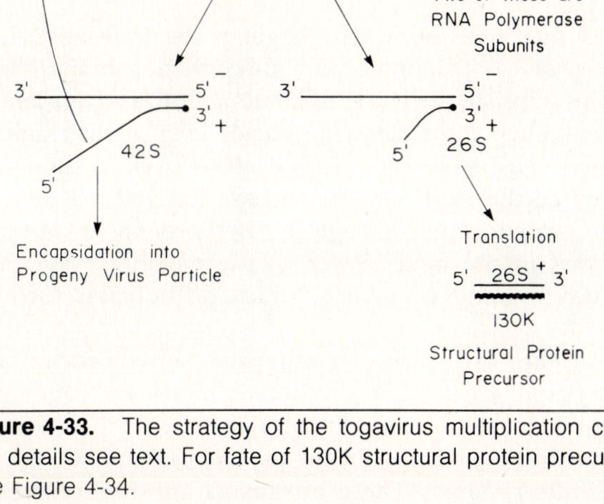

Figure 4-33. The strategy of the togavirus multiplication cycle. For details see text. For fate of 130K structural protein precursor, see Figure 4-34.

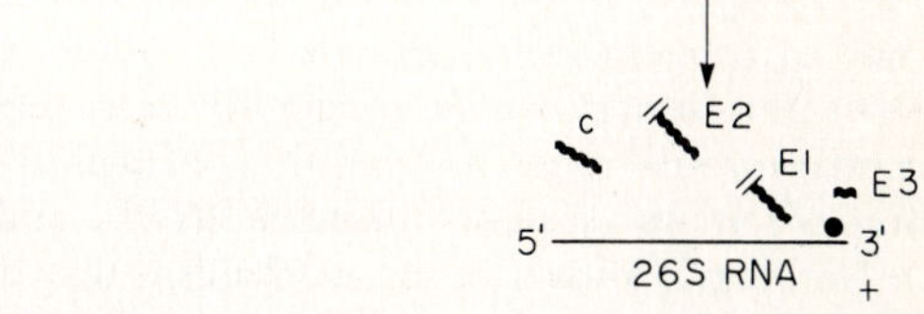

Figure 4-34. The processing of the togavirus 130K structural protein precursor. The precursor only accumulates to a significant extent within cells if its processing is inhibited by protease inhibitors. Under normal conditions, the C or nucleocapsid protein is cleaved off the amino-terminal end of the growing precursor chain, and at the same time the newly generated amino terminus of the E2 precursor (PE2) is inserted into membrane. PE2 is then cleaved off the growing precursor chain, and the amino terminus of E1 is inserted into membrane in similar manner. E3 is cleaved from PE2 during virus maturation. The protease activity is located on the C protein.

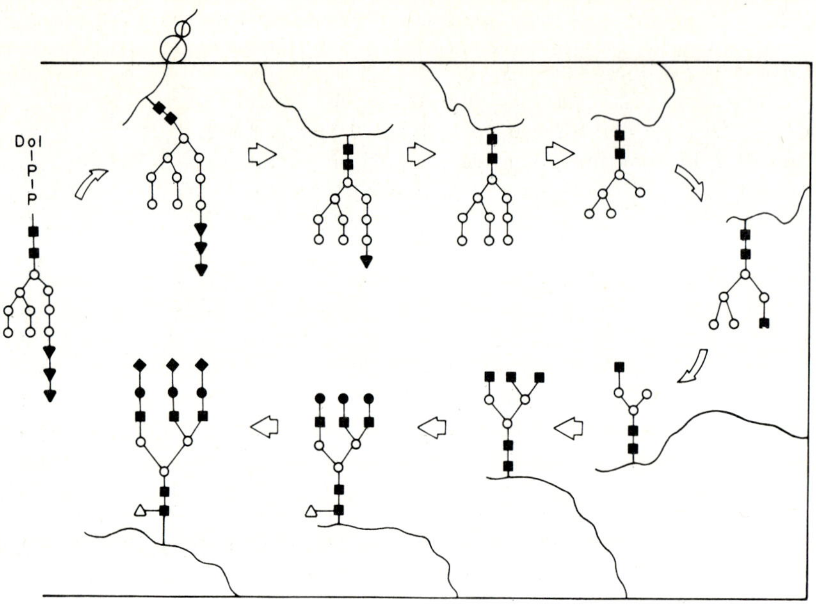

Figure 4-35. Proposed sequence of reactions for the synthesis of the oligosaccharide subunit of the G spike protein of vesicular stomatitis virus. The first step is the transfer of a mannose-rich precursor from dolichol pyrophosphate to an asparagine residue of the G protein; this precursor is then processed to yield the final oligosaccharide unit. Dol, dolichol; ■, N-acetylglucosamine; ○, mannose; ▲, glucose; ●, galactose; ◆, sialic acid (N-acetylglucosamine acid-galactose); △, fucose. *(From Kornfeld et al.: J Biol Chem 253:7771, 1978.)*

the N gene. At the end of its coding region, an intragenic sequence is encountered—the first 11 residues of which act as a polyadenylation signal. Accordingly, about 250 adenine residues are added by a process such as reiterative copying or slippage polymerization. The polymerase then resumes transcription of the next gene, the preceding sequence is cleaved off at the end of the poly (A) sequence, and this process is repeated until messenger RNAs corresponding to all five genes have been synthesized. Interestingly, there is a sixth transcript: the extreme 3′-terminal region of VSV RNA, preceding gene N, is transcribed into a 48-nucleotide long RNA, the so-called leader sequence, which migrates to the nucleus of infected cells where it may help shut down host RNA and DNA synthesis.

Transcription of parental minus strands into plus-stranded RNA molecules is referred to as primary transcription; because the nucleocapsid contains the polymerase, it proceeds without requiring newly synthesized protein. Transcription of plus strands into progeny minus strands, and of progeny minus strands into additional genome-length plus strands or messenger RNAs is referred to as secondary transcription and requires the synthesis of newly synthesized nucleocapsid proteins (N, L, and NS proteins). Nothing is known of the mechanism that determines whether a minus strand is to be transcribed into a genome-length plus strand, or into messenger RNAs.

The five VSV proteins are synthesized in about the same molar ratios as those in which they exist in virus particles; for example, about 30 times as many N as L protein molecules are synthesized. These ratios appear to be controlled at the level of transcription rather than translation. This presents a paradox, for the manner in which VSV RNA is transcribed implies that equal numbers of all five species of messenger RNA molecules should be formed. It seems, however, that there is a polarity effect (attenuation); that is, as the polymerase transcribes the RNA it tends to "fall off," so that the further a gene is situated from the origin of transcription, the less likely it is to be transcribed. Indeed, the gene order 3′-N-NS-M-G-L-5′ in the VSV RNA minus strand parallels the frequency, in a decreasing sense, of the transcription of each gene into messenger RNA.

Like other enveloped viruses, VSV has a special mechanism for being liberated from cells, namely, budding. Enveloped viruses code for two types of structural proteins, nucleocapsid proteins and envelope proteins. The nucleocapsid proteins (the N, NS, and L proteins in the case of VSV) are assembled into nucleocapsids either in the nucleus (in the case of orthomyxoviruses) or in the cytoplasm (in all other enveloped RNA viruses), where they are often found in large numbers. The envelope proteins (the membrane-associated M protein and the G glycoprotein, in the case of VSV) follow a different pathway. The glycoproteins are synthesized on ribosomes that either are attached to membranes, or become attached to membranes very soon after they begin to be translated. Like other proteins that must pass through membranes, viral glycoproteins possess hydrophobic amino acid leader sequences some 15- to 20-amino acids long at their amino-terminal ends, which are cleaved off as soon as they have penetrated the lipid bilayer and have led and fed the rest of the protein chain through it. Glycoproteins are usually anchored in the lipid bilayer of the membrane via their carboxyl-terminus sequences, which do not pass through it.

As they are being synthesized, glycoproteins are glycosylated. Glycosylation proceeds in several stages, the first of which is the transfer of a mannose-rich precursor oligosaccharide from dolichol pryrophosphate to specific asparagine residues. These precursors are then processed to the final prosthetic group in a series of reactions depicted in Figure 4-35. As discussed in Chapter 2, the precise nature of the final oligosaccharide is determined in part by the nature and relative amounts of the various cellular glycosyl transferases, and in part, particularly beyond the mannose fork, by the nature of the protein that is being glycosylated. While glycosylation is proceeding, the glycoproteins are transported through the cell membrane system to patches on the plasma membrane and membranes lining intracytoplasmic vacuoles, where they replace host-specified membrane proteins. Nucleocapsids then migrate to these modified areas, which they recognize with great specificity; align themselves with them; and then bud through them, becoming coated by them in the process (Figs. 4-36 and 4-37). The M protein is incorporated into virus particles immediately prior to budding.

Interestingly, actin-containing microfilaments may play a role in the release of budding viruses, because treatment of cells with cytochalasin B, a drug that disrupts such filaments, inhibits the release of viruses such as measles virus.

Whereas budding is very efficient in some strains of cells, it is very inefficient in others. This sometimes leads to the accumulation in the cytoplasm of very large numbers of nucleocapsids (Fig. 4-38).

The budding process itself does not harm the host cell significantly. Many cells persistently infected with enveloped viruses (see Chap. 5) remain normal in appearance and continue to multiply for many generations while viruses bud from their surfaces. This is not to say that many enveloped viruses are not cytopathic; it merely says that budding per se is not a factor in cytopathogenicity.

Paramyxoviruses

Paramyxovirus RNA (mol wt 5.4×10^6) encodes six proteins, all of which have counterparts among the rhabdovirus structural proteins; there are three nucleocapsid proteins (NP, P, and L), and three envelope proteins (the M [matrix] protein and two glycoproteins, F and HN). Together, these proteins account for most of the coding capacity of the paramyxovirus genome. Their order, from the 3′-terminus of the minus strand, is NP-P-F-M-HN-L.

Paramyxoviruses enter cells by fusing with plasma cell membranes, with resultant liberation of their nucleocapsids into the cytoplasm. The very pronounced ability of the envelopes of these viruses to fuse with cell membranes is a function of one of the two paramyxovirus glycoproteins spikes, namely, that which is made up of the F (fusion) protein (see Chap. 2).

The strategy of the paramyxovirus multiplication cycle resembles that of the rhabdovirus multiplication cycle.

A remarkable feature of the two paramyxovirus glycoproteins, F and HN, which form the two types of spikes on the virus particle surface—the former being responsible for the fusion and hemolytic, and the latter for the hemagglutinin and neuraminidase activities (see Chap. 2)—is that they must be cleaved once, and once only, for virus particles to be infectious. The resultant fragments are not lost, but remain covalently bound via -SS- bonds to the other fragment of each molecule, which is anchored in the lipid bilayer like the VSV G glycoprotein. The cleavage is accomplished by a protease that is present in some cells but not in others, which therefore produce noninfectious virus particles. Cleavage can also be accomplished by certain proteases in vitro, which results in the activation of noninfectious virus particles.

Orthomyxoviruses—Influenza Virus

The influenza viruses are enveloped helical nucleocapsids. Their envelope consists of a lipid bilayer derived from the plasma membrane of the host cell, to which two types of spikes are attached. One is the hemagglutinin spike, of which there are about 350 per virus particle, each composed of a trimer of two -SS-linked proteins, HA1 and HA2, that are formed by cleavage of the hemagglutinin protein. Both are glycosylated, and HA2 is also esterified with fatty acid in a hydrophobic region at its carboxyl terminus, which is anchored in the lipid bilayer of the envelope, with about 10 amino acids penetrating into the interior of the virus particle.

The second type of spike is the neuraminidase. There are about 50 of these per virus particle, each made up of a tetramer of the neuraminidase protein, which is also glycosylated and may also be acylated. It is anchored in the lipid bilayer not by its carboxyl terminus, but by its amino terminus.

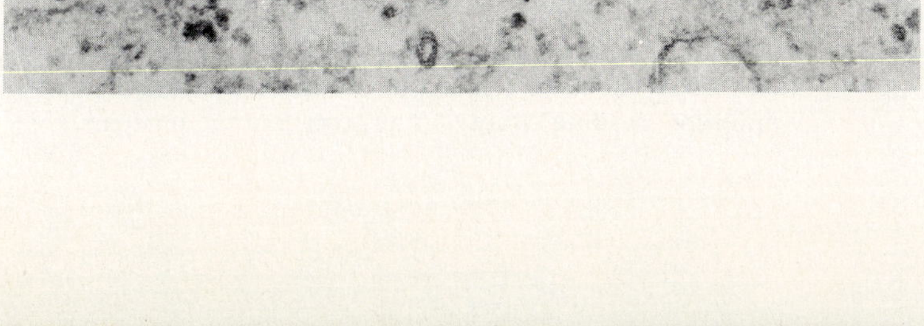

Figure 4-36. Modification of the plasma membrane of a monkey kidney cell infected with SV5. A layer of dense material resembling the spikes present on viral envelopes is present on the outer surface of the membrane. Nucleocapsid strands, many seen in cross-section, are aligned immediately beneath modified patches of the cell membrane. In due course they will bud through these membrane patches, becoming enveloped by them in the process. × 76,000. *(From Compans et al.: Virology 30:411, 1966.)*

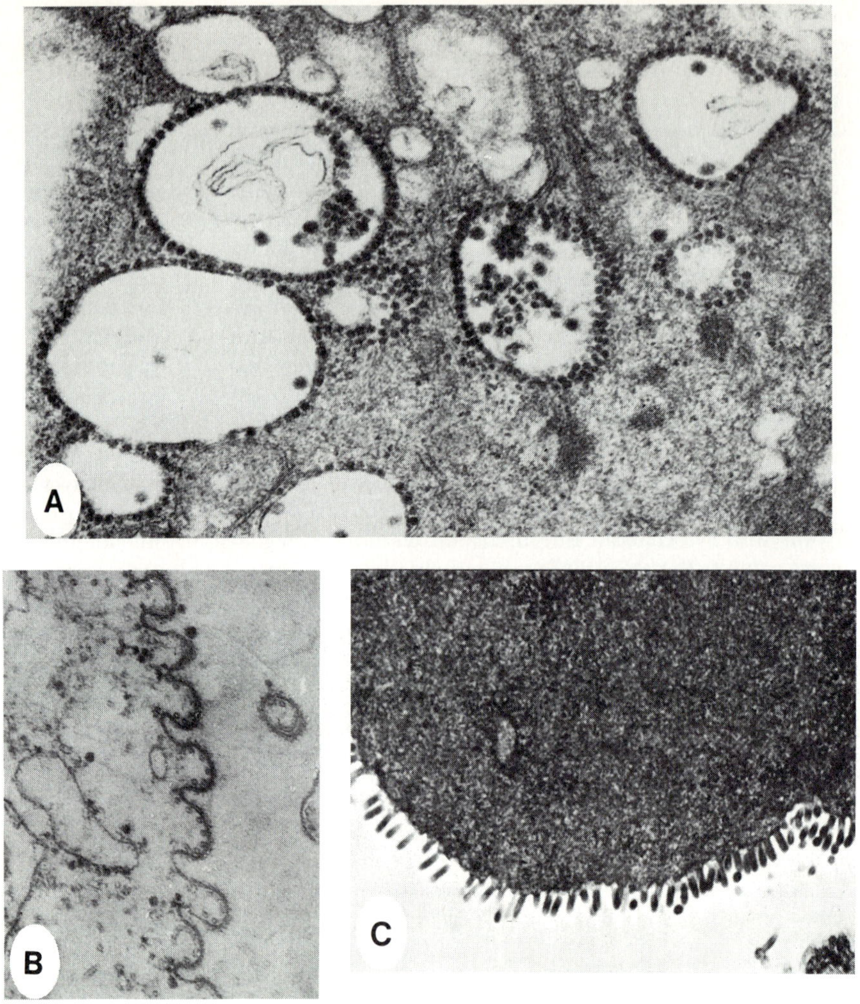

Figure 4-37. Budding of enveloped viruses. **A.** A chick embryo cell infected with the togavirus Semliki Forest virus (SFV). Numerous nucleocapsids lining cytoplasmic vacuoles prior to budding into them can be seen. × 22,000. **B.** A row of SV5 particles budding from the plasma membrane of a monkey kidney cell, showing many cross-sections of nucleocapsids. × 50,000. **C.** Vesicular stomatitis virus (VSV) budding from the plasma membrane of a mouse L cell. In L cells, the majority of VSV particles bud from the plasma membrane; in other cells, such as chick embryo fibroblasts and pig kidney cells, VSV buds mostly into cytoplasmic vacuoles. × 21,500. *(**A,** from Grimley et al.: J Virol 2: 1326, 1968; **B,** from Compans et al.: Virology 30:411, 1966; **C,** from Zee et al.: J Gen Virol 7:95, 1970.)*

Within the lipid envelope lies the M (matrix) protein, and within the matrix shell are eight negative-stranded RNA molecules, the influenza virus genes, associated in helical nucleocapsid structure with the NP (nucleocapsid) protein, and several molecules of three large proteins, namely P1, P2, and P3. The RNA accounts for about 2.5 percent of the virus particle mass.

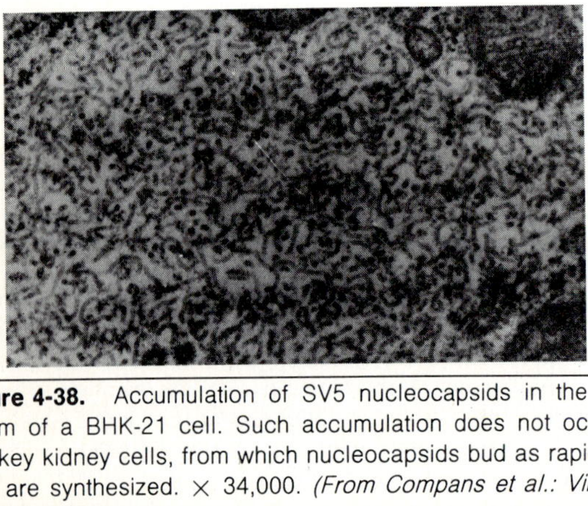

Figure 4-38. Accumulation of SV5 nucleocapsids in the cytoplasm of a BHK-21 cell. Such accumulation does not occur in monkey kidney cells, from which nucleocapsids bud as rapidly as they are synthesized. × 34,000. *(From Compans et al.: Virology 30:411, 1966.)*

Table 4-5 summarizes current information concerning the eight genes of influenza virus and the proteins encoded by them, and Figure 4-39 shows electropherograms of the proteins encoded by the genes of two influenza virus A strains. The three large proteins are present in few copy numbers only and appear to function in RNA transcription and replication: P1 and P3 initiate transcription and elongation, respectively, whereas P2 appears to be the cap-binding protein that causes short capped 5′-terminal sequences from host cell messenger RNA molecules to be used as primers to initiate the transcription of influenza virus genes into messenger RNAs (see below).

The two smallest genes are fascinating. Each codes not for one protein, but for two—each encodes a major protein in about three quarters of its sequences, and a smaller one in about one third. These smaller proteins are encoded by messenger RNAs that are either spliced or the transcription of which is initiated at an internal site, and whose coding sequences overlap those of the messenger RNA of the major proteins, but are read in a different reading frame. The two minor proteins, M2

TABLE 4-5. THE EIGHT INFLUENZA VIRUS GENES AND THE PROTEINS THEY ENCODE

	Size of Gene						
Gene	Mol Wt	No. of Nucleotides	Protein	Size of Protein Mol Wt	Approx. No. of Protein Molecules per Virus Particle	Approx. Percent of Virus Particle Protein	Function of Protein
1	750,000	2341	P1	96,000	16	1	Initiation of transcription
2	730,000	2300	P2	87,000	16	1	Cap-binding protein
3	715,000	2233	P3	85,000	16	1	Elongation of transcription
4	565,000	1765	HA → HA1	36,000	750	25	Hemagglutinin spike. The size of the carbohydrate groups on HA1 and HA2 are 11,500 and 1400 daltons, respectively
			HA → HA2	27,000	750		
5	500,000	1565	NP	56,000	1000	30	Structural protein of helical nucleocapsid
6	450,000	1413	NA	50,000	160	4	Neuraminidase
7	330,000	1027	M1	27,000	3000	38	Matrix protein
			M2	11,000	0		Nonstructural protein of unknown function
8	285,000	890	NS1	26,000	0		Nonstructural protein of unknown function
			NS2	12,000	0		Nonstructural protein of unknown function

and NS2, are both nonstructural proteins of unknown function.

Influenza viruses are classified into three types, A, B, and C, on the basis of their antigenic properties. Protein NP and M possess antigenic determinants common to all strains of influenza virus. Type A influenza virus strains are subdivided into subtypes based on the antigenic characteristics of their surface antigens, namely, the hemagglutinin and the neuraminidase, each of which possesses four major antigenic determinants. Thirteen distinct hemagglutinin subtypes and nine neuraminidase subtypes are currently recognized. Human influenza A strains contain hemagglutinins of three subtypes (H1, H2, or H3), and neuraminidases of two subtypes (N1 and N2); the other hemagglutinin and neuraminidase subtypes are present in influenza virus strains of other animal species (horses, swine, birds, etc.). The nature of the extensive antigenic variations of influenza virus that cause the emergence of the virus strains responsible for successive pandemics is discussed in Chapter 6.

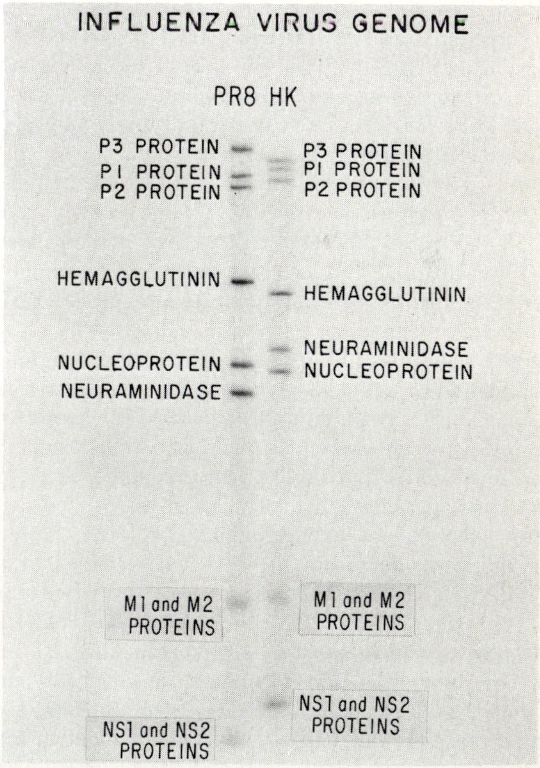

Figure 4-39. Electropherogram of a polyacrylamide gel of the eight negative-stranded genes of influenza A (strains PR8 and HK), together with the proteins that they encode. Proteins P1, P2, and P3 function in RNA replication and transcription; the nucleoprotein NP is the nucleocapsid protein; the M1 protein is associated with the internal side of the envelope membrane; the hemagglutinin (HA) and neuraminidase (NA) are the two spike glycoproteins; and MS2, NS1, and NS2 are nonstructural proteins of unknown function. *(From Ritchey et al.: J Virol 20:307, 1976.)*

Influenza Virus Multiplication Cycle

Influenza virus probably enters cells via coated vesicles. It has recently been found that the hemagglutinin possesses cell membrane-fusing activity, and this activity may also play a role in influenza virus penetration and uptake. The liberated nucleocapsids do not remain in the cytoplasm, but migrate to the nucleus, where they are transcribed and replicate. The overall strategy of the influenza virus multiplication cycle resembles that of rhabdoviruses and paramyxoviruses, with primary transcription catalyzed by parental nucleocapsids leading to the formation of plus-stranded templates for the transcription of progeny minus strands, followed by secondary transcription of both plus and minus strands catalyzed by newly synthesized polymerase. A remarkable feature of influenza virus RNA transcription is that it is primer dependent; and the primers that are used are 10- to 15-residues long, capped oligonucleotides from the 5′-ends of host transcripts. Apparently these 5′-terminus sequences are recognized by P2, cleaved by a virus-encoded endonuclease, and then transcription of influenza virus RNA is initiated on them. As a result, all influenza transcripts possess a heterogeneous assortment of host-derived sequences at their 5′-end. These transcripts are of two types. First, there are the messenger RNAs. These are incomplete transcripts because transcription of them stops about 40-nucleotide residues before the polymerase reaches the 5′-ends of the minus-strand templates being transcribed. All messenger RNA species are polyadenylated at their 3′-termini. The second type of transcripts, formed mostly during the later stages of the multiplication cycle, are faithful plus-stranded nonpolyadenylated copies of the negative-stranded genes. They, in turn, serve as the templates for the synthesis of progeny minus strands.

The morphogenesis of influenza virus proceeds as described above for VSV, but there are some unique features. The first is that in order for influenza progeny virus to be infectious, its hemagglutinin must be cleaved three times. The hemagglutinin of one typical strain is synthesized in the cytoplasm as one polypeptide chain, 566-amino acids long. It is processed as a glycoprotein and passes through the plasma cell membrane by virtue of the presence of a 16-amino acid long hydrophobic leader sequence at its amino terminus, which is cleaved off by a cellular protease on the outer cell surface. The protein remains anchored to the lipid bilayer by virtue of a hydrophobic region at its carboxyl terminus end. As in many other viral glycoproteins, such as paramyxovirus, rhabdovirus, togavirus, and coronavirus glycoproteins, the carboxyl terminus is esterified with fatty acid. At about the time when influenza virus nucleocapsids bud through what has by now become the viral envelope, the hemagglutinin protein is cleaved by a cellular trypsin-like protease, and a virus-associated carboxypeptidase B (either loosely associated or an intrinsic activity of the hemagglutinin/HA1/HA2) removes one arginine residue from the carboxyl terminus of the distal (HA1) fragment. The result is that the hemagglutinin is converted to HA1 (328 amino acids) plus HA2 (221 amino acids), which remain linked covalently by -SS-bonds. In some cells, the protease is inactive and virus with uncleaved hemagglutinin is released. Such virus is noninfectious, but can be activated by treatment in vitro with trypsin, the arginine being removed immediately thereafter by an enzyme activity intrinsic to the virus.

A second unique feature concerns the function of the influenza virus neuraminidase. It seems that the primary function of this enzyme is to remove neuraminic acid from the oligosaccharide moieties of the hemagglutinin protein. If this function is prevented (either by the addition of inhibitors or by the use of appropriate mutants), the neuraminic acid-containing hemagglutinin serves as the receptor for virus about to bud from the cell surface, with resultant inhibition of virus liberation. It is also known that hemagglutinin cannot be cleaved to HA1 plus HA2, unless neuraminic acid is first removed from its obligosaccharides.

FURTHER READING

Books and Reviews

GENERAL

Dimmock NJ: Initial stages in infection with animal viruses. J Gen Virol 59:1, 1982

Simons K, Garoff H: The budding mechanisms of enveloped animal viruses. J Gen Virol 50:1, 1980

Lenard J, Miller DK: Uncoating of enveloped viruses. Cell 28:5, 1983

Doerfler W: DNA methylation—A regulatory signal in eukaryotic gene expression. J Gen Virol 57:1, 1981

Shatkin AJ (ed): Initiation signals in viral gene expression. Curr Top Microbiol Immunol 93, 1981

Broker TR: Animal virus RNA processing. In Apirion D (ed): RNA Processing. Boca Raton, Fla, CRC Press, 1983

Challberg MD, Kelly TJ: Eukaryotic DNA replication: Viral and plasmid model systems. Ann Rev Biochem 51:901, 1982

Klenk H, Rott R: Cotranslational and posttranslational processing of viral glycoproteins. Curr Top Microbiol Immunol 90:19, 1980

Simons K, Garoff H, Helenius A: How an animal virus gets into and out of its host cell. Sci Am 246/2:58, 1982

Ward DC, Tattersall P (eds): Replication of Mammalian Parvoviruses. New York, Cold Spring Harbor Laboratory, 1978

Becht H: Infectious bursal disease virus. Curr Top Microbiol Immunol 90:107, 1980

Mahy BWJ, Barry RD (eds): Negative Strand Viruses and the Host Cell. London, Academic Press, 1978

Pedersen IR: Structural components and replication of arenaviruses. Adv Virus Res 24:277, 1979

Howard CR, Simpson DIH: The biology of the arenaviruses. J Gen Virol 51:1, 1980

Siddell S, Wege H, ter Meulen V: The biology of coronaviruses. J Gen Virol 64:761, 1983

Siddell S, Wege H, ter Meulen V: The structure and replication of coronaviruses. Curr Top Microbiol Immunol 100:131, 1982

PAPOVAVIRUSES

Cremisi C: Chromatin replication revealed by studies of animal cells and papovaviruses (simian virus 40 and polyoma virus). Microbiol Rev 43:297, 1979

Elder JT, Spritz RA, Weissman SM: Simian virus 40 as a eukaryotic cloning vehicle. Annu Rev Genet 15:295, 1981

Ziff EB: Transcription and RNA processing by the DNA tumor viruses. Nature 287:491, 1980

ADENOVIRUSES

Logan JS, Shenk T: Transcriptional and translational control of adenovirus gene expression. Microbiol Rev 46:377, 1982

Nevins JR: Adenovirus gene expression: Control at multiple steps in RNA biogenesis. Cell 28:1, 1982

Nevins JR, Chen-Kiang S: Processing of adenovirus nuclear RNA to mRNA. Adv Virus Res 26:1, 1981

Persson H, Philipson L: Regulation of adenovirus gene expression. Curr Top Microbiol Immunol 97:157, 1982

HERPESVIRUSES

Roizman B: The structure and isomerization of herpes simplex virus genomes. Cell 16:481, 1979

Ben-Porat T: Replication of herpesvirus DNA. Curr Top Microbiol Immunol 91:81, 1981

POXVIRUSES

Moss B: Poxviruses. In Nayak DP (ed): The Molecular Biology of Animal Viruses, New York, Marcel Dekker, 1978, vol 2, p 849

Holowczak JA: Poxvirus DNA. Curr Top Microbiol Immunol 97:27, 1982

REOVIRUSES

Joklik WK: Structure and function of the reovirus genome. Microbiol Rev 45:483, 1981

PICORNAVIRUSES

Crowell RL, Landau DJ: Receptors in the initiation of picornavirus infections. In Fraenkel-Conrat H, Wagner RR (eds): Comprehensive Virology. New York, Plenum, vol 18, p 1

Sangar DV: The replication of picornaviruses. J Gen Virol 45:1, 1979

Putnak RJ, Phillips BA: Picornaviral structure and assembly. Microbiol Rev 45:287, 1981

MacNaughton MR: The structure and replication of rhinoviruses. Curr Top Microbiol Immunol 97:1, 1982

TOGAVIRUSES

Kaariainen L, Soderlund H: Structure and replication of alphaviruses. Curr Top Microbiol Immunol 82:15, 1978

Garoff H, Kondor-Koch C, Riedel H: Structure and assembly of alphaviruses. Curr Top Microbiol Immunol 100:1, 1982

Schlesinger RW (ed): The Togaviruses: Biology, Structure, and Replication. New York, Academic Press, 1980

BUNYAVIRUSES

Bishop DHL: Genetic potential of bunyaviruses. Curr Top Microbiol Immunol 86:1, 1979

RHABDOVIRUSES

Bishop DHL (ed): The Rhabdoviruses. Boca Raton, Fla, CRC Press, 1979

PARAMYXOVIRUSES

Morgan EM, Rapp F: Measles virus and its associated diseases. Bacteriol Rev 41:636, 1977

Wechler SL, Meissner HC: Measles and SSPE viruses: Similarities and differences. Prog Med Virol 28:65, 1982

MYXOVIRUSES

Choppin PW, Richardson CD, Merz DC, et al.: The functions and inhibition of the membrane glycoproteins of paramyxoviruses and myxoviruses and the role of the measles virus M protein in subacute sclerosing parencephalitis. J Infect Dis 143:352, 1981

Hinshaw VS, Webster RG, Rodriguez RJ: Influenza A viruses: Combinations of hemagglutinin and neuraminidase subtypes isolated from animals and other sources. Arch Virol 67:191, 1981

Lamb RA, Choppin PW: The gene structure and replication of influenza viruses. Ann Rev Biochem 52:467, 1983

Skehel JJ, Hay AJ: Influenza virus transcription. J Gen Virol 39:1, 1978

Ward CW: Structure of the influenza virus hemagglutinin. Curr Top Microbiol Immunol 94/95:1, 1981

Selected papers

PAPOVAVIRUSES

Reddy VB, Thimmappaya B, Dhar R, et al.: The genome of Simian virus 40. Science 200:494, 1978

Wasylyk B, Wasylyk C, Augereau P, et al.: The SV40 72bp repeat preferentially potentiates transcription starting from proximal natural or substitute promoter elements. Cell 32:503, 1983

Laimonis LA, Khoury G, Gorman C, et al.: Host specific activation of transcription by tandem repeats from simian virus 40 and Moloney sarcoma virus. Proc Natl Acad Sci USA 79:6453, 1982

Frisque RJ: Nucleotide sequence of the region encompassing the JCV origin of DNA replication. J Virol 46:170, 1983

ADENOVIRUSES

Chow LT, Gelinas RE, Broker TR, et al.: An amazing sequence arrangement at the 5′ ends of adenovirus 2 messenger RNAs. Cell 12:1, 1977

Chow LT, Lewis JE, Broker TR: RNA transcription and splicing at early and intermediate times after adenovirus-2 infection. Cold Spring Harbor Symp Quant Biol 44:401, 1980

Nevins JR, Darnell JE Jr: Steps in the processing of ad2 mRNA: poly $(A)^+$ nuclear sequences are conserved and poly (A) addition precedes splicing. Cell 15:1477, 1978

Wilson MC, Fraser NW, Darnell JE: Mapping of RNA initiation sites by high doses of UV irradiation: Evidence for three independent promoters within the left 11% of the Ad-2 genome. Virology 94:175, 1979

Shaw AR, Ziff EB: Transcripts from the adenovirus-2 major late promoter yield a single early family of 3′ coterminal mRNAs and five late families. Cell 22:905, 1980

Stillman BW, Lewis JB, Chow LT, et al.: Identification of the gene and mRNA for the adenovirus terminal protein precursor. Cell 23:497, 1981

Friefeld BR, Lichy JH, Hurwitz J, et al.: Evidence for an altered adenovirus DNA polymerase in cells infected with the mutant H5ts149. Proc Natl Acad Sci USA 80:1589, 1983

Challberg MD, Desiderio SV, Kelly TJ Jr: Adenovirus DNA replication in vitro: Characterization of a protein covalently linked to nascent DNA strands. Proc Natl Acad Sci USA 77:5105, 1980

Cepko CL, Sharp PA: Assembly of adenovirus major capsid protein is mediated by a nonviron protein. Cell 31:407, 1982

HERPESVIRUSES

Parris DS, Dixon RAF, Schaffer PA: Physical mapping of herpes simplex virus type 1 ts mutants by marker rescue: Correlation of the physical and genetic maps. Virology 100:275, 1980

DeLuca N, Zik DJ, Bond VC, et al.: Nucleotide sequences of herpes simplex virus 1 (HSV-1) affecting virus entry, cell fusion, and production of glycoprotein gB (VP7). Virology 122:411, 1982

Honess RW, Roizman B: Regulation of herpesvirus macromolecular synthesis: Sequential transition of polypeptide synthesis requires functional viral polypeptides. Proc Natl Acad Sci USA 72:1276, 1975

Mackem S, Roizman B: Differentiation between α promoter and regulator regions of herpes simplex virus 1: The functional domains and sequence of a movable α regulator. Proc Natl Acad Sci USA 79:4917, 1982

Poffenberger KL, Tabares E, Roizman B: Characterization of a viable, noninverting herpes simplex virus 1 genome derived by insertion and deletion of sequences at the junction of components L and S. Proc Natl Acad Sci USA 80:2690, 1983

Post LE, Norrild B, Simpson T, et al.: Chicken ovalbumin gene fused to a herpes simplex virus α promoter and linked to a thymidine kinase gene is regulated like a viral gene. Mol Cell Biol 2:233, 1982

Lee GT-Y, Para MF, Spear PG: Location of the structural genes for glycoproteins gD and gE and for other polypeptides in the S component of herpes simplex virus type 1 DNA. J Virol 43:41, 1982

Stringer JR, Holland LE, Wagner EK: Mapping early transcripts of herpes simplex virus type 1 by electron microscopy. J Virol 27:56, 1978

Mocarski ES, Roizman B: Structure and role of the herpes simplex virus DNA termini in inversion, circularization and generation of virion DNA. Cell 31:89, 1982

POXVIRUSES

Ichihashi Y, Oie M: Proteolytic activation of vaccinia virus for the penetrationphase of infection. Virology 116:297, 1982

Oda K, Joklik WK: Hybridization and sedimentation studies on "early" and "late" vaccinia messenger RNA. J Mol Biol 27:395, 1967

Cooper JA, Moss B: In vitro translation of immediate early, early, and late classes of RNA from vaccinia virus-infected cells. Virology 96:368, 1979

Isle HB, Venkatesan S, Moss B: Cell-free translation of early and late mRNAs selected by hybridization to cloned DNA fragments derived from the left 14 million to 72 million daltons of the vaccinia virus genome. Virology 112:306, 1981

Weir JP, Moss B: Nucleotide sequence of the vaccinia virus thymidine kinase gene and the nature of spontaneous frameshift mutations. J Virol 46:530, 1983

Hiller G, Weber K, Schneider L, et al.: Interaction of assembled progeny pox viruses with the cellular cytoskeleton. Virology 98:142, 1979

Krempien U, Schneider L, Hiller G, et al.: Conditions for pox virus-specific microvilli formation studied during synchronized virus assembly. Virology 113:556, 1981

REOVIRUSES

Schonberg M, Silverstein SC, Levin DH, et al.: Asynchronous synthesis of the complementary strands of the reovirus genome. Proc Natl Acad Sci USA 68:505, 1971

Silverstein SC, Schonberg M, Levin DH, et al.: The reovirus replicative cycle: Conservation of parental RNA and protein. Proc Natl Acad Sci USA 67:275, 1970

Zweerink HJ, McDowell MJ, Joklik WK: Essential and nonessential noncapsid reovirus proteins. Virology 45:716, 1971

McCrae MA, Joklik WK: The nature of the polypeptide encoded by each of the ten double-stranded RNA segments of reovirus type 3. Virology 89:578, 1978

Huismans H, Joklik WK: Reovirus-coded polypeptides in infected cells: Isolation of two native monomeric polypeptides with affinity for single-stranded and double-stranded RNA, respectively. Virology 70:411, 1976

Antczak JB, Chmelo R, Pickup DJ, et al.: Sequences at both termini of the 10 genes of reovirus serotype 3 (strain Dearing). Virology 121:307, 1982

Cashdollar LW, Esparza J, Hudson GR, et al.: Cloning the double-stranded RNA genes of reovirus: Sequence of the cloned S2 gene. Proc Natl Acad Sci USA 79:7644, 1982

Lee PWK, Hayes EC, Joklik WK: Characterization of anti-reovirus immunoglobulins secreted by cloned hybridoma cell lines. Virology 108:134, 1981

PICORNAVIRUSES

Nomoto A, Omata T, Toyoda H, et al.: Complete nucleotide sequence of the attenuated poliovirus Sabin 1 strain genome. Proc Natl Acad Sci USA 79:5793, 1982

Adler CJ, Elzinga M, Wimmer E: The genome-linked protein of picornaviruses. VIII. Complete amino acid sequence of poliovirus VPg and carboxy-terminal analysis of its precursor, P3-9. J Gen Virol 64:349, 1983

Summers DF, Maizel JV, Darnell JE: Evidence for virus-specific noncapsid proteins in poliovirus-infected HeLa cells. Proc Natl Acad Sci USA 56:505, 1965

Larsen GR, Anderson CW, Dorner AJ, et al.: Cleavage sites within the poliovirus capsid protein precursors. J Virol 41:340, 1982

Korant B, Chow N, Lively M, et al.: Virus specified protease in poliovirus infected HeLa cells. Proc Natl Acad Sci USA 76:2992, 1979

Palmenberg AC, Rueckert RR: Evidence for intramolecular self-cleavage of picornaviral replicase precursors. J Virol 41:244, 1982

Dasgupta A, Baron MH, Baltimore D: Poliovirus replicase: A soluble enzyme able to initiate copying of poliovirus RNA. Proc Natl Acad Sci USA 76:2679, 1979

TOGAVIRUSES

Garoff H, Frischauf A-M, Simons K, et al.: Nucleotide sequence of cDNA coding for Semliki Forest virus membrane glycoproteins. Nature 288:236, 1980

Rice CM, Strauss JH: Nucleotide sequence of the 26 S mRNA of Sindbis virus and deduced sequence of the encoded virus structural proteins. Proc Natl Acad Sci USA 78:2062, 1981

Fuller FJ, Marcus PI: Sindbis virus. 1. Gene order of translation in vivo. Virology 107:441, 1980

Huggins JW, Jahrling PB, Rill W, Linden CD: Characterization of the binding of the TC-83 strain of Venezuelan equine encephalitis virus to BW-J-M, a mouse macrophage-like cell line. J Gen Virol 64:149, 1983

RHABDOVIRUSES

Schlegel R, Tralka TS, Willingham ME, et al.: Inhibition of VSV binding and infectivity by phosphatidylserine: Is phosphatidylserine a VSV-binding site? Cell 32:639, 1983

Ball LA, White CN: Order of transcription of genes of vesicular stomatitis virus. Proc Natl Acad Sci USA 73:442, 1976

Emerson SU: Reconstitution studies detect a single polymerase entry site on the vesicular stomatitis virus genome. Cell 31:635, 1982

Herman RC, Schubert M, Keene JD, et al.: Polycistronic vesicular stomatitis virus RNA transcripts. Proc Natl Acad Sci USA 77:4662, 1980

Schubert M, Keene JD, Herman RC, et al.: Site on the vesicular stomatitis virus genome specifying polyadenylation and the end of the L gene mRNA. J Virol 34:550, 1980

Keene JD, Schubert M, Lazzarini RA: Intervening sequence between the leader region and the nucleocapsid gene of vesicular stomatitis virus RNA. J Virol 33:789, 1980

Villarreal LP, Breindl M, Holland JJ: Determination of molar ratios of vesicular stomatitis virus-induced RNA species in BHK_{21} cells. Biochemistry 15:1663, 1976

Toneguzzo F, Ghosh HP: In vitro synthesis of vesicular stomatitis virus membrane glycoprotein and insertion into membranes. Proc Natl Acad Sci USA 75:715, 1978

Jacobs BL, Penhoet EE: Assembly of vesicular stomatitis virus: Distribution of the glycoprotein on the surface of infected cells. J Virol 44:1047, 1982

Rose JK, Welch WJ, Sefton BM, et al.: Vesicular stomatitis virus glycoprotein is anchored in the viral membrane by a hydrophobic domain near the COOH terminus. Proc Natl Acad Sci USA 77:3884, 1980

Schlesinger MJ, Malfer C: Cerulenin blocks fatty acid acylation of glycoproteins and inhibits vesicular stomatitis and Sindbis virus particle formation. J Biol Chem 257:9887, 1982

Birdwell CR, Strauss JH: Maturation of vesicular stomatitis virus: Electron microscopy of surface replicas of infected cells. Virology 59:587, 1974

Zee YC, Hackett AJ, Talens L: Vesicular stomatitis virus maturation sites in six different host cells. J Gen Virol 7:95, 1970

PARAMYXOVIRUSES

Markwell MA, Svennerholm L, Paulson JC: Specific gangliosides function as host cell receptors for Sendai virus. Proc Natl Acad Sci USA 78:5406, 1981

Peeples M, Levine S: Respiratory syncytial virus polypeptides: Their location in the virion. Virology 95:137, 1979

Collins PL, Hightower LE, Ball LA: Transcriptional map for Newcastle disease virus. J Virol 35:682, 1980

Glazier K, Raghow R, Kingsbury DW: Regulation of Sendai virus transcription: Evidence for a single promoter in vivo. J Virol 21:863, 1977

Huang YT, Wertz GW: Respiratory syncytial virus mRNA coding assignments. J Virol 46:667, 1983

Stallcup KC, Raine CS, Fields BN: Cytochalasin B inhibits maturation of measles virus. Virology 124:59, 1983

MYXOVIRUSES

Jones KL, Huddlestone JA, Brownlee GG: The sequence of RNA segment 1 of influenza virus A/NT/60/68 and its comparison with the corresponding segment of strains A/PR/8/34 and A/WSN/33. Nucleic Acids Res 11:1555, 1983

Mowshowitz SL: P1 is required for initiation of cRNA synthesis in WSN influenza virus. Virology 91:493, 1978

Blaas D, Patzelt E, Kuechler E: Cap-recognizing protein of influenza virus. Virology 116:339, 1982

Kaptein N, Nayak DP: Complete nucleotide sequence of the polymerase 3 gene of human influenza virus A/WSN/33. J Virol 42:55, 1982

Palese P, Ritchey MB, Schulman JL: P1 and P3 proteins of influenza virus are required for complementary RNA synthesis. J Virol 21:1187, 1977

Allen H, McCauley J, Waterfield M, et al.: Influenza virus RNA segment 7 has the coding capacity for two polypeptides. Virology 107:548, 1980

Briedis DJ, Lamb RA, Choppin, PW: Influenza B virus RNA segment 8 codes for two nonstructural proteins. Virology 112:417, 1981

Bouloy M, Plotch SJ, Krug RM: Globin mRNAs are primers for the transcription of influenza viral RNA in vitro. Proc Natl Acad Sci USA 75:4886, 1978

Garten W, Bosch FX, Linder D, et al.: Proteolytic activation of the influenza virus hemagglutinin: The structure of the cleavage site and the enzymes involved in cleavage. Virology 115:361, 1981

Varghese JN, Laver WG, Colman PM: Structure of the influenza virus glycoprotein antigen neuraminidase at 2.9 Å resolution. Nature 303:35, 1983

CORONAVIRUSES

Lai MMC, Brayton PR, Armen RC, et al.: Mouse hepatitis virus A59: Messenger RNA structure and genetic localization of the sequence divergence from hepatotropic strain MHV-3. J Virol 39:823, 1981

Siddell S: Coronavirus JHM: Coding assignments of subgenomic mRNAs. J Gen Virol 64:113, 1983

GENERAL

Darnell JE Jr: Implications of RNA : RNA splicing in evolution of eukaryotic cells. Science 202:1257, 1978

Fan DP, Sefton BM: The entry into host cells of Sindbis virus, vesicular stomatitis virus and Sendai virus. Cell 15:985, 1978

Schmidt MFG: Acylation of viral spike glycoproteins: A feature of enveloped RNA viruses. Virology 116:327, 1982

CHAPTER 5

The Effect of Virus Infection on the Host Cell

The effect of virus infection on host cells is far more difficult to study in molecular terms than the process of virus multiplication. Study of the multiplication process requires merely the ability to recognize and measure virus-specified macromolecules; study of the effect on host cells requires a detailed knowledge of the functioning of the normal host cell. In fact, studies that have focused attention on the effect of virus infection on host cells have broadened our knowledge of the functioning of uninfected cells, and the acquisition of such knowledge has been one of the important spinoffs of the study of virus–cell interactions.

Whatever the reason that lytic viruses destroy their host cells, several causes can be ruled out. One is that virus synthesis creates an excessive demand for protein and nucleic acid precursors, so that competition causes a shortage of building blocks that prevents synthesis of host cell macromolecules. This is unlikely, since the amount of viral material that is synthesized rarely exceeds 10 percent of total host cell material. Considerations of this nature also rule out the necessity for breakdown of host cell material in order to provide precursors for the synthesis of viral macromolecules.

Since both nucleic acid and protein synthesis are absolutely dependent on the supply of energy, the largest virus yields would be expected in cells that are damaged least for the longest periods of time. Many highly lytic viruses are, however, very successful. This is primarily because they take over the host cell's synthetic apparatus very rapidly and multiply extensively in the brief period of time for which the apparatus can function.

Cytopathic Effects

The most easily detected effects of infection with lytic viruses are the cytopathic effects, which can be observed both macroscopically and microscopically. Plaque formation is due to the cytopathic effect of viruses; viruses kill the cells in which they multiply, and plaques are the areas of killed cells. The light microscope, as well as the electron microscope, often reveals changes in a variety of cell organelles soon after infection. Frequently the nucleus is affected first, with pyknosis, changes in nucleolar structure, and margination of the chromatin. Changes in the cell membrane usually follow; cells gradually lose their ability to adhere to supporting surfaces and therefore round up and sometimes develop a strong tendency to fuse with one another (see below). This is then often followed by the appearance, either in the nucleus or in the cytoplasm, of distinct spreading foci that are generally composed of fibrillar material. These are the classic inclusion bodies that have long been described by cytologists, and they represent the sites of virus-directed biosynthesis and morphogenesis. Finally, at about the time when structural viral protein synthesis proceeds at its maximum rate, necrotic and grossly degradative changes become noticeable. They may be attributed to at least three causes. First, by this time interference with host cell macromolecular biosynthesis is generally complete (see below). It is known that all host cell macromolecules turn over to a greater or lesser extent—that is, they are continually broken down and resynthesized by a mechanism that operates no matter whether the cells grow or not. Inhibition of resynthesis in the presence of continuing breakdown could clearly lead to structural and functional failure. Second, plasma membrane function declines, probably because host protein and lipid synthesis ceases and because patches of host membrane protein are replaced by virus-coded ones. Certainly, permeability increases soon after infection, and before long loss of plasma membrane function results in failure to maintain the proper intracellular ionic environment and in diminished transport of essential nutrients into the cell and of waste products out of it. Third, the membranes lining lysosomes also begin to fail, and as a result the degradative hydrolytic enzymes that they contain begin to leak out into the cytoplasm, thereby exacerbating the effects caused by the other mechanisms.

The net result of cell necrosis is the release of those viruses that do not bud from the cell membrane. In general, the smaller the virus, the more readily it is released. Large viruses, such as poxviruses, are often retained in the ghosts of infected cells for considerable periods of time. In the body, the situation may be different, for damaged cells may become phagocytized, thereby providing an additional mechanism for the dissemination of viral progeny.

Whereas the reasons for the necrotic and degradative changes that occur during the late phases of the virus multiplication cycle are reasonably well understood, it is not as obvious why some viruses cause cytopathic effects soon after infection. For some viruses, it is likely that early cytopathic effects are caused by early viral proteins—that is, proteins that are synthesized after infection; for others, it seems that such effects are caused by components of the invading virus particles. It is interesting in this regard that the adenovirus fiber is known to be cytotoxic, that the surface tubule protein of vaccinia virus inhibits protein synthesis, and that the vesicular stomatis virus (VSV) glycoprotein inhibits cellular DNA and RNA synthesis. On the other hand, it is also known that empty reovirus particles—that is, particles that contain no RNA—cause no cytopathic effects, even at very high multiplicities.

Inhibition of Host Macromolecular Biosynthesis

The induction of cytopathic effects early after infection may be intimately related to the more or less rapidly developing inhibition of host protein, DNA and RNA synthesis, which is a fundamentally important factor in the lytic virus–cell interaction.

Host protein synthesis is inhibited first. This effect is often missed if only the overall rate of protein synthesis is measured, since viral protein synthesis generally takes over as host protein synthesis declines. Inhibition of host protein synthesis then quickly causes inhibition of host DNA replication, which is known to depend on the activity of several short-lived proteins. Host RNA synthesis also soon ceases, probably not as a result of any direct effect on DNA-dependent RNA polymerases but because of changes in the physical state of the DNA (margination of chromatin, changes in nucleolar structure—see above) that prevent it from acting as a template for transcription. As a result, not only is progressively less and less host cell messenger RNA synthesized, but also the supply of new ribosomes is quickly interrupted. In fact, the only ribosomes that are usually available for protein synthesis during the virus multiplication cycle are those that are present in the cytoplasm at the time of infection.

The reasons why infection with viruses inhibits host protein synthesis have been studied extensively but are not well understood. Sometimes the reason may be that less and less host cell messenger RNA reaches the cytoplasm. However, it is clear that in many virus infections the rate of host protein synthesis decreases far more rapidly than would be expected on the basis of the decay rate of messenger RNA in uninfected cells; for example, infection with high multiplicities of vaccinia virus inhibits host protein synthesis by well over 90 percent within 2 hours (Fig. 5-1). This is not a general toxic effect on the host cell, since viral proteins are already being synthesized vigorously at this time; nor is inhibition of host protein synthesis usually due to destruction of host cell messenger RNA, since the continued existence of undiminished amounts of fully functional messenger RNA can often be demonstrat-

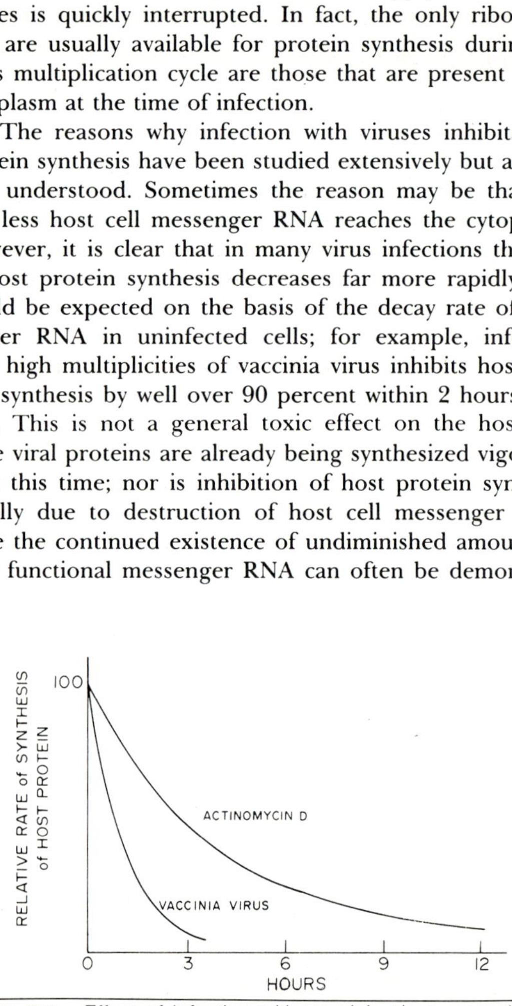

Figure 5-1. Effect of infection with vaccinia virus, as well as of actinomycin D, on cellular protein synthesis in mouse L fibroblasts. Actinomycin D inhibits RNA transcription; the decrease in the rate of host protein synthesis in its presence, therefore, reflects the stability of cellular messenger RNA, whose average half-life is about 3 hours. Infection with vaccinia virus inhibits host protein synthesis much more rapidly. Presumably the infection either causes host messenger RNA to be inactivated, or it actively prevents host messenger RNA from being translated.

ed by its ability to be translated in in vitro protein-synthesizing systems prepared from uninfected cells. Rather, shortly after infection a mechanism apparently develops that actively prevents from being translated the cellular messenger RNA that is present in the cytoplasm at the time of infection.

There is probably not one but several such mechanisms, depending on the nature of the virus. As pointed out above, the plasma cell membrane is often damaged soon after infection, and as a result the Na^+–K^+ gradient collapses, which causes the Na^+ concentration to rise and the K^+ concentration to fall. There is evidence that these changes inhibit the translation of host cell messenger RNAs more than that of viral messenger RNAs. Further, soon after infection with some viruses such as poliovirus, cap binding protein, essential for the translation of capped messenger RNAs such as most cellular messenger RNAs, is inactivated, while translation of uncapped poliovirus RNA is of course not affected. However, it is known that not *all* uncapped messenger RNAs can be translated in poliovirus-infected cells. This finding is in line with earlier observations that suggested that viral messenger RNAs may, in general, be more efficient messenger RNAs than host cell messenger RNAs; thus, in vitro protein-synthesizing systems presented with mixtures of host and viral messenger RNAs usually translate the latter preferentially. The most important reason that viral messenger RNAs are translated almost exclusively once the late period has begun is simply that by that time viral messenger RNA molecules greatly outnumber host cell messenger RNA molecules; by that time transcription of host messenger RNAs is greatly reduced for the reasons discussed above, and large amounts of viral messenger RNAs are being transcribed. Even if virus messenger RNAs were not translated preferentially, simple competition would cause host protein synthesis to be almost completely shut down.

While the hypothesis that inhibition of host DNA and RNA synthesis is secondary to inhibition of host protein synthesis is probably correct for most virus infections, several exceptions have been reported. Thus VSV and Sindbis virus rapidly shut off host RNA and DNA synthesis, respectively, by mechanisms that do not appear to involve protein-synthesis inhibition; a component of parental poxvirus particles has been reported to inhibit host DNA synthesis; and the isolated G glycoprotein of VSV inhibits cell DNA, but not protein synthesis.

Changes in the Regulation of Gene Expression

Virus infection may also affect the regulation of host genome expression. Thus, the activity of enzymes on the pathway of nucleic acid biosynthesis often increases after infection; for example, infection with the papovaviruses polyoma and SV40 causes increases in the activity of at least six enzymes. One of these enzymes is a deoxypyrimidine kinase that phosphorylates both deoxyuridine and deoxycytidine. Cells possess two forms of this enzyme, one of which is synthesized in resting cells, the other in growing cells. When resting cells are infected with SV40 or adenovirus, it is the latter form of the enzyme whose formation is induced. Further, infection with almost all viruses leads to the synthesis of a new protein, interferon (Chap. 7). All this evidence suggests that infection may upset the mechanisms that usually prevent the expression of a large portion of cellular DNA and that during the early part of the infection cycle more of the cell's genome may be expressed in infected than in uninfected cells.

Appearance of New Antigenic Determinants on the Cell Surface

Sooner or later following infection, the outer cell membrane is modified. This manifests itself in a variety of ways: the cells' morphology changes, they become more agglutinable by the lectin concanavalin A (Chap. 8), permeability increases, and new antigenic determinants appear on the cell surface. When the infecting virus is an enveloped virus, these new determinants are likely to be viral envelope proteins that have become incorporated into the cell membrane, but new antigenic determinants also appear on the surfaces of cells that are infected with nonenveloped viruses. The presence of these determinants serves to alert the immune mechanism to the fact that the cells are infected and should be eliminated (Fig. 5-2). These new antigens are discussed further in Chapter 8 in relation to tumor and transplantation antigens.

Cell Fusion

Several viruses, particularly paramyxoviruses such as Sendai virus and herpesviruses, cause cells to fuse with one another, which results in the formation of giant syncytia, masses of cytoplasm bounded by one membrane that may contain hundreds and even thousands of nuclei. Fusion seems to be caused by changes induced in cell membranes as a result of interaction with certain glycoproteins in viral envelopes (glycoproteins gB and gD in herpesvirus envelopes and the F spike glycoprotein of paramyxoviruses). It is therefore caused not only by active but also by inactivated virus particles. Further, it can be induced not only among identical but also among different cells. The products of fusion are either heterokaryons—cells containing several nuclei of different types (Fig. 5-3)—or hybrid cells that contain the fused nuclei of the parents. Hybrid cells are frequently viable and have become widely used

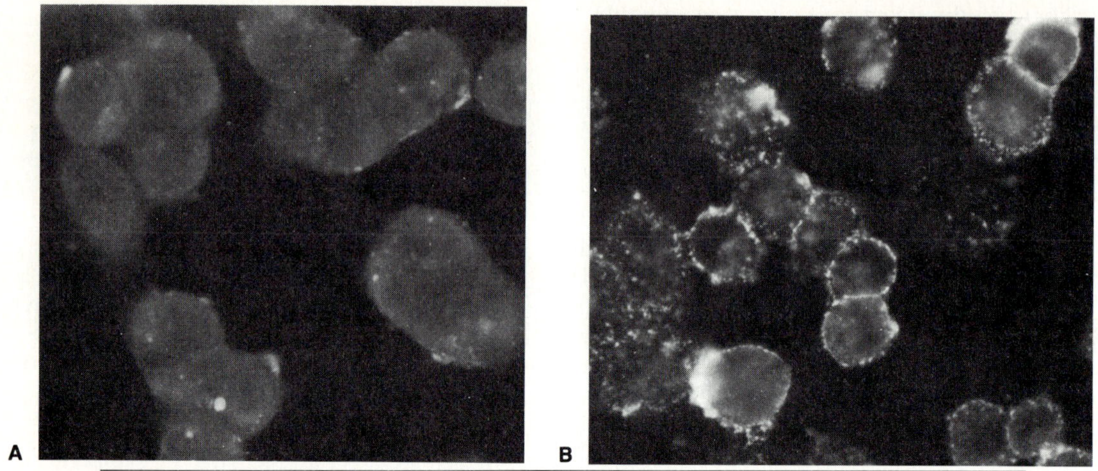

Figure 5-2. Virus-specified surface antigen on HeLa cells infected with vaccinia virus. A. Uninfected cells. B. Cells infected for 8 hours. The cells were stained with rabbit antiserum to rabbit cells infected with vaccinia virus. *(Courtesy of Dr. Yoshiaki Ueda.)*

for studies in somatic cell genetics. They are produced by fusing mixtures of the two cell lines to be hybridized with inactivated Sendai virus or, more commonly nowadays, by treatment with polyethylene glycol, and are then cloned. They are particularly useful for determining the chromosomal location of specific genes; as hybrid cells multiply, they often lose chromosomes, and one can readily correlate the loss of a particular gene function with loss of a specific chromosome. In recent years, many human genes have been assigned to chromosomes in this manner, using human–mouse hybrid cells that lose human chromosomes. The genetic factors that control susceptibility to virus infection and the expression of tumorigenicity can also be studied with the aid of somatic cell hybrids. The technique has also become very important in immunology for the production of hybridomas that produce individual species of antibodies (monoclonal antibodies).

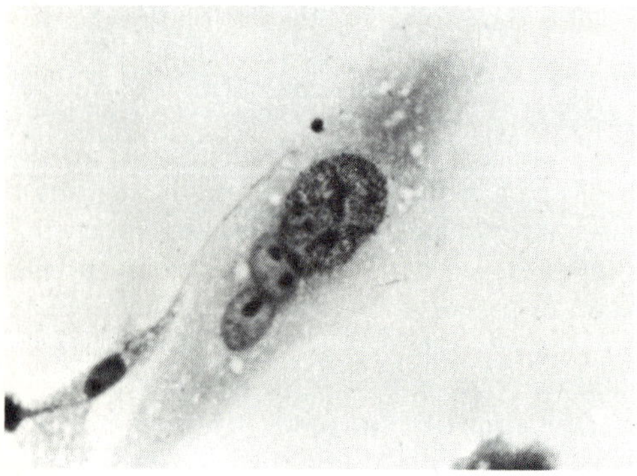

Figure 5-3. Cell fusion induced by UV-inactivated Sendai virus. Three chick embryo fibroblasts have fused to yield the heterokaryon shown here, which contains three nuclei. The two small ones are normal chick nuclei; the large one is from a chick cell transformed with Rous sarcoma virus. × 400. *(From Svoboda and Dourmashkin: J Gen Virol 4:523, 1969.)*

Abortive Infection

Most of the changes described so far relate to the lytic multiplication cycle under conditions of productive infection, that is, when a virus multiplies to high titer in permissive cells. However, viruses can also infect cells that are not fully permissive and even cells that are nonpermissive. In such cells, viruses cannot multiply because some essential step of the multiplication cycle cannot proceed. Examples of this type are the abortive infection of HeLa cells by influenza virus, of dog kidney cells by herpes simplex virus, of pig kidney cells by certain mutants of rabbitpox virus, of monkey cells by human adenovirus, and many others. The infection of permissive cells in the presence of antiviral agents (Chap. 7) is also abortive. In almost all such cases the viral genome begins to express itself, the alterations in the host cell that were described above occur, and the cells die.

Persistent Infections

As a rule, the infection of permissive cells with lytic viruses leads to productive infection and cell death. Occasionally, however, cell cultures are observed that, while multiplying more or less normally, nevertheless release significant amounts of virus. Such cultures are said to be persistently infected. Stable relationships between cell growth and virus multiplication, which occur not only in vitro but also in vivo, are of two kinds.

The first involves infection by viruses that cause a minimum of the type of cell damage discussed above. A good example is provided by the paramyxovirus SV5. This virus interacts with many cells by means of a lytic, cytocidal interaction. However, when it infects monkey kidney cells, it causes practically no cell damage and permits the infected cells to grow freely while multiplying itself. In such cultures, all cells multiply, all cells are infected, and all cells produce virus. Infection of new cells plays no role in this situation; consequently, this type of infection cannot be cured by the addition of neutralizing antibody.

The second situation is quite different. Here the virus–cell interaction is lytic—that is, the cells that are infected always die—but the extent of virus multiplication is limited, so that the yield is small. In addition, various factors reduce the probability of reinfection, so that the proportion of infected cells in the total cell population is kept small and constant. The factors that induce and maintain this type of persistent infection are as follows: First, this type of infection occurs most readily in cells that are almost, but not quite, nonpermissive and that, therefore, produce only small amounts of virus. Second, it occurs in situations where factors in the medium, such as antibody or interferon, prevent the majority of released progeny virus from infecting new cells. The role of small amounts of interferon is sometimes not readily apparent but becomes obvious if antibody to interferon is added, when persistent infections become lytic infections. Third, many of the virus strains that have been isolated from persistently infected cells and animals are less virulent, less cytopathic, and, interestingly enough, temperature-sensitive with respect to their ability to multiply. This has now been found for foot-and-mouth disease virus, Coxsackie virus, Sindbis virus and WEE, influenza virus, Newcastle disease virus, Sendai virus, mumps and measles virus, VSV and herpesvirus, and others. Attempts to isolate viruses from the tissues of patients with suspected chronic and persistent virus infections should take account of the possibility that they may grow better at 31C to 33C than at 37C.

The fact that virus strains recovered from persistently infected cells are frequently temperature-sensitive has aroused considerable interest, and, indeed, persistent virus infection can be established readily by infecting cells with temperature-sensitive mutants. However, the important fact is not that virus strains present in persistently infected cells are temperature-sensitive but rather that they are not cytopathogenic. Although temperature-sensitive virus strains are usually much less cytopathogenic than wild-type virus, presumably because much less viral protein causing cytopathogenicity is synthesized in cells infected with them (Chap. 6), virus strains do not have to be temperature-sensitive to cause persistent infection. For example, a strain of VSV, isolated from persistently infected cells, is not temperature-sensitive (except above 40C) but transcribes much less of its minus strand into messenger RNAs relative to complete plus strands than does wild-type virus (Chap. 4). This, in turn, results in less viral protein being synthesized and the virus strain being relatively noncytopathogenic.

Finally, virus yields from persistently infected cells sometimes contain, in addition to infectious virus, deletion mutants, that is, virus particles that lack a portion of their genome (Chap. 6). These virus particles, which are unable to multiply on their own, are nevertheless capable of interfering with the multiplication of infectious virus and are, therefore, known as defective interfering or DI particles. Their presence dampens the effect of virus infection, that it, it reduces both cell damage and the amount of infectious virus that is produced. Their role in initiating and maintaining persistent infection is readily demonstrated as follows: if DI particles of VSV, the so-called T particles (Chap. 6), are inoculated into animals together with normal, infectious VSV, an otherwise fatal disease is converted to a slowly progressing persistent infection; and if cultured cells are infected with wild-type virus together with DI particles, persistent infection is readily established. The formation of DI particles has now been implicated in persistent and chronic infections with influenza virus, Sendai virus, NDV and measles, lymphocytic choriomeningitis virus, Sindbis virus, Semliki Forest virus, WEE, and rubella, as well as VSV. The nature of the deletions in the DI particles of various viruses and the nature of the mechanisms that cause such particles to inhibit the multiplication of wild-type virus is discussed in Chapter 6.

In summary, the replacement of virulent by less virulent virus strains and the inhibition of virus multiplication by DI particles are major factors in the establishment and maintenance of persistent virus infections. Persistent infections of this class are important in the intact organism, where the presence of antiviral antibody and interferon in amounts too low to eliminate virus may provide conditions favoring low-level persistent infections. It should be noted that this kind of persistent infection can be cured by the addition of large amounts of neutralizing antibody.

Latency

We have so far considered only persistently infected cell populations that release significant amounts of virus. However, there are also persistently infected cells that release virus only rarely. In such cells virus multiplication can start but is arrested at some stage or other. The best known infections of this type are caused by herpesviruses. Most herpesviruses have a pronounced tendency to infect cells in which their development is normally blocked but from which they can be released in infectious form if conditions are right. The released virus particles can then initiate productive infection in some other type of cell. This is the phenomenon of latency, the best known example of which is the latent herpes simplex virus type 1 infection of the neurons of sensory ganglia, from which the virus emerges to cause infections of the skin, such as fever blisters (Chap. 13). The form in which herpesvirus persists in ganglion cells is not known. An interesting recent observation that may explain why viral DNA is transcribed minimally, if at all, in latent infections is that latent herpesvirus DNA is heavily hypermethylated, and hypermethylation is known to reduce gene expression very significantly.

This type of persistent infection, whether by herpes simplex virus or varicella-zoster virus, generally does not cause progressive disease; that is, the virus multiplies for some time, then becomes latent, and then reinitiates productive infection. Other persistent infections of this type tend to cause progressive disease. Examples are subacute sclerosing panencephalitis (SSPE), an infection of the central nervous system by a virus closely related to measles virus, in which large amounts of viral nucleocapsids are present in infected cells (Chap. 4); and progressive multifocal leukoencephalopathy (PML), a papovavirus infection (Chap. 15).

Modification of Cellular Permissiveness

Occasionally, virus infection can alter to an amazing degree the permissiveness of cells for completely unrelated viruses. The effects are always highly specific. Thus, adeno-associated virus (AAV) can multiply only in cells infected with adenovirus; SV40 enables human adenovirus to grow in monkey cells; and poxviruses, such as vaccinia and fibroma virus, enable VSV to multiply in rabbit cells. The helper functions appear always to involve translation of messenger RNA, that is, protein synthesis. For example, in rabbit cornea cells infected with VSV, viral messenger RNA is made and forms polyribosomes, but no VSV proteins are synthesized; VSV protein synthesis is inhibited at the stage of elongation. If such cells are also infected with vaccinia virus, VSV multiplies normally. Apparently vaccinia virus modifies the protein-synthesizing mechanism of these cells in such a way that VSV messenger RNA can be translated normally. The ability of SV40 to correct the inability of human adenoviruses to multiply in monkey cells appears to have a similar basis. However, other mechanisms may also be involved. For example, the reason why VSV cannot multiply in rabbit kidney cells appears to be the fact that it is not adsorbed, that is, an absence of VSV receptors. If such cells are first infected with Shope fibroma virus, the plasma membrane is modified, VSV adsorbs normally and, as a result, is able to replicate.

FURTHER READING

Books and Reviews

GENERAL

Ehrenfeld E: Poliovirus-induced inhibition of host-cell protein synthesis. Cell 28:435, 1982

Holland JJ, Kennedy SIT, Semler BL, et al.: Defective interfering RNA viruses and the host-cell response. In Fraenkel-Conrat H, Wagner RR (eds): Comprehensive Virology. New York, Plenum, 1980, vol 16, p 137

Maltzman W, Levine AJ: Viruses as probes for development and differentiation. Adv Virus Res 26:65, 1981

PATHOGENESIS

Ennis A: Some newly recognized aspects of resistance against and recovery from influenza. Arch Virol 73:207, 1982

Fields BN: Molecular basis of reovirus virulence. Arch Virol 71:95, 1982

Johnson RT (ed): Viral Infections of the Nervous System. New York, Raven, 1982

Klein RJ: The pathogenesis of acute, latent and recurrent herpes simplex virus infections. Arch Virol 72:143, 1982

Rott R: Molecular basis of infectivity and pathogenicity of myxovirus. Arch Virol 59:285, 1979

Sever JL, Madden DL (eds): Polyomaviruses and Human Neurological Disease. New York, Liss, 1983

ter Meulen V, Stephenson JR, Kreth HW: Subacute sclerosing panencephalitis. In Fraenkel-Conrat H, Wagner RR (eds): Comprehensive Virology. New York, Plenum, 1983, vol 18, p 105

Wege H, Siddell S, ter Meulen V: The biology and pathogenesis of coronaviruses. Curr Top Microbiol Immunol 100:165, 1982

Wolinsky JS, Johnson RT: Role of viruses in chronic neurological diseases. In Fraenkel-Conrat H, Wagner RR (eds): Comprehensive Virology. New York, Plenum, 1980, vol 16, p 257

PERSISTENT INFECTIONS

Norkin LC: Papovaviral persistent infections. Microbiol Rev 46:384, 1982

Porter DD, Cho HJ: Aleutian disease of mink: A model for persistent infection. In Fraenkel-Conrat H, Wagner RR (eds): Comprehensive Virology. New York, Plenum, 1980, vol 16, p 233

Rapp F: Persistence and transmission of cytomegaloviruses. In Fraenkel-Conrat H, Wagner RR (eds): Comprehensive Virology. New York, Plenum, 1980, vol 16, p 193

Stevens JG, Todaro DJ, Fox CF (eds): Persistent Viruses. New York, Academic Press, 1978

Streissle G: Persistent viral infections as models for research in virus chemotherapy. Adv Virus Res 26:37, 1981

Stroop WG, Baringer JR: Persistent, slow and latent viral infections. Prog Med Virol 28:1, 1982

Youngner JS, Preble OT: Viral persistence: Evolution of viral populations. In Fraenkel-Conrat H, Wagner RR (eds): Comprehensive Virology. New York, Plenum, 1980, vol 16, p 73

Selected Papers

INHIBITION OF MACROMOLECULAR BIOSYNTHESIS

Abreu SL, Lucas-Lenard J: Cellular protein synthesis shutoff by mengovirus translation of nonviral and viral mRNAs in extracts from uninfected and infected Ehrlich ascites tumor cells. J Virol 18:182, 1976

Bablanian R, Esteban M, Baxt B, et al.: Studies on the mechanisms of vaccinia virus cytopathic effects. I. Inhibition of protein synthesis in infected cells is associated with virus-induced RNA synthesis. J Gen Virol 39:391, 1978

Brown D, Jones CL, Brown BA, et al.: Translation of capped and uncapped VSV mRNAs in the presence of initiation factors from poliovirus-infected cells. Virology 123:60, 1982

Castiglia CL, Flint SJ: Effects of adenovirus infection on rRNA synthesis and maturation in HeLa cells. Mol Cell Biol 3:662, 1983

Coppola G, Bablanian R: Discriminatory inhibition of protein synthesis in cell-free systems by vaccinia virus transcripts. Proc Natl Acad Sci USA 80:75, 1983

Ebina T, Satake M, Ishida N: Involvement of microtubules in cytopathic effects of animal viruses: Early proteins of adenovirus and herpesvirus inhibit formation of microtubular paracrystals in HeLa-S3 cells. J Gen Virol 38:535, 1978

Eggleton KH, Norkin LC: Cell killing by simian virus 40: The sequence of ultrastructural alterations leading to cellular degeneration and death. Virology 110:73, 1981

Ehrenfeld E, Lund H: Untranslated vesicular stomatitis virus messenger RNA after poliovirus infection. Virology 80:297, 1977

Etchison D, Milburn SC, Eldery I, et al.: Inhibition of HeLa cell protein synthesis following poliovirus infection correlates with the proteolysis of a 220,000-dalton polypeptide associated with eucaryotic initiation factor 3 and a cap binding protein complex. J Biol Chem 257:14, 806, 1982

Fields BN, Greene MI: Genetic and molecular mechanisms of viral pathogenesis: Implications for prevention and treatment. Nature 300:19, 1982

Golini F, Thach SS, Birge CH, et al.: Competition between cellular and viral mRNAs in vitro is regulated by a messenger discriminatory initiation factor. Proc Natl Acad Sci USA 73:3040, 1976

Jaye MC, Godchaux W III, Lucas-Lenard J: Further studies on the inhibition of cellular protein synthesis by vesicular stomatitis virus. Virology 116:148, 1982

Jen G, Detjen BM, Thatch RE: Shutoff of HeLa cell protein synthesis by encephalomyocarditis virus and poliovirus: A comparative study. J Virol 35:150, 1980

Kauffman RS, Wolf JL, Finberg R, et al.: The $\sigma 1$ protein determines the extent of spread of reovirus from the gastrointestinal tract of mice. Virology 124:403, 1983

Koizumi S, Simizu B, Hashimoto K, et al.: Inhibition of DNA synthesis in BHK cells infected with Western equine encephalitis virus. 1. Induction of an inhibitory factor of cellular DNA polymerase activity. Virology 94:314, 1979

Marcus PI, Sekellick MJ: Cell killing by viruses. 1. Comparison of cell-killing, plaque-forming, and defective-interfering particles of vesicular stomatitis virus. Virology 57:321, 1974

Mbuy GN, Morris RE, Bubel HC: Inhibition of cellular protein synthesis by vaccinia virus surface tubules. Virology 116:137, 1982

McSharry JJ, Choppin PW: Biological properties of the VSV glycoprotein. I. Effects of the isolated glycoprotein or host macromolecular synthesis. Virology 84:172, 1978

Nishioka Y, Jones G, Silverstein S: Inhibition by vesicular stomatitis virus of herpes simplex virus-directed protein synthesis. Virology 124:238, 1983

Ray BK, Brendler TG, Adya S, et al.: Role of mRNA competition in regulating translation: Further characterization of mRNA discriminatory initiation factors. Proc Natl Acad Sci USA 80:663, 1983

Rose JK, Trachsel H, Leong K, et al.: Inhibition of translation by poliovirus: Inactivation of a specific initiation factor. Proc Natl Acad Sci USA 75:2732, 1978

Schaefer A, Kuhne J, Zibirre R, et al.: Poliovirus-induced alterations in HeLa cell membrane functions. J Virol 44:444, 1982

Schnitzlein WM, O'Banion MK, Poirot MK, et al.: Effect of intracellular vesicular stomatitis virus mRNA concentration on the inhibition of host cell protein synthesis. J Virol 45:206, 1983

Sharpe AH, Fields BN: Reovirus inhibition of cellular RNA and protein synthesis: The role of the S4 gene. Virology 122:381, 1982

Stenberg RM, Pizer LI: Herpes simplex virus-induced changes in cellular and adenovirus RNA metabolism in an adenovirus type 5-transformed human cell line. J Virol 42:474, 1982

Thomas JR, Wagner RR: Inhibition of translation in lysates of mouse L cells infected with vesicular stomatitis virus: Presence of a defective ribosome-associated factor. Biochemistry 22:1540, 1983

CELL FUSION

Ege T, Krondahl U, Ringertz NR: Introduction of nuclei and micronuclei into cells and enucleated cytoplasms by Sendai virus induced fusion. Exp Cell Res 88:428, 1974

Lee GT-Y, Spear PG: Viral and cellular factors that influence cell fusion induced by herpes simplex virus. Virology 107:402, 1980

Manservigi R, Spear PG, Buchan A: Cell fusion induced by herpes simplex virus is promoted and suppressed by different viral glycoproteins. Proc Natl Acad Sci USA 74:3913, 1977

Tedesco TA, Diamond R, Orkwiszewski KG, et al.: Assignment of the human gene for hexose-1-phosphate uridylyltransferase to chromosome 3. Proc Natl Acad Sci USA 71:3483, 1974

PERSISTENT AND LATENT INFECTIONS

Barrett PN, Atkins GJ: Establishment of persistent infection in mouse cells by Sindbis virus and its temperature-sensitive mutants. J Gen Virol 54:57, 1981

Frey TK, Youngner JS: Novel phenotype of RNA synthesis expressed by vesicular stomatitis virus isolated from persistent infection. J Virol 44:167, 1982

Galloway DA, Fenoglio C, Shevchuk M, et al.: Detection of herpes simplex RNA in human sensory ganglia. Virology 95:265, 1979

Gerdes JC, Marsden HS, Cook ML, et al.: Acute infection of differentiated neuroblastoma cells by latency-positive and latency-negative herpes simplex virus ts mutants. Virology 94:430, 1979

Newton SE, Short NJ, Dalgarno L: Bunyamwera virus replication in cultured *Aedes aldopictus* (mosquito) cells: Establishment of a persistent viral infection. J Virol 38:1015, 1981

Preble OT, Youngner JS: Temperature-sensitive defects of mutants isolated from L cells persistently infected with Newcastle disease virus. J Virol 12:472, 1973

Price RW, Schmitz J: Route of infection, systemic host resistance, and integrity of ganglionic axons influence acute and latent herpes simplex virus infection of the superior cervical ganglion. Infect Immun 23:373, 1979

Rock DL, Fraser NW: Detection of HSV-1 genome in central nervous system of latently infected mice. Nature 302:523, 1983

Thacore HR, Youngner JS: Persistence of vesicular stomatitis virus in interferon-treated cell cultures. Virology 63:345, 1975

Williams MP, Brawner TA, Riggs HG Jr, et al.: Characteristics of a persistent rubella infection in a human cell line. J Gen Virol 52:321, 1981

Yoshida T, Hamaguchi M, Naruse H, et al.: Persistent infection by a temperature-sensitive mutant isolated from a Sendai virus (HVJ) carrier culture: Its initiation and maintenance without aid of defective interfering particles. Virology 120:329, 1982

Youngner JS, Preble OT, Jones EV: Persistent infection of L cells with vesicular stomatitis virus: Evolution of virus populations. J Virol 28:6, 1978

PERMISSIVENESS

Chen C-Y, Crouch NA: Shope fibroma virus-induced facilitation of vesicular stomatitis virus adsorption and replication in nonpermissive cells. Virology 85:43, 1978

Jones EV, Whitaker-Dowling PA, Youngner JS: Restriction of vesicular stomatitis virus in a nonpermissive rabbit cell line is at the level of protein synthesis. Virology 121:20, 1982

CHAPTER 6

The Genetics of Animal Viruses

The genetic approach to studying the virus–cell interaction in general and the virus multiplication cycle in particular has long been recognized as being extremely powerful in the bacteriophage field (Chap. 9). During the last two decades it has become very useful in animal virology as well. The principal techniques of viral genetics are the isolation of mutants in the various genes, their characterization, and identification of the proteins that they encode. These techniques permit dissection of the complex series of interactions that is initiated when viruses infect cells into its individual components.

Types of Virus Mutants

Viruses are encapsidated segments of genetic material, and like other genetic systems, viral genomes are not invariate but are subject to change by mutation. Spontaneous mutations occur constantly in the course of virus multiplication, and while many mutations are lethal, others are not. Virus populations may thus be regarded as genetically heterogeneous, since they are likely to contain mutants, at an average rate of 10^{-6}, at each locus. This value refers to DNA-containing viruses. It is sometimes suggested that the error rate for RNA-containing viruses is much higher, since RNA polymerases appear to lack the proofreading mechanism that some DNA polymerases possess. However, RNA-containing viruses are not inherently unstable genetic systems. In fact, many genes of RNA-containing viruses exhibit sequence conservation as extensive as those of DNA-containing viruses.

Mutant virus strains can also be generated in the laboratory as a result of mutagenesis, and it is from mutagenized virus populations that mutant isolation is usually undertaken. Among the procedures for mutagenizing RNA-containing viruses are treatment of virus particles with nitrous acid, hydroxylamine, N-methyl-N-nitro-N-nitrosoguanidine (NTG) or ethane methane sulfonic acid, and propagation in the presence of 5-fluorouracil, 5-azacytidine, or proflavine (for the double-stranded RNA-containing reovirus). For DNA-containing viruses, treatment of virus particles with nitrous acid, hydroxylamine, or ultraviolet irradiation, and growth in the presence of 5-bromodeoxyuridine, NTG, or proflavine are used most commonly.

There are two principal types of virus mutants: point mutants, in which there is a change in a single nucleotide base, and deletion mutants, in which a whole sequence or region of nucleic acid has been deleted. Deletion mutants will be considered below when defective virus particles are discussed. The most important point mutants are the conditional lethal mutants.

Conditional Lethal Mutants

Conditional lethal mutants, as the name implies, can multiply under some conditions but not under others that will, however, still permit the multiplication of wild-type virus. There are two classes of such mutants. The first comprises mutants that are temperature-sensitive (ts) with respect to their ability to multiply. Wild-type animal viruses can generally multiply over a temperature range that extends from a lower limit of about 20C to 24C to an upper limit of about 39.5C for mammalian viruses and 40C to 41C for avian ones. In ts mutants there is a nucleic acid base substitution that causes an amino acid replacement in some virus-coded protein, as a result of which it cannot assume or maintain the structural conformation necessary for activity at elevated or nonpermissive (restrictive) temperatures, though still able to do so at lower or permissive temperatures. The typical ts mutation causes the formation of an enzyme or a structural protein that cannot function in a temperature range (typically from about 36C to 41C) where the corresponding protein of the wild-type strain can function.

The second class of conditional lethal mutants is the host-dependent mutants, which have been extremely useful in the bacterium/bacteriophage fields. In these mutants, the codon for some amino acid is changed to a termination codon (UAG, UAA or UGA), and, as a result, proteins are formed that are shorter than those specified by wild-type virus and therefore cannot function. However, mutant bacterial strains exist that contain mutated tRNA molecules that recognize these termination codons as the codon for some amino acid (generally different from the original one), which is therefore inserted into the amino acid sequence, thereby again permitting a full-length protein to be formed. If the amino acid change is such that the altered protein can still function, the effect of the original nonsense mutation is therefore suppressed. The mutated tRNA molecules are known as suppressor tRNAs and the mutant bacterial strains as suppressor strains. The mutations that give rise to UAG, UAA, and UGA are known as *amber, ochre,* and *opal* respectively. Recent work has shown that this type of mutation also exists in mammalian cells/viruses.

The reason that conditional lethal mutants are so important in studies seeking to define the reactions essential for virus multiplication is that they permit study of the virus multiplication cycle with one, and only one, reaction unable to proceed. Use of such mutants permits both the assessment of the role of any particular known reaction during the course of virus multiplication and also the detection of hitherto unknown functions.

Mutants with Other Commonly Observed Phenotypes

In addition to temperature-sensitive and host-dependent mutants, several other mutant phenotypes are commonly observed, primarily because selection for them is easy and they are therefore readily observed and isolated.

Plaque-size Mutants

Many virus strains give rise to spontaneous mutants that form smaller plaques than wild-type virus because their adsorption is inhibited by sulfated polysaccharides present in agar (Fig. 6-1). Large plaque mutants are also known, and in this case the ability of wild-type virus to adsorb is inhibited by the polysaccharides, whereas that of the mutants is not. In either case, the site of the mutation is in a capsid protein that functions in adsorption.

Host Range Mutants

Host range mutants of several animal viruses are known. The best characterized are those of adenoviruses, papovaviruses, and poxviruses. Adenovirus *hr* mutants map in the

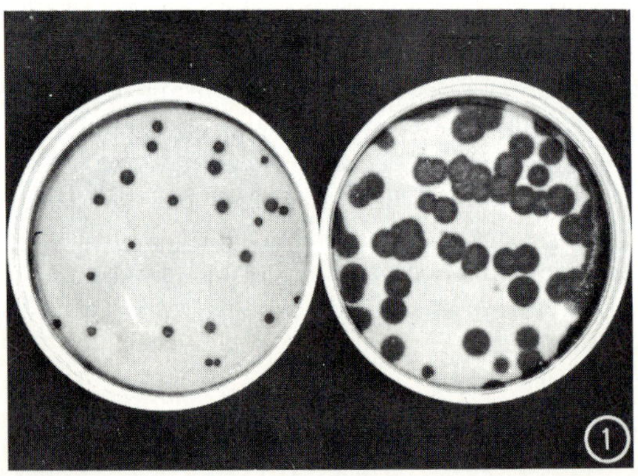

Figure 6-1. Comparative sizes of two Mengovirus plaque size variants, S-Mengo (left) and L-Mengo (right). The plaques are 48 hours old. The L mutant is more virulent in animals and more cytopathic in cell cultures. *(From Amako and Dales: Virology 32: 184, 1967.)*

leftmost portion of the viral genome, the region that also contains the genetic information required for transformation. Not surprisingly, these adenovirus *hr* mutants tend to be defective in their ability to transform cells.

Drug-resistant Mutants

Drugs capable of inhibiting the multiplication of certain viruses are known (Chap. 7), and mutants exist that are resistant to these drugs. Examples are poliovirus mutants resistant to guanidine, herpesvirus mutants resistant to phosphonoacetic acid, and vaccinia virus mutants resistant to rifampicin and IBT. Poliovirus mutants dependent on guanidine and vaccinia virus mutants dependent on IBT also exist.

Enzyme-deficient Mutants

Viruses code for several enzymes essential for virus multiplication, and mutations that result in loss of this ability are obviously lethal. Some viruses also code for enzymes that are not essential, and mutants lacking the ability to code for them are viable. For example, poxviruses and herpesviruses code for enzymes that phosphorylate thymidine (thymidine kinases). Virus mutants that are deficient in the ability to induce the synthesis of these enzymes are known. They multiply well, which suggests that the survival advantage conferred by the ability to code for them is small.

Hot Mutants

These are mutants that can grow well at temperatures higher than can wild-type virus. For example, whereas 41C is near the upper limit of the temperature growth range of wild-type poliovirus, mutant strains exist that grow as well at 41C as at 37C, or even better. Not surprisingly, such strains are very virulent, since they can multiply rapidly in patients with high fever, when the multiplication of wild-type virus is at least partially inhibited.

Interactions Among Viruses

Under conditions of multiple infection, cells may become infected with two or more virus particles with different genomes. If they are sufficiently closely related—that is, if they belong to the same genus or virus family—they can even interact. There are several types of such interactions.

Recombination

The detection of recombination between two virus strains depends on the availability of techniques that permit recombinants to be detected in the presence of a large excess of the two parents. If the two parents are single-step mutants of some wild-type strain, each differing from it in some recognizable manner, some of the recombinants will have the wild-type genotype and phenotype and be easily detectable. The detection of other recombinants, such as the reciprocal recombinants or recombinants between viruses that differ in several loci, is usually more difficult.

Viruses differ greatly in the ease with which they undergo recombination, the principal relevant factor being the nature of their genomes. With the exception of poliovirus and foot-and-mouth-disease virus, viruses that possess a single molecule of single-stranded RNA do not recombine. By contrast, viruses that contain double-stranded DNA recombine efficiently, most probably by a mechanism that is analogous to that by which the genomes of bacteria and higher organisms recombine.

The important point here is that viruses must be reasonably closely related for recombination to occur: only viruses in the same genus recombine, and ability to recombine may well become a useful taxonomic criterion. (Note, however, the infectious adenovirus-SV40 recombinants, which present a very special case, see below.)

Genome Segment Reassortment

The most efficiently recombining viruses are those whose genomes consist of several nucleic acid segments. In such cases recombination proceeds not by classic recombination involving breakage and reformation of covalent bonds but by simple reassortment of segments into new sets (Fig. 6-2). Both single-stranded and double-stranded RNA segments participate in this type of recombination, as shown by the fact that pairs of reovirus and influenza virus mutants with mutations in different genome segments generate wild-type virus with high frequency. For reoviruses and rotaviruses, bunyaviruses, and arenaviruses, genome segment reassortment does not appear to play a major role under natural conditions: although reassortants can readily be detected among the viruses that circulate in populations infected with two virus strains, such reassortants tend to die out, perhaps because some of their structural proteins are specified by one virus strain, others by the other, and the resulting heterologous capsids are less stable than homologous capsids. However, genome segment reassortment is very important in generating new influenza virus strains. It is very likely that such reassortment is the cause of the major antigenic shifts that have occurred in human influenza virus during the last half-century. The influenza viruses that exist in nature each possess one of 13 different kinds (subtypes) of hemagglutinin (H1 to H13) and one of 9 different subtypes of neuraminidase (N1 to N9). These different subtypes differ markedly in amino acid sequence and possess quite different antigenic determinants. Before 1957 the influenza virus strains that circulated in humans had the constitution H1N1; in 1957 they were replaced by Asian influenza, which was H2N2; in 1968 the

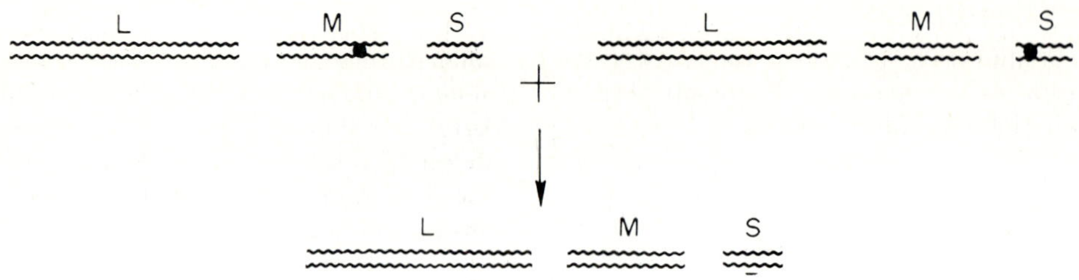

Figure 6-2. Generation of wild-type genomes by reassortment of damaged genome segments. Two genomes, each consisting of three segments of double-stranded nucleic acid, are shown. One carries a mutation in an M segment, the other in an S segment. When they are introduced into the same cell, sets of undamaged segments are generated by reassortment. This type of mechanism can account for the generation of new genotypes among reoviruses, influenza viruses, bunyaviruses, and arenaviruses.

Hong Kong virus appeared, which is H3N2 and is still circulating; and in 1977 H1N1 human influenza virus reappeared after an absence of 20 years. All these major antigenic shifts occurred in China. The most likely mechanism for the appearance and reappearance of these new subtypes is the introduction of new genome segments into human influenza virus from some animal influenza virus by genome segment reassortment. For example, the Hong Kong influenza virus strain of 1968 most probably derived its H3 hemagglutinin gene from an equine or duck influenza virus.

Multiplicity Reactivation

Viruses that contain double-stranded nucleic acid frequently exhibit multiplicity reactivation after being subjected to ultraviolet radiation. Ultraviolet radiation damages nucleic acids. In particular, it causes the formation of covalent bonds between adjacent pyrimidines, thereby giving rise to cyclobutane derivatives. In DNA, the most commonly formed pyrimidine dimers are those between adjacent thymine rings. In RNA, dimers are formed between any adjacent uracil and cytosine rings. Dimer formation inactivates viral genomes by preventing replication and probably also transcription and translation.

Dimers are removed from DNA by several mechanisms. These have been studied mainly in bacteria, but there is evidence that they operate in animal cells as well. One involves an enzyme system that utilizes radiation of longer wavelengths, particularly those of visible light, for dissociating dimers. This is the so-called photoreactivating repair system. Another mechanism (the dark or excision repair mechanism) involves nucleases that recognize dimers and excise them, the gaps then being repaired by a DNA polymerase acting in conjunction with polynucleotide ligase. This is the host cell reactivating system.

Ultraviolet radiation also induces crosslinking of the two strands of double-stranded DNA by a mechanism that is not clear. No doubt this also contributes to virus inactivation.

Ultraviolet radiation also causes the addition of water molecules across the C5—C6 double bond of pyrimidines in both DNA and RNA, which results in the formation of photohydrates (6-hydroxy-5,6-dihydro derivatives). These photohydrates represent a major portion of the lethal damage caused by ultraviolet light in many RNA-containing viruses.

The most radiation-sensitive property of a virus is its infectivity. The reason is that infectivity requires expression of the genome's entire information content and thus presents the largest target. Sometimes virus particles that have lost the ability to reproduce can still express some special function or group of functions that originate from cistrons that have not sustained radiation damage. Examples of such functions are the ability to synthesize early enzymes and the ability to transform cells. At very high radiation doses, damage to capsid proteins becomes important. This causes loss of the ability to interfere with the multiplication of related viruses, loss of ability to hemagglutinate, and loss of antigenicity.

Multiplicity reactivation is recognized by the fact that the frequency of viral survivors increases sharply with multiplicities of infection above 1. It is due to cooperation between viral genomes that have been damaged by the radiation and that can, therefore, no longer multiply on their own. The nature of the cooperation is recombination, that is, the damaged genomes recombine until an intact genome arises, which can then replicate and form progeny.

Complementation

Viral genomes can also interact indirectly by means of complementation. A typical example of this type of interaction is provided by infection of cells at the restrictive temperature with two virus mutants that bear temperature-sensitive mutations in different cistrons and neither of which can multiply alone. If complementation occurs, progeny comprising both mutants is produced. The explanation of this phenomenon is that each mutant produces functional gene products of all cistrons except that bearing the temperature-sensitive mutation, so that in cells infected with both mutants all gene products necessary for virus multiplication are formed, and both mutants can therefore multiply. Complementation plays a major role in permitting the survival of viruses with genomes that contain damaged or nonfunctional genes.

Phenotypic Mixing and Phenotypic Masking

The dual phenomena of phenotypic mixing and phenotypic masking represent a special case of complementation. When two closely related viruses, for example, poliovirus type 1 and poliovirus type 3, infect the same cell, the two types of progeny genomes may become encapsidated not only by their own capsids but also by hybrid capsids—that is, capsids composed of proteins encoded by both genomes (phenotypic mixing)—or even by capsids entirely specified by the other genome (phenotypic masking or transcapsidation) (Fig. 6-3). This situation is mostly readily detected by antigenic analysis, for the former class of virus particles is neutralized by antiserum to either parent, whereas virus particles of the latter class are neutralized by antiserum to one of the parents, while their progeny is neutralized by antiserum to the other.

A similar phenomenon occurs among enveloped viruses, but here it involves not only viruses that are related but also viruses that are completely unrelated. In particular, the nucleocapsid of the rhabdovirus vesicular stomatitis virus (VSV) possesses a remarkable ability to become encapsidated in envelopes that are only partially, or not at all, specified by it. For example, among the yield from cells simultaneously infected with both VSV and the paramyxovirus SV5, there are bullet-shaped particles that contain VSV nucleocapsids encased in envelopes that bear not only VSV-specified glycoprotein spikes but also both types of SV5-specified spikes. Another example is provided by VSV nucleocapsids completely encased in RNA tumor virus envelopes. Since such particles are easily and rapidly quantitated (because VSV causes plaques rapidly on cell monolayers), they are useful for studies on RNA tumor virus host range (which is specified by the envelope) and for detecting the presence of RNA tumor virus-specified envelope proteins, particularly in connection with the search for human tumor viruses (Chap. 8). Finally, VSV nucleocapsids can even be encased in herpesvirus envelopes. Nucleocapsids of one virus enclosed in envelopes specified by another are known as "pseudotypes." Viruses differ in their propensity to form pseudotypes; those that do so most readily are VSV and RNA tumor viruses.

Defective Virus Particles

There are several types of virus particles that cannot multiply on their own but can multiply in cells simultaneously infected with some infectious "helper" virus. They can be subdivided into two classes; those that interfere extensively with the multiplication of their helper virus, and those that do not.

Defective Interfering (DI) Virus Particles

When viruses are passaged repeatedly at high multiplicity, the progeny frequently includes, in addition to mature virus particles, defective virus particles that are capable of interfering with the multiplication of homologous virus. Such virus particles have the following properties: (1) they contain the normal structural capsid proteins, (2) they contain only a part of the viral genome—that is, they are de-

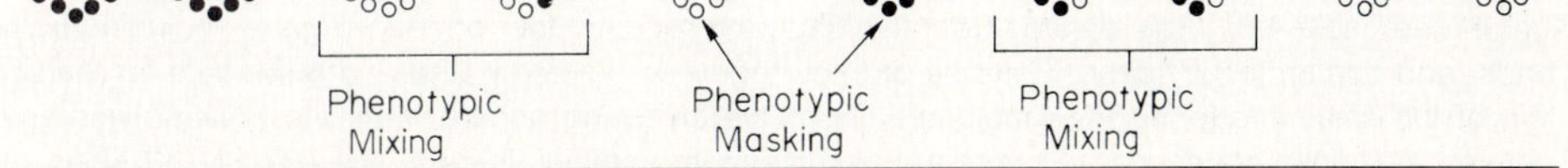

Figure 6-3. Phenotypic mixing and phenotypic masking. Simultaneous infection with two related viruses is illustrated. Either genome can be encapsidated in capsids that are composed exclusively of homologous capsomers or mixed capsomers (phenotypic mixing) or of exclusively heterologous capsomers (phenotypic masking). The method of detecting the latter two classes of particles is described in the text.

letion mutants, (3) they can reproduce only in cells infected with homologous virus, which acts as helper, (4) although unable to reproduce on their own, they can nevertheless express a variety of functions in the absence of helper, such as inhibition of host biosynthesis, transformation of cells, and synthesis of viral proteins, and (5) they specifically interfere with the multiplication of homologous virus.

The following are some examples of defective interfering virus particles that have been characterized in some detail.

Defective Interfering Influenza Virus Particles

Under conditions of repeated passaging at high multiplicity, the infectivity of successive yields of influenza virus gradually decreases a million-fold or even more, though the total number of virus particles that is produced remains roughly the same. In other words, noninfectious, defective virus particles gradually replace virions in the yields. This phenomenon was first described in 1952 by von Magnus and bears his name. Defective particles are not formed if influenza virus is passaged at low multiplicity, and they are readily eliminated from virus stocks by passaging at a multiplicity of less than 1, which shows that defective particles cannot multiply on their own. The ability of the defective particles to inhibit the multiplication of infectious virus is demonstrated by the fact that the addition of defective particles to influenza virus preparations free of them immediately reduces the yield of infectious virus in most types of cells.

The essential difference between infectious and defective influenza virus particles is that the latter have lost most of their three large RNA segments (Chap. 4) and acquired instead several new RNA segments that are smaller than the smallest segment of wild-type virus and that are derived from the three largest segments. The loss of infectivity is a consequence of the deletions; the ability to interfere with the multiplication of wild-type virus is due to the presence of the new small RNA segments. The nature of several small influenza interfering RNA species is shown in Figure 6-4. The mechanism of the interference and the reason that these deletion mutants compete successfully with wild-type virus are discussed below.

Defective Interfering Particles of Other Viruses

DI particles of such rhabdoviruses as VSV contain RNA that is about one-third as long as genome RNA. As a result, they are about one-third as long as infectious virus particles, which makes them very nearly spherical (Fig. 6-5). The interfering RNA molecules are, like those of influenza virus, the result of aberrant transcription: for rea-

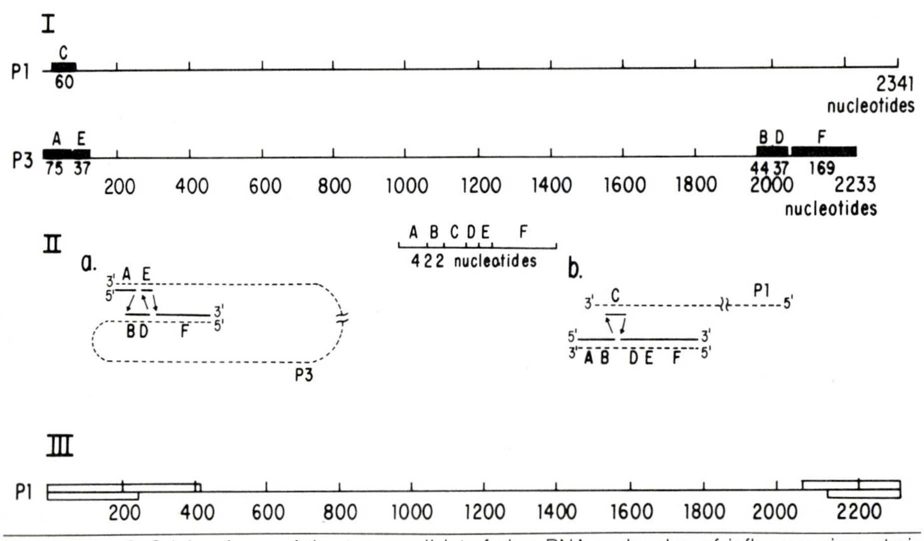

Figure 6-4. I. Origin of one of the two small interfering RNA molecules of influenza virus strain A/NT/60/68. It is 422 nucleotides long, a little less than one-half as long as the smallest influenza gene (see Table 4-5). It is derived from five separate regions, four on the *P3* gene, including both ends, and one on the *P1* gene. The size of each region is indicated. **II. a** and **b.** Models for the origin of the small interfering RNA molecule. Template switching occurs when the RNA polymerase pauses at U-rich sequences and reinitiates synthesis at another site. **III.** The A/WSN/33 strain of influenza virus gives rise to two different interfering RNA molecules; each is derived from gene *P1* via a single large deletion. The larger and smaller RNA species (composed of the two terminal sequences indicated above and below the gene, respectively) are 683 and 441 nucleotides long, respectively. Note that all small interfering influenza RNA molecules contain both ends of influenza virus genes. *(From Fields and Winter: Cell 28:303, 1982; Nayak et al.: Proc Natl Acad Sci USA 79: 2216, 1982.)*

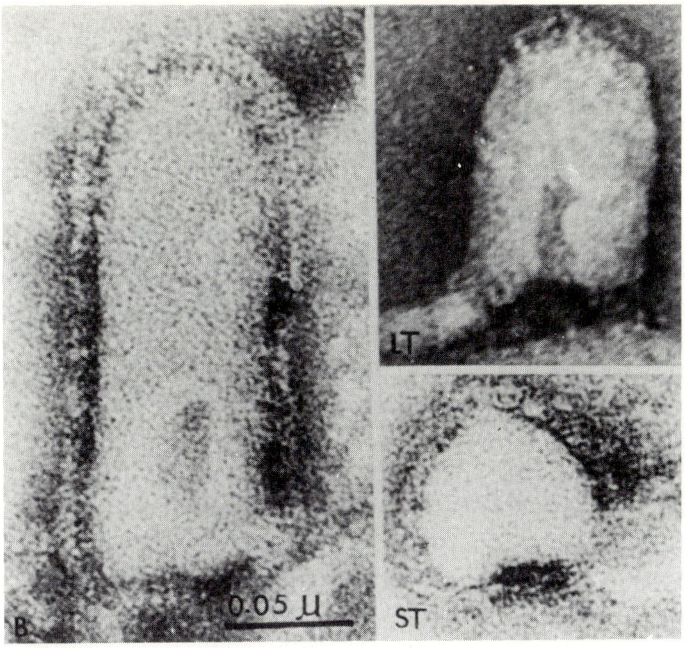

Figure 6-5. Defective interfering particles of VSV. B, a bullet-shaped normal virus particle; LT, a long truncated particle; ST, a short truncated particle. LT particles are about half as long as normal virus particles; ST particles, which are round, are about one-third as long. The defective particles contain RNA molecules that are proportionately shorter than the RNA molecules in normal virus particles. *(Courtesy of Dr C.Y. Kang.)*

sons that are poorly understood, the RNA polymerase suddenly switches transcription from one template sequence to another, causing deletions if reinitiation occurs downstream on the same template, or the synthesis of sequences complementary to portions of the strand being synthesized if reinitiation occurs on it. As a result, interfering VSV RNA molecules may possess either both ends of normal viral RNA or complementary copies of one end. The nature of small interfering VSV RNA molecules is shown in Figure 6-6. Small interfering RNA molecules of paramyxoviruses, such as Sendai virus, are quite similar.

DI particles of togaviruses, such as Semliki Forest virus and Sindbis virus, contain small interfering RNA molecules one-sixth to one-half as long as full-length RNA. They are generated by a mechanism in which template switching is carried to the nth degree. They tend to comprise a short region derived from one end of the genome, two or three tandemly arranged copies of regions 500 to 800 nucleotides long composed of regions transcribed from several portions of the viral genome, regions that may themselves be repeated, and a unique sequence derived from the other end of the viral genome. All regions from the 3′-terminal one-third of the viral genome, which comprises the structural togavirus genes (Chap. 4), are usually completely deleted. The generation of these molecules requires very extensive template switching, with the RNA polymerase disengaging from the template it is transcribing and, while remaining attached to the transcript that it is in the process of synthesizing, reinitiating transcription elsewhere on the same strand, either upsteam or downstream, or on a different strand, which may be the transcript to which it is attached.

DI particles also occur in high passage yields of polioviruses, reoviruses, bunyaviruses, herpesviruses such as pseudorabies virus, and probably most other viruses. All are deletion mutants that require the presence of wild-type virus as helpers but outgrow them quickly. DI polioviruses tend to be simple deletion mutants, the deletions being only 4 to 15 percent of the genome, and DI mutants of reovirus simply lack one or two genes.

General Observations on the Significance of DI Particles

The basic attributes of DI particles are that they outgrow infectious virus particles and that they interfere very successfully with the multiplication of wild-type virus. No doubt these two properties are connected. Small interfering RNA molecules are heterogeneous populations, but they must all possess two regions: the recognition site(s) for RNA polymerase and the recognition site(s) for encapsidation. Since these recognition sites are at the termini of viral RNAs, all small interfering RNAs contain at least one end of intact viral RNA. All available evidence indicates that small interfering RNAs are encapsidated and serve as template for RNA polymerase at least as efficiently as intact RNA, if not more so. Since, in addition, they are formed much more rapidly than intact RNA because they are smaller, very soon most RNA polymerase and encapsidation recognition sites will be on small interfering RNA molecules, not on intact RNA molecules. Interestingly, the host cell can influence profoundly both the extent to which DI particles are formed and their nature. Thus, a single clonal isolate of influenza virus or VSV will produce different types of small interfering RNA molecules in different cell types and will produce DI particles in different cell types after different numbers of passages (that is, at different passage levels). Sometimes DI particles are not

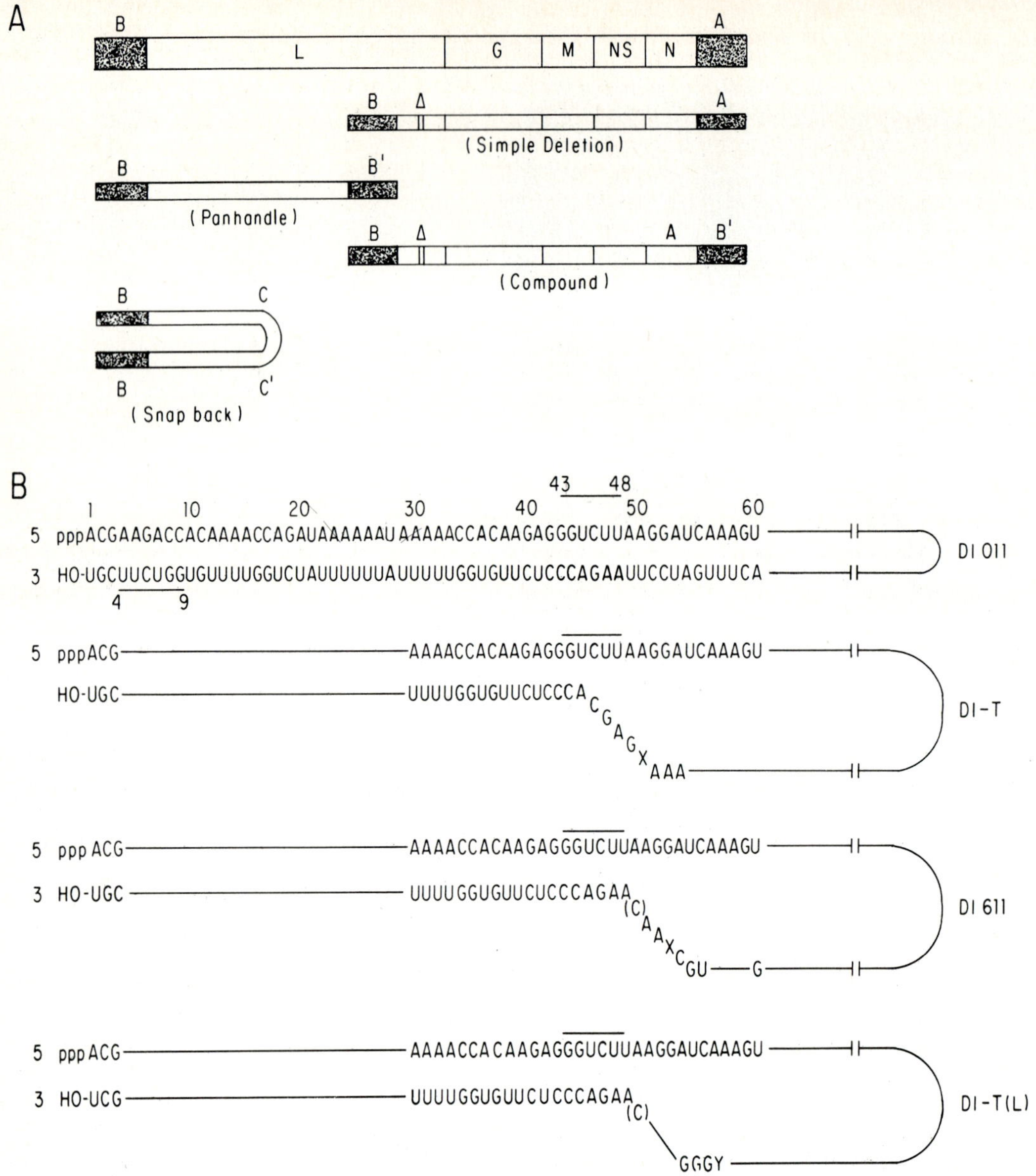

Figure 6-6. A. The nature of four types of small interfering RNAs of VSV. The structure of intact VSV RNA is shown at the top; *A* and *B* serve to identify the sequences at its two ends, and *L, G, M, NS,* and *N,* refer to the five VSV genes. The first interfering RNA is a simple deletion mutant, with most of the *L* gene deleted. Small interfering Sendai virus RNA molecules have been described in which genes *other* than the *L* gene are deleted (although some of the *L* gene is deleted also). To generate the second small interfering RNA, the RNA polymerase transcribes part of the *L* gene, then stops, reinitiates on the transcript that it is in the process of synthesizing about 45 nucleotides from the end, and transcribes it back to the end. B′ and B are complementary to each other. This process is described in more detail in **B.** Many panhandle molecules of this type are generated in which the length of the *L* gene sequences that are transcribed are all different, but the polymerase always starts transcribing backwards at the same position, where there is the sequence UUCUGG (overlined), which is also present near the 3′-end (underlined) and which is probably an RNA polymerase recognition sequence. Thus all RNA molecules of this type contain an identical panhandle and varying lengths of *L* gene sequences. The third type of small interfering RNA is a combination of the first and the second, while in the fourth the polymerase transcribes the *L* gene for a certain distance and then immediately transcribes it backwards, probably using as a template not the strand it is synthesizing but the strand that is being transcribed by the polymerase molecule immediately in front of it (note that one template can be transcribed by many RNA polymerase molecules at the same time). *(From Schubert et al.: Cell 18:749, 1979; Lazzarini et al.: Cell 26:145, 1981.)*

formed at all; for example, VSV will not form DI particles in cells treated with actinomycin D, which inhibits host cell transcription, or in cells simultaneously infected with fibroma virus. All this evidence suggests that host factors are required for the generation of DI particles, but whether they function in the *generation* of small interfering RNAs (by decreasing fidelity of transcription and/or promoting template switching) or by increasing the efficiency with which DI particles are formed is not known.

Finally, a word about the role of DI particles in the establishment and maintenance of persistent infections in nature. There is no question that persistent infections can be established readily in animals by infecting them with mixtures of infectious and DI particles and that DI particles are often present in persistently infected cells. However, it seems that, in general, persistent infections are caused by viral variants that are less cytopathogenic than wild-type virus. Often such variants are also temperature-sensitive with respect to the ability to grow, but they need not be so (Chap. 5). Perhaps the generation and propagation of DI particles is a mechanism for ensuring the survival of viruses by permitting them to establish persistent infections. If this is true, DI RNA should not only be smaller than wild-type RNA, possess higher affinity for RNA polymerase, and replicate more rapidly but should also preferably not code for structural viral proteins (so as to minimize cytopathic effects). Small interfering RNAs appear to fulfill all of these criteria.

Adenovirus and Papovavirus Deletion Mutants

When repeatedly passaged at high multiplicity, adenoviruses and papovaviruses give rise to a variety of deletion mutants, among which are the following:

1. Viable adenovirus deletion mutants. A sizable region of the adenovirus genome centered around map position 83 (in early transcription region 3) is not essential for the ability to replicate. Mutants that lack more than 2200 base pairs in this region have been isolated and are viable.
2. Adenovirus and papovavirus particles that contain DNA molecules that are almost the same size as the viral genome but comprise only a small fraction of it, the remainder being cellular DNA. These particles are called "evolutionary variants" because they evolve over the course of repeated passages from a variety of simple deletions or substitutions to more complex reiterations. Usually they acquire a selective growth advantage (but do not interfere significantly with the multiplication of wild-type virus) and become a significant fraction of the virus yield, and they require infectious virus as helper. Like the nucleic acids in DI particles, their DNA must contain recognition sites for the initiation of viral DNA replication and encapsidation. Extreme examples of adenovirus evolutionary variants are

   (a) one that contains only the leftmost 3 percent of the viral DNA and host DNA corresponding to 93 percent of the viral DNA and another that contains about 6 percent of each end of viral DNA and host DNA corresponding to 80 percent of the viral DNA, and
   (b) one that contains a deletion comprising only about 10 percent of the viral DNA that is partially substituted to the extent of about 3 percent by host DNA.

   Among extreme SV40 evolutionary variants is one with a DNA molecule that comprises a sequence of about 150 base pairs that includes the SV40 origin of replication and is repeated tandemly three times, linked to about 1500 base pairs of host cell DNA.

Adenovirus-SV40 Hybrid Particles

Human adenovirus cannot multiply in monkey cells but will do so in the presence of the simian papovavirus SV40, which performs some helper function related to the ability of viral messenger RNA to be translated. The progeny of such mixed infections sometimes includes particles that contain, within an adenovirus capsid, a hybrid DNA molecule that contains both adenovirus and SV40 DNA sequences but does not contain all the sequences of either. One well-known example of such particles is the E46+ strain of adenovirus serotype 7, which was generated during attempts to adapt human adenovirus to grow in monkey kidney cells for vaccine production. It turned out that the monkey kidney cells contained SV40, which recombined with the adenovirus type 7 to produce genomes that contain covalently linked sequences of both adenovirus and SV40 DNA. These genomes lack the adenovirus DNA sequences between map positions 5 and 21 and contain instead two SV40 DNA sequences joined end to end—namely, those between map positions 0.50 and 0.71 and between 0.11 and 0.66. These particles cannot, of course, multiply on their own, since they contain neither a complete adenovirus genome nor a complete SV40 genome, but they can perform that function that enables human adenoviruses to multiply in monkey cells. They are, therefore, called "PARA" (particles aiding the replication of adenovirus). Further, they can themselves multiply in the presence of the human adenovirus, which presumably supplies the function(s) coded by the piece of adenovirus DNA that is missing in the hybrid particle DNA. Thus, here are two types of virus particles, human adenovirus and hybrid PARA particle, neither of which can multiply in monkey cells by itself but both of which multiply if they infect monkey cells simultaneously. The significance of this system is that viruses that can multiply only in cells also harboring other viruses may be of great importance in causing human diseases of as yet undefined etiology. These situations are very difficult to detect, but detailed studies such as those described above may provide valuable clues in the search for others of clinical relevance. Another interesting class of adenovirus-SV40 hybrids is the infectious adenovirus type 2-SV40 hybrids, five of which have been characterized in detail (Table 6-1). In these hybrids, a portion of the adenovirus genome is deleted from a region that is not essential for virus multiplication. This region comprises 4 to 7 percent of the adenovirus genome and ends at map position 86 in all hybrids (see above). In its place is inserted a portion of SV40 DNA that codes for early functions. This portion varies from 7 to 43 percent of the SV40 genome and starts at map position 0.11 in all five hybrids. The largest piece (43 percent) of SV40 DNA expresses all early SV40 functions, while the smallest piece (7 percent) can code for no more than 10,000 to 15,000 daltons of protein. Yet this is sufficient to endow even this hybrid with the ability to multiply in monkey cells.

Interference Between Viruses

It has been known for a long time that when two different viruses infect the same cell, they may interfere with each other and diminish each other's yield. Although the precise nature of the inhibition is usually not known, it appears that there are two primary causes of interference. First, the first virus may inhibit the ability of the second virus to adsorb, either by blocking its receptors (certain pairs of enteroviruses) or by destroying its receptors (certain pairs of myxoviruses). Second, one virus may prevent the messenger RNA of the second virus from being translated. Thus, just as poliovirus inhibits the translation of host-cell messenger RNA by inactivating the cap-dependent mRNA recognition mechanism (Chap. 5), so does it inhibit the translation of VSV messenger RNA and interfere with the ability of VSV to multiply. Similarly, the translation of vaccinia virus messenger RNA is prevented in cells infected with adenoviruses. The ability of Sindbis virus to interfere with the multiplication of VSV and NDV and of rubella virus to interfere with the multiplication of NDV may also be due to interference with the ability of viral messenger RNA to be translated. This mechanism of interference would account for the marked specificity of such inhibitory effects. Thus, whereas cells infected with rubella virus become resistant to NDV, they remain susceptible to a variety of other viruses.

Yet another mechanism may operate in cells infected with VSV and herpesvirus. VSV inhibits host cell protein synthesis by inhibiting transcription; herpesvirus inhibits host cell protein synthesis by causing polyribosomes to dissociate (an effect of a capsid protein) and host cell messenger RNA to be degraded (a function of an early herpesvirus protein). In cells infected with both these viruses, VSV is dominant, as it inhibits herpesvirus transcription. In cells infected with both herpesvirus and adenovirus, however, transcription of adenovirus messenger RNAs is inhibited, a function, apparently, of yet another early herpesvirus protein.

Studies that are directed specifically at determining how certain pairs of viruses interfere with each other's ability to multiply may possess great potential for defining how viruses interfere with host cell protein and RNA and DNA synthesis (Chap. 5).

Evolution of Viruses

The advent of recombinant DNA technology and the development of rapid nucleic acid sequencing techniques during the last decade have yielded a rapidly increasing body of information concerning the genetic relationship between and the relatedness of virus strains that circulate in natural host populations. They have also provided insight into the process of viral evolution. For example, there are three serotypes of mammalian reovirus, two of which, serotypes 1 and 3, are related to the extent of about 70 percent, while serotype 2 is related to the other

TABLE 6-1. NONDEFECTIVE ADENOVIRUS TYPE 2-SV40 HYBRIDS

	Portion of Adenovirus DNA Deleted		Portion of SV40 DNA Inserted	
Hybrid	Map Position*	Mol Wt	Map Position	Mol Wt
$Ad2^+ ND_1$	80.6–86.0	1.24×10^6	0.11–0.39	0.58×10^6
$Ad2^+ ND_2$	79.9–86.0	1.40×10^6	0.11–0.43	1.02×10^6
$Ad2^+ ND_3$	80.7–86.0	1.22×10^6	0.11–0.18	0.22×10^6
$Ad2^+ ND_4$	81.5–86.0	1.04×10^6	0.11–0.54	1.38×10^6
$Ad2^+ ND_5$	78.9–86.0	1.63×10^6	0.11–0.39	0.90×10^6

*According to convention, the adenovirus and SV40 maps are referred to as being 100 and 1.00 map units long, respectively.

two to the extent of only about 10 percent. Interestingly, the antigenic determinants on the proteins specified by most of their genes have been highly conserved during evolution, as demonstrated by the fact that antisera against any one serotype cannot readily differentiate between the proteins encoded by any of the three serotypes, even the distantly related (in genetic terms) serotype 2. The only exception is provided by the proteins encoded by the *S1* gene; the three *S1* genes are related only about one-quarter as closely as the other genes. Thus, we have an ancestral set of genes that diverged along three pathways to yield three gene pools, two closely and one by now only slightly related, and nine of the ten genes evolved more or less together, while the tenth diverged markedly.

This type of analysis is also applicable to viruses of other families, particularly influenza viruses. Influenza viruses, particularly influenza A viruses, exhibit a large degree of antigenic variation. Minor antigenic variants cause new epidemics every 1 or 2 years, and major antigenic variants cause new pandemics every 10 to 15 years. The marked degree of antigenic variation of influenza viruses, that is, their rapid evolution, cannot be explained by an enhanced capacity to produce mutant viruses, for the frequencies with which antigenic variants in Sendai virus, VSV, and influenza A virus arise are about the same, namely, $10^{-4.5}$ to $10^{-4.7}$. Rather, it is due to the fact that many antigenic variants of the two influenza spike proteins, the neuraminidase and especially the hemagglutinin, are functional, presumably because they are not structural proteins in the sense of having to fit into a capsid structure. It is also due to the fact that influenza A virus is a ubiquitous virus to which humans are constantly exposed, so that new antigenic variants are constantly being selected by an immune system that has multiple prior experiences with previously encountered variants.

Antigenic variation of influenza A virus is of two types. The first is antigenic drift, minor antigenic changes that occur continuously in partially immune host populations during intrapandemic periods and that sporadically lead to the emergence of new epidemic virus strains. These minor antigenic changes are caused by the selective growth advantage that new antigenic variants possess in the presence of antibodies capable of neutralizing the previous, parental virus strains. The second type of antigenic variation is antigenic shift, the emergence of new major antigenic variants, primarily in the hemagglutinin (H) but also to a lesser extent in the neuraminidase (N). These new antigenic variants are genetic reassortants that are generated when an *H* or an *N* gene from an influenza virus of some animal species is introduced into the gene set of an influenza virus pathogenic for humans. For example, the *H3* gene of the Hong Kong strain of human influenza A virus that emerged in 1968 and that caused the most recent human pandemic was probably derived from an equine or a duck influenza virus strain. Both equine and duck influenza virus A strains contain *H3* genes that are very closely related to that now present in human H3N2 influenza virus strains (Chap. 5).

Mapping of Genomes of Animal Viruses

The basic aims of virologists are (1) to characterize the various functions involved in virus multiplication and (2) to identify the portions of the viral genome that encode these functions. The first of these aims depends primarily on the availability of mutants. As pointed out above, mutants permit the virus multiplication cycle to be examined when one of its component reactions fails to function. These reactions can, therefore, be identified and characterized one by one.

Great strides have recently been made in mapping animal virus genomes, that is, in identifying the regions or genes that encode specific proteins. A brief summary follows of the techniques that are most useful for mapping the genes of DNA- and RNA-containing viruses.

DNA-containing Viruses

1. Recombination analysis. This has been described on page 70.
2. Restriction endonuclease analysis of the DNA of recombinants of pairs of mutants in different genes, using related viruses. This was described in Figure 4-10.
3. Marker rescue. Cells are infected with a ts mutant together with individual restriction endonuclease fragments of wild-type virus DNA. The fragments will recombine with the mutant genome, generating a wild-type recombinant if they contain the gene, or portion of the gene, that contained the original mutation. If the location on the genome of the restriction endonuclease fragment is known, the location of the mutated gene is known.
4. Virus-coded messenger RNAs can be isolated from infected cells and translated in cell-free protein-synthesizing systems, and the proteins for which they code identified. Since the origin of these messenger RNAs can be specified by determining with which restriction endonuclease fragment they can hybridize, the regions of the viral genomes that code for specific viral proteins can be identified. Another version of this analysis is described on page 69.

RNA-containing Viruses

The gene order on viral genomes that consist of RNA can be identified as follows.

UV-transcriptional Mapping

UV irradiation damages RNA (page 106) and inactivates it as a template for transcription. Since transcription of such viral RNA as paramyxovirus and rhabdovirus RNA is initiated from a single site (at its 3′ terminus), the effect of irradiation is to interfere differentially with the transcription of the various genes; transcription of those farthest from the transcription initiation site is inhibited most, while transcription of those closest to it is inhibited least. Since the relative amount of each species of messenger RNA that is transcribed can be determined readily by measuring the amount of protein that is translated from it, the gene order can be determined (Chap. 4).

Pactamycin Translation Inhibition Mapping

This technique is capable of mapping the gene order of viral genomes that act as messenger RNAs (such as the genomes of picornaviruses). The technique depends on the fact that these genomes are multigenic but monocistronic, that is, there is a single site (at their 5′ terminus) where translation is initiated, but it comprises several cistrons (genes), the RNA being translated into a large precursor protein, the polyprotein, which is then cleaved into the various functional proteins (Chap. 4). Pactamycin inhibits initiation of translation but not elongation. Thus, if pactamycin is added to infected cells and a radioactively labeled amino acid is then added at various times thereafter, its incorporation into the region of polyprotein closest to the 5′ end will be inhibited first, and its incorporation into the region of the polyprotein that is furthest from the 5′ end will be inhibited last. It has been found in this way that the 5′ terminal half of poliovirus RNA codes for the structural proteins, while the 3′ terminal half codes for nonstructural proteins, such as the polymerase.

Identification of Genes in Segmented Genomes

Identification of the genes of reovirus and influenza virus can be accomplished in two ways. The first is the direct one: it is possible to translate the individual RNA species in cell-free protein-synthesizing systems and to identify the proteins for which they code. The second way takes advantage of the fact that the individual RNA and protein species of different serotypes of reovirus and influenza virus can be identified because they possess different migration rates when electrophoresced in polyacrylamide gels (Fig. 6-7). By crossing pairs of virus strains that belong to different serotypes and examining the RNA and protein patterns of the reassortants that are produced, one can determine which RNA segment codes for each individual protein. In the simplest case, one would look for recombinants in which all RNA segments except one are derived from one parent. Then there would be one, and only one, protein that would be characteristic of the other parent. This technique also permits ts mutations to be assigned to RNA segments. To do this, ts mutants of one serotype are crossed with the wild-type strain of another serotype, progeny are then plaqued at the restrictive (normal) temperature, and the pattern of RNA segments of several

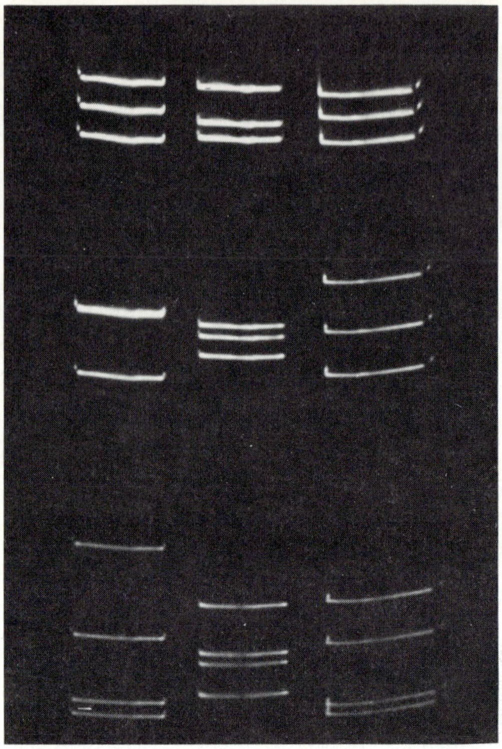

Figure 6-7. Separation by electrophoresis in polyacrylamide gels (Maizel Tris-glycine system) of the 10 double-stranded RNA-containing genes of reovirus serotype 3, 2, and 1. Note that two genes in the reovirus serotype 3 genome overlap in this system (but can be readily separated in others). The cognate segments differ slightly but significantly in electrophoretic mobility and can therefore be identified. Similar patterns are obtained if the protein species of these strains are compared by electrophoresis in SDS-containing polyacrylamide gels. *(Courtesy of Dr. R. Gaillard.)*

plaque isolates is then examined by polyacrylamide gel electrophoresis. Since recombination in reovirus and influenza virus occurs by random assortment of RNA segments (p. 105), one would expect that all RNA segments would be randomly derived from either one parent or the other, except one—namely, that which bears the ts lesion. That segment will always be derived from the wild-type parent.

FURTHER READING

Books and Reviews

Boettiger D: Animal virus pseudotypes. Prog Med Virol 25:37, 1979

Bratt MA, Hightower LE: Genetics and paragenetic phenomena of paramyxoviruses. In Fraenkel-Conrat H, Wagner RR (eds): Comprehensive Virology. New York, Plenum, 1977, vol 9, p 457

Cooper PD: Genetics of picornaviruses. In Fraenkel-Conrat H, Wagner RR (eds): Comprehensive Virology. New York, Plenum, 1977, vol 9, p 133

Fields BN: Genetics of reovirus. Curr Top Microbiol Immunol 91:1, 1981

Gorman BM: Variation in orbiviruses. J Gen Virol 44:1, 1979

Halliburton IW: Intertypic recombinants of herpes simplex viruses. J Gen Virol 48:1, 1980

Holland J. Spindler J, Horodyski F, et al.: Rapid evolution of RNA genomes. Science 215:1577, 1982

Lazzarini RA, Keene JD, Schubert M: The origins of defective interfering particles of negative-strand RNA viruses. Cell 26:145, 1981

Nayak DP: Defective interfering influenza viruses. Annu Rev Microbiol 34:619, 1980

Palese P, Young JF: Variation of influenza virus A, B and C viruses. Science 215:1468, 1982

Patch CT, Levine AS, Lewis AM Jr: The adenovirus-SV40 hybrid viruses. In Fraenkel-Conrat H, Wagner RR (eds): Comprehensive Virology. New York, Plenum, 1979, vol 13, p 459

Pfefferkorn ER: Genetics of togaviruses. In Fraenkel-Conrat H, Wagner RR (eds): Comprehensive Virology. New York, Plenum, 1977, vol 9, p 209

Pringle CR: The genetics of vesiculoviruses. Arch Virol 72:1, 1982

Reanney DC: The evolution of RNA viruses. Annu Rev Microbiol 36:47, 1982

Sambrook J, Sleigh M, Engler JA, et al.: The evolution of the adenoviral genome. Ann NY Acad Sci 354:426, 1980

Webster RG, Laver WG, Air GM, et al.: Molecular mechanisms of variation in influenza viruses. Nature 296:115, 1982

Selected Papers

MUTANTS, VARIANTS, AND RECOMBINANTS

Desselberger U, Nakajima K, Alfina P, et al.: Biochemical evidence that "new" influenza virus strains in nature may arise by recombination (reassortment). Proc Natl Acad Sci USA 75:3341, 1978

Drayna A, Fields BN: Genetic and biochemical studies on the mechanism of chemical and physical inactivation of reovirus. J Gen Virol 63:149, 161, 1982

Dubbs DR, Kit S: Isolation and properties of vaccinia mutants deficient in thymidine kinase inducing activity. Virology 22:214, 1964

Gaillard RK Jr, Joklik WK: Quantitation of the relatedness of reovirus serotypes 1, 2, and 3 at the gene level. Virology 123:152, 1982

Hinshaw VS, Webster RG, Bean WJ: Swine influenza-like viruses in turkeys: Potential source of virus for humans? Science 220:206, 1983

Klessig DF, Hassel JA: Characterization of a variant of human adenovirus type 2 which multiplies efficiently in simian cells. J Virol 28:945, 1978

Larsen SH: Evolutionary variants of mouse adenovirus containing cellular DNA sequences. Virology 116:573, 1982

Laver WG, Air GM, Webster RG, et al.: Amino acid sequence changes in antigenic variants of type A influenza virus N2 neuraminidase. Virology 122:450, 1982

Lee TNH, Nathans D: Evolutionary variants of simian virus 40: Replication and encapsidation of variant DNA. Virology 92:291, 1979

Portner A, Webster RG, Bean WJ: Similar frequencies of antigenic variants in Sendai, vesicular stomatitis, and influenza A viruses. Virology 104:235, 1980

Ramig RF, Ahmeed R, Fields BN: A genetic map of reovirus: Assignment of the newly defined mutant groups H, I, and J to genome segments. Virology 125:299, 1983

Sambrook JF, Padgett BL, Tomkins JKN: Conditional lethal mutants of rabbitpox virus. 1. Isolation of host-cell dependent and temperature-dependent mutants. Virology 25:592, 1966

Schuerch AR, Matsuhisa T, Joklik WK: Temperature-sensitive mutants of reovirus. VI. Mutant ts447 and ts556 particles that lack either one or two genome RNA segments. Intervirology 3:36, 1974

Smith GL, Mackett M, Moss B: Infectious vaccinia virus recombinants that express hepatitis B virus surface antigen. Nature 302:490, 1983

Werner G, zur Hausen H: Deletions and insertions in adenovirus type 12 DNA after viral replication in vero cells. Virology 86:66, 1978

NONGENETIC INTERACTIONS AMONG VIRUSES

Chen C, Crouch NA: Shope fibroma virus induced facilitation of vesicular stomatitis virus adsorption and replication in nonpermissive cells. Virology 85:43, 1978

Choppin PW, Compans RW: Phenotypic mixing of envelope proteins of the parainfluenza virus SV5 and vesicular stomatitis virus. J Virol 5:609, 1970

Huang AS, Palma El, Hewlett N, et al.: Pseudotype formation between enveloped RNA and DNA viruses. Nature 252:743, 1974

Joklik WK, Abel P, Holmes IH: Reactivation of poxviruses by a nongenetic mechanism. Nature 186:992, 1960

Joklik WK, Woodroofe GM, Holmes IH, et al.: The reactivation of poxviruses. I. The demonstration of the phenomenon and techniques of assay. Virology 11:168, 1960

Trautman R, Sutmoller P: Detection and properties of a genomic masked viral particle consisting of foot-and-mouth disease virus nucleic acid in bovine enterovirus protein capsid. Virology 44:537, 1971

Zavadova Z, Zavada J: Unilateral phenotypic mixing of envelope antigens between togaviruses and vesicular stomatitis virus or avian RNA tumor virus. J Gen Virol 37:557, 1977

GENE MAPPING

Ball A: Transcriptional mapping of vesicular stomatitis virus in vivo. J Virol 21:411, 1977

Frost E, Williams J: Mapping temperature-sensitive and host-range mutations of adenovirus type 5 by marker rescue. Virology 91:39, 1978

Greenberg HB, Flores J, Kalica AR, et al.: Gene coding assignments for growth restriction, neutralization and subgroup specificities of the W and DS-1 strains of human rotavirus. J Gen Virol 64:313, 1983

Halliburton IW, Morse LS, Roizman B, et al.: Mapping of the thymidine kinase genes of type 1 and type 2 herpes simplex viruses using intertypic recombinants. J Gen Virol 49:235, 1980

Mustoe TA, Ramig RF, Sharpe AH, et al.: A Genetic map of reovirus. III. Assignment of the double-stranded RNA-positive mutant groups A, B, and G to genome segments. Virology 85:545, 1978

Palese P, Ritchey MB, Schulman JL: Mapping of the influenza virus genome. II. Identification of the P1, P2, and P3 genes. Virology 76:114, 1977

Ramig, RF, Fields BN: Revertants of temperature-sensitive mutants of reovirus: Evidence for frequent extragenic suppression. Virology 92:155, 1979

Wilson MC, Fraser NW, Darnell JE Jr: Mapping of RNA initiation sites by high doses of UV irradiation: Evidence for three independent promoters within the left 11% of the Ad-2-genome. Virology 94:175, 1979

DEFECTIVE AND DEFECTIVE INTERFERING VIRUS PARTICLES

Amesse LS, Pridgen CL, Kingsbury DW: Sendai virus DI RNA species with conserved virus genome termini and extensive internal deletions. Virology 118:17, 1982

Ben-Porat T, Demarchi JM, Kaplan AS: Characterization of defective interfering viral particles present in a population of pseudorabies virions. Virology 61:29, 1974

Fields S, Winter G: Nucleotide sequences of influenza virus segments 1 and 3 reveal mosaic structure of a small viral RNA segment. Cell 28:303, 1982

Huang AS, Greenawalt JW, Wagner RR: Defective T particles of vesicular stomatitis virus. Virology 30:161, 173, 1966

Huang AS, Baltimore D: Defective viral particles and viral disease processes. Nature 226:325, 1970

Lehtovaara P, Söderlund H, Keränen S, et al.: Extreme ends of the genome are conserved and rearranged in the defective interfering RNAs of Semliki Forest virus. J Mol Biol 156:731, 1982

McClure MA, Holland JJ, Perrault J: Generation of defective interfering particles in picornaviruses. Virology 100:408, 1980

Nayak DP, Sivasubramanian N, Davis AR, et al.: Complete sequence analyses show that two defective interfering influenza viral RNAs contain a single internal deletion of a polymerase gene. Proc Natl Acad Sci USA 79:2216, 1982

Nomoto A, Jacobson A, Lee YF, et al.: Defective interfering particles of poliovirus; mapping of the deletion and evidence that the deletions in the genomes of DI(1), (2), and (3) are located in the same region. J Mol Biol 128:179, 1979

Schubert M, Keene JD, Lazzarini RA: A specific internal RNA polymerase recognition site of VSV RNA is involved in the generation of DI particles. Cell 18:749, 1979

Sivasubramanian N, Nayak DP: Defective interfering influenza RNAs of polymerase gene 3 contain single as well as multiple internal deletions. Virology 124:232, 1983

Winship TR, Thacore HR: Inhibition of vesicular stomatitis virus-defective interfering particle synthesis by Shope fibroma virus. Virology 93:515, 1979

INTERFERENCE BETWEEN VIRUSES

Aubertin A, Guir J, Kirn A: The inhibition of vaccinia virus DNA synthesis in KB cells infected with frog virus 3. J Gen Virol 8:105, 1970

Dubovi EJ, Youngner JS: Inhibition of pseudorabies virus replication by vesicular stomatitis viruses. J Virol 18:526, 1976

Ehrenfeld E, Lund H: Untranslated vesicular stomatitis virus messenger RNA after poliovirus infection. Virology 80:297, 1977

Hunt JM, Marcus PI: Mechanism of Sindbis virus-induced intrinsic interference with vesicular stomatitis virus replication. J Virol 14:99, 1974

Marcus PI, Carver DH: Intrinsic interference; a new type of viral interference. J Virol 1:334, 1967

CHAPTER 7

Antiviral Chemotherapy, Interferon, and Vaccines

Rational Approach to Antiviral Chemotherapy

Virus multiplication consists of the synthesis of viral nucleic acids and proteins and their assembly into virus particles. A rational approach to antiviral chemotherapy should examine whether and where these processes can best be interrupted without detriment to the host. The following is a relevant brief analysis.

Replication of Viral Nucleic Acids

The replication of the nucleic acids of many viruses is catalyzed by enzymes that do not exist in uninfected cells. This is true for all RNA-containing viruses, as well as for poxviruses, herpesviruses, and adenoviruses. It should be possible to isolate and characterize these enzymes and find specific inhibitors for them.

Synthesis of Viral Proteins

Several lines of evidence suggest that viral messenger RNAs differ in some fundamental way from host messenger RNAs. Viral messenger RNAs are generally translated in preference to host cell messenger RNAs. Furthermore, translation to host messenger RNAs often ceases entirely several hours after infection, when translation of viral messenger RNAs proceeds rapidly and extensively. This suggests that viral messenger RNAs differ in some recognizable manner from host messenger RNAs, and this difference should be exploitable. In fact, two antiviral agents, isatin-β-thiosemicarbazone and interferon, act by preventing viral messenger RNAs from being translated. A promising avenue of approach, therefore, is analysis of the features in which viral messenger RNAs differ from host cell messenger RNAs.

Viral Morphogenesis

Viral morphogenesis proceeds at several levels. Many viral capsid proteins are now known to be synthesized in the form of precursors that are cleaved to furnish the actual proteins used for the formation of virus particles. The nature of the enzymes that cleave these precursors is not known. It may be fruitful to characterize them and design inhibitors for them. In fact, recent experiments indicate that peptide analogs of amino acid sequences in the regions where viral proteins are cleaved possess antiviral activity.

No means of specifically inhibiting the assembly of virus particles exists. It may be possible to prevent budding when more is known about the properties of cell membranes, but it seems that cell membranes are such important organs that it may be unwise to attempt to prevent virus particle formation at this stage. By the same token, inhibition of the uptake and penetration of virus particles at the beginning of the multiplication cycle has not been attempted seriously. As will be discussed below, the drug α-adamantanamine does inhibit the uptake of certain myxoviruses, but it does not do so by directly affecting the functioning of the cell membrane. In summary, the two most promising avenues of approach for specifically inhibiting virus multiplication are inhibition of viral genome replicases and exploitation of the differences between viral and host cell messenger RNAs.

Mode of Action of Certain Antiviral Chemotherapeutic Agents

An appreciable number of compounds inhibit virus multiplication very efficiently in cultured cells and have no adverse effect on the growth of uninfected cells. Unfortunately, many of these compounds either inhibit virus multiplication in the body much less efficiently or have unacceptable toxic side effects. They are therefore not suitable for antiviral chemotherapy in man. However, clinical trials currently underway have revealed several compounds of great promise. Most of them act via one of the mechanisms discussed above.

Before considering individually the mode of action of successful and promising antiviral agents, it is well to examine which viral pathogens of humans present the most suitable targets for chemotherapy at the present time. It is reassuring to note that the incidence of many severe virus-caused diseases, such as smallpox, poliomyelitis, yellow fever, and measles, has decreased dramatically in recent decades, owing to the success of vaccination campaigns. Other important virus-caused diseases fall into two classes. First, there are those that, although severe and life-threatening, are rare in most parts of the world; such diseases are rabies, the encephalitides, and the African and South American hemorrhagic fevers (Marburg disease, Ebola fever, Lassa fever, and Machupo). Second, there are diseases that are usually no more than mild to moderate but may become life-threatening; such diseases are caused by influenza virus and the various herpesviruses. In fact, herpesviruses may well be regarded as the primary targets for antiviral chemotherapy at this time, closely followed by influenza virus and the rare severe diseases mentioned above.

Isatin-β-thiosemicarbazone (IBT)

IBT is a potent inhibitor of poxvirus multiplication (Fig. 7-1). At a concentration of 3 mg per liter, it inhibits vaccinia virus multiplication in cultured cells by over 90 percent without having any detectable effect on the host cells themselves. In the presence of IBT, the early period of the poxvirus multiplication cycle, viral DNA replication, and transcription of late messenger RNA all proceed normally. However, the translation of late messenger RNA is inhibited. The synthesis of late proteins, which include most of the viral capsid proteins, is therefore prevented, and no progeny virus particles are formed.

A derivative of IBT, N-methyl-IBT (Marburan), was administered by mouth to known smallpox contacts in field trials in India and Pakistan, and beneficial results of this prophylactic treatment were observed.

2-Hydroxybenzylbenzimidazole (HBB) and Guanidine

These two reagents (Fig. 7-2) inhibit the multiplication of many picornaviruses, such as poliovirus, echoviruses, Coxsackie viruses, and foot-and-mouth disease virus. They are examples of reagents that interfere with the replication of viral RNA, either by preventing initiation of the synthesis of progeny plus strands or by preventing progeny plus strands from separating from the replicative form-replicase complex (Chap. 4). The precise manner in which this is accomplished is not known. Although both drug-resistant and drug-dependent virus mutants quickly emerge, HBB has been used with some success in controlling enterovirus infections in animals.

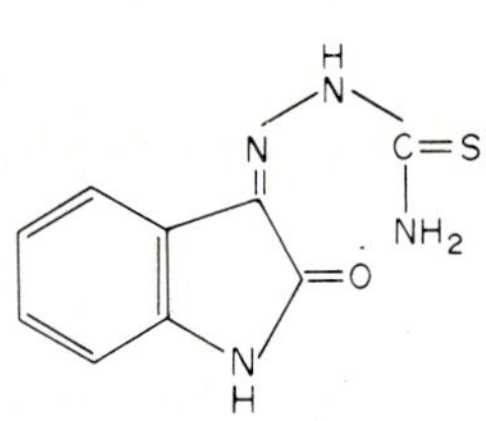

Figure 7-1. Isatin-β-thiosemicarbazone (IBT).

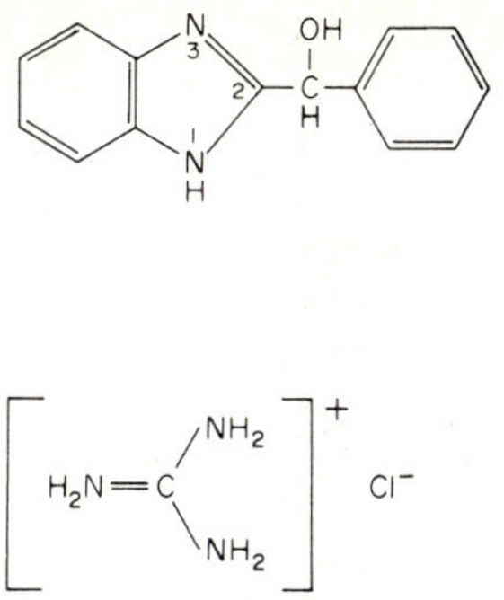

Figure 7-2. 2-Hydroxybenzylbenzimidazole (HBB) and guanidine hydrochloride.

Rifampin

Rifampin and related rifamycin derivatives bind to bacterial RNA polymerases, thereby preventing the initiation of transcription. Rifampin does not bind to animal RNA polymerases, but it does inhibit the multiplication of poxviruses and adenoviruses. The mechanism by which it achieves this has been studied most intensively in vaccinia virus-infected cells. Inhibition of viral RNA polymerase is not involved, since both early and late messenger RNAs are transcribed normally. Rather, the mechanism involves some event in viral morphogenesis, for in the presence of the drug immature virus particles of the type illustrated in Figure 4-25 accumulate. The specific nature of the step that is inhibited is not known. However, it is clear that it involves a diffusible product, most probably a protein, since wild-type virus sensitive to rifampin matures normally in its presence in cells simultaneously infected with mutants resistant to it. Presumably the mutants code for a protein that is unaffected by the drug and can thus function when the normal wild-type protein cannot. As a result, resistant mutants rescue sensitive virus.

Although rifampin does not inhibit the vaccinia DNA-dependent RNA polymerase, the RNA-dependent DNA polymerase of RNA tumor viruses (the reverse transcriptase, Chap. 8) is very sensitive to it and to certain of its derivatives.

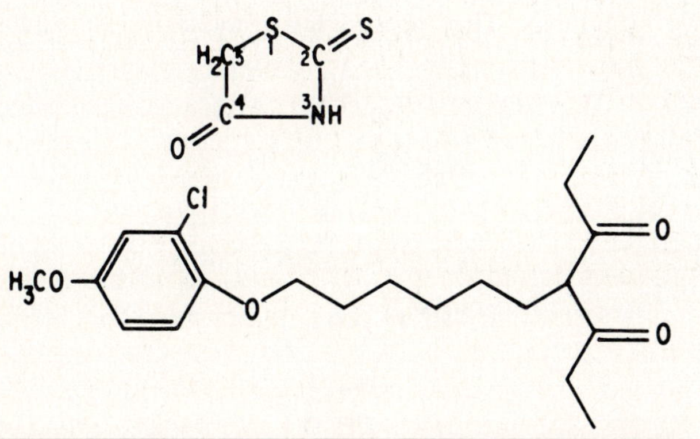

Figure 7-3. Top. Rhodanine (2-thio-4-oxothiazol idine). **Bottom.** Arildone (4-[6-(2-chloro-4-methoxyphenoxyl)hexyl]-3,5-heptanedione).

Arildone and Rhodanine

Arildone (4-[6-(2-chloro-4-methoxyphenoxy)hexyl]-3,5-heptanedione) and rhodanine (2-thio-4-oxothiazolidine) (Fig. 7-3) inhibit the uncoating of poliovirus and Echovirus 12, respectively. Neither drug affects adsorption or penetration, but both interact with the capsids of these viruses, increasing their stability to such an extent that active virus can be recovered from cells 4 hours after infection with treated virus. The mechanism by which arildone and rhodanine increase the stability of poliovirus and Echovirus capsids is not known.

α-Adamantanamine

α-Adamantanamine (Amantadine, Symmetrel) (Fig. 7-4), a substance with a remarkably rigid structure, inhibits an early event in the multiplication cycle of influenza virus (and also of arenaviruses). It does not inhibit adsorption and penetration but completely inhibits primary transcription. It is thought, therefore, that it inhibits uncoating. Drug-resistant mutants exist, which are mutants in the M protein gene. It is conceivable, therefore, that the drug interacts with the M protein.

On the basis of large-scale trials that demonstrated that it had a significant prophylactic effect, α-adamantanamine has been recommended for the prevention of disease caused by influenza virus type A. It has been used extensively in the Soviet Union and is presently the only drug for virus respiratory disease that is licensed in the United States. However, it is not used extensively in this country because it seems impractical to control, through chemoprophylaxis, a disease that is generally mild and that the individual patient has a good chance of avoiding anyway. As for the problem of protecting individuals at high risk and in whom the disease may be potentially dangerous, there is a choice between this drug and the influenza vaccine (p. 125). At least at this time, the vaccine would seem to be preferred.

Phosphonoacetic Acid (PAA)

Phosphonoacetic acid (Fig. 7-5) is a potent inhibitor of herpesvirus-coded DNA polymerase but not of cellular DNA polymerases. Unfortunately it has undesirable side effects, and drug-resistant mutants emerge rapidly. It is conceivable that modification of the structure of this drug will yield compounds to which resistance will develop less readily and that will be less toxic. The closely related

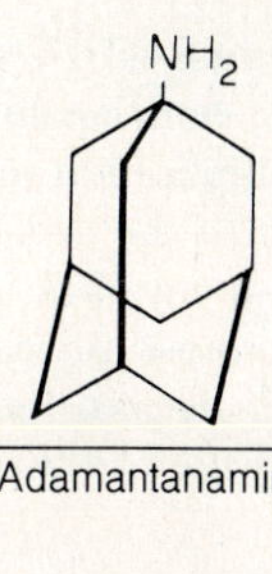

Figure 7-4. α-Adamantanamine (Amantadine).

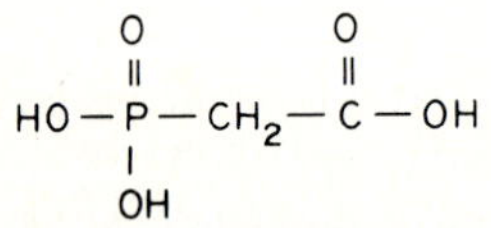

Figure 7-5. Phosphonoacetic acid (PAA).

phosphonoformic acid is also an inhibitor of herpesvirus DNA polymerase and is effective in treating cutaneous herpes simplex virus infections in guinea pigs.

Analogs of Ribonucleosides and Deoxyribonucleosides

The agents that have been discussed so far inhibit virus multiplication very well in cultured cells, but only IBT and α-adamantanamine are suitable antiviral agents in humans. The class of compounds that appears to have the greatest potential for antiviral chemotherapy in humans is the analogs of ribo- and deoxyribonucleosides. These substances consist of nucleic acid bases or derivatives of them, linked to either ribose or analogs of ribose.

The mechanism of action of these compounds is twofold. First, all become phosphorylated to mono-, di-, and triphosphates, the final precursors of nucleic acids. The analog-containing phosphorylated nucleosides may inhibit to a greater or lesser extent the various enzymes on the nucleic acid biosynthetic pathway and interfere competitively with the metabolism of normal phosphorylated nucleosides; indeed, many of the analogs of ribo- and deoxyribonucleosides with antiviral activity were designed and first tested as anticancer agents. Their importance as antiviral agents lies in the fact that if the virus that is to be inhibited codes for its own enzyme(s) on the nucleic acid biosynthetic pathway, such as a deoxyribonucleoside kinase or a DNA polymerase, this enzyme may be inhibited to a greater extent by the analog-containing phosphorylated nucleosides than the corresponding host cell enzyme, thus causing a specific antiviral effect. Further, the analog-containing nucleoside triphosphates are incorporated into nucleic acids and may then interfere with the functioning of such nucleic acids. For example, if the analog is 5′-iodouracil (IU), which is an analog of thymine, IU does not pair with adenine as faithfully as thymine, and mismatching occurs during both the replication and the transcription of the substituted DNA. This causes the formation of defective progeny DNA strands and defective messenger RNAs and inhibits virus multiplication.

Among the most promising analogs that have been studied are the following:

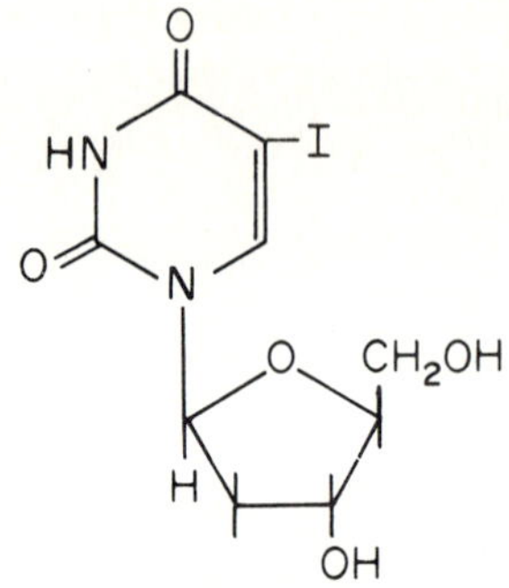

Figure 7-6. 5′-Iododeoxyuridine (IDU). In trifluorothymidine (F_3T), I is replaced by CF_3.

1. 5′-Iododeoxyuridine (IDU) and trifluorothymidine (F_3T) (Fig. 7-6), both analogs of thymidine. Both inhibit the multiplication of herpesviruses. IDU, applied topically to the eye, has been used successfully in the treatment of herpetic conjunctivitis. Although IDU is most probably incorporated into host cell as well as into viral DNA, it reaches so few host cells in the eye that no serious damage is caused. At worst, damaged corneal cells regenerate after virus multiplication has been inhibited and infected cells have been eliminated.
2. Cytosine arabinoside (ara-C), adenosine arabinoside (ara-A or vidarabine), and ara-AMP. All these substances have had more or less extensive clinical trials as antiherpesvirus agents. They are inhibitors of DNA polymerases, and one of their effects is to act as chain terminators. The reason that they are antiviral agents is that herpesvirus DNA polymerase is more sensitive to them than are host cell DNA polymerases.
3. Ribavirin or virazole (Fig. 7-7), an analog of the purine precursor 5′-aminoimidazole-4-carboxamide. This substance inhibits the biosynthesis of guanine nucleotides. Its antiviral target is probably virus-coded enzymes that have a higher affinity for its phosphorylated derivatives than have normal cellular enzymes. It has a wide antiviral spectrum and is effective against RNA- as well as DNA-containing viruses.
4. (E)-5-(2-bromovinyl)-2′-deoxyuridine (BVdU) and E-5-(2-iodovinyl)-2′-deoxyuridine (IVdU); 5-vinyl-2′-deoxyuridine and 5-vinyl-2′-deoxycytidine; 1-(2′-deoxy-2′-F-β-D-arabinofuranosyl)-5′-iodocytosine (FIAC); and 9-[(1,3-dihydroxy-2-propoxy)- methyl]-guanine (DHPG) (Fig. 7-8). These compounds are the most recent and powerful antiherpesvirus compounds. They possess low cytotoxicity. All inhibit

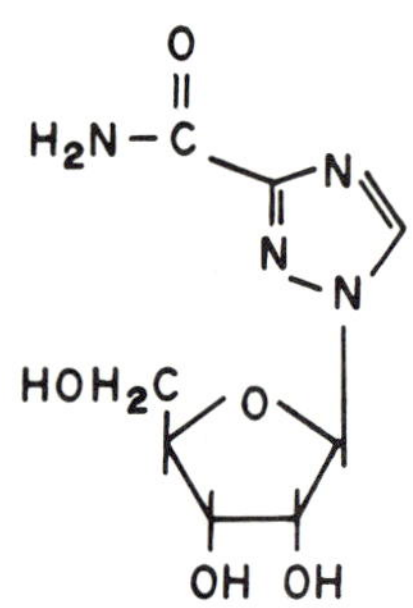

Figure 7-7. Ribavirin (1-β-D-ribofuranosyl-1,2,4-triazole-3-carboxamide).

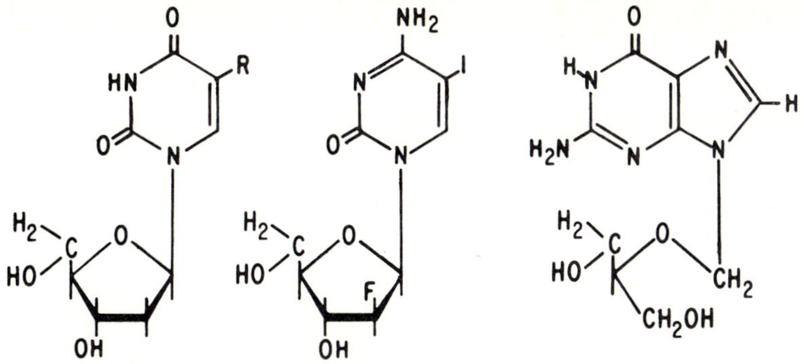

Figure 7-8. **Left**. R = $-CH = CH_2$, 5-vinyl-2'-deoxyuridine; R = $-CH{=}CHBr$, (E)-5-(2-bromovinyl)-2'-deoxyuridine. **Center**. FIAC. **Right**. DHPG.

the herpesvirus DNA polymerase much more powerfully than do cellular DNA polymerases (see also below).

Target Cell Approach

It has long been realized that the most successful strategy in antiviral chemotherapy would be to use drugs that could enter, or would be activated in, only virus-infected cells—in other words, a strategy that focused on the infected cell as the target cell.

Several approaches to the target cell strategy are as follows. The first takes advantage of the fact that one of the early herpesvirus-coded enzymes is a deoxypyrimidine kinase capable of phosphorylating compounds that cannot be phosphorylated by any cellular enzyme. It is, therefore, possible to use as highly specific antiherpesvirus agents analogs of nucleosides that are phosphorylated only in cells infected with herpesviruses. Examples of such compounds are acycloguanosine or acyclovir [9-(2-hydroxyethoxymethyl)-guanine] (Fig. 7-9), IVdU, and DHPG (Fig. 7-8). These drugs are converted to their triphosphates and incorporated into DNA much more extensively in herpesvirus-infected cells (by the herpesvirus-encoded deoxypyrimidine kinase) than in uninfected cells. They are now undergoing clinical trials against several herpesviruses.

The second approach takes advantage of the fact that infection with viruses often changes the permeability properties of cell membranes (Chap. 5). This provides the opportunity for introducing into infected cells antiviral agents that would not be taken up by uninfected cells. In fact, this approach should permit the administration of drugs that are quite toxic to normal cells.

The third approach is to couple powerful antiviral agents that may be so toxic that they could not be used on their own to monoclonal antibodies directed against virus-coded antigens on the surfaces of infected cells (Chap. 5). The monoclonal antibodies would, in effect, be used as homing devices. Once the coupled antibodies reached their target cells, they would presumably be internalized, and the antiviral drug would inhibit virus multiplication. Like the second, this approach still requires a great deal of research before becoming a practical reality.

Interferon

The antiviral agent on which interest is currently focused most intensely is one that is elaborated by living cells themselves. Animal cells infected with viruses very often produce a protein that, when added to uninfected cells, protects them against virus infection or, more precisely, greatly decreases the chance that subsequent virus infection will initiate a productive multiplication cycle. This substance is called "interferon." Interferon provides the first line of defense against virus infection: in animals treated with antiserum to interferon, virus infections progress much more rapidly and cause much more severe disease than in untreated animals.

Interferons are host-coded proteins. Normal cells do not as a rule contain detectable amounts of interferon. The formation of interferon is induced by a variety of agents, the best known of which is infection with a virus (see below). Since it is a cellular protein, interferon is host cell species-specific but not virus-specific. Sometimes this specificity is very narrow. For example, chick and duck interferons exhibit little if any cross-protective activity, nor do mouse and rat interferons. However, not unexpectedly, there are exceptions; for example, human interferon protects bovine cells even better than does bovine interferon.

There is not one type of human interferon but three: IFN-α and IFN-β, produced predominantly by leukocytes and fibroblasts, respectively, in response to virus infection, and IFN-γ, formerly called "immune" or type 2 interferon, which is produced by unsensitized lymphoid cells in re-

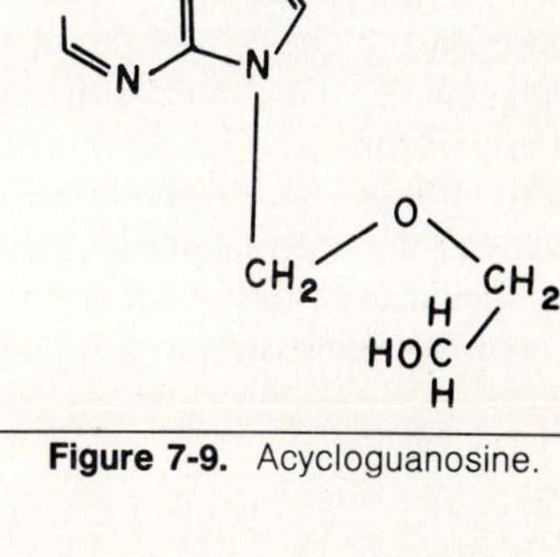

Figure 7-9. Acycloguanosine.

TABLE 7-1. CHARACTERISTICS OF HUMAN INTERFERONS

Type	Alpha (Leukocyte)	Beta (Fibroblast)	Gamma (Immune or class 2)
Produced by	Peripheral leukocytes	Fibroblasts	Lymphocytes
Inducing agent	Virus infection, dsRNA	Virus infection, dsRNA	Mitogens (nonsensitized lymphocytes), specific antigen (sensitized lymphocytes)
Number of genes	14	At least 2, possibly 5	1
Presence of introns	No	No	Yes
Chromosomal location	9	9,2,5	12
Size of primary protein (number of amino acids)	166	166	166
Length of signal sequence (number of amino acids)	23	21	20
Size of actual protein (number of amino acids)	143	145	146
Molecular weight	17,000	17,000	17,000
Glycoprotein	No	Yes	Yes
Stability at pH 2	Yes	Yes	No
Activity in the presence of SDS	Yes	Yes	No

sponse to mitogens and by sensitized lymphocytes when stimulated with specific antigens (Table 7-1).

Nature of Interferon Genes

Recombinant DNA technology (cloning of some species of interferon, and the use of cloned genes to search through human gene libraries) has demonstrated that there are at least 14 different human IFN-α genes, from 2 to 5 IFN-β genes, and 1 IFN-γ gene. All these genes encode proteins 166 amino acids long with 20 to 23 amino acid long N-terminal signal sequences, which are necessary because interferons are secreted proteins. These signal sequences are not present in normal interferon molecules.

The various IFN-α genes are 80 to 90 percent related to each other. The coding sequences of the IFN-α and IFN-β gene families are about 30 percent related to each other, which indicates that they diverged at least 500 million years ago, before the emergence of vertebrates. The IFN-γ gene exhibits essentially no homology to the other interferon genes but codes for a similar sized protein in which certain single amino acids occupy the same positions as in α and β interferons.

Most if not all IFN-α genes are arranged tandemly on chromosome 9. IFN-β genes are dispersed throughout the genome, one also being located on chromosome 9 and the others on chromosomes 2 and 5, and the IFN-γ gene is located on chromosome 12. The latter is the only interferon gene that possesses introns.

In addition to all these genes, the human genome also contains at least six interferon pseudogenes whose sequences are very similar but which contain alterations or deletions that prevent the expression of full length interferon proteins.

Induction and Production of Interferons

The formation of interferons can be induced by a variety of conditions and agents other than infectious virus. Among these are:

1. Viruses inactivated by heat or ultraviolet irradiation. Among such viruses are influenza virus, NDV, reovirus, rotavirus, and bovine enterovirus.
2. Double-stranded RNA, such as reovirus RNA, and synthetic double-stranded polyribonucleotides, such as poly (I):poly (C). The amount of interferon that is induced by poly (I):poly (C) can often be increased greatly by *superinduction.* This is a phenomenon that is elicited when cells are treated with poly (I):poly (C) together with the protein synthesis inhibitor, cycloheximide. If, after 5 hours, actinomycin D is added, followed 1 hour later by reversal of the inhibition of protein synthesis, about 50 times more interferon is produced than if cycloheximide had not been added initially. The basis of this phenomenon is thought to be the existence of an unstable regulator of the expression of the interferon gene. During the first 5-hour period, both interferon and regulator messenger RNA would accumulate. After the addition of actinomycin D, both interferon and regulator messenger RNA would decay, the latter more rapidly than the former. Upon the release of the protein synthesis block, only interferon would then be formed in the presence of greatly reduced levels of regulator.
3. Single-stranded RNA and single-stranded or double-stranded DNA are inactive as interferon inducers, as are double-stranded RNA-DNA hybrid molecules. However, certain synthetic polycarbo-

xylic acids and pyran copolymers are inducers of interferon formation at relatively high concentrations, as is bacterial endotoxin. The feature common to all these substances, including the polyribonucleotides, is that they are polyanions.

4. The preceding agents induce IFN-α and IFN-β. IFN-γ is induced by stimulation of lymphocytes, as described above.

The mechanism by which interferon formation is induced is not clear, nor is it known why substances as diverse as double-stranded RNA and endotoxin can induce interferon, whereas a substance as similar to double-stranded RNA as double-stranded DNA cannot.

In practice, IFN-α is usually prepared from leukocytes, obtained as the buffy coat layer by low-speed centrifugation of human blood. Since IFN-α genes are located close to each other, they are generally induced coordinately. IFN-β species are prepared from fibroblasts grown in monolayer culture, induced with poly (I):poly (C) and superinduced with inhibitors of RNA and protein synthesis (see above). Since IFN-β genes are dispersed, they tend to be expressed in a noncoordinate manner, that is, different strains of diploid fibroblasts express different relative amounts of the various IFN-β genes.

The disadvantages of these methods of producing interferon are (1) interferon is produced in small amounts only (typically about 1 mg interferon per 10 liters of tissue culture supernatant medium), and (2) they are destructive, that is, the induced cells produce interferon for 48 to 72 hours and then die.

Recently two advances have enormously improved methods of producing and purifying interferon. First, the cloned IFN-α, IFN-β, and IFN-γ genes have been inserted into expression vectors by genetic engineering technology, and interferons can now be produced in large amounts in either procaryotic or eucaryotic cells that synthesize them constitutively. Second, monoclonal antibodies to all classes of interferon have been obtained and are now being used to purify interferons efficiently and rapidly by means of immunoaffinity chromatography. The biologic properties of the cloned interferons are the same as those of naturally occurring interferons.

Assay of Interferons

Interferons are commonly assayed by exposing cells to serially diluted interferon preparations for about 12 hours and then infecting them with a standard amount of virus known to produce a certain number of plaques. The titer of an interferon preparation is the reciprocal of that dilution that reduces this number by 50 percent. The specific activity of pure interferons is 5 to 10 $\times 10^8$ PRD_{50} (50 percent plaque reduction doses) per milliliter. This astonishingly high biologic activity means that in some very sensitive cell-virus systems interferon activity is detectable at concentrations as low as 10^{-14} *M*.

Nature of Interferons

The IFN-β and IFN-γ species are glycoproteins; the IFN-α species are not. IFN-α and IFN-β species, but not IFN-γ species, are remarkably resistant to low pH—both are quite stable at pH 2 at 4C—and retain activity in the presence of sodium dodecylsulfate, an unusual property that is very useful in the final stages of purification.

There is evidence for two highly conserved domains in the interferon molecule: one, in the aminoterminal half of the molecule, probably contains the site that binds to the cell surface receptor, and the other, in the other half of the molecule, appears to modulate such binding and mediate other biologic functions.

As isolated from cells and organs, interferons sometimes appear to be larger than the 17,000 dalton molecules specified by their genes. There are several possible reasons for this. First, some interferons are glycoproteins; second, some naturally occurring interferon species may be dimers; and third, under certain conditions interferons may associate or complex with other proteins.

The three classes of human interferon are immunologically quite distinct, that is, antisera raised against any one class do not inactivate heterologous interferons.

Finally, interferons possess two types of biologic activity: antiviral activity and anticellular activity. Both types of activity vary markedly with the nature of the cell. The antiviral activity of all three classes of interferon is comparable, but the anticellular activity of IFN-γ seems to be far greater than that of IFN-α and IFN-β.

Antiviral Activity of Interferons

Interferons interfere with virus multiplication; this is the property for which they are named. Interferons themselves are not the proteins that actually inhibit virus multiplication, but rather, interferons are inducers that cause cells to synthesize proteins that are the actual effectors of the antiviral state. In fact, interferons do not induce the antiviral state if messenger RNA or protein synthesis is inhibited. The antiviral state usually lasts for several days and then decays. Expression of the antiviral state is controlled by a gene on chromosome 21 that probably codes for a specific interferon receptor on the cell surface. Interferons do not enter cells; they express themselves via second messengers that are activated at the cell surface. Interferon injected into cells fails to induce the antiviral state.

It seems clear that the basic mechanism by which interferons inhibit virus multiplication involves interference with the ability of parental or early viral messenger RNA molecules to be translated. As a result, no virus-specified proteins are synthesized, no progeny viral genomes are formed, and infection is aborted.

The precise mechanism by which interferon inhibits viral protein synthesis is under intense investigation. It has been found that treatment with interferon—and all three classes of interferon act similarly—induces the synthesis of several cellular proteins. One is an enzyme, 2′,5′-oligo (A)

TABLE 7-2. EFFECT OF INTERFERONS ON CELL FUNCTIONS

Effect	Dose Required (PRD_{50}/ml)	Description
Inhibition of cell growth	0.2–1000	Most cell types are sensitive but differ widely in sensitivity; tumor cells may be somewhat more sensitive than normal cells; molecular basis not known
Enhancement of differentiation	1–1000	Seen most strongly in functioning effector cells of the immune system
Inhibition of differentiation	100–1000	Observed when induced RNA and protein synthesis is required for expression of differentiation
Effects on the immune system	10–1000	Inhibition of proliferative responses, such as primary and secondary antibody response, mitogen- and antigen-induced lymphocyte blastogenesis, and delayed-type hypersensitivity
		Enhancement of differentiated responses, such as a natural killer cell activation, T cell cytotoxicity, macrophage phagocytosis and cytotoxicity, and IgE-mediated histamine release
Increased expression of histocompatibility antigens (HLA-A, B, and C) and β microglobulin	1–1000	May lead to increased susceptibility of infected and malignant cells to cell killing by effector cells that use these antigens for cell recognition; this effect is far stronger for IFN-γ than for IFN-α or IFN-β

synthetase, which, in the presence of double-stranded RNA, converts ATP to 2′-5′-linked oligo (A) molecules up to 15 residues long, the trimer being the most abundant. This 2′,5′-oligo (A) then activates an endoribonuclease, RNase L, that is present in normal cells in widely varying amounts and the level of which increases in some types of cells in response to interferon treatment. It is hypothesized that this enzyme hydrolyzes viral messenger RNAs, thereby inhibiting viral protein synthesis.

The principal problems with this explanation of the mechanism of interferon action are: (1) What is the source of the double-stranded RNA (especially for DNA-containing viruses)? (2) Can it account for the selectivity of interferon action? (Note that interferon prevents the synthesis of viral proteins but not of host cell proteins, yet RNase L hydrolyzes both viral and host cell RNAs.), (3) In certain cells the antiviral state is established without 2′,5′-oligo (A) synthetase being induced, while in others the synthesis of 2′,5′-oligo (A) synthetase is induced, but the antiviral state is not established.

Another effect of interferon is that it causes the phosphorylation of a 67,000 dalton membrane-associated protein that is itself a protein kinase, and in the presence of double-stranded RNA, phosphorylates the α subunit of protein synthesis initiation factor eIF-2, thereby inactivating it. The problems with this explanation of how interferon inhibits viral protein synthesis are similar to those enumerated above. It remains to be seen whether either or neither of these mechanisms is the basis of the antiviral state.

Anticellular Activity of Interferons

In addition to their antiviral activity, interferons also affect a variety of cell functions, summarized in Table 7-2. It is conceivable that all these functions are mediated by messenger RNAs that share certain sequences and that the primary function of interferon is to regulate the expression of these *cellular* messenger RNAs rather than those of viral messenger RNAs (which may be inhibited because they are structurally similar). Thus interferon may have evolved as a cellular regulator rather than as an antiviral defense mechanism.

Their remarkable and varied effects on immunoregulatory mechanisms have recently focused intense attention on interferons as lymphokines, soluble effectors of immune reactions. This, coupled with their cell multiplication inhibitory activity (CMI), the molecular basis of which is not known and which is often greater against tumor than against normal cells, has given rise to hopes that interferons may be useful as anticancer agents in humans, and numerous clinical trials are currently underway to test this possibility. All classes of interferons are under investigation, but expectations are highest for IFN-γ, for which the ratio of anticellular to antiviral activity is much higher than for IFN-α and IFN-β. Such clinical trials were impossible until recently because of the very large amounts of interferon that are required. Daily injections of 1 to 5 million PRD_{50} are generally regarded as necessary for obtaining a therapeutic effect. Such large amounts of interferon could not be prepared from leukocytes or cultured fibroblasts except for only a very few patients. However, the situation is now changing radically as large amounts of cloned interferons are becoming available.

Prospects for Clinical Use

Extensive clinical trials are currently underway to evaluate interferons as anticancer agents (for the treatment of breast cancer, lung cancer, brain tumors, osteogenic sarcoma, myeloma, lymphoma, hepatoma, and others) and as antiviral agents (in such life-threatening infections as rabies, hemorrhagic fevers, and herpesvirus-caused encephalitis, as well as in persistent infections, such as hepatitis B, herpesvirus zoster, wart viruses, and cytomegalovirus infections). Interferon treatment does cause some undesirable side effects, such as fever, hypotension, myalgia, tachycardia, and impaired liver function, but such side effects may be acceptable in the context of life-threatening disease. The primary need at this time is large-scale well-controlled clinical investigations. There is no doubt that the availability of large amounts of cloned interferon species will usher in a new era in the employment of interferon as an antiviral and as an anticancer agent. In particular, as the characteristics of the functional domains on interferon molecules become defined, recombinant DNA technology may permit the construction of nontoxic interferon molecules tailor-made for the treatment of specific infections or tumors.

Vaccines

The only currently feasible means of preventing diseases caused by viruses is through mobilization of the immune mechanism by means of vaccines. There are two types of antiviral vaccines: inactivated virus and attenuated active virus.

Inactivated Virus Vaccines

The primary requirements for an effective vaccine of this type are complete inactivation of infectivity coupled with minimum loss of antigenicity. These requirements are not easily met simultaneously, since few reagents are available that inactivate viral genomes, the source of infectivity, without also affecting viral protein, the source of antigenicity. Ultraviolet irradiation could accomplish this best but is inapplicable because virus inactivated in this manner is capable not only of expressing the function of those genes that have not received a lethal hit but also of undergoing multiplicity reactivation (Chap. 6). Photodynamic inactivation, in which virus is treated with such dyes as neutral red dyes that are capable of intercalating between adjacent nucleic acid bases, and is then irradiated with white light, inactivates viral nucleic acids efficiently and irreversibly without damaging viral proteins, but suffers from similar drawbacks in that genome segments that have not received a hit remain potentially functional. For example, herpesvirus inactivated in this manner can still transform cultured cells in vitro and may be tumorigenic. Beta-propiolactone is a potentially useful inactivating agent but is a potent carcinogen. The best reagent for inactivating viral nucleic acid without compromising antigenicity is formaldehyde, which destroys infectivity primarily by reacting with those amino groups of adenine, guanine, and cytosine that are not involved in hydrogen bond formation. Viruses that contain single-stranded nucleic acid are therefore inactivated readily, while those that contain double-stranded nucleic acid are resistant to formaldehyde. It also reacts with amino groups of proteins, forming addition compounds of the Schiff's base type and crosslinking polypeptide chains without, however, significantly disturbing protein conformation. Reaction with protein is most probably responsible for the occasional generation of a formaldehyde-resistant infectious virus fraction, which appears to be caused by such extensive crosslinking of capsid proteins that formaldehyde cannot reach and inactivate the viral nucleic acid. Careful control of reaction conditions and rigorous checks for residual infectious virus are mandatory for the preparation of formaldehyde-inactivated virus vaccines.

Attenuated Active Virus Vaccines

The second method of immunizing against viral pathogens is by administering attenuated virus strains, antibody to which is capable of neutralizing the pathogen (Chap. 3). This is the principle on which Jenner's vaccination procedure against smallpox in 1798 was based. He inoculated with cowpox virus to induce antibodies against the highly virulent smallpox virus. Since then many attenuated virus vaccine strains have been developed, among them Theiler's yellow fever virus vaccine strain, the attenuated Sabin poliovirus vaccine strains, and attenuated measles and rubella virus strains. The most commonly used method of producing such attenuated virus strains is by repeated passage of the human pathogen in other host species, which results in the selection of multistep variants with drastically reduced virulence for humans.

Attenuated virus vaccines are effective in very small amounts, since the attenuated virus can multiply. This provides a powerful amplification effect: the viral progeny, rather than the virus in the inoculum, acts as the antigen. The attenuated vaccines also possess the advantage of stimulating the formation of all the correct types of antibody molecules (i.e., IgA, etc., as well as IgG).

Immunization with Chemically Synthesized Antigenic Determinants

An entirely new perspective for the development of antiviral vaccines has opened recently as a result of recombinant DNA technology. Numerous viral genomes are now being cloned and sequenced, and as a result the amino acid sequences of many proteins, including those of the proteins that elicit neutralizing antibodies, have become known. Antibodies are made against relatively short sequences at the antigenic determinant sites of proteins. Therefore, knowing the amino acid sequence of a type-specific, neutralizing- antibody-eliciting viral antigen, peptides about 10 amino acids long that correspond to its antigenic determinants can be synthesized chemically, and these peptides will elicit the formation of fully functional, high-affinity neutralizing antibodies. Such synthetic peptide vaccines should be economical to produce and safe. They are the ideal vaccines, presenting the minimum amount of antigen. Several such vaccines are under development at this time and appear to be effective in containing, limiting, and eliminating viral infections. No doubt such vaccines will soon be developed against influenza virus and paramyxoviruses, hepatitis B, herpesviruses, rotaviruses, arenaviruses, togaviruses, and others.

FURTHER READING

Books and Reviews

CHEMOTHERAPEUTIC AGENTS

Gauri KK (ed): Anti-herpes Virus Chemotherapy: Experimental and Clinical Aspects. New York, Karger, 1979

Grunert RR: Search for antiviral agents. Annu Rev Microbiol 33:335, 1979

Hann FE (ed): Virus Chemotherapy. New York, Karger, 1980

INTERFERON

Billiau A: Interferon therapy: Pharmacokinetic and pharmacological aspects. Arch Virol 67:121, 1981

De Maeyer E, De Maeyer-Guignard J: Interferons. In Fraenkel-Conrat H, Wagner RR (eds): Comprehensive Virology. New York, Plenum, 1979, vol 15, p 205

Gordon J, Minks MA: The interferon renaissance: Molecular aspects of induction and action. Microbiol Rev 45:244, 1981

Gresser I (ed): Interferon 1979. New York, Academic Press, 1979

Gresser I, Tovey MG: Antitumor effect of interferon. Biochim Biophys Acta 516:231, 1978

Hayes TG: Differences between human α (leukocyte) and β (fibroblast) interferons. Arch Virol 67:267, 1981

Lengyel P: Biochemistry of interferons. Annu Rev Biochem 51:251, 1982

Rubinstein M: The structure of human interferons. Biochim Biophys Acta 695:5, 1982

Sehgal PB: The interferon genes. Biochim Biophys Acta 695:17, 1982

Stewart WE II: The Interferon System. New York, Springer-Verlag, 1979

Taylor-Papadimitriou J, Balkwill FR: Implications for clinical application of new developments in interferon research. Biochim Biophys Acta 695:49, 1982

VACCINES

Arnon R: Chemically defined antiviral vaccines. Annu Rev Microbiol 34:593, 1980

Chanock RM: Strategy for development of respiratory and gastrointestinal tract viral vaccines in the 1980s. J Infect Dis 143:364, 1981

Lerner RA, Sutcliffe JG, Shinnick TM: Antibodies to chemically synthesized peptides predicted from DNA sequences as probes of gene expression. Cell 23:309, 1981

Melnick JL: Viral vaccines. Prog Med Virol 23:158, 1977

Sutcliffe JG, Shinnick JM, Green N, et al.: Antibodies that react with predetermined sites on proteins. Science 219:660, 1983

Selected Papers

CHEMOTHERAPEUTIC AGENTS

Allaudeen HS, Descamps J, Sehgal PK, et al.: Selected inhibition of DNA replication in herpes simplex virus infected cells by 1-(2′-deoxy-2′-fluoro-β-D-arabinofuranosyl)-5-iodocytosine. J Biol Chem 257:11879, 1982

Benedetto A, Rossi GB, Amici C, et al.: Inhibition of animal virus production by means of translation inhibitors unable to penetrate normal cells. Virology 106:123, 1980

Carrasco L: Membrane leakiness after viral infection and a new approach to the development of antiviral agents. Nature 272:694, 1978

Cheng Y-C, Huang E-H, Lin J-C, et al.: Unique spectrum of activity of 9-[(1,3-dihydroxy-2-propoxy)methyl]-guanine against herpesviruses in vitro and its mode of action against herpes simplex virus type 1. Proc Natl Acad Sci USA 80:2767, 1983

Descamps J, DeClercq E: Specific phosphorylation of E-5-(2-iodovinyl)-2′-deoxyuridine by herpes simplex virus-infected cells. J Biol Chem 256:597, 1981

Katz E, Moss B: Formation of a vaccinia virus structural polypeptide from a higher molecular weight precursor: Inhibition by rifampicin. Proc Natl Acad Sci USA 66:677, 1970

Korant BD: Poliovirus coat protein as the site of guanidine action. Virology 81:25, 1977

Lubeck MD, Schulman JL, Palese P: Susceptibility of influenza A viruses to amantadine as influenced by the gene coding for the M protein. J Virol 28:710, 1978

Richardson CD, Scheid A, Choppin PW: Specific inhibition of paramyxovirus and myxovirus replication by oligopeptides with amino acid sequences similar to those at the N-terminal of the F_1 or HA_2 viral polypeptides. Virology 105:205, 1980

Schlegel R, Dickson RB, Willingham ME, et al.: Amantadine and dansylcadaverine inhibit vesicular stomatitis virus uptake and receptor-mediated endocytosis of α_2-macroglobulin. Proc Natl Acad Sci USA 79:2291, 1982

Whitley RJ, Alford CA: Developmental aspects of selected antiviral chemotherapeutic agents. Annu Rev Microbiol 32:285, 1978

Willis RC, Carson DA, Seegmiller JE: Adenosine kinase initiates the major route of ribavirin activation in a cultured human cell line. Proc Natl Acad Sci USA 75:3042, 1978

Woodson B, Joklik WK: The inhibition of vaccinia virus multiplication by isatin -β-thiosemicarbazone. Proc Natl Acad Sci USA 54:946, 1965

INTERFERON

Creasey AA, Eppstein DA, March YV, et al.: Growth regulation of melanoma cells by interferon and (2′-5′)oligoadenylate synthetase. Mole Cell Biol 3:780, 1983

Friedman RM, Sonnabend JA: Inhibition of interferon action by *p*-fluorophenylalanine. Nature 203:366, 1964

Jacobsen H, Czarnieck CW, Krause D, et al.: Interferon-induced synthesis of 2-5A-dependent RNase in JLS-V9R cells. Virology 125:496, 1983

Joklik WK, Merigan TC: Concerning the mechanism of action of interferon. Proc Natl Acad Sci USA 56:558, 1966

Kerr IM, Brown RE: pppA2′p5′A2′p5′A: An inhibitor of protein synthesis synthesized with an enzyme fraction from interferon-treated cells. Proc Natl Acad Sci USA 75:256, 1978

Krust B, Rivière Y, Hovanessian AG: p67K kinase in different tissues and plasma of control and interferon-treated mice. Virology 119:240, 1982

Le J, Vilcek J, Saxinger C, et al.: Human T cells hybridomas secreting immune interferon. Proc Natl Acad Sci USA 79:7857, 1982

Miyata T, Hayashida H: Recent divergence from a common ancestor of human IFN-α genes. Nature 295:165, 1982

Rehbert E, Kelder B, Hoal EG, et al.: Specific molecular activities of recombinant and hybrid leukocyte interferons. J Biol Chem 257:11497, 1982

Samuel CE, Knutson GS: Mechanism of interferon action. J Biol Chem 257:11791, 1982

Shaw GD, Boll W, Taira H, et al.: Structure and expression of cloned mouse IFN-α genes. Nucl Acid Res 11:555, 1983

Slate DL, D'Eustachio P, Pravtcheva D, et al.: Chromosomal location of a human α interferon gene family. J Exp Med 155:1019, 1982

Stewart WE II, Gosser LB, Lockhart RZ: Priming: A nonantiviral function of interferon. J Virol 7:792, 1971

Stewart WE II, de Somer P, Edy VG, et al.: Human interferons: Requirements for stabilization and reactivation of human leukocyte and fibroblast interferon. J Gen Virol 26:327, 1975

Tanaka S, Oshima T, Ohsuye K, et al.: Expression in *Escherichia coli* of chemically synthesized gene for the human immune interferon. Nucl Acid Res 11:1707, 1983

Virelizier J, Gresser I: Role of interferon in the pathogenesis of viral diseases of mice as demonstrated by the use of anti-interferon serum. J Immunol 120:1616, 1978

Wallach D, Fellous M, Revel M: Preferential effect of γ-interferon on the synthesis of HLA antigens and their mRNAs in human cells. Nature 299:833, 1982

Wiebe ME, Joklik WK: The mechanism of inhibition of reovirus replication by interferon. Virology 66:229, 1975

Zilberstein A, Kimichi A, Schmidt A, et al.: Isolation of two interferon-induced translational inhibitors: a protein kinase and an oligo-isoadenylate synthetase. Proc Natl Acad Sci USA 75:4734, 1978

VACCINES

Bittle JL, Houghten RA, Alexander H, et al.: Protection against foot-and-mouth disease by immunization with a chemically synthesized peptide predicted from the viral nucleotide sequence. Nature 298:30, 1982

Neurath AR, Kent SBH, Strick N: Specificity of antibodies elicited by a synthetic peptide having a sequence in common with a fragment of a virus protein, the hepatitis B surface antigen. Proc Natl Acad Sci USA 79:7871, 1982

CHAPTER 8

Tumor Viruses

Viruses are at the forefront of a large effort that is being devoted to discovering how normal cells are turned into cancer cells; they are at the cutting edge of studies of the mechanisms of tumorigenesis. There are two reasons for this. First, infection with tumor viruses transforms *all* cells in a population into potential tumor cells; with all other agents the frequency of transformation is far lower. As a result, studies at the biochemical and molecular level are possible on virus-induced transformation but are not possible on transformation caused by other agents. Second, mutants of tumor viruses exist that are incapable of transforming cells or maintaining the transformed state at nonpermissive temperatures (typically 38C or above), but capable of doing so at permissive temperatures (typically 35C or below). Transformation of cells is therefore a function of a *single* virus-coded protein. Clearly, it should be possible to isolate such proteins, determine what their function is, identify their targets, and thereby gain insight into the basic reactions that cause normal cells to be converted into tumor cells. This is impossible with any other carcinogenic agent.

Both RNA-containing and DNA-containing viruses can cause various types of neoplasms in animals, and most probably also in humans. Awareness of the principles of tumor virology is, therefore, important for the medical practitioner.

Origins of Tumor Virology

Tumor etiology, the study of the causes of tumors, has brought to light a bewildering variety of tumorigenic agents that fall into three classes: chemical substances, physical stimuli, and biologic agents. The chemical substances include compounds of the most diverse constitution, ranging from polycyclic hydrocarbons, such as methylcholanthrene, benzo(a)pyrene, and dimethylbenzanthracene, on the one hand, to such multifunctional compounds as dimethylnitrosamine, nitrosomethylurea, and 4-nitroquinoline-1-oxide, on the other. The physical agents include both x-rays and ultraviolet irradiation, and the most important biologic agents are viruses.

The concept that infectious agents might be involved etiologically in the cancer process was advanced as early as 1908 by Ellerman and Bang, who observed that the mode of transmission of leukemia in the fowl was similar to that of an infectious disease. Shortly thereafter, Rous demonstrated that the infectious agent in avian sarcomas could pass through filters that would not permit passage of bacteria. For many years this discovery remained an isolated finding, until in 1932 Shope discovered in wild cottontail rabbits a viral agent that transmitted a wart-like growth not only to cottontails but also to domestic rabbits. While most warts in cottontails remained benign or regressed, those in domestic rabbits sometimes developed into highly malignant carcinomas. Then, in 1938, Bittner discovered, in mammary gland tumors of mice, the mammary tumor virus or milk factor, a virus that is passed from mother to offspring through suckling. The finding that, more than any other, elicited the upsurge of interest in viruses as carcinogenic agents was the discovery by Gross in 1951 of a virus that induced leukemia in mice, a disease that is remarkably similar to leukemia in humans. Efforts to develop animal models applicable to the human disease have resulted in the isolation of a large number of viruses that cause many kinds of cancers in every major group of animals.

Characteristics of Virus-transformed Cells

Discussion of the virus–cell interaction up to this point has been focused on the lytic interaction, which involves multiplication of the virus and destruction of the host cell. However, certain DNA viruses can interact with cells not only by means of the lytic interaction but also by means of an interaction in which virus multiplication is repressed and the host cell is not destroyed. In this type of interaction the viral DNA is either integrated into the genome of the host cell, or it replicates as a plasmid. In either case a new entity, the transformed or tumor cell, is created that can multiply indefinitely.

In addition, a family of RNA-containing viruses, the RNA tumor viruses (oncornaviruses or retroviruses), can also transform cells and cause tumors. At first, the problem of how viral RNA could be integrated into the host genome presented a major conceptual hurdle. This has now been overcome by the discovery in RNA tumor viruses of a DNA polymerase that can transcribe RNA into DNA; this is the so-called reverse transcriptase. It is the DNA transcribed from viral RNA by this enzyme that is integrated into the cellular genome.

Transformed or tumor cells differ from normal cells in several important respects. Since these changes are at the genetic level, they are passed on to the cells' descendants. The principal properties in which virus-transformed cells differ from normal ones are as follows.

Possession of the Viral Genome

Transformed cells contain either the whole or part of the genome of the virus that causes the transformation. More often than not, this genome is integrated into the cell DNA, but in some transformed cell nuclei it may exist as a free plasmid-like entity. The extent to which viral genetic information is expressed in transformed cells varies widely, from full expression, with resultant formation of progeny virus particles, to complete silence, as judged by the absence of messenger RNA transcribed from it or proteins encoded by it.

Tumorigenicity

Transformed cells generally give rise to tumors when injected into animals, particularly immunosuppressed or immunologically deficient animals, such as athymic nude mice. Like naturally occurring tumors, different lines of virus-transformed cells exhibit wide variation in invasiveness. Even large numbers of some types of transformed cells produce only benign tumors at the site of infection, while even small numbers of others give rise to highly invasive cancers.

Morphology

Normal and transformed cells differ in morphology. There are two major differences. First, transformed cells are usually more rounded and refractile than are normal cells. Second, normal and transformed cells differ in the orientation of cells relative to one another. Normal cells usually arrange themselves in regular patterns, while transformed cells tend to orient themselves randomly (Fig. 8-1). These morphologic changes are often virus-specific. There are variants of Rous sarcoma virus and polyoma virus that give rise to transformed cells with morphologies that differ from those induced by the corresponding wild-type viruses.

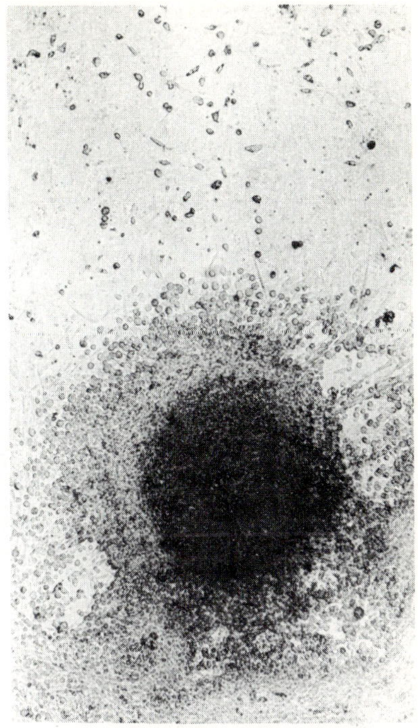

Figure 8-1. Focus of chick embryo fibroblasts transformed with Rous sarcoma virus. The transformed cells are densely piled on top of one another in the center of the focus. *(Courtesy of Dr. P.K. Vogt.)*

Changes in Growth Patterns

Most types of untransformed cells grow in vitro to a certain cell density. Cell division stops (or almost stops) when a monolayer of uniformly spread cells has formed. Under the same conditions, transformed cells continue to divide so that very much higher cell densities are attained. This alteration of growth patterns is due primarily to two factors.

Loss of Contact Inhibition. When an untransformed cell comes into contact with another cell, there is cessation of the rapid movement of pseudopodia (ruffles) that are constantly extended and retracted, and forward movement is arrested. At the same time the cell stops dividing. This dual phenomenon is known as "contact inhibition." The ability to respond to contact with other cells ensures that any given cell grows only in its appropriate location within the complete organism and does not proliferate unless it receives a signal that more of its kind are needed for the organism's orderly growth or maintenance.

While cell strains differ appreciably in their susceptibility to contact inhibition, transformed cells are always much less susceptible than their untransformed counterparts. This loss of contact inhibition represents release from one of the normal controls over multiplication, and it may account in part for their unregulated growth in the organism. Some transformed cells, such as cells of benign tumors, have lost only the ability to respond to contact with each other but are still inhibited by contact with other cell types. Others, such as those of metastasizing tumors, respond to contact neither with each other nor with other types of cells.

Reduction in Requirement for Serum. Contact inhibition is not the only factor that limits cell growth. The addition of serum to a nondividing contact-inhibited monolayer of untransformed cells results in further rounds of division, so that cells may actually pile up on top of one another. Virus transformation markedly reduces cellular serum dependence, and transformed cells require much less serum to initiate division than do untransformed cells. For example, 3T3 cells, a line of mouse fibroblasts, will not grow optimally unless the serum concentration is greater than 5 percent. By contrast, 3T3 cells transformed with SV40 can divide to a small but significant extent in serum concentrations as low as 0.5 percent. The nature of the serum factors that are required by cells and how these factors act is not known. It is hoped that studying them will hasten the deciphering of the signals that guide cells through their growth cycles.

Ability to Form Colonies in Soft Agar Suspension. Untransformed cells of fibroblast origin must attach to a solid surface before they can divide; this requirement is known as "anchorage dependence of multiplication." By contrast, transformed cells will divide in suspension culture. In particular, ability to grow and form colonies when

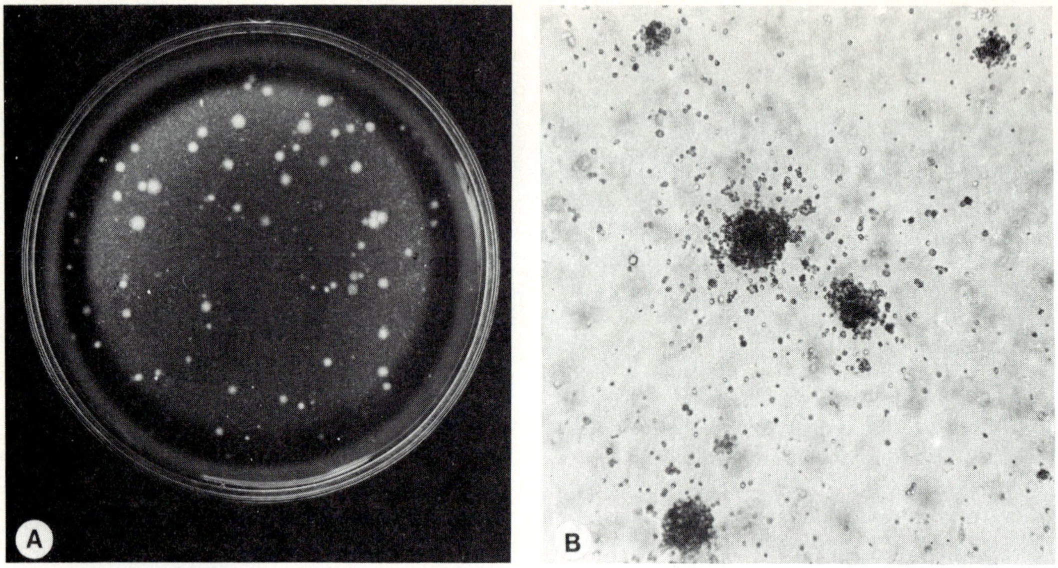

Figure 8-2. Suspension colonies in soft agar of chick embryo fibroblasts transformed with Rous sarcoma virus. **A.** Appearance of a Petri dish with numerous colonies (14 days after infection and plating). **B.** Enlargement of several colonies (8 days after infection and plating). *(Courtesy of Dr. Thomas Graf.)*

suspended in soft (0.5 percent) agar (Fig. 8-2) provides not only a very useful test for the stably transformed state but also the basis for a selective procedure that permits the isolation of transformed cells from populations of predominantly untransformed ones.

Changes in Membrane Transport Properties

Simple sugars and other nutrients are transported several times more rapidly across the plasma membrane of transformed than of untransformed cells. This is generally the earliest observable change following transformation. It is conceivable that increased sugar transport into transformed cells is responsible, at least in part, for the increased rate of glycolysis that is generally observed in transformed cells.

Acquisition of New Surface Antigens

The surfaces of virus-transformed cells possess antigenic determinants not present on untransformed cells. These new surface antigens can be detected by immunofluorescence (Fig. 8-3) or by tests for cytotoxic and cell-mediated immunologic response. Indeed, their presence causes transformed cells to be recognized as foreign and therefore subject to immunologic surveillance. Most of these new antigenic determinants are virus-specified; some may be coded by the host genome. Among the mechanisms that may cause new host-specified antigens to manifest themselves following transformation are derepression of genes that do not ordinarily express themselves and unmasking or exposure of determinants that are not normally apparent.

Increased Agglutinability by Lectins

Many animal cells are agglutinated by certain glycoproteins and proteins that are present in plant seeds, snails, crabs, and some fish and that possess affinity for sugars in general and glycoproteins in particular. They are collectively known as lectins (or agglutinins). Some of these lectins preferentially agglutinate tumor cells. The two lectins that best discriminate between normal and transformed cells are the jack bean agglutinin concanavalin A (con A) and wheat germ agglutinin (WGA). At first it was thought that transformed cells are agglutinated more readily than nontransformed ones because they bind more lectin molecules. However, it is now known that this is not so. Rather the reason seems to lie in the arrangement of the lectin-binding sites, which are dispersed in untransformed cells and clustered in transformed ones. Further, it is now known that both con A and WGA can agglutinate untransformed cells under certain conditions—they will agglutinate cells in metaphase and cells exposed briefly to proteases, such as trypsin. Interestingly, contact-inhibited protease-treated cells escape from growth control for brief periods of time, probably until the proteins that are removed by protease are regenerated. The reason why treatment with proteases renders cells more agglutinable is not known. One explanation is that proteases split off surface

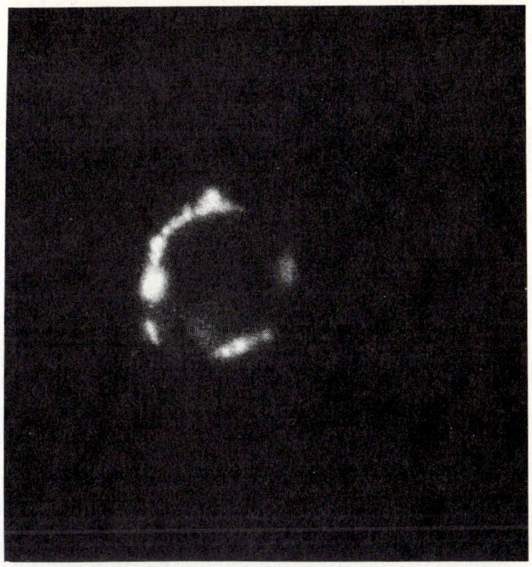

Figure 8-3. Demonstration, by means of immunofluorescence, of the tumor-specific transplantation antigen (TSTA) on a cell derived from a tumor induced in hamsters with adenovirus type 12. The cell was treated first with a hamster antiserum to such cells and then with rabbit antihamster immunoglobulin conjugated with fluorescein isothiocyanate. The hamster antiserum was prepared by repeated injection of adenovirus type 12, followed by one injection of tumor cells. Note the annular pattern of specific fluorescence on the cell membrane. TSTA on cells transformed with papovaviruses can be demonstrated by analogous procedures. *(From Vascencelos-Costa: J Gen Virol 8:69, 1970.)*

glycopeptides, thereby increasing membrane fluidity and facilitating clustering of lectin receptor sites.

Changes in Chemical Composition of Plasma Cell Membrane Components

Whereas the protein composition of plasma membranes appears to be fairly constant, their lipid, glycolipid, and glycoprotein carbohydrate components are notoriously variable. They are exquisitely sensitive to changes in the medium, changes in the cell growth rate, and changes in growth conditions in general. It is difficult, therefore, to pick out changes attributable to transformation, but the following appear to be significant.

1. When untransformed cells become density (contact) inhibited, their glycolipids become larger and more complex. Apparently, glycosyl transferases that are not expressed in rapidly growing cells are expressed in contact-inhibited cells. Transformed cells do not exhibit this cell density-dependent glycolipid extension response. Fucose-containing, galactose-containing, and NANA(N-acetylneuramic acid)-containing glycolipids are present in transformed cells in smaller amounts than in untransformed cells and are smaller in size.
2. Strangely, changes of a similar but opposite nature occur in the oligosaccharides of glycoproteins. In transformed cells these groups are larger than in untransformed cells, and they contain more NANA (which always occupies a terminal position).
3. One of the major components of plasma membranes of normal cells is fibronectin, a large polymorphic glycoprotein (subunit mol wt 200,000 to 250,000). Fibronectin possesses affinity for collagen, fibrin, heparin, and cell surfaces. Transformed cells usually, but not always, lack this protein, which is therefore also known as LETS (large external transformation-sensitive) protein. Its absence may decrease cell-cell and cell-tissue matrix interactions and may also increase membrane fluidity, thereby facilitating access to nutrients (thus lowering the requirement for serum) as well as lateral movement of membrane components (which would explain the increased agglutinability by lectins).

Decreased Levels of Cyclic AMP

In normal cells the level of cyclic AMP increases as they reach confluency. Lowering the concentration of serum in the medium has a similar effect. Transformed cells generally possess lower levels of cyclic AMP than normal ones, and lowering the serum concentration fails to elevate these levels.

Increased Secretion of Plasminogen Activator

Most cells produce small amounts of a protease, commonly known as plasminogen activator, that converts plasminogen to plasmin, the protease that digests fibrin. Many, but not all, transformed cells produce very much more plasminogen activator than their normal counterparts. The significance of this increased level of protease production is not clear. Since normal cells produce less plasminogen activator when contact-inhibited than when growing and since tumor cells are less subject to contact inhibition than normal cells, production of high levels of plasminogen activator may have a role in cell growth stimulation.

Chromosomal Changes

Transformation generally results in changes in karyotype. Among the most common changes are deletion of portions of some chromosomes, duplication/amplification of portions of others, translocation of material from one chromosome to another, and duplication of entire chromosomes.

Members of six virus families are known to be tumorigenic and capable of transforming cells in culture. The manner in which transformation by these viruses is established, maintained, transmitted, and detected will now be described.

DNA Tumor Viruses

Papillomaviruses

Papillomaviruses cause both benign and malignant tumors in a wide variety of animals. There are good reasons for considering human papillomaviruses (HPV) as candidate etiologic agents of cancer in humans:

1. Human papillomaviruses are ubiquitous.
2. They are epitheliotropic, which is important because most human cancers are carcinomas.
3. HPVs are the only viruses known to induce tumors (warts or papillomas) naturally in humans.
4. Papillomaviruses are the natural causes of cancer in animals. For example, Shope papilloma virus induces skin warts in cottontail rabbits, and these warts transform into squamous cell carcinomas in about 25 percent of animals. Further, bovine papilloma viruses induce upper alimentary tract papillomas in cattle that convert to carcinomas, as well as adenomas and adenocarcinomas of the intestine, urinary bladder tumors, meningiomas, fibropapillomas, penile and esophageal papillomas, and urinary bladder papillomas. Bovine papilloma viruses may also be involved in naturally occurring equine connective tissue tumors.

In humans, at least 15 distinct types of HPV cause a variety of lesions (see Table 2-4). Many HPVs cause benign warts, but in about 25 percent of patients with epidermodysplasia verruciformis, a rare hereditary disease involving generalized degeneration of flat warts, malignant transformation occurs. Human genital warts (condylomata acuminata) tend to convert to squamous cell carcinomas of the penis, vulva, and the perianal region, and recurrent laryngeal warts also sometimes convert to malignant tumors.

The various HPVs are surprisingly diverse. Their genomes possess quite distinct restriction endonuclease maps, and most of them exhibit very little homology; for example, the DNA of HPV-1 hybridizes to the DNAs of HPV-2 and HPV-7 only to the extent of about 6 and 0.6 percent, respectively. Not surprisingly, the proteins encoded by the various types of HPV are serologically quite distinct. As a result, individual patients may be simultaneously infected with numerous HPV types.

Little is known concerning the interaction of HPV with cells because they are extremely fastidious and have not yet been grown in cells cultured in vitro. It is clear, however, that HPV DNA tends to persist in the cells that it infects and transforms in stable episomal, rather than in integrated, form. From 5 to 200 copies of it per cell have been detected. Further, there is evidence that papilloma virus DNA in transformed cells is heavily hypermethylated. Active gene sequences are generally undermethylated, while inactive genes show a high degree of methylation. The hypermethylation of papilloma virus DNA would, therefore, suggest that it is transcribed sparingly in infected cells, which agrees with the finding that transcripts corresponding to only about 10 percent of the papilloma virus genome are present in infected cells, and these only in small amounts. Thus papilloma virus genomes express themselves only minimally in transformed cells.

Polyomaviruses

Polyoma virus was isolated from mouse cell extracts used for the transmission of leukemia. It is only rarely responsible for tumors in nature. When infected into newborn mice or hamsters, it produces a wide variety of histologically distinguishable tumors, hence its name.

SV40 was first isolated from apparently normal cultures of monkey kidney cells. The only host in which it causes tumors is the baby hamster. Lymphocytic leukemia, lymphosarcoma, reticulum cell sarcoma, and osteogenic sarcoma are all produced.

There are also two human polyomaviruses, BK virus and JC virus (BK and JC are the initials of the persons from whom they were isolated in 1971). Both are more closely related to SV40 than to polyoma virus. For example, the amino acid sequences of the proteins encoded by SV40 and BKV are about 80 percent homologous, and the antigenic determinants on their T antigens are almost completely cross-reactive. However, BKV and JCV are quite distinct from each other; and there are only weak immunologic cross-reactions between them.

BKV was isolated from the urine of an immunosuppressed renal transplant patient, while JCV was isolated from the brain of a patient with progressive multifocal leukoencephalopathy (PML). Both viruses are very widespread in humans. Infection occurs in childhood, and most adults have antibodies to them. Apparently primary infection is asymptomatic and is followed by a low-grade lifelong persistent infection that is activated when the immune system is compromised. The viruses then establish silent foci of infection in the urinary tract, which causes them to be excreted in the urine, and in a very few individuals JCV reaches oligodendrocytes in the brain and causes PML, a chronic, fatal demyelinating disease. Interestingly, a very similar disease occurs in rhesus monkeys, the natural host of SV40; and two human PML cases have yielded SV40, rather than JCV.

Both BKV and JCV possess oncogenic potential. Both transform cultured cells and cause tumors in a variety of animals. Both are markedly neurotropic. Thus, JCV induces brain tumors in owl monkeys, and most of the tumors caused by BKV in Syrian hamsters are ependymomas, while JCV shows a predilection for neuroectodermal cells. However, neither virus is associated with any form of cancer in humans.

SV40 and polyoma virus are moderately closely related. Their proteins share some antigenic determinants, and their amino acid sequences are about 40 percent homologous (that is, they possess the same amino acids in equivalent positions).

Transformation by Polyomaviruses

Polyomaviruses not only interact with cells by means of the lytic pathway (Chap. 4) but also transform cells. Cells are transformed if they are nonpermissive—that is, if the virus cannot multiply in them—or if they are permissive, they can be transformed if they are infected with defective virus particles, such as the deletion mutants that arise upon repeated passage at high multiplicity (Chap. 6), or if they are infected with inactivated virus particles (for example, by photodynamic inactivation). In other words, if a polyomavirus can multiply in a cell, that cell will generally not be transformed; if it cannot multiply, the cell will often be transformed. The establishment of the transforming papovavirus-cell interaction requires high multiplicities of infection (10^6 to 10^7 particles per cell). There is evidence that the frequency of transformation is enhanced, by some as yet unknown mechanism, by treating cells with chemical carcinogens, such as 4-nitroquinoline-1-oxide. The essential feature of the transforming polyomavirus-cell interaction is that viral DNA becomes stably integrated into the DNA of the host cell. As a result it cannot multiply, except as a cellular gene, and no progeny virus is produced. Not all infected cells are transformed in this manner; the majority are transformed abortively—that is, they escape from growth control for a few cell generations but then revert to the normal uninfected state for reasons that are not understood.

Polyomavirus DNA can integrate at many sites in the cellular genome. The number of integrated viral genomes generally varies from 1 to 3 but can be as high as 20 to 50. Transformation by one polyomavirus does not preclude transformation by another nor by unrelated viruses. Thus, double transformants of SV40 and polyoma, as well as of SV40 and adenovirus and SV40 and various RNA tumor viruses, have been isolated and studied.

Function of Polyomavirus Tumor Antigens

Although viral DNA in transformed cells does not replicate except as part of the host genome, it does express itself. In fact, substantial amounts of messenger RNA are generally transcribed from it by the α-amanitin-sensitive cellular RNA polymerase II. However, not the entire viral genome is transcribed but only that portion of it that encodes the early functions, that is, the various tumor antigens [large T and small t in the case of SV40, and large T, middle t, and small t antigens in the case of polyoma virus (see Chap. 4)]. It is the presence of these proteins that is responsible for the induction and maintenance of the transformed state, and a very large amount of work has been done to define their functions. Clearly, knowledge of these presumably complementary functions would provide fundamentally important clues concerning the mechanisms by which normal cells are transformed into cancer cells. The most important approach has been examination of the characteristics of cells infected with SV40 and polyoma virus mutants that contain well-defined deletions—in other words, cells in which either large T, middle t, or small t antigen cannot be made. This work has permitted the following conclusions:

1. Large T antigen (Fig. 8-4) is responsible for stimulating host cell DNA synthesis, a function that is inseparable from ability to transform. It is also responsible for the ability to form colonies in soft agar and proliferate in the presence of low serum concentrations. Further, at least a portion of it is exposed on the transformed cell surface as the *transplantation antigen,* the antigen that elicits antibodies and sensitizes lymphocytes that protect against subsequent challenge with polyomavirus-induced tumor cells or with polyomavirus particles.
2. Small t antigen complements the functions of large T antigen. The presence of functional small t antigen is also usually necessary for the ability to form colonies in soft agar, produce plasminogen activator (p. 133), and cause dissolution of the intracel-

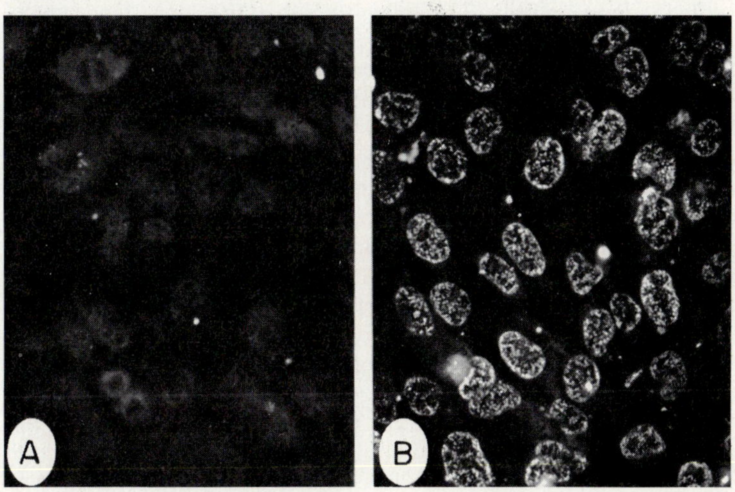

Figure 8-4. Demonstration of the SV40 T antigen by means of immunofluorescence. Cells from a tumor induced by SV40 in a hamster were exposed to fluorescein-conjugated serum from a nontumor-bearing hamster (**A**) and a tumor-bearing hamster (**B**). × 280. *(From Rapp, et al.: Proc Soc Exp Biol Med 116:1131, 1964.)*

lular actin cable network, absence of which is a hallmark of fully transformed cells. Maintenance of the transformed state and tumor progression are also dependent on the continued presence of small t antigen.

3. In cells transformed with polyoma virus, middle t antigen plays an additional role in enhancing full expression of the transformed phenotype and transformed cell growth in general and membrane alterations in particular. It is located in the plasma cell membrane and is associated with a protein kinase activity that phosphorylates tyrosine residues in middle t antigen itself. Phosphorylation of tyrosine residues in proteins also occurs in cells transformed with RNA tumor viruses (see below), and a great deal of research is currently directed at determining the significance of tyrosine phosphorylation in the cancer process. The reason for the excitement is that most phosphoproteins in normal cells are phosphorylated in serine and threonine residues, not in tyrosine residues.
4. SV40 does not code for a middle t antigen. Instead, intracellular large T antigen is tightly associated with a cellular phosphoprotein, the p53 protein, whose formation it stimulates some 25- to 50-fold over normal cell levels. The p53 protein is also present in cells transformed by other agents, such as chemicals or irradiation, and in spontaneously arising carcinoma cells. It is also induced in nondividing lymphocytes when stimulated with mitogens, which suggests that it functions somehow in cell division.

Rescue of Transforming Genome

Whereas viral DNA in transformed cells never expresses itself in its entirety, it is nevertheless the entire viral DNA that is integrated, not portions or segments of it, as can be proved by several types of experiments. For example, the genome of SV40 can be rescued from transformed cells by fusing them with uninfected permissive cells. Fusion may be effected by simple cocultivation or, much more efficiently, by treatment with inactivated Sendai virus (Chap. 5). Apparently only the cytoplasm of permissive cells is necessary, since fusion with enucleated cells has been shown to rescue SV40. This rescue of virus can be effected from cells that have been transformed for many generations and many years. Presumably the mechanism involves excision and/or recombination to generate free circular viral genomes.

Transformed cells can also be shown to harbor the entire SV40 genome because infectious SV40 DNA can be extracted from them.

Revertants of Transformed Cells

Numerous attempts have been made to isolate revertants of transformed cells. Among the techniques that have led to the selection of revertant cell lines that exhibit growth control comparable to that of normal cells are selection for serum dependence, passage at high dilution, resistance to nucleic acid-base analogs at high cell density (i.e., inability to multiply at high cell density), and resistance to con A. All these methods yield cells that display contact inhibition of growth and resemble normal cells morphologically. However, almost always they still synthesize the tumor antigens, display unaltered virus-specific transcription patterns, and contain the entire viral genome. Therefore, reversion is due to a change in the cellular rather than in the viral genome. Revertants cannot be retransformed with the virus whose genome they already harbor, but they can be retransformed with other tumor viruses. Finally, revertant cell lines often contain more chromosomes than their transformed antecedents. This has suggested a hypothesis that the cell phenotype is modified as a result of changes in the relative amounts of chromosomes with genes that promote and genes that oppose transformation.

Adenoviruses

Adenoviruses also can transform animal cells in vitro, and some but not all cause tumors in animals.

Human adenoviruses can be divided into three groups on the basis of their oncogenicity. Serotypes 12, 18, and 31 are highly oncogenic: when injected into newborn hamsters, they cause tumors rapidly and with high frequency. Serotypes 3, 7, 14, 16, and 21 are weakly oncogenic: they produce tumors in newborn hamsters with low frequency and after a long latent period. Most of the remaining serotypes, exemplified by serotypes 2 and 5, are nononcogenic, but even they can transform rodent cells in culture.

Adenovirus-transformed cells display many of the properties described above for cells transformed by polyomaviruses, but there are also important differences. For example, in contrast to integrated SV40 and polyoma virus DNA, adenovirus DNA integrated into the genomes of transformed cells cannot be rescued by fusion with permissive cells. This suggests either that only a portion of adenovirus DNA is integrated or that it is integrated in the form of fragments. Analysis of the nature of viral DNA sequences present in a variety of cells transformed by several adenoviruses has shown that (1) none of them contained the complete adenovirus genome, (2) all contained at least the left-hand 8 percent of the viral genome (which agrees with the finding that cells can be transformed with its leftmost restriction endonuclease fragments), and (3) some contain most of the viral genome but in fragmented form. To take specific examples, one rat embryo cell line transformed by adenovirus type 2 contains three copies of the sequence comprising the leftmost 17 percent of the adenovirus genome, another contains about 13 copies of the leftmost 70 percent of the viral DNA, 3 of which are linked covalently to the sequence between map units 98 and 96.5 *inverted* with respect to its normal orientation in the viral DNA, and a hamster cell line transformed by adenovirus type 12 contains about 8 copies of fragments that together comprise virtually the entire viral genome.

Virus-specific proteins were first detected in cells transformed by adenoviruses by immunologic means, such as immunofluorescence or complement fixation, using antisera from hamsters bearing tumors induced by adenoviruses. Such proteins were designated "adenovirus T antigen." It is clear now that various adenovirus-transformed cell lines contain very different amounts of viral DNA and that a variety of viral proteins, all early region proteins, are formed in them. The term "adenovirus T antigen" should be reserved for those proteins that are encoded by the minimal segment of adenovirus DNA capable of transforming cells, that is, its leftmost 4.5 percent, which corresponds to early region E1A (Chap. 4). This region codes for about four proteins, one of which has recently been highly purified and appears to be a true T antigen that is present in all adenovirus-transformed cells and is therefore diagnostic of adenovirus transformation.

The demonstrated oncogenicity of human adenoviruses in rodents raises the possibility that they may cause neoplasia in humans. This has been investigated using exquisitely sensitive hybridization techniques that have been refined to the extent that one part of viral DNA can be detected in the presence of 10^6 parts of host DNA, which corresponds to less than one adenovirus genome per cell. So far no human neoplasms have been found that contain adenovirus DNA.

Herpesviruses

Numerous herpesviruses either are oncogenic, are associated with tumors, or can transform cells in vitro. Eight are oncogenic in animals (Table 8-1); they include herpesviruses of primates and other mammals, birds, and amphibians. In humans, no fewer than three herpesviruses may be involved in tumorigenesis: Epstein–Barr virus (EBV), the genome of which is often present in cultured Burkitt's lymphoma and nasopharyngeal carcinoma cells and which can transform human B lymphocytes; herpes simplex virus type 2 (HSV 2), which seroepidemiologic evidence suggests may be associated with carcinoma of the cervix and which can transform a variety of cells, especially when inactivated with ultraviolet irradiation so as to preclude the productive or lytic virus-cell interaction; and human cytomegalovirus (HCMV), which may play a role in the etiology of Kaposi's sarcoma and which, after exposure to ultraviolet irradiation, can also transform cultured cells.

Epstein–Barr Virus

Burkitt's lymphoma is a tumor that is relatively common in East Africa and New Guinea but rare in other parts of the world. It occurs chiefly in children 5 to 12 years of age. In the body, the tumor cells contain no virus, but a small proportion of lymphoblastoid cells established in vitro from tumor tissue produce a herpesvirus that is antigenically distinct from all known herpesviruses and is known as Epstein–Barr virus (EBV) after its discoverers. EBV is very widely distributed; 80 percent of adults worldwide possess antibodies to it. Thus, even in regions where Burkitt's lymphoma is endemic, only a very small proportion of infected individuals develop the tumor. Interestingly, a small proportion of African Burkitt's lymphomas and most American and European Burkitt's lymphomas contain no trace of EBV infection.

EBV is one of three tumorigenic B lymphotropic herpesviruses of humans and primates, the others being herpesvirus papio (baboons) and herpesvirus pan (chimpanzees), the DNAs of which share about 40 percent sequence homology. All cause lymphoproliferative disease in primates, such as marmosets. Their host range is very narrow; only B lymphocytes possess receptors for them, and they transform these cells into lymphoblastoid cells with an infinite life span. All cells infected with EBV or cell lines isolated from EBV-induced tumors contain EBV DNA and a tumor antigen known as EBNA (Epstein–Barr nuclear antigen), but productive virus multiplication occurs in only a very small proportion of them, possibly because EBV DNA is unusually hypermethylated (hypermethylation being an attribute of genetically silent genome regions). The proportion of cells in which EBV multiplies can be in-

TABLE 8-1. ONCOGENIC HERPESVIRUSES

Virus	Host	Host Cell	Malignancy
Epstein–Barr virus	Humans	B lymphocytes	Burkitt's lymphoma, nasopharyngeal carcinoma
Herpesvirus pan	Primates	B lymphocytes	Lymphoma
Herpesvirus papio	Primates	B lymphocytes	Lymphoma
Marek's disease virus	Chicken	T lymphocytes	Lymphoma
Herpesvirus saimiri	Primates	T lymphocytes	Lymphoma
Herpesvirus ateles	Primates	T lymphocytes	Lymphoma
Herpesvirus sylvilagus	Rabbits	B lymphocytes (?)	Lymphoma
Cytomegalovirus	Humans		Kaposi's sarcoma (?)
Lucké frog herpesvirus	Frogs		Adenocarcinoma of the kidney

creased by arginine deprivation or treatment with bromodeoxyuridine, TPA (12-O-tetradecanoylphorbol-13-acetate, a tumor promoter), 5-azacytidine, or dimethylsulfoxide. The last three reagents are demethylating agents. More than 80 messenger RNAs and 50 proteins have been characterized in cells infected with EBV.

The number of EBV DNA molecules (Fig. 8-5) present in transformed or tumor cells ranges from 2 to more than 200, mostly as free episomal closed circles. Only a few are integrated into the host genome. They are present not only in Burkitt's lymphoma cells but also in the cells of nasopharyngeal (postnasal) carcinoma, which occurs with rather high frequency among Southern Chinese and, to a lesser extent, among Algerians.

It is impossible to say, at present, whether the relationship between EBV and Burkitt's lymphoma and nasopharyngeal carcinoma is casual or causal. On the one hand, there is no doubt that EBV possesses oncogenic potential in vivo and in vitro, its target cells being cells of the B lymphocytic lineage. Further, the cells of most of the Burkitt's tumors that arise in Africa and some of the tumors that arise elsewhere contain EBV DNA and EBV antigens. However, some such tumors do not, and if EBV has an etiologic role in Burkitt's lymphoma and nasopharyngeal carcinoma, other cofactors must also be involved.

EBV and Infectious Mononucleosis. The majority of the normal adult population of the United States possesses antibodies against EBV. Conversion from the seronegative to the seropositive state occurs during the acute phase of infectious mononucleosis. Apparently, therefore, EBV is the etiologic agent of infectious mononucleosis. Presumably, most infections with EBV are subclinical, that is, so mild as to go unnoticed. Some can cause overt infectious mononucleosis, and, very rarely in most populations but more frequently in others where special factors may be operative, Burkitt's lymphoma and nasapharyngeal carcinoma ensues. The nature of these factors and their mode of action are not known.

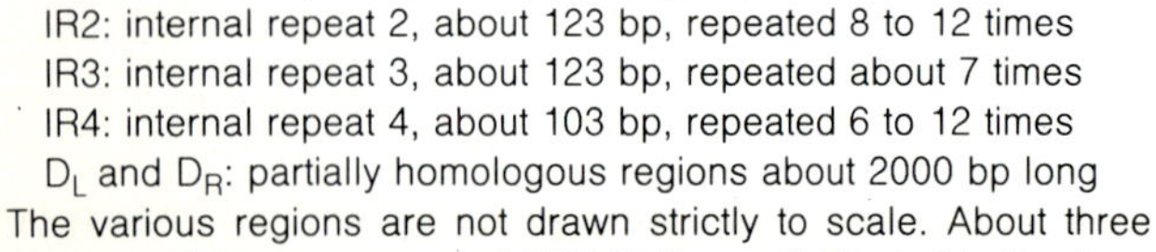

Figure 8-5. Schematic representation of the DNA of EBV. Its size is similar to that of herpes simplex virus [about 100×10^6 or 170,000 base pairs (bp)].

TR: terminal repeat, about 500 bp, repeated 6 to 12 times
IR1: internal repeat 1, about 3000 bp, repeated 6 to 12 times
IR2: internal repeat 2, about 123 bp, repeated 8 to 12 times
IR3: internal repeat 3, about 123 bp, repeated about 7 times
IR4: internal repeat 4, about 103 bp, repeated 6 to 12 times
D_L and D_R: partially homologous regions about 2000 bp long

The various regions are not drawn strictly to scale. About three quarters of the sequences of EBV DNA are distributed in 5 unique regions, while about one quarter are present in the form of repeated sequence elements. IR1 is transcribed very extensively into messenger RNA, but the proteins that it encodes have not yet been identified. IR2 appears to contain the origin of replication. IR3 is also transcribed very actively and appears to encode the EBNA, a 380 amino acid long protein with a remarkable composition: more than two thirds of its amino acids are alanine and glycine, which no doubt causes EBNA to possess a unique structure.

Herpes Simplex Virus

Two types of herpes simplex virus infect humans: type 1, which causes primarily oral lesions, and type 2, which is associated with genital infections. Several lines of epidemiologic and serologic evidence suggest that infection with herpes simplex virus type 2 is associated with carcinoma of the cervix. In particular, women with genital herpetic infections have a higher than average incidence of cervical carcinoma, and women with cervical carcinoma have a higher than average incidence of antibodies to herpes simplex virus type 2.

Although suggestive, this evidence is not sufficient to establish a definitive causal relationship between herpes simplex virus and malignant disease in humans. In fact, such a relationship will be difficult to establish because herpesviruses are ubiquitous and tend to establish latent and persistent infections. Since experimentation with humans is not feasible, the most direct evidence is likely to be provided by a vaccine that markedly reduces the incidence of some form of cancer.

Poxviruses

Two poxviruses are tumorigenic: fibroma virus, including the classic Shope fibroma virus which is pathogenic for rabbits, as well as several closely related viruses pathogenic for deer, squirrels, and hares, and Yaba monkey tumor virus, which is pathogenic for several species of monkeys and for humans. Both produce benign tumors that soon regress.

The interest in poxvirus tumorigenicity derives from the fact that poxviruses are DNA-containing viruses that have always been thought to multiply exclusively in the cytoplasm. Recently acquired evidence suggests, however, that while vaccinia virus does not appear to have an obligatory nuclear phase in its multiplication cycle, some viral DNA and RNA are often present in the nucleus. Poxvirus DNA may therefore have the opportunity to become integrated into the host cell genome or to become otherwise stably associated with it, and when that happens, cell transformation may result. When fibroma virus transforms cells, host DNA replication is first arrested, and viral DNA replication is initiated. However, it quickly ceases, host DNA replication recommences, and the cells become transformed. They then multiply more rapidly than before, exhibit an altered morphology, are less sensitive to contact inhibition, and display new antigens on their surface. While the precise nature of the association of fibroma DNA and the host cell genome is not known, it is clear that the association is not a stable one, since the tumors often regress and contain fibroma virus particles when they do so.

Hepatitis B Virus

The only known hosts of hepatitis B virus are humans. About 200 million humans are currently infected with this virus, which causes hepatitis B or serum hepatitis. Many of them are carriers in whom the virus established a chronic or persistent infection manifested by the circulation for months or years of relatively high concentrations of HBsAg particles, defective or incomplete viral forms that consist predominantly of hepatitis B surface antigen, as well as small amounts of infectious virus. In other individuals the virus establishes a highly virulent, often fatal disease (Chap. 25). What has recently caused great excitement is evidence that infection with this virus is strongly associated not only with cirrhosis of the liver but also with the most common fatal cancer of humans, primary hepatic carcinoma.

The complete hepatitis B virus particle, known as the "Dane" particle, consists of an outer layer, the so-called HBsAg, and an inner core, the HBcAg. In the serum of patients and carriers, most HBsAg and HBcAg exists in free form, not in the form of intact virus particles. Both consist of several protein species. Hepatitis B DNA in Dane particles is *partially* double-stranded; it consists of a complete 3200 nucleotide long minus strand, but the plus strand is on the average only about two thirds of full length. The virus contains a DNA polymerase, and if it is incubated in vitro with nucleoside triphosphates, plus strand synthesis is completed.

Efforts to understand its life cycle have been hindered by the failure of hepatitis B virus to grow in cultured cells. Current evidence suggests that hepatitis B virus multiplies as depicted in Figure 8-6. It appears that soon after infection the minus strand of its genome is transcribed into plus-stranded RNA, which after being translated becomes encapsidated in hepatitis B core-like particles and is then reverse-transcribed into DNA in maturing progeny virus particles. The fascinating feature of this sequence of reactions is that it is a temporally permuted version of the retrovirus multiplication cycle (see below), where infectious virus particles contain RNA that is reverse-transcribed into double-stranded DNA soon after infection and, after integration into the host genome, is used as the template for the repeated synthesis of genome RNA later in infection.

As pointed out above, chronic hepatitis B infection is associated with increased risk of primary hepatic carcinoma. The question then arises as to whether hepatitis B virus causes cancer the same way retroviruses do, namely, by integrating their DNA into that of the cell. Little is known yet concerning the integration of hepatitis B DNA into the human genome, but preliminary evidence indicates that it does occur and that the DNA is not integrated intact, as is the DNA provirus of retroviruses, but that integration is accompanied by complex rearrangements within multimeric inserts and loss of genetic material. It seems, however, that one particular region of the hepatitis B genome is always retained, and it is conceivable that it contains a super promoter like polyoma and SV40 DNA (Chap. 4) and the LTR of retroviruses (p. 144). As a result, promoter insertion may play a role in transformation by hepatitis B virus, just as it does for certain retroviruses.

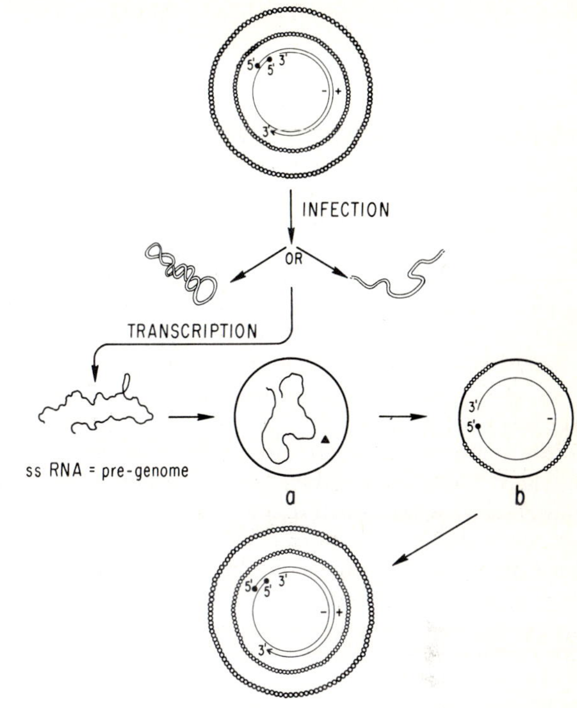

Figure 8-6. The multiplication cycle of hepatitis B virus. Following infection and uncoating, the viral DNA is transcribed into plus-stranded RNA—the pre-genome. After being translated, the pre-genome is encapsidated into immature cores (**a**) and reverse-transcribed into negative-stranded DNA, while the RNA pre-genome is degraded (**b**). The outer virus particle coat is then added, the minus DNA strand is partially transcribed into its plus strand, and the virus is liberated.

RNA Tumor Viruses

The most intensively investigated tumor viruses are the RNA tumor viruses. There are three primary reasons for this. First, in many animal species they cause leukemias and solid tumors that are often strikingly similar to human neoplasms. This raises the question of their role in the genesis of cancer in humans. Second, the genomes of RNA tumor viruses are integrated into the genomes of many species of animals ranging from reptiles to higher apes. Why not also into that of humans? Third, the transforming genes of RNA tumor viruses are very closely related to genes that are present in the genomes of all animals, genes that may function during embryonic development. Thus RNA tumor viruses seem to provide the best chance for solving the basic secret of cancer, namely, why genes are switched on inappropriately and out of context and how they are switched on. In other words, since cancer undoubtedly has a genetic basis, our best hope of unraveling its molecular mechanisms lies in studying the nature of the interaction of tumor virus genomes with those of the host cells, and RNA tumor viruses provide a far wider spectrum of viruses than any of the DNA tumor virus families.

Since the term "RNA tumor virus" is cumbersome and since viruses exist that, while exhibiting the same strategy of genome structure and expression, are not tumorigenic (Table 4-4), attempts have been made to devise a more concise and/or generally applicable designation. Among the proposed names are oncornavirus (oncoRNA), oncovirus, and retrovirus. The latter term has found wide acceptance and is used in the discussion that follows.

Nature of Retrovirus Particles

Retrovirus particles possess an electron-dense nucleoid or core surrounded by two shells (Figs. 8-7 and 8-8). The inner shell, which appears to possess icosahedral symmetry, is the nucleocapsid shell, while the outer shell consists of a lipid bilayer membrane to which glycoprotein spikes are attached. Retrovirus particles comprise seven structural proteins (Table 8-2). Two are glycoproteins that make up the envelope spikes, the larger forming the knobs, the smaller the stalks. They are linked by covalent-SS-bonds. The larger, glycoprotein gp85 in the case of avian retroviruses and gp70 in the case of mammalian ones, is the antigen that gives rise to neutralizing antibodies and is responsible for host range specificity. These envelope proteins are encoded by the *env* gene. The other structural proteins, p27, p19, p15, p12, and p10 in the case of avian retroviruses, and p30, p15, p12, p12E and p10 in the case of mammalian ones, are nucleocapsid components. The p27 and p30 proteins make up the nucleocapsid shells and are the principal virus particle components; p12 and p10 in avian and mammalian viruses, respectively, are intimately associated with the RNA. All these nucleocapsid proteins are derived by cleavage of a precursor that is the primary protein product of one of the three retrovirus genes, the so-called *gag* protein gene (see below). The order of these proteins in the precursors is NH_2-p19-p10-p27-p12-p15-COOH and NH_2-p15-p12-p30-p10-COOH for avian and mammalian retroviruses, respectively. There is evidence that in the avian system the protease that effects the cleavages is p15. Retrovirus particles also contain about 10 molecules of an RNA-dependent DNA polymerase, the reverse transcriptase, which is coded by the *pol* gene (see below).

All these proteins exhibit a multiplicity of antigenic determinants. There are type-specific antigenic determinants private to individual virus strains, group-specific determinants common to groups of viruses with common hosts, and interspecies-specific determinants that are common to all mammalian or avian retroviruses.

Three Morphologic Types of Retrovirus Particles

There are three morphologic types of retrovirus particles: C-type particles characteristic of most leukemia and sarcoma viruses; B-type particles characteristic of mammary tumor viruses that differ from C-type particles in the eccentric rather than central location of their nucleocapsid in thin sections, their more prominent glycoprotein spikes, and in the fact that their nucleoids can often be seen in the cytoplasm of infected cells (these are the so-called *intracytoplasmic* A-type of particles); and D-type particles isolated from a variety of primates, the properties of which are intermediate between those of C-type and B-type retrovirus particles.

Retrovirus Genome

The retrovirus genome consists of two identical plus-stranded RNA molecules that are 5,000 to 10,000 nucleotides long (mol wt 1.5 to 3×10^6) and hydrogen-bonded to each other via palindromic sequences some 15 nucleotides long that are centered about 60 nucleotides from their 5′ ends (Fig. 8-9).

The essential features of the basic retrovirus genome, that is the genome of nondefective avian and mammalian (particularly murine) leukosis or leukemia viruses (ALV and MLV), also sometimes called lymphoid leukosis viruses (LLV) are shown in Figure 8-10. It possesses sequences with regulatory features at each end flanking the coding sequences of three intronless genes: the *gag* gene that encodes the four or five nucleocapsid proteins, the *pol* gene that encodes the RNA-dependent DNA polymerase (the so-called reverse transcriptase), and the *env* gene that encodes the glycoprotein spike components. Other important features are the presence of direct terminal repeats (the R regions), the PB (-) region where a tRNA molecule binds to act as primer for the transcription of the RNA into DNA, the fact that the 5′ terminus untranslated region [R-U5-PB(-)-L] serves as a leader for subgenomic mRNA species (for example, the *env* proteins are transcribed from a messenger RNA that is derived from a complete genomic plus strand by splicing out the *gag-pol* coding sequences), and the presence of a strong promoter of transcription in the U3 region.

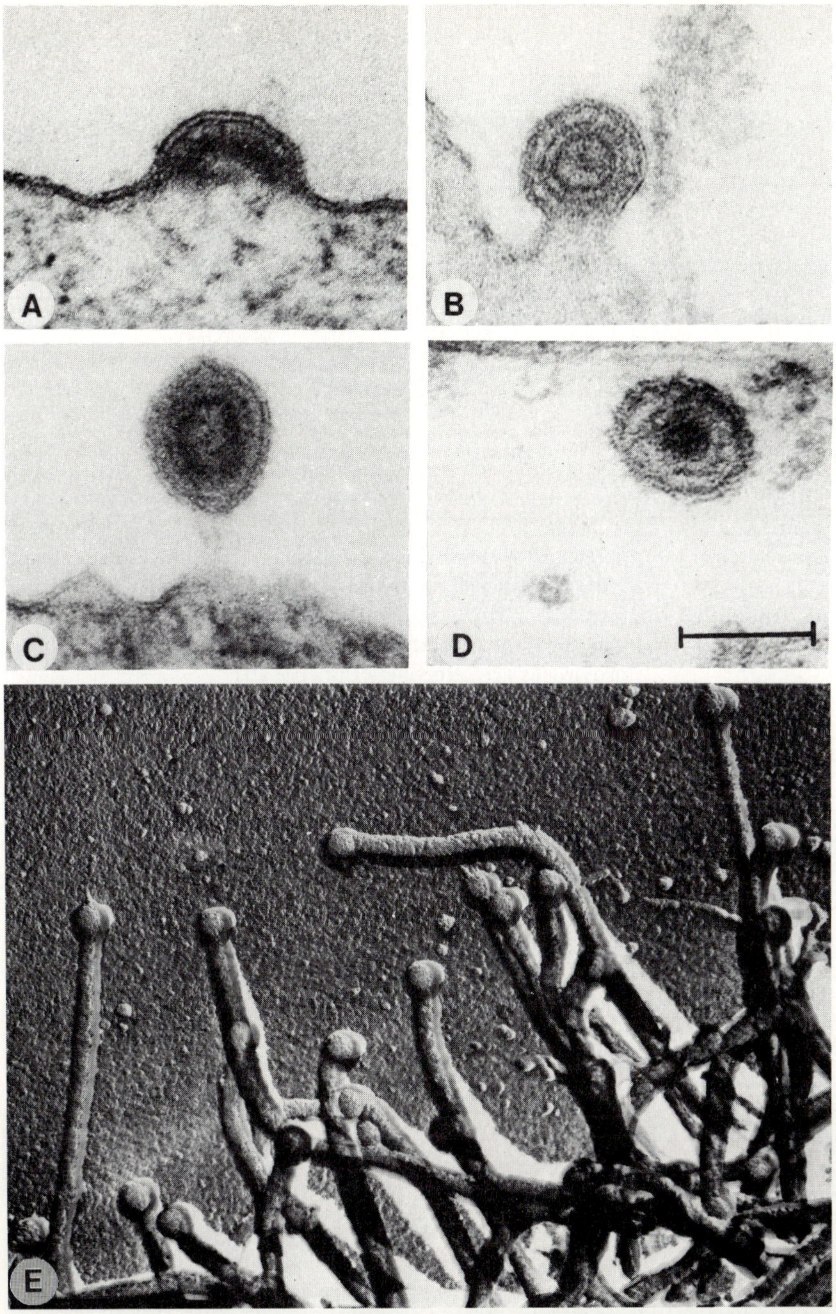

Figure 8-7. The morphogenesis and structure of RNA tumor viruses. **A-D**. Four stages in the budding of a C-type (avian) retrovirus. Note the electron-lucent center or core in immature particles (**B** and **C**) and the electron-dense core in mature particles (**D**). **E**. A micrograph of a surface replica of a GR cell that is producing murine mammary tumor virus (MMTV) particles (B-type retrovirus). The micrograph shows the cell margin with microvilli, from the tips of which the virus buds. (***A** through **D**, courtesy of Dr. Heinz Bauer; **E**, courtesy of Dr. J.B. Sheffield.*)

Molecular Biology of Retroviruses

There has long existed a conceptual difficulty concerning the role of retroviruses as oncogenic agents. Transformation represents a heritable alteration of cellular biosynthetic patterns that is most plausibly accounted for by a change in genetic capabilities. Conceivably there are mechanisms whereby a viral DNA genome might cause such changes after being integrated, but how could a viral RNA genome achieve this? Furthermore, many cells transformed by retroviruses produce virus for generation after generation. What type of mechanism could ensure that host and viral genome replication would proceed in step? In 1964 Temin advanced a revolutionary hypothesis: he proposed that upon infection the viral RNA genome is transcribed into DNA by a reversal of the usual flow of information transfer, that this DNA is then integrated into the host genome, and that progeny viral genomes are tran-

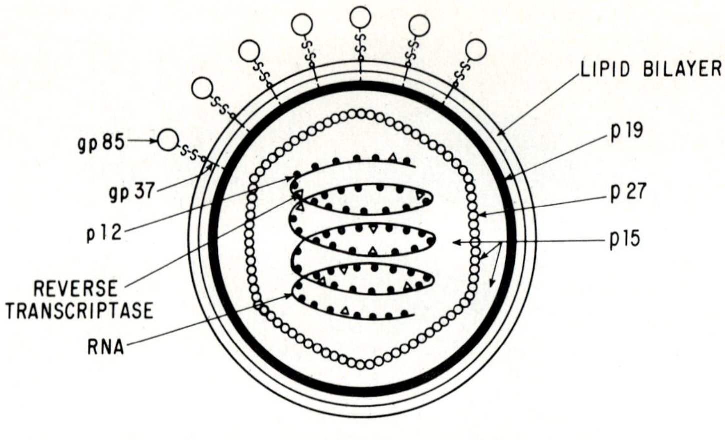

Figure 8-8. Model of an avian C-type retrovirus particle. For further details, see text and Table 8-2.

scribed from it just as all other RNA is normally transcribed. In essence, the hypothesis implied that the RNA present in retroviruses is not the genome but rather the messenger RNA of a genome that exists only intracellularly.

The discovery of reverse transcriptase independently by Temin and Baltimore in 1970 proved Temin's hypothesis correct.

Formation and Integration of Proviral DNA

Following adsorption and penetration into the cell, the RNA in parental nucleocapsids is transcribed by the reverse transcriptase into linear double-stranded DNA, the proviral DNA. The exact mechanism by which transcription is accomplished is not known, but it probably proceeds approximately as depicted in Figure 8-11. Linear proviral DNA then moves to the nucleus, circularizes to form supercoiled circles, and is integrated into the genome of the host cell.

The structure of the integrated provirus is shown in Figure 8-12. As a consequence of the transcription process described in Figure 8-11, its coding sequences are flanked by long terminal repeats (LTRs) composed of the U3, R, and U5 regions of retrovirus RNA. Their significance lies in the fact that they contain strong promoters of transcription. The integrated provirus is flanked by short inverted repeats of viral sequences (IR) and direct repeats (DR) of host cell sequences. This suggests that the mechanism of provirus integration is formally analogous to the insertion into bacterial DNA of transposable elements: proviruses are effectively transposons.

All available evidence indicates that integration can occur anywhere into cellular DNA. There are no preferred insertion loci. However, once integrated, a provirus is a stable genetic element; it is a gene. The number of integrated proviruses per haploid host genome may be as low as 1 or as high as 100, depending on the virus and on the cell.

Transcription of Integrated Proviral DNA

Integrated proviral DNA is transcribed by cellular RNA polymerase II into transcripts that are capped at their 5′ termini and polyadenylated at their 3′ termini. They are used in one of three ways. They may be encapsidated into progeny virus particles, or they may be translated either into the *gag* gene product, a protein with a molecular weight of

TABLE 8-2. RETROVIRUS STRUCTURAL PROTEINS*

Protein†				
Avian	Murine	Percent of Total Protein‡	Coded by	Location and Properties
p10	p12E	5,9	*gag*	Envelope
p12	p10	14,6	*gag*	Core, RNA-associated, phosphoprotein
p15		6	*gag*	Between core and envelope, protein-cleaving activity
p19		20	*gag*	Between core and envelope, phosphoprotein, hydrophobic
	p15	14	*gag*	Between core and envelope, hydrophobic
	p12	8	*gag*	Between core and envelope, phosphoprotein
p27	p30	36,50	*gag*	Core shell, major virus particle component
gp85	gp70	13,11	*env*	Major envelope protein, spike knob
gp37	gp15E	6,2	*env*	Minor envelope protein, spike stalk

*The structure of B-type retroviruses is similar to that of the C-type viruses. The major B-type internal *gag*-coded protein is p28; the major surface *env*-coded glycoprotein is gp52.

†p, protein; gp, glycoprotein. The number indicates the approximate size in daltons $\times\ 10^{-3}$. In addition to the seven proteins listed, each virus particle also contains about 10 molecules of the RNA-dependent DNA polymerase (reverse transcriptase).

‡Approximate percentages in avian and murine retroviruses, respectively.

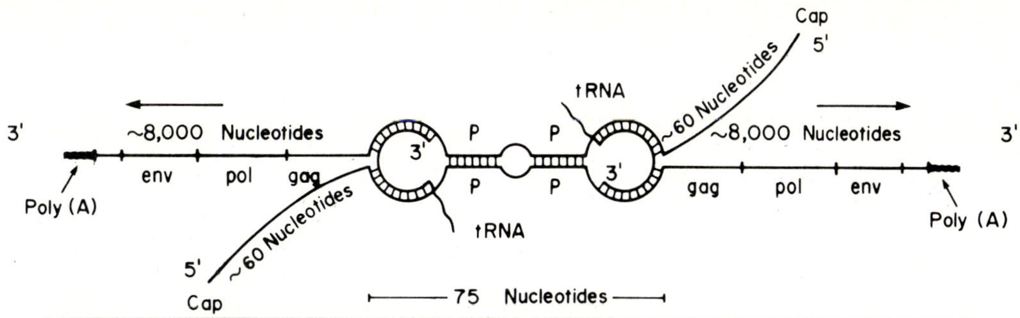

Figure 8-9. The avian retrovirus genome. Its two RNA subunits are held together by base pairing between the palindromic sequences P and by base pairing with tRNA molecules. *(Adapted from Haseltine et al.: Proc Natl Acad Sci USA 74:989, 1977.)*

about 70,000 that is cleaved into the 4 or 5 *gag* proteins, or, infrequently, into a *gag-pol* readthrough product, a large protein, P180, that is cleaved to the *pol* gene product (the reverse transcriptase) as well as the *gag* proteins. This mode of synthesizing the *pol* gene product (that is, without a messenger RNA of its own and by infrequent readthrough from another gene) provides a convenient mechanism for ensuring that it will not be synthesized in excessive amounts (clearly far more *gag* gene products are required for viral morphogenesis than *pol* gene product). Finally, provirus transcripts may have the *gag* and *pol* gene sequences spliced out, thereby providing messenger RNA molecules that are translated into the *env* gene product. If a transforming gene is also present in the provirus (see below), the *env* gene sequences may also be spliced out to provide messenger RNA for the transforming gene product.

Proviruses as Transposable Elements

All available evidence suggests that there are no specific integration sites for proviruses in animal genomes, but that they can be integrated in very many sites, perhaps anywhere. Since an RNA transcribed from one proviral site can, after being encapsidated, be transferred via a virus particle to another cell only to be reverse-transcribed and inserted into another site, proviruses are transposable elements. The essential features of this aspect of retroviruses are (1) the fact that their DNA genomes are transcribed into RNA, in which form their genetic information is transported, and (2) the fact that transcription of proviral DNA into RNA and RNA into proviral DNA generates unique structures at the provirus termini, the LTRs—these are the structures that permit integration. LTRs possess two essential functions: they are necessary for integration, and they possess strong promoters for transcription (see below).

Endogenous Retroviruses: Leukemia and Leukosis Viruses

Retroviruses enjoy an unusually intimate relationship with their hosts. They exist in proviral form in numerous, perhaps all, animal species. These proviruses are transmitted

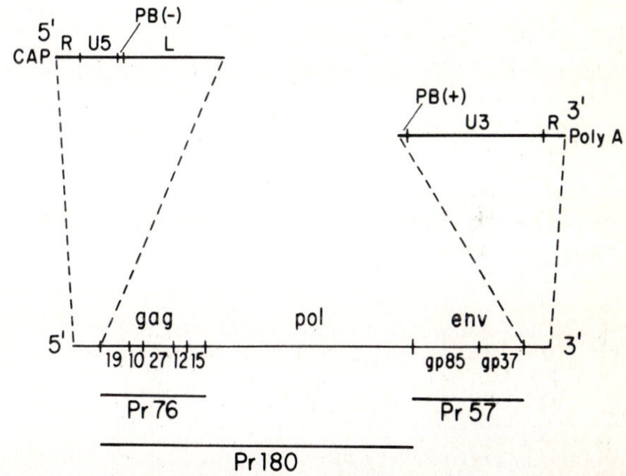

Figure 8-10. The structure of the basic retrovirus genome: the genome of nondefective avian or murine leukemia/leukosis viruses. Note that the RNA is capped at its 5′ terminus and polyadenylated at its 3′ terminus.

R: 20 to 80 nucleotides repeated at both ends

U5: 80 to 100 nucleotide unique sequence

PB(−): A sequence complementary to the 16-19 3′ terminal residues of $tRNA_{trp}$, $tRNA_{pro}$, or $tRNA_{lys}$ in avian leukosis viruses (ALVs), murine leukemia viruses (MLVs) and murine mammary tumor viruses (MMTVs), respectively. The tRNAs bind at these primer binding (hence PB) sites to serve as primers for the transcription of the RNA into complementary DNA (cDNA).

L: An untranslated region about 250 nucleotides long that precedes the coding sequences of the *gag* gene.

gag, pol, and *env*: The genes that encode the nucleocapsid (*gag*) proteins, the RNA-dependent DNA *pol*ymerase (the so-called reverse transcriptase), and the *env*elope proteins or spike components.

Pr76: The precursor of the ALV *gag* proteins. The precursor of MLV *gag* proteins is a Pr65.

Pr180: The infrequently formed readthrough product of the *gag* and *pol* genes, cleavage of which provides the RNA-dependent DNA polymerase.

Pr57: The precursor of gp85 and gp37, the knob and stalk proteins of the spikes of ALVs. The corresponding MLV precursor protein is a Pr80.

PB(+): A short, highly conserved sequence upstream from the initiation site for *positive* strand DNA synthesis. Its primer is not known.

U3: A unique region 200 to 1,000 nucleotides long. It is thought to contain a powerful transcriptional promoter.

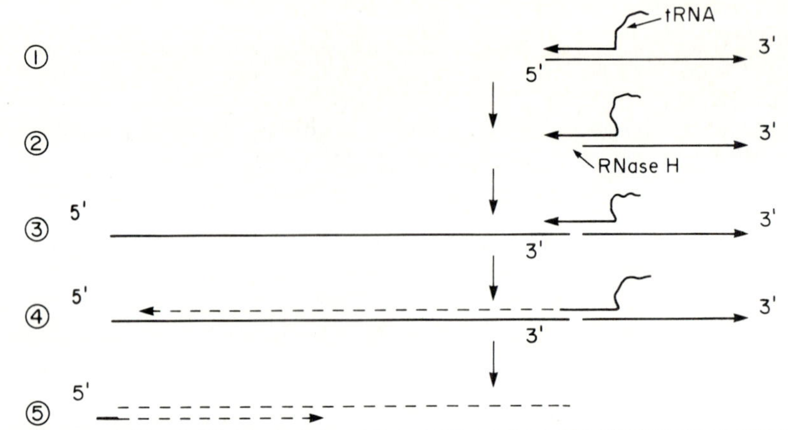

Figure 8-11. Scheme for the transcription of retrovirus RNA into DNA. Step 1. Using tRNA as primer, the 100 or so nucleotides at the 5′ terminus are transcribed. Step 2. The terminally redundant (R) RNA sequence is removed by the action of ribonuclease H, another enzymic activity of the reverse transcriptase. Step 3. The DNA transcript region of the R sequence pairs with an R sequence at the 3′ terminus of another RNA subunit, or it could also be on the same subunit that has just been transcribed at its 5′ terminus. Step 4. The new RNA subunit is transcribed into minus-strand DNA. There may be another strand switch at the 5′ end. Step 5. Transcription of minus-strand into plus-strand DNA proceeds, perhaps using viral RNA as primer, to yield a double-stranded DNA transcript of RNA. *(Adapted from Bishop: Annu Rev Biochem 47:35, 1978.)*

vertically as dominant genetic traits, like cellular genes, and their expression is controlled by individual specific regulatory controls that no doubt involve repression/derepression at the DNA transcription level. These are the endogenous retroviruses. In feral animal populations the expression of these proviruses as virus particles is greatly repressed. However, breeding programs for mice and chickens in particular have produced many strains of inbred animals in which the mechanisms that control endogenous provirus expression have been dissociated from the proviruses themselves, with the result that in these animals RNA tumor viruses are produced continuously and often throughout the animal's life. For example, there are mice, such as the albino AK and the C58BL mice, that have large numbers of leukemia virus particles in their bloodstream and develop leukemia between 6 and 12 months of age with high frequency. These mice are high-incidence-of-leukemia mouse strains. In other mice, such as in BALB/c and DBA strain mice, endogenous proviruses express themselves during embryonic life, even to the extent of virus particle formation, but then become repressed, so that the virus is generally undetectable in young adults. Later in life, however, the proviruses again begin to express themselves and leukemia may result, albeit with low frequency. Mice that harbor such endogenous proviruses are known as low-incidence-of-leukemia mouse strains. Finally, some mice, such as NIH Swiss and NZB mice, do not develop leukemia at all, because the endogenous proviruses capable of producing spontaneous leukemia have been bred out of them.

In addition to the spontaneously inducible endogenous viruses described above, which generally exist in the animal genome in the form of 1 to about 100 copies, mice and chickens, as well as other rodents, cats, monkeys, and primates, contain endogenous viruses that do not normally express themselves but can be induced to do so by treatment with a variety of substances, including inhibitors of protein synthesis, inhibitors of nucleic acid synthesis, such as halogenated deoxyribonucleosides, inhibitors of glycosylation, and B lymphocyte mitogens. Different inducers induce different viruses, which indicates that the nature of the cellular controls that regulate their ability to express themselves are diverse. That proviruses are indeed under the control of *cis*-acting control elements is suggested by transfection experiments. Proviral DNA is infectious, even when integrated, but proviruses have been found that are not infectious unless the cellular DNA in which they reside is reduced in size to approximate provirus size, a proce-

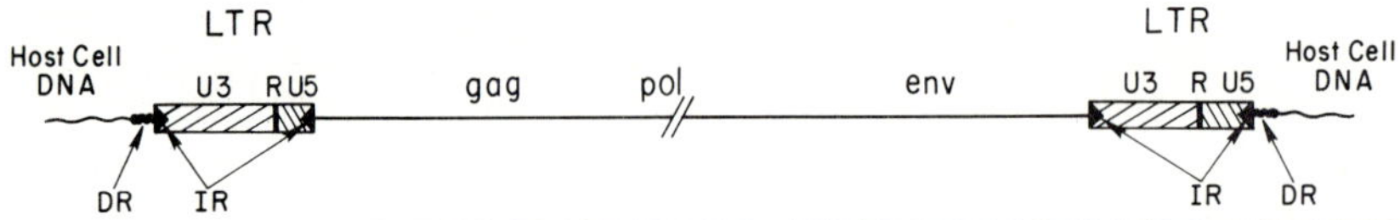

Figure 8-12. Structure of the integrated provirus. The coding sequences of the *gag, pol,* and *env* genes are flanked by long terminal repeats (LTRs) from 250 to 1200 bp long, depending on the virus, each composed of the U3, R, and U5 regions (Fig. 8-10), which are themselves flanked by short (5 to 22 bp) inverted repeat regions (IR). The entire provirus is flanked by direct repeats (DR) 4 to 6 bp long that are of host cell origin.

dure that would be expected to remove control elements linked to proviruses.

Ecotropic and Xenotropic Endogenous Viruses

There are two groups of endogenous viruses which differ in host range, interference patterns, and antigenic determinants. The first group comprises viruses that multiply readily in cells of the species in which they were induced; these are the ecotropic viruses. The second group comprises viruses that cannot infect cells of the species in which they were induced but can infect cells of other species; these are the xenotropic viruses. The host range is determined by the *env* gene.

Many ecotropic and xenotropic viruses have now been isolated from numerous animal species, including primates. For example, chickens contain at least 16 proviruses that have been mapped and that differ with respect to how readily they express themselves (some do not express themselves at all and are noninducible, others only express their *env* gene, still others form infectious virus particles), as well as in the structure of their LTRs. Mice also contain numerous proviruses in their genomes. It is probably conservative to estimate that wild-type mice, that is, mice that have not been inbred for provirus repression or derepression, harbor as many as 10 different proviruses of both types, each present to the extent of an average of 10 copies.

Most of these viruses are related to each other, as judged by nucleotide sequence analysis, and some fascinating evolutionary relationships have emerged from studies to determine whether proviruses in germline cells of various animal species are more closely related to each other than are their genes. If they are, this may indicate horizontal transmission and insertion of virus into germline cells. For example, the avian reticuloendotheliosis virus (REV) is much more closely related to murine viruses than to endogenous or exogenous (see below) chicken viruses, which suggests that a murine provirus was transferred from mice to birds many millions of years ago. The exogenous primate simian sarcoma virus and gibbon ape leukemia virus are derived from a murine xenotropic virus, and the cat xenotropic virus RD114 was acquired in the Pliocene from a monkey. Further, the diversity of integration sites (see above) suggests that vertebrate species experience a continual accretion of new endogenous proviruses in their germlines. This is the case for the high-incidence-of-leukemia AKR mouse strain in which new germline provirus integrations are accumulating at a rate of about 1 per 30 generations.

Expression and Significance of Endogenous Retroviruses

The expression of endogenous retroviruses appears to be under controls similar to those of developmentally regulated genes. Activation of an endogenous virus in a given tissue apparently reflects transcriptional activity of the insertion site. This may explain the occasional expression of endogenous viruses during early development and in some tissues of the adult, which has led to speculation that they may play a role in cellular differentiation. However, this is unlikely. Not only is provirus gene expression idiosyncratic with respect to tissue and age in different mouse strains, which is not compatible with provirus expression playing an essential functional role in ontogeny, but healthy chickens that lack all endogenous proviruses have been bred. However, it is conceivable that possession of endogenous proviruses may confer some form of survival advantage under natural conditions, such as protection against infectious retrovirus particles (see below). Beyond that, it is clear that endogenous proviruses represent a mode of persistence developed by retroviruses.

Retroviruses as Exogenous Viruses

Retroviruses not only exist as endogenous viruses that are passed on vertically from generation to generation, occasionally causing tumors in the animals in which they are activated, but also they can infect animals horizontally, as any other infectious agent. In fact, several natural populations suffer from retrovirus infections that cause tumors: examples are household cats infected with feline leukemia virus, cattle infected with bovine leukemia virus, and feral mice infected with murine leukemia viruses. The ability of endogenous viruses to act as exogenous viruses is demonstrated best by using, as hosts, animals such as AKR strain mice that have been bred to remove many of the alleles that protect normal mice against virus-induced leukemia.

There is also another class of retroviruses which only exist as exogenous viruses. Endogenous proviruses occasionally incorporate cellular genes that seem to play a role in development and differentiation into their sequences. As a result, they acquire the ability to transform cells and cause cancer. However, these chimeric viruses, the sarcoma/acute leukemia viruses (see below), are not integrated into germline cells, and they are therefore not endogenous viruses. Nor are they transmitted horizontally in nature with any frequency because most of them cannot multiply on their own, the acquired cellular gene having replaced one or other of the *gag, pol,* or *env* genes. The only exception is the group of avian sarcoma viruses whose prototype is Rous sarcoma virus (see below). As a result, these viruses arise occasionally in viremic animals and can be isolated and propagated in the laboratory but very probably die out in nature with the afflicted host.

Viruses with and without Transforming Genes: Nondefective and Defective Viruses

C-type retroviruses can be divided into two groups—those that can transform fibroblasts as well as certain other cells in vitro and rapidly cause tumors in animals, and those that cannot do so. It turns out that the difference lies in whether the viruses encode transforming genes or not.

Leukemia Viruses

Leukemia viruses possess the three genes, *gag, pol,* and *env,* that are essential for their multiplication; they are nondefective. However, they do not transform fibroblasts or any other cells in vitro, and while they are widely distributed and the animals that they infect are generally viremic throughout life, they cause tumors (lymphocytic, myeloid, and erythroblastic leukemias, osteopetrosis, nephroblastoma, and thymic and generalized lymphosarcomas) only late in life. When injected in large amounts into animals, they cause neoplasms only after a prolonged latent period.

Sarcoma/Acute Leukemia Viruses

The viruses in this group possess high oncogenic potential. They transform fibroblasts and hematopoietic cells in vitro and rapidly cause a wide variety of tumors of the hematopoietic system as well as sarcomas, endotheliomas, neurolymphomatosis, and splenomegaly. The reason for this is that their genomes contain an additional gene, a transforming gene or oncogene, that encodes a protein that triggers the transformation of normal cells into cancer cells. The first viruses of this group to be discovered and studied were several avian sarcoma viruses, the prototype of which is Rous sarcoma virus. These viruses possess four genes: *gag, pol, env,* and *src* (for sarcoma), which encodes a phosphoprotein, pp60^{src}, that possesses protein kinase activity. The *src* gene is the transforming gene, because viral mutants with temperature-sensitive lesions in this gene are temperature-sensitive with respect to ability to transform or maintain transformation. These viruses are nondefective, since they possess all three genes necessary for multiplication.

The other sarcoma/acute leukemia viruses include avian sarcoma viruses such as the Fujinami sarcoma virus, avian leukemia viruses such as MC29 (avian myelocytomatosis virus), avian erythroblastosis virus (AEV), and avian myeloblastosis virus (AMV), murine leukemia viruses such as Abelson murine leukemia virus, murine sarcoma viruses such as the Moloney, Kirsten, and Harvey murine sarcoma viruses, feline sarcoma viruses, and simian sarcoma virus. All these viruses possess genomes that are deficient in the genes that encode their structural proteins; many lack part of the *gag* and *pol* genes, and some lack part of the *env* gene. They are therefore defective. They can only multiply in the presence of a helper virus, typically a leukemia virus, that encodes the missing nucleocapsid, polymerase, or envelope proteins. Strains of these viruses consist of two types of particles, the helper virus particles and particles specified by the helper virus that contain the genome of the defective sarcoma/acute leukemia virus. These particles are known as "pseudotype particles" and are denoted thus: Mo-MSV(Mo-MLV) for Moloney murine sarcoma virus, the virus in parentheses denoting the helper virus that is generally present in large excess. Usually any one of numerous leukemia viruses can serve as helper.

The part of the viral genome that is missing in these viruses is replaced by sequences like the *src* gene, sequences that are unrelated to normal retrovirus genetic information. These sequences are specific for each defective sarcoma/acute leukemia virus and represent their transforming genes. Usually, the amount of genetic material that is deleted exceeds that which replaces it, so that the genomes of defective sarcoma/acute leukemia viruses are generally smaller than, and sometimes only one-half the size of, standard leukemia virus genomes.

Transforming Genes

The reason that sarcoma/acute leukemia viruses transform cells readily in vitro and rapidly induce cancer in animals is that they possess special genes, transforming genes or oncogenes. About 20 transforming genes have been discovered thus far on the basis of the presence in retrovirus genomes of specific nucleic acid sequences and the detection in cells transformed by them of proteins of specific size, possessing specific antigenic determinants and specialized functions. Ten of the best characterized of these oncogenes are identified in Table 8-3, and their physical maps are illustrated in Figure 8-13. Some of these transforming proteins are encoded by specific transforming genes, such as pp60$^{v\text{-}src}$ of Rous sarcoma virus (RSV), P45$^{v\text{-}myb}$ of avian myeloblastosis virus (AMV), P45$^{v\text{-}erb\text{-}B}$ of avian erythroblastosis virus (AEV), P37$^{v\text{-}mos}$ of Moloney murine sarcoma (Mo-MSV), pp21$^{v\text{-}ras}$ of Harvey and Kirsten murine sarcoma virus (Ha-MSV and Ki-MSV), and P28$^{v\text{-}sis}$ of simian sarcoma virus (SiSV). Others are fusion proteins in which the N-terminal portion of the transforming gene product is the N-terminal portion of the *gag*-encoded protein, while the remainder is encoded by the specific oncogene.

Recently, transforming genes have also been detected in human cancer cells. This finding is of enormous potential significance as it affords yet another avenue for studying the basic mechanisms underlying tumorigenesis. The basic finding is that when DNA from a variety of human cancers is added to NIH 3T3 cells, an established strain of mouse cells, the cells become transformed and form readily identifiable foci. Table 8-4 lists some human tumors that have been shown to contain dominant transforming or cancer genes by this transfection technique, and the list is growing. There are several such genes, as can be shown by testing their sensitivity to various restriction endonucleases. All except one are related to the *ras* oncogenes in Harvey and Kirsten murine sarcoma virus; that in human breast cancer is closely related to the oncogene in mammary carcinomas induced by mouse mammary tumor virus (MMTV). Interestingly, *c-Ki-ras* is the oncogene that is frequently activated in fibrosarcomas and skin carcinomas induced in the mouse by chemical carcinogenes.

TABLE 8-3. VIRAL ONCOGENES

Oncogene	Virus	Type of Tumor	Animal	Protein Product	Cellular Proto-oncogene Product
v-src	Rous sarcoma virus, B77 ASV	Sarcoma	Chicken	$pp60^{v\text{-}src}$	$pp60^{c\text{-}src}$
v-myb	Avian myeloblastosis virus (AMV)	Leukemia	Chicken	$P45^{v\text{-}myb}$	$P75^{c\text{-}myb}$
v-myc	Avian myelocytomatosis virus (MC29)	Carcinoma, sarcoma, leukemia	Chicken	$P110^{v\text{-}gag\text{-}myc}$	*c-myc*
v-erb-B	Avian erythroblastosis virus (AEV)	Leukemia, sarcoma	Chicken	$P45^{v\text{-}erb\text{-}B}$	*c-erb*
v-fps	Fujinami sarcoma virus (FSV)	Sarcoma	Chicken	$pp140^{v\text{-}gag\text{-}fps}$	$P98^{c\text{-}fps}$
v-mos	Moloney murine sarcoma virus (Mo-MSV)	Sarcoma	Mouse	$P37^{v\text{-}mos}$	*c-mos*
v-ras	Kirsten murine sarcoma virus	Sarcoma	Rat	$pp21^{v\text{-}ras}$	$pp21^{c\text{-}ras}$
	Harvey murine sarcoma virus	Leukemia	Rat		
v-abl	Abelson murine leukemia virus	Leukemia	Mouse	$pp120^{v\text{-}gag\text{-}abl}$	$pp150^{c\text{-}abl}$
v-fes	Feline sarcoma virus (FeSV)	Sarcoma	Cat	$pp85^{v\text{-}gag\text{-}fes}$	$pp92^{c\text{-}fes}$
v-sis	Simian sarcoma virus	Sarcoma	Wooly monkey	$P28^{v\text{-}sis}$	*c-sis*

Protooncogenes

The fact that human cancers harbor transforming genes and that some of these transforming genes are very similar to genes in sarcoma/acute leukemia viruses, although not predictable, was not totally unexpected since a most surprising discovery had been made shortly before: namely that retrovirus transforming genes are closely related to genes present in the genomes of most animals. As indicated in Table 8-3, each of the viral oncogenes has a cellular counterpart, or homolog. The degree of relatedness of the viral oncogenes with their cellular counterparts is often surprisingly close; for example, *v-myb* and *c-myb* differ in only 15 nucleotides out of 1197. The major difference between the viral oncogenes and their cellular counterparts is that the latter possess introns, whereas the viral oncogenes do not.

These transforming genes, or protooncogenes, are extraordinarily widespread in animals. They are present not only in all vertebrates but probably also in all metazoan genomes. The presence of *src* sequences is, for example, easily recognizable in the *Drosophila* genome. Clearly, these genes have survived more than a thousand million years; they exhibit extraordinary evolutionary conservation. Presumably the cellular genes arose first, since they are distributed throughout innumerable animal genomes, whereas the viral oncogenes are restricted to a very few sarcoma/acute leukemia viruses. The fact that retroviruses do indeed possess the ability to acquire these cellular protooncogenes has been demonstrated conclusively as follows. When mutants of RSV with large deletions in their *src* gene are injected into chickens, virus can be recovered that can again cause tumors (which the deletion mutant could not do) because the *src* gene has been reconstituted in them by pirating the chicken *c-src* gene. This indirect evidence that cellular protooncogenes possess, under appropriate conditions, the same oncogenic potential as viral oncogenes was soon supplemented by direct and conclusive proof. It was shown that whereas cellular protooncogenes do not transform cells in transfection experiments of the type described above (p. 146), at least some of them do so when linked by genetic engineering to LTR regions of proviruses, which, as pointed out above, contain strong promoters (p. 142).

Exactly how protooncogenes are incorporated into retrovirus genomes is not known. Presumably the protooncogene first recombines with and is inserted into the provirus, and its introns are lost when the transcripts of this new recombinant provirus are spliced to yield the RNA genome of the new transforming virus. This insertion of cellular material into the retrovirus genome provides the opportunity for further recombination with homologous regions within the host cell genome. Thus, the provirus of a murine sarcoma virus has been shown to contain a *ras* gene flanked by sequences derived not only from mouse but also from rat DNA, which suggests that it was generated as a result of numerous recombination events.

Functions of Oncogenes/Protooncogenes

The first retrovirus transforming gene to be studied in detail was the *src* gene of RSV. The protein encoded by this gene, $pp60^{v\text{-}src}$, is a phosphoprotein that either possesses protein kinase activity itself or is very closely associated with a protein kinase. Phosphorylation of proteins has for some time been recognized as a mechanism for modifying protein function. The excitement occasioned by the discovery of the protein kinase activity of $pp60^{v\text{-}src}$ was that it phosphorylates tyrosine residues rather than serine or threonine residues, which are the amino acids phosphorylated by most other protein kinases. Further, it is itself phosphorylated on a serine and on a tyrosine residue. Phosphorylation of tyrosine residues in proteins is much more common in tumor cells than in normal cells, although it does occur in normal cells. For example, it oc-

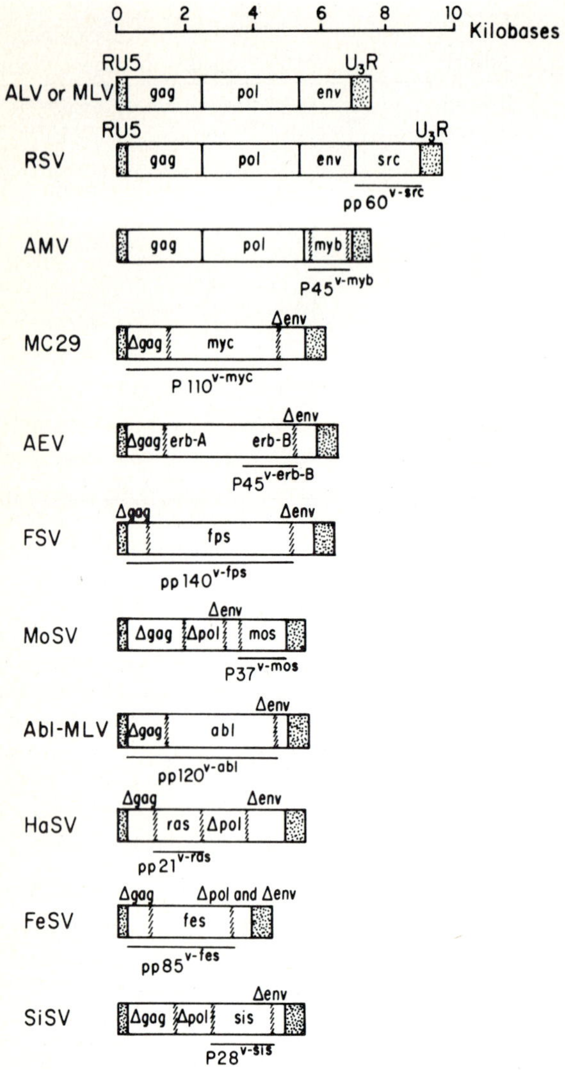

Figure 8-13. The genomes, transforming genes, and transforming gene products of acute leukemia/sarcoma viruses. The genomes of avian and murine leukemia viruses (ALV and MLV) and of Rous sarcoma virus (RSV), which are nondefective, are shown for comparison. The transforming proteins are indicated beneath the RNA sequences that encode them. Phosphoproteins are denoted by the prefix pp, other proteins by the prefix P. Note that some transforming proteins are fusion proteins with portions of *gag* proteins (the v-myc, v-fps, v-abl, and v-fes gene products), while others (the v-src, v-myb, v-erb-B, v-mos, v-ras, and v-sis gene products) are not. Note that in all cases, except RSV, the transforming gene replaces a very substantial portion of the normal retrovirus genome, leaving only partially deleted genes (Δ*gag*, Δ*pol*, and Δ*env*), which are not large enough to encode functional proteins/enzymes. ALV and MLV, avian and murine leukemia virus, respectively; RSV, Rous sarcoma virus; AMV, avian myeloblastosis virus; MC29 is a strain of avian myelocytomatosis virus; AEV, avian erythroblastosis virus; FSV, Fujinami sarcoma virus; MoSV, Moloney murine sarcoma virus; Abl-MLV, Albelson murine leukemia virus; HaSV, Harvey murine sarcoma virus; FeSV, feline sarcoma virus; SiSV, simian sarcoma virus.

TABLE 8-4. PROTOONCOGENES/ONCOGENES IN HUMAN TUMORS DEMONSTRATED WITH THE NIH 3T3 CELL TRANSFECTION ASSAY

Tumor	Gene
Bladder carcinoma	*c-Ha-ras*
Lung cancer	*c-Ki-ras*
Colon cancer	*c-Ki-ras*
Neuroblastoma	*c-N-ras**
Pancreatic carcinoma	As yet unidentified
Wilms' tumor	As yet unidentified
Testicular tumors	As yet unidentified
Breast cancer	As yet unidentified

**c-N-ras* is related to both *c-Ha-ras* and *c-Ki-ras* but is not identical with them.

curs when cells are stimulated with growth factors, such as epidermal growth factor (EGF) whose binding to the surface of cells stimulates DNA synthesis and cell division.

The protein $pp60^{v\text{-}src}$ appears to be localized mainly in adhesion plaques, specialized regions of the plasma membrane that adhere to solid surfaces and that are dismantled in cancer cells. Interestingly, the protein kinase activity of $pp60^{v\text{-}src}$ phosphorylates a tyrosine residue in vinculin, a protein that is a constituent of adhesion plaques and becomes dispersed throughout the cell following transformation by RSV. It seems reasonable to suggest that the phosphorylation of vinculin precipitates the dismantling of adhesion plaques, but the actual importance of this event in cell transformation remains to be established, especially since other cellular proteins, in particular the glycolytic enzymes enolase, phosphoglycerate mutase, and lactic dehydrogenase, as well as several other as yet unidentified proteins, also become phosphorylated very soon after infection with RSV.

The proteins encoded by three other retrovirus oncogenes also possess or are very closely associated with tyrosine-phosphorylating protein kinase activity (Table 8-5), but the proteins encoded by several other viral oncogenes do not. For example, $pp21^{v\text{-}ras}$ is also a protein kinase, but it phosphorylates threonine residues; $P45^{v\text{-}erb\text{-}B}$ is a glycoprotein that becomes associated with dense intracytoplasmic membrane; $P110^{v\text{-}gag\text{-}myc}$ is a DNA-binding protein that localizes in the nucleus, which is where $P45^{v\text{-}myb}$ is also found; and $P37^{v\text{-}mos}$ is a soluble protein in the cytoplasm.

Thus, proteins encoded by retrovirus oncogenes cellular protooncogenes are a heterogeneous group of proteins with a plethora of functions. It is interesting to compare them with the tumor antigens that are expressed by DNA-containing tumor viruses: the middle t antigen of polyoma virus, which also possesses tyrosine-phosphorylating protein kinase activity, and the large T antigens of SV40, polyoma virus, and adenovirus, which are nuclear DNA-binding proteins, as is the EBNA of EBV.

The picture that emerges is that all vertebrate cells

TABLE 8-5. FUNCTIONS OF ONCOGENES/PROTOONCOGENES

Gene	Species of Origin	Protein Kinase	GTP-binding Activity	Glyco-protein	DNA-binding Protein	Intracellular Location
v-src	Chicken	+ tyr				Plasma membrane
v-myb	Chicken	−				Nucleus
v-myc	Chicken	−			+	Nucleus
v-erb-B	Chicken	−		+		Intracytoplasmic membrane
v-fps	Chicken	+ tyr				Plasma membrane
v-mos	Mouse	−				Cytoplasm
v-ras	Rat	+ thre	+			Plasma membrane
v-abl	Mouse	+ tyr				Plasma membrane
v-fes	Cat	+ tyr				?
v-sis	Monkey	?				?

contain at least one copy of about 20 distinct genes, the protooncogenes, the messenger RNAs of which may on occasion be incorporated into retrovirus genomes. The chromosomal location of many of these protooncogenes in the human genome is known: thus *c-myb* is located on chromosome 6, *c-myc* and *c-mos* are on chromosome 8, *c-ras* is on chromosomes 6, 11, 12, and X (the human genome contains two *c-Ha-ras* genes and two *c-Ki-ras* genes, genes that are incorporated into the Harvey and Kirsten strains of MSV, respectively), *c-N-ras* (Table 8-4) is on chromosome 1, *c-fes* is on chromosome 15, and *c-sis* is on chromosome 22.

Most of these protooncogenes express themselves to a certain extent in normal cells and presumably fulfill specific essential functions. The nature of these functions is not clear, though clues are provided by examining the functions of their viral homologs. It is known that *c-ras* is transcribed extensively during liver regeneration, that *c-abl* and *c-ras* are transcribed during prenatal and early postnatal development of the mouse, and that *c-myc, c-erb* and *c-src* are transcribed in a variety of chick cells and tissues. Further, *c-myb* is transcribed in immature lymphoid and erythroid hematopoietic cells, and *c-ras* is transcribed at elevated levels in a human hematopoietic precursor cell line.

Interestingly, the various protooncogenes are related to a most surprising degree. It is clear, for example, partly from studies of their nucleic acid sequences and partly from studies of the amino acid sequences of their gene products, that *src, fps, abl, fes, mos,* and *erb,* of which some are tyrosine phosphorylating protein kinases while others are not, are all quite closely related and that they exhibit homology not only with certain cellular serine phosphorylating cyclic nucleotide-dependent protein kinases but also with the β-subunit of mitochondrial and bacterial ATP-synthetase, primarily in the region that is believed to contribute to nucleotide binding. It may be noted, in this regard, that $pp21^{v\text{-}ras}$ is also a GTP-binding protein (see Table 8-5). It seems that all these protooncogenes are derived from a common ancestor that arose before the emergence of metazoan phyla.

Whereas in normal cells several protooncogenes are usually transcribed simultaneously to greater or lesser extent, only one protooncogene is transcribed in large amounts in cancer cells. For example, the HL-60 cell line, derived from a patient with acute promyelocytic leukemia, expresses high levels of *c-myc,* the gene that is also expressed at high levels in most lymphomas; a human bladder cancer cell line expresses high levels of *c-Ha-ras*; avian erythroleukemia cells express high levels of *c-erb*; and a murine plasmacytoma cell line expresses high levels of *c-mos.* Thus, each type of tumor is associated with high transcriptional activity of one particular oncogene. This target cell specificity is not due to the host range of the virus that carries the oncogene. Thus MC29 virus transforms both fibroblasts and macrophages in culture but not erythroblasts, though the *myc* gene expresses itself in such cells, and RSV infects both macrophages and fibroblasts and $pp60^{src}$ is synthesized in both, but only fibroblasts are transformed. Rather, target cell specificity is a property of the oncogene/protooncogene itself, and these genes appear to be tissue-specific regulators of cellular growth and development. This conclusion is supported by the finding that different transforming genes are activated in neoplasms representative of different stages of normal B and T cell differentiation, which suggests that an excess of oncogene or protooncogene products inhibits the maturation of the various hematopoietic precursor cells from one compartment to the next.

How Do Retroviruses that Lack Oncogenes Transform Cells?

This brings us to the two most central questions concerning the role of retroviruses and oncogenes/protooncogenes in transforming cells and causing cancer. There is no conceptual hurdle concerning how sarcoma/acute leukemia viruses accomplish this, since they possess oncogenes, and following provirus integration, these genes are presumably brought under the control of provirus LTRs and express themselves vigorously so that large amounts of the proteins encoded by them are formed. But how do leukemia/leukosis viruses that do not possess

TABLE 8-6. CELLULAR GENES ACTIVATED IN NONVIRAL HUMAN AND MURINE TUMORS

Gene	Tumor	Activated by
c-myc	Burkitt's lymphoma	Translocation
c-mos	Plasmacytoma	Translocation
c-myc	Myeloid leukemia	Amplification
c-abl	Myeloid leukemia, erythroid leukemia	Translocation, amplification

oncogenes cause cancer, as they all do late in life, and why do protooncogenes, most of which are expressed all the time, suddenly transform cells?

There may be several mechanisms (Table 8-6).

Insertional Mutagenesis

Leukemia/leukosis provirus can probably become integrated anywhere in the animal genome, and in most cases no noticeable change will result. If, however, insertion occurs in the vicinity of a protooncogene, it will come under the influence of the proviral LTR and be stimulated to be expressed vigorously, with resultant cell transformation. Indeed, it is known that the *c-myc* gene is expressed to a high degree in many of the lymphomas caused by infection of chickens with avian leukosis viruses and that it takes no more than a 5-fold increase in the amount of *src* gene product to transform a cell.

Gene Amplification

Many tumor cells display abnormalities in their chromosomes due to the presence of excess amounts of amplified DNA. The general progression is as follows. A region of a chromosome, usually encompassing many genes, begins to replicate excessively, up to 1000-fold and beyond, for reasons that are not known, probably because of a rare spontaneous event. Sooner or later, the amplified DNA departs the chromosome and exists in the form of a ring chromosome and then in the form of double minute chromosomes. Finally, it reenters chromosomes as homogeneously staining regions. These homogeneously staining regions have been shown to contain protooncogenes, *c-myc* and *c-Ki-ras* among them in different tumor cells, which therefore exist in such cells in the form of far more copies than in normal cells, that is, in highly amplified form. They then give rise to very large amounts of messenger RNA and of the proteins that they encode. Once again, cell transformation is associated with enhanced protooncogene expression.

Mutation

The two preceding mechanisms invoke increased *dosage* of protooncogene products as the cause of transformation. Another mechanism involves a *qualitative alteration* of the protooncogene product. Such an alteration could be caused by a point mutation in the protooncogene. Indeed, it has been found that the *c-Ha-ras* protooncogene that is activated in a human bladder carcinoma to the point that it becomes able to transform NIH 3T3 cells in the transfection assay differs in one nucleotide residue from the *c-Ha-ras* protooncogene that is present in normal human cells. This change causes a single amino acid substitution in the $pp21^{ras}$ protein that is expressed in the cancer cell. It seems clear that it is this change that triggers cell transformation.

Translocation

Finally, many cancer cells display chromosomal abnormalities caused by translocations, where one portion of a chromosome breaks away and exchanges position with another portion of another chromosome. Some of these translocations involve DNA sequences that contain protooncogenes. For example, in Burkitt's lymphoma a portion of chromosome 8 is transferred to chromosome 14, and the transferred DNA includes *c-myc*. Murine plasmacytomas also often exhibit translocations in which the translocated chromosome portion includes *c-myc*. Such translocations may have two effects: they may affect the extent to which a protooncogene is transcribed, and altered protooncogenes may be produced as a result of recombination, the gene products of which, like that of the mutated gene discussed above, may trigger cell transformation.

Naturally, we are only considering here the very first of a series of steps that culminate in the generation of fully fledged cancer cells. It is conceivable, and indeed likely, that various oncogenes may act sequentially in the same cell. It is known, for example, that in B cell lymphomas of chickens induced by infection with avian leukemia viruses (ALVs), not only is the expression of the *c-myc* gene enhanced but another gene is also activated, a gene that can transform NIH 3T3 cells in the transfection assay described above. This second gene has been cloned and found to encode a protein that is homologous to the N-terminal portion of transferrin (although it is much smaller than transferrin). Interestingly, a related gene is also activated in Burkitt's lymphoma cells. This second gene may well act during a later stage in tumorigenesis. However this may be, it is clear that recognition of the relationship between viral oncogenes and cellular protooncogenes has provided a most powerful tool with which to probe the reactions fundamental to the initiation of the cancer process.

Recombinant Endogenous Viruses: MCF Viruses

As pointed out above, mice, and no doubt other vertebrates as well, harbor retrovirus proviruses in their genomes that cause leukemia at some stage of their life. In the numerous inbred mouse strains that have been developed over the years, the actual ability of these proviruses to cause leukemia has been separated from some of the elements that control their ability to express themselves. Very likely, some of the factors that cause leukemia are those that were discussed in the preceeding section, that is, protooncogene activation or protooncogene alteration. However, it appears that other factors may also be involved. For example, the development of spontaneous leukemia tends to be associated with the generation of a new class of retroviruses. Such new viruses have been isolated from the thymuses of late preleukemic or leukemic AKR and preleukemic C58 mice and from the lymphomas that develop in NIH Swiss mice. These viruses are recombinants in the *env* gene between ecotropic and xenotropic endogenous viruses. They possess the *gag* and *pol* genes of ecotropic viruses, but their *env* genes comprise sequences from both ecotropic and xenotropic endogenous viruses. They multiply not only in mouse cells but also in cells of other species and are, therefore, said to be dualtropic. They also induce focal morphologic alterations in a mink lung cell line and are therefore often referred to as mink cell focus (MCF)-inducing viruses. They are *not* endogenous viruses, since they are not present in germline cells.

The emergence of MCF viruses from lymphoid tissue in the preleukemic and leukemic state indicates that they may be involved in the pathogenesis of leukemia. It remains to be established whether the recombinant *env* glycoproteins themselves are the transforming proteins or whether their role is host range modification/expansion.

Expression of *env* Gene of Endogenous Viruses

While endogenous viruses usually do not express themselves to the extent of virus particle formation, they do frequently express their *env* gene. The first indication in this direction was the discovery that a strain of RSV whose RNA contains a deletion in the *env* gene (the Bryan strain) is incapable of growing in some chick cells but is capable of growing in others, which were therefore said to possess a "chick-helper-factor" (chf). This factor turned out to be the spontaneously expressed glycoprotein encoded by the *env* gene of the endogenous chick RNA tumor virus RAV-O. Thus RAV-O does not express itself at all in chick cells that are chf^-; it expresses its *env* gene in cells that are chf^+; and there are one or two inbred strains of chickens in which it expresses itself completely, to the extent of infectious virus particle formation (and causing leukemia infrequently late in life).

The situation is similar in the mouse. It has long been known that a differentiation alloantigen designated G_{IX} (since it appeared to be specified by a gene in linkage group IX of the mouse) is present in the thymocytes of certain mouse strains. It is also present in the serum of some mouse strains (particularly strain 12A), in epithelia associated with the digestive tract, and in the epithelial lining of the male reproductive tract and, therefore, in seminal fluid. It was then found that the G_{IX} antigen could be induced in rats by infection with murine leukemia virus and that it represents the gp70 glycoprotein specified by the *env* gene of a provirus that expresses itself irrespective of *gag* and *pol* gene expression, just as does chf. Mice harbor numerous proviruses, all of which may express their *env* genes independently of each other in the form of gp70 molecules located on the surface of cells of various organs. Thus in mouse strains such as the 129/J mouse, from which no C-type virus has ever been isolated, the gp70s of four different endogenous viruses are expressed in different developmental compartments—one in the serum, one on thymus and spleen cells, one on bone marrow cells, and one on cells lining the male genital tract. This polymorphism may benefit the mouse through the various gp70s acting as differentiation antigens.

Mouse Mammary Tumor Viruses (MMTV)

Mouse mammary tumor virus, the prototype of B-type RNA tumor viruses, exists in the form of numerous endogenous proviruses that express themselves to varying degrees in different strains of mice. The most familiar is the milk factor of Bittner, a virus strain that is resident in C3H and A strain mice (high-incidence strains), expresses itself in all cells of its hosts, and is present in particularly large amounts in lactating mammary tissue and, therefore, in milk. As a result, it is passed on readily to progeny animals, in which it produces mammary adenocarcinomas with high frequency early in life (generally between age 6 and 12 months). It is also passed on to animals of low-incidence strains when they are reared by foster mothers of the C3H and A strains and, with high frequency, produces tumors in them also.

The other MMTV strains express themselves less readily. They are not present in large amounts in milk and are transmitted vertically through the gametes. They are also much less oncogenic and cause tumors with low frequency late in life.

These various endogenous proviruses express themselves to very different degrees in different mouse tissues. In virus-producing tumors and lactating mammary tissue of high-incidence mouse strains there are from 100 to 1000 genome equivalents of MMTV RNA per cell; in tumors of low-incidence mouse strains only 1 to 2; and in livers and spleens from either high- or low-incidence mouse strains (that is, in cells that never become transformed and never produce MMTV), there is only 0.1 to 1 genome equivalent of viral RNA per cell.

The factors that regulate the transcription of MMTV proviruses are both genetic and hormonal. Estrogens enhance the development of mammary cancer (which normally occurs only in female mice but can also be induced in male mice of high-incidence strains); and glucocorticoids greatly increase the degree of MMTV formation in lactating mammary tissue cells and mammary tumor cells, but do not effect significant increases in other mouse cells.

The hormone-sensitive control element for MMTV provirus expression appears to reside in its LTR sequences, which are about five times as long as those of C-type retroviruses.

A transforming gene active in the NIH 3T3 cell transfection assay has been detected in the DNA of MCF7 cells, a human breast cancer cell line, and this gene retains its hormone inducibility. This human gene is very closely related to the transforming gene of MMTV. Thus, in both mice and humans, breast cancer appears to involve the activation and functioning of an oncogene/protooncogene. Whether the human gene is also part of a retrovirus provirus remains to be determined.

Retrovirus-like DNA Sequences and Particles

Three types of DNA sequences that share certain basic features with the proviruses of retroviruses have been detected in animal genomes. They are:

Intracisternal A-type Particles (IAP)

Mouse cells often contain particles some 60 to 80 nm in diameter that consist of toroidal (ring-shaped) nucleoids enclosed by a membrane (Fig. 8-14). These particles are found budding abundantly into the cisternae of the rough endoplasmic reticulum in all murine plasmacytomas, as well as in a variety of other murine tumors (rhabdomyosarcoma and neuroblastoma) and in normal murine embryos at certain stages of development but only rarely in normal adult murine tissues. Usually they remain attached to the rough endoplasmic reticulum membrane, but in many myelomas they are released in extracellular form.

Like retrovirus particles, IAP contain two identical molecules of RNA about 7000 nucleotides long (mol wt about 8×10^6) and possess an RNA-dependent DNA polymerase. They possess no infectivity, but their major structural protein is encoded by their RNA. Their RNA is not related to the RNA of any retrovirus of the common mouse *Mus musculus* but is closely related (about 25 percent homology and similarly situated restriction endonuclease sites) to the RNA of M432, an endogenous retrovirus of the Asian mouse *Mus cervicolor.* Amazingly, the genome of *M. musculus* contains about 1000 dispersed copies of the IAP provirus, while the genome of *M. cervicolor* contains only about 20 copies. These two mouse species diverged about 5 million years ago. Clearly, the evolution of *M. musculus* was accompanied by a striking amplification of IAP proviral DNA, which now makes up about 0.3 percent of the total cellular DNA. Recently, IAP-related sequences have also been detected in moderate copy number in the hamster and in low copy number in other rodents. The extent of sequence divergence indicates that they have been resident in the hamster genome for millions of years.

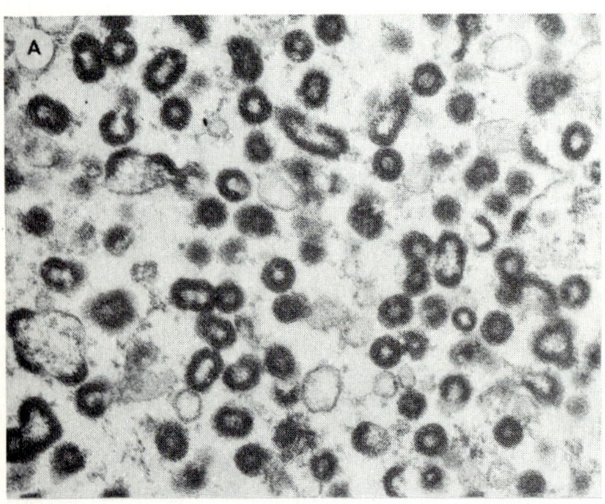

Figure 8-14. Intracisternal A-type particles (IAP) extracted from mouse plasma cell tumor MOPC 104E and partially purified by sucrose density gradient centrifugation. × 70,000. *(Courtesy of Dr. N.A. Wivell.)*

Examination of mouse gene libraries has revealed that the 1000 or so IAP proviruses in the mouse genome are a strikingly heterogeneous population of sequences. About a quarter of the IAP provirus, near one end, is highly conserved, but varying lengths of its central portion are often deleted; and the other end is highly variable. Thus, while there is a common provirus pattern, there is also very extensive sequence switching, which is no doubt the result of recombination and sequence deletion. One feature common to all IAP proviruses is possession of LTRs with the same structure as retrovirus LTRs and flanking short direct repeats of cellular DNA. IAP proviruses are thus integrated into cellular DNA just as are retrovirus proviruses and, like them, they are transposable elements.

The relatedness of IAP to retrovirus M432 indicates that they have evolved from a C-type retrovirus. They are nonfectious, which is not surprising in view of the obviously degenerate form of their RNA; and although they appear regularly in early mouse embryos, they have no as yet defined physiologic role. In view of the fact that IAP proviruses are so abundant and widely dispersed in the *M. musculus* genome, they may have assumed in this species some function beyond coding for the particles themselves. It is conceivable, for example, that they can activate cellular genes and possess regulatory functions controlling other genetic elements of the mouse.

VL30 DNA Sequences

Recently, two fascinating extensions of this work have come to light. First, it has been found that many species of mice contain yet another set of dispersed reiterated DNA sequences about the same size as IAP or retrovirus proviruses, the so-called VL30 (for virus-like) sequences. They possess the following properties: (1) some mouse species contain only 1 to 2 copies of them, whereas others, such as *M. musculus,* contain about 200; (2) like retrovirus and IAP proviruses, VL30 sequences are flanked by LTRs, attributes of transposable elements; (3) in certain mouse cells they are transcribed extensively into 30S polyadenylated RNA that tends to exist in dimeric form like retrovirus RNA and is efficiently encapsidated into noninfectious C-type retrovirus particles which provide a means for transferring them from cell to cell; (4) they are not related to any retrovirus or IAP provirus; (5) certain portions of VL30 sequences appear to exist in the mouse genome in a form that is not part of intact VL30 sequences; and (6) more or less related sequences are also present in the DNAs of other animals, such as rats and humans.

VL30 sequences clearly have a long evolutionary history, part of which they may share with IAP and retroviruses. If their LTRs contain promoters of transcription like the LTRs of retroviruses, they may function as portable promoters and play a significant role in differentiation and cellular regulation.

The *copia* Element of *Drosophila*

The *copia* element is a transposable element found throughout the *Drosophila* genome. Usually 100 to 200 DNA sequences are present, and they constitute about 5 percent of the total DNA. Like retrovirus and IAP proviruses and VL30 sequences, *copia* sequences are flanked by LTRs several hundred base pairs long, short inverted repeats, and very short direct repeats of cellular DNA (p. 144), and they are transcribed into long polyadenylated RNA molecules. Virus-like particles have now been found in *Drosophila* that contain *copia* RNA sequences and RNA-dependent DNA polymerase activity. Like IAPs they are not infectious, and, further, like retrovirus and IAP RNA but unlike VL30 RNA, *copia* RNA encodes what appears to be the major structural component of the *copia* virus-like particles.

The existence of yet another class of these large transposable genetic elements intensifies still further the question of their biologic role, which may be fundamentally important in view of the extraordinary extent to which they have been conserved during evolution. It may also be asked, are *copia* elements evolving toward retroviruses, or are they descended from them?

Do Viruses Cause Cancer in Humans?

Many viruses transform cells, and many viruses cause cancer in animals. But which viruses cause cancer in humans?

In most cases, it is impossible to demonstrate a direct causal relationship; but there are four groups of viruses that seem to play a very important role in carcinogenesis in humans.

Human Papillomaviruses. As described on page 134 and in Chapter 15, several types of HPV cause lesions that progress to malignant carcinomas.

EBV. This virus plays a very important role in the genesis of Burkitt's lymphoma and nasopharyngeal carcinoma. The role of human herpes simplex virus type 2 in cervical cancer is less well defined.

Hepatitis B Virus. The DNA of this virus is known to be integrated into the human genome, where its presence correlates strongly with the incidence of hepatoma.

Retroviruses. An enormous amount of work has been devoted to attempts to find and isolate a human retrovirus. Only one, HTLV, has so far been isolated (see below). This is remarkable for two reasons. First, most animal species harbor endogenous retroviruses that express themselves more or less frequently during the animal's life. This includes the closest relatives of humans, namely, gorillas, orangutans, chimpanzees, and baboons. Second, all animals contain protooncogenes, cellular genes that can be incorporated into retrovirus genomes and thereby transferred from cell to cell. The human genome also contains these protooncogenes, and, as described above, they are known to be activated in human cancer cells. Extensive searches for human retroviruses during the last decade or so, which took the form of searches in normal and cancerous human tissues for RNA, DNA, and protein sequences related to primate, feline, or murine retroviruses, yielded results that were sometimes tantalizingly close to being convincingly positive. Yet they were never sufficiently regular, frequent, and reproducible to provide conclusive evidence for the existence of human retroviruses.

Human T Cell Leukemia Virus (HTLV)

Recently a human retrovirus has been isolated that does indeed appear to play a role in a human cancer. This is *human T cell leukemia virus (HTV)*, which has been isolated from peripheral blood T lymphocytes of patients with adult T cell leukemia (ATL). It is not an endogenous retrovirus, and its provirus is not present in human germline cells. Not surprisingly, the distribution of ATL is that of a disease caused by an infectious agent: it occurs most frequently in Southwest Japan and in the Caribbean basin (where the disease is called T cell lymphosarcoma cell leukemia). About 10 percent of the population in Southwest Japan possess antibodies to the major components of HTLV particles. Such antibodies are absent in humans in parts of the world where the disease is not endemic. Recent evidence suggests that there may be at least three types of HTLV that are related but substantially different serologically. HTLV is not closely related to any known retrovirus, but its major core protein, p24, displays some relatedness to the p24 of bovine leukemia virus.

The evidence suggests, therefore, that HTLV is a unique novel retrovirus, exogenous for humans and of unknown origin, that is capable of causing T cell leukemia in humans. It is the only retrovirus so far associated with any human neoplasm.

FURTHER READING

Books and Reviews

GENERAL

Bishop JM: Cancer genes come of age. Cell 32:1018, 1983

Cairns J: The origins of human cancers. Nature 289:353, 1981

Doerfler W: DNA methylation and gene activity. Annu Rev Biochem 52:93, 1983

Ponder BAJ: Genetics and cancer. Biochim Biophys Acta 605:369, 1980

DNA TUMOR VIRUSES

Tooze J: DNA Tumor Viruses. New York, Cold Spring Harbor Laboratory, 1980

Klein G (ed): DNA-virus Oncogenes and their Action. New York, Raven P, 1983

Ziff EBl: Transcription and RNA processing by the DNA tumor viruses. Nature 287:491, 1980

Doerfler W: Uptake, fixation and expression of foreign DNA in mammalian cells: The organization of integrated adenovirus DNA sequences. Curr Top Microbiol Immunol 101:127, 1982

Papovaviruses

Lancaster WD, Olson C: Animal papillomaviruses. Microbiol Rev 46:191, 1982

Benjamin TL: The hr-t gene of polyoma virus. Biochim Biophys Acta 695:69, 1982

Hand R: Functions of T antigens of SV40 and polyomavirus. Biochim Biophys Acta 651:1, 1981

Levine AJ: The nature of the host range restriction of SV40 and polyoma viruses in embryonal carcinoma cells. Curr Top Microbiol Immunol 101:1, 1982

Klein G (ed): The Transformation-associated Cellular p53 Protein. New York, Raven, 1982

Norkin LC: Papovaviral persistent infections. Microbiol Rev 46:384, 1982

Walker DL, Padgett BL: Progressive multifocal leukoencephalopathy. In Fraenkel-Conrat H, Wagner RR (eds): Comprehensive Virology. New York, Plenum, 1983, vol 18, p 161

Herpesviruses

Fleckenstein B: Oncogenic herpesviruses of non-human primates. Biochim Biophys Acta 560:301, 1979

Kieff E, Danbaugh T, Heller M, et al.: The biology and chemistry of Epstein–Barr virus. J Infect Dis 146:506, 1982

Knipe DM: Cell growth transformation by herpes simplex virus. Prog Med Virol 28:114, 1982

Nazerian K: Marek's disease lymphoma of chicken and its causative herpesvirus. Biochim Biophys Acta 560:375, 1979

Vonka V, Hirsch I: Epstein–Barr-virus nuclear antigen. Prog Med Virol 28:145, 1982

zurHausen H, Fresen K: Heterogeneity of Epstein–Barr virus. Biochim Biophys Acta 560:343, 1979

Hepatitis B Virus

Maupas P, Melnick JL (eds): Hepatitis B virus and primary hepatocellular carcinoma. Prog Med Virol 27, 1980 and 1981

Tiollais P, Charney P, Vyas GN: Biology of hepatitis B virus. Science 213:406, 1981

RNA TUMOR VIRUSES

General

Weiss R, Teich N, Varmus H, et al.: RNA Tumor Viruses. New York, Cold Spring Harbor Laboratory, 1982

Bishop JM: Cellular oncogenes and retroviruses. Annu Rev Biochem 52:301, 1983

Coffin JM: Structure, replication and recombination of retrovirus genomes: Some unifying hypotheses. J Gen Virol 42:1, 1979

Eisenman RN, Vogt VM: The biosynthesis of oncovirus proteins. Biochim Biophys Acta 473:188, 1978

Gilden RV, Rabin H: Mechanisms of viral tumorigenesis. Adv Virus Res 27:281, 1982

Ihle JN, Enjuanes L, Lee JC, et al.: The immune response to C-type viruses and its potential role in leukemogenesis. Curr Top Microbiol Immunol 101:31, 1982

Jaenisch R: Endogenous retroviruses. Cell 32:5, 1983

Levy JA: Xenotropic type C viruses. Curr Top Microbiol Immunol 79:111, 1978

Montelaro RC, Bolognesi DP: Structure and morphogenesis of type C retroviruses. Adv Cancer Res 28:63, 1978

Nooter K, Bentvelzen P: Primate type-C oncoviruses. Biochim Biophys Acta 695:461, 1980

O'Connor TE, Rauscher FJ Jr (eds): Oncogenes and Retroviruses: Evaluation of Basic Findings and Clinical Potential. New York, Alan R. Liss, 1983

Risser R: The pathogenesis of Abelson virus lymphomas of the mouse. Biochim Biophys Acta 651:213, 1981

Scolnick EM: Hyperplastic and neoplastic erythroproliferative diseases induced by oncogenic murine retroviruses. Biochim Biophys Acta 651:273, 1982

Stephenson JR (ed): Molecular Biology of RNA Tumor Viruses. New York, Academic Press, 1980

Varmus H (ed): Readings in Tumor Virology. New York, Cold Spring Harbor Laboratory, 1983

Temin HM: Origin of retroviruses from cellular moveable genetic elements. Cell 21:599, 1980

Troxler DH, Ruscetti Sk, Scolnick EM: The molecular biology of Friend virus. Biochim Biophys Acta 605:305, 1980

Weinberg RA: Origins and roles of endogenous retroviruses. Cell 22:643, 1980

Oncogenes/Protooncogenes

Bishop JM: Enemies within: The genesis of retrovirus oncogenes. Cell 23:5, 1981

Fine D, Schochetman G: Type D primate retroviruses: A review. Cancer Res 38:3123, 1978

Dalla-Favera R, Martinotti S, Gallo RC: Translocation and rearrangements of the c-myc oncogene locus in human undifferentiated B-cell lymphomas. Science 219:963, 1983

Erikson RL: The transforming protein of avian sarcoma viruses and its homologue in normal cells. Curr Top Microbiol Immunol 92:25, 1981

Hayman MJ: Transforming proteins of avian retroviruses. J Gen Virol 52:1, 1981

Hayward WS, Neel DG: Retroviral gene expression. Curr Top Microbiol Immunol 91:217, 1981

Huebner RJ, Todaro GJ: Oncogenes of RNA tumor viruses as determinants of cancer. Proc Natl Acad Sci USA 64:1087, 1969

Graf T, Stéhelin D: Avian leukemia viruses: Oncogenes and genome structure. Biochim Biophys Acta 651:245, 1982

Klein G (ed): Oncogene Studies. New York, Raven, 1982

Klein G: Specific chromosomal translocations and the genesis of B-cell-derived tumors in mice and men. Cell 32:311, 1983

Temin HM: Function of the retrovirus long terminal repeat. Cell 28:3, 1982

Varmus HE: Form and function of retroviral proviruses. Science 216:812, 1982

Weinberg RA: Use of transfection to analyze genetic information and malignant transformation. Biochim Biophys Acta 651:25, 1981

Weinberg RA: Fewer and fewer oncogenes. Cell 30:3, 1982

Weinberg RA, Steffen DL: Regulation of expression of the integrated retrovirus genome. J Gen Virol 54:1, 1981

Mammary Tumor Viruses

Bentvelzen P: Interaction between host and viral genomes in mouse mammary tumors. Ann Rev Genet 16:173, 1982

Hynes NE, Groner B: Mammary tumor formation and hormonal control of mouse mammary tumor virus expression. Curr Top Microbiol Immunol 101:51, 1982

Ringold GM: Glucocorticoid regulation of mouse mammary tumor virus gene expression. Biochim Biophys Acta 560:487, 1979

Selected Papers

DNA TUMOR VIRUSES

Papovaviruses

Carmichael CG, Schaffhausen BS, Dorsky DI, et al.: Carboxy terminus of polyoma middle-sized tumor antigen is required for attachment to membranes, associated protein kinase activities, and cell transformation. Proc Natl Acad Sci USA 79:3579, 1982

Chandrasekaran K, McFarland VW, Simmons DT, et al.: Quantitation and characterization of a species-specific and embryo stage-dependent 55-kilodalton phosphoprotein also present in cells transformed by simian virus 40. Proc Natl Acad Sci USA 78:6953, 1981

Eckhart W, Hutchinson MA, Hunter T: An activity phosphorylating tyrosine in polyoma T-antigen immunoprecipitates. Cell 18:925, 1979

Gissmann L, Wolnik L, Ikenberg H, et al.: Human papillomavirus types 6 and 11 DNA sequences in genital and laryngeal papillomas and in some cervical cancers. Proc Natl Acad Sci USA 80:560, 1983

Ito Y, Spurr N: Polyoma virus T-antigens expressed in transformed cells: Significance of middle T-antigen in transformation. Cold Spring Harbor Symp Quant Biol 44:149, 1980

Kahn P, Topp WC, Shin S-I: Tumorigenicity of SV40-transformed human and monkey cells in immunodeficient mice. Virology 126:348, 1983

Kremsdorf D, Jablonska S, Favera M, et al.: Biochemical characterization of two types of human papillomaviruses associated with epidermodysplasia verruciformis. J Virol 43:436, 1982

Oren M, Reich NC, Levine AJ: Regulation of the cellular p53 tumor antigen in teratocarcinoma cells and their differentiated progeny. Mol Cell Biol 2:443, 1982

Rubin H, Figge J, Bladon MT, et al.: Role of small t antigen in the acute transforming activity of SV40. Cell 30:469, 1982

Topp WC, Rifkin DB: The small-t protein of SV40 is required for loss of actin cable networks and plasminogen activator synthesis in transformed rat cells. Virology 106:282, 1980

Volckart G, van de Voorde A, Fiers W: Nucleotide sequence of the simian virus 40 small-t gene. Proc Natl Acad Sci USA 75:2160, 1978

Adenoviruses

Gallimore PH, Sharp PA, Sambrook J: Viral DNA in transformed cells. II. A study of the sequences of adenovirus 2 DNA in nine lines of transformed rat cells using specific fragments of the viral genome. J Mol Biol 80:49, 1974

Houweling A, van den Elsen PJ, van der EB AJ: Partial transformation of primary rat cells by the leftmost 4.5% fragment of adenovirus 5 DNA. Virology 105:337, 1980

Sarnow P, Ho YS, Williams J, et al.: Adenovirus Elb-58kd tumor antigen and SV40 large tumor antigen are physically associated with the same 54 kd cellular protein in transformed cells. Cell 28:387, 1982

Herpesviruses

Duff R, Rapp F: Oncogenic transformation of hamster embryo cells after exposure to inactivated herpes simplex virus type 1. J Virol 12:209, 1973

Henle G, Henle W, Diehl V: Relation of Burkitt's tumor-associated herpes-type virus to infectious mononucleosis. Proc Natl Acad Sci USA 59:94, 1968

Hummel M, Kieff E: Mapping of polypeptides encoded by the Epstein–Barr virus genome in productive infection. Proc Natl Acad Sci USA 79:5698, 1982

Klein G, Giovanella BV, Lindahl T, et al.: Direct evidence for the presence of Epstein–Barr virus DNA and nuclear antigen in malignant epithelial cells from patients with poorly differentiated carcinoma of the nasopharynx. Proc Natl Acad Sci USA 71:4737, 1974

Hepatitis B Virus

Summers J, Mason WS: Replication of the genome of a hepatitis B-like virus by reverse transcription of an RNA intermediate. Cell 29:403, 1982

RNA TUMOR VIRUSES

Endogenous Retroviruses

Elder JH, Gautsch JW, Jensen FC, et al.: Multigene family of endogenous retroviruses: Recombinant origin of diversity. J Natl Cancer Inst 61:625, 1978

Gardner MB: Type C viruses of wild mice: Characterization and natural history of amphotropic, ecotropic and xenotropic MuLV. Curr Top Microbiol Immunol 79:215, 1978

Herr W, Schwarz D, Gilbert W: Isolation and mapping of DNA hybridization probes specific for ecotropic and nonecotropic murine leukemia proviruses. Virology 125:139, 1983

Igel HJ, Heubner RJ, Turner RC, et al.: Mouse leukemia virus activation by chemical carcinogens. Science 166:1624, 1969

Weiss RA, Friis PR, Vogt PK: Induction of avian tumor viruses in normal cells by physical and chemical carcinogens. Virology 46:920, 1971

Recombinants between Endogenous Viruses

Bryant ML, Roy-Burman P, Gardner MB, et al.: Genetic relationship of wild mouse amphotropic virus to murine ecotropic and xenotropic viruses. Virology 88:389, 1978

Chattopadhyay SK, Cloyd MW, Linemeyer DR, et al.: Cellular origin and role of mink cell focus-forming viruses in murine thymic lymphomas. Nature 295:25, 1982

Chien Y-H, Verma IM, Shih TY, et al.: Heteroduplex analysis of the sequence relations between the RNAs of mink cell focus-inducing and murine leukemia viruses. J Virol 25:352, 1978

Cloyd MW: Characterization of target cells for MCF viruses in AKR mice. Cell 32:217, 1983

Coffin JM, Tsichlis PN, Conklin KF, et al.: Genomes of endogenous and exogenous avian retroviruses. Virology 126:151, 1983

Hartley NW, Wolford NK, Old LJ, et al.: A new class of murine leukemia virus associated with development of spontaneous lymphomas. Proc Natl Acad Sci USA 74:789, 1977

Hoffman PM, Davidson WF, Ruscetti SK, et al.: Wild mouse ecotropic murine leukemia virus infection of inbred mice: Dualtropic virus expression precedes the onset of paralysis and lymphoma. J Virol 39:597, 1981

Rapp UR, Todaro GJ: Generation of oncogenic type C viruses: Rapidly leukemogenic viruses derived from C3H mouse cells in vivo and in vitro. Proc Natl Acad Sci USA 75:2468, 1978

Thomas CY, Coffin JM: Genetic alterations of RNA leukemia viruses associated with the development of spontaneous thymic leukemia in AKR/J mice. J Virol 43:416, 1982

Troxler DH, Lowy D, Howk R, et al.: Friend strain of spleen focus-forming virus is a recombinant between ecotropic murine type C virus and the *env* gene region of xenotropic type C virus. Proc Natl Acad Sci USA 74:467, 1977

Acute Leukemia/Sarcoma Viruses

Devare SD, Reddy EP, Law JD, et al.: Nucleotide sequence of the simian sarcoma virus genome: Demonstration that its acquired cellular sequences encode the transforming gene product $p28^{sis}$ Proc Natl Acad Sci USA 80:731, 1983

Duesberg PH, Bister K, Vogt PK: The RNA of avian acute leukemia virus MC29. Proc Natl Acad Sci USA 74:4320, 1977

East JL, Amesse LS, Kingsbury DW, et al.: Sequence relationships between Kirsten retrovirus genomes and the genomes of other murine retroviruses. Virology 126:126, 1983

Goff SP, Gilboa E, Witte ON, et al.: Structure of the Abelson murine leukemia virus genome and the homologous cellular gene: Studies with cloned viral DNA. Cell 22:777, 1980

Graf T, Beug H: Avian leukemia viruses: Interaction with their target cells in vivo and in vitro. Biochim Biophys Acta 516:269, 1978

Hu SSF, Vogt PK: Avian oncovirus MH2 is defective in gag, pol, and env. Virology 92:278, 1979

Reddy EP, Smith MJ, Aaronson SA: Complete nucleotide sequence and organization of the Moloney sarcoma virus genome. Science 214:445, 1981

Schwartz DE, Tizard R, Gilbert W: Nucleotide sequence of Rous sarcoma virus. Cell 32:853, 1983

Shibuya M, Hanafusa H: Nucleotide sequence of Fujinami sarcoma virus: Evolutionary relationship of its transforming gene with transforming genes of other sarcoma viruses. Cell 30:787, 1982

Wong TC, Lai MMC, Hu SSF, et al.: Class II defective avian sarcoma viruses: Comparative analysis of genome structure. Virology 120:453, 1982

Retrovirus Provirus

Barbacid M, Stephenson JR, Aaronson SA: Evolutionary relationships between gag gene-coded proteins of murine and primate endogenous type C RNA viruses. Cell 10:641, 1977

Hizi A, Joklik WK: RNA-dependent DNA polymerase of avian sarcoma virus B77. I. Isolation and partial characterization of the α, β_2, and $\alpha\beta$ forms of the enzyme. J Biol Chem 252:2281, 1977

McLellan WL, Ihle JN: Purification and characterization of a murine tumor cell surface glycoprotein of 75,000 daltons that is related to the major envelope glycoprotein of murine leukemia virus. Virology 89:547, 1978

Vogt VM, Wight A, Eisenman R: In vitro cleavage of avian retrovirus gag proteins by viral protease p15. Virology 98:154, 1979

Nature of Oncogenes/Protooncogenes

Alitalo K, Bishop JM, Smith DH, et al.: Nucleotide sequence of the v-myc oncogene of avian retrovirus MC29. Proc Natl Acad Sci USA 80:100, 1983

Capon DJ, Chen EY, Levinson AD, et al.: Complete nucleotide sequence of the T24 human bladder carcinoma oncogene and its normal homolog. Nature 302:33, 1983

Collett MS, Brugge JS, Erikson RL: Characterization of a normal avian cell protein related to the avian sarcoma virus transforming gene product. Cell 15:1363, 1978

Cooper JA, Reiss NA, Schwarz RJ, et al.: Three glycolytic enzymes are phosphorylated at tyrosine in cells transformed by Rous sarcoma virus. Nature 302:218, 1983

Dhar R, Ellis RW, Shih TY, et al.: Nucleotide sequence of the p21 transforming protein of Harvey sarcoma virus. Science 217:934, 1982

Fung YT, Crittenden LB, Fadley AM, et al.: Tumor induction by direct injection of cloned v-src DNA into chickens. Proc Natl Acad Sci USA 80:353, 1983

Gay NJ, Walker JE: Homology between human bladder carcinoma oncogene product and mitochondrial ATP-synthase. Nature 301:262, 1983

Gondo TJ, Bishop JM: Structure and transcription of the cellular homolog (c-myb) of the avian myeloblastosis virus transforming gene (v-myb). J Virol 46:212, 1983

Groffen J, Heisterkamp N, Shibuya M, et al.: Transforming genes of avian (v-fps) and mammalian (v-fes) retroviruses correspond to a common cellular locus. Virology 125:480, 1983

Hayman MJ, Ramsay GM, Graf T, et al.: Identification and characterization of the avian erythroblastosis virus erbB gene product as a membrane glycoprotein. Cell 32:579, 1983

Hirano A, Neil JC, Vogt PK: ts transformation mutants of avian sarcoma virus PRCII: Lack of strict correlation between transforming ability and properties of the P105-associated kinase. Virology 125:219, 1983

Iwashita S, Kitamura N, Yoshida M: Molecular events leading to fusiform morphological transformation by partial src deletion mutant of Rous sarcoma virus. Virology 125:419, 1983

Kloetzer WS, Maxwell SA, Arlinghaus RB: $P85^{gag\text{-}mos}$ encoded by ts110 Moloney murine sarcoma virus has an associated protein kinase activity. Proc Natl Acad Sci USA 80:412, 1983

Langbeheim H, Shih TY, Scolnick EM: Identification of a normal vertebrate cell protein related to the p21 src of Harvey murine sarcoma virus. Virology 106:292, 1980

Levinson AD, Opermann H, Levintow L, et al.: Evidence that the transforming gene of avian sarcoma virus encodes a protein kinase associated with a phosphoprotein. Cell 15:561, 1978

Maness PF, Levy BT: Highly purified $pp60^{src}$ induces the actin transformation in microinjected cells and phosphorylates selected cytoskeletal proteins in vitro. Mol Cell Biol 3:102, 1983

Parker RC, Varmus HE, Bishop JM: Cellular homolog (c-src) of the transforming gene of Rous sarcoma virus: Isolation, mapping, and transcriptional analysis of c-src and flanking regions. Proc Natl Acad Sci USA 78:5842

Shi TY, Papageorge AG, Stokes PE, et al.: Guanine nucleotide-binding and autophosphorylating activities associated with the p21^{src} protein of Harvey murine sarcoma virus. Nature 287:686, 1980

Shimizu K, Goldbarb M, Suard Y, et al.: Three human transforming genes are related to the viral ras oncogene. Proc Natl Acad Sci USA 80:2112, 193

Snyder MA, Bishop JM, Colby WW, et al.: Phosphorylation of tyrosine-416 is not required for the transforming properties and kinase activity of pp60$^{v\text{-}src}$. Cell 32:891, 1983

Takeya T, Hanafusa H: Structure and sequence of the cellular gene homologous to the RSV src gene and the mechanism for generating the transforming virus. Cell 32:881, 1983

Vennstrom B, Sheiness D, Zapielski J, et al.: Isolation and characterization of c-myc, a cellular homolog of the oncogene (v-myc) of avian myelocytomatosis virus strain 29. J Virol 42:773, 1982

Watson R, Oskarsson M, Vande Woode GF: Human DNA sequence homologous to the transforming gene (mos) of Moloney murine sarcoma virus. Proc Natl Acad Sci USA 79:4078, 1982

Transfection of Oncogenes

Balmain A, Pragnell ID: Mouse skin carcinomas induced in vivo by chemical carcinogens have a transforming Harvey-ras oncogene. Nature 303:72, 1983

Chang EH, Furth ME, Scolnick EM, et al.: Tumorigenic transformation of mammalian cells induced by a normal gene homologous to the oncogene of Harvey murine sarcoma virus. Nature 297:479, 1982

Der CJ, Cooper GM: Altered gene products are associated with activation of cellular ras^{k} genes in human lung and colon carcinomas. Cell 32:201, 1983

Der CJ, Krontiris TG, Cooper GM: Transforming genes of human bladder and lung carcinoma cell lines are homologous to the ras genes of Harvey and Kirsten sarcoma viruses. Proc Natl Acad Sci USA 79:3637, 1982

Parada LF, Tabin CJ, Shih C, et al.: Human EJ bladder carcinoma oncogene is homologue of Harvey sarcoma virus ras gene. Nature 297:474, 1982

Activation of Oncogenes

PROMOTER INSERTION

Hayward WS, Neel BG, Astrin SM: Activation of a cellular onc gene by promoter insertion in ALV-induced lymphoid leukosis. Nature 290:475, 1981

Joyner A, Yamamoto Y, Bernstein A: Retrovirus long terminal repeats activate expression of coding sequences for the herpes simplex virus thymidine kinase gene. Proc Natl Acad Sci USA 79:1573, 1982

Kuff EL, Feenstra A, Lueders K, et al.: Homology between an endogenous viral LTR and sequences inserted in activated cellular oncogene. Nature 302:547, 1983

AMPLIFICATION

Alitalo K, Schwab M, Lin CC, et al.: Homogeneously staining chromosomal regions contain amplified copies of an abundantly expressed cellular oncogene (c-myc) in malignant neuroendocrine cells from a human colon carcinoma. Proc Natl Acad Sci USA 80:1707, 1983

Collins S, Groudine M: Amplification of endogenous myc-related DNA sequences in a human myeloid leukemia cell line. Nature 298:679, 1982

Favera RD, Wong-Staal F, Gallo RC: Onc gene amplification in promyelocytic leukemia cel line HL-60 and primary leukemic cells of the same patient. Nature 299:61, 1982

TRANSLOCATION

Erikson J, Ar-Rushdi A, Drwinga HL, et al.: Transcriptional activation of the translocated c-myc oncogene in Burkitt lymphoma. Proc Natl Acad Sci USA 80:820, 1983

Mushinski JF, Bauer SR, Potter M, et al.: Increased expression of myc-related oncogene mRNA characterizes most BALB/c plasmacytomas induced by pristane or Abelson murine leukemia virus. Proc Natl Acad Sci USA 80:1073, 1983

MUTATIONS

Reddy EP, Reynolds RK, Santos E, et al.: A point mutation is responsible for the acquisition of transforming properties by the T24 human bladder carcinoma oncogene. Nature 300:149, 1982

STAGE-SPECIFIC ACTIVATION

Groffen J, Heisterkamp N, Blennerhassett G, et al.: Regulation of viral and cellular oncogene expression by cytosine methylation. Virology 126:213, 1983

Lane M-A, Sainten A, Cooper GM: Stage-specific transforming genes of human and mouse B- and T-lymphocyte neoplasms. Cell 28:873, 1983

Muller R, Slamon DJ, Tremblay JM, et al.: Differential expression of cellular oncogenes during pre- and postnatal development of the mouse. Nature 299:640, 1982

Chromosomal Location

Chang EH, Gonda MA, Ellis RM, et al.: Human genome contains four genes homologous to transforming genes of Harvey and Kirsten murine sarcoma viruses. Proc Natl Acad Sci USA 79:4848, 1982

Favera RD, Gallo RC, Giallongo A, et al.: Chromosomal localization of the human homolog (c-sis) of the simian sarcoma virus onc gene. Science 218:686, 1982

Neel BG, Jhanwar SC, Chaganti RSK, et al.: Two human c-onc genes are located on the long arm of chromosome 8. Proc Natl Acad Sci USA 79:7842, 1982

Retrovirus env Gene Products as Differentration Antigens

del Villano BC, Lerner RA: Relationship between the oncornavirus gene product gp70 and a major protein secretion of the mouse genital tract. Nature 259:497, 1976

Elder JH, Jensen FC, Bryant ML, et al.: Polymorphism of the major envelope glycoprotein (gp70) of murine C-type viruses: Virion associated and differentiation antigens encoded by a multigene family. Nature 267:23, 1977

Hesselink WG, van der Kemp ACM, Bloemers HPJ: Moloney cell surface antigen (MCSA) has properties of the env gene products of the Moloney strain of murine leukemia virus. Virology 110:375, 1981

Mammary Tumor Viruses

Calahan R, Drohan W, Tronick S, et al.: Detection and cloning of human DNA sequences related to the mouse mammary tumor virus genome. Proc Natl Acad Sci USA 79:5503, 1982

Diggelman H, Vessaz AL, Buetti E: Cloned endogenous mouse mammary tumor virus DNA is biologically active in transfected mouse cells and its expression is stimulated by glucocorticoid hormones. Virology 122:332, 1982

Huang AL, Ostrowski MC, Berard D, et al.: Glucocorticoid regulation of the Ha-MuSV p21 gene conferred by sequences from mouse mammary tumor virus. Cell 27:245, 1981

Morrios VL, Medeiros E, Ringold GM, et al.: Comparison of mouse mammary tumor virus-specific DNA in inbred, wild and Asian mice, and in tumors and normal organs from inbred mice. J Mol Biol 114:73, 1977

Parks WP, Ransom JC, Young HA, et al.: Mammary tumor virus induction by glucocorticoids. Characterization of specific transcriptional regulation. J Biol Chem 250:3330, 1975

Ringold GM, Yamamoto KR, Bishop JM, et al.: Glucocorticoid-stimulated accumulation of mouse mammary tumor virus RNA: Increased rate of synthesis of viral RNA. Proc Natl Acad Sci USA 74:2879, 1977

Ucker DS, Firestone GL, Yamamoto K: Glucocorticoids and chromosomal position modulate murine mammary tumor virus transcription by affecting efficiency of promoter utilization. Mol Cell Biol 3:551, 1983

Human T Cell Leukemia Virus (HTLV)

Gallo RC, Mann D, Broder S, et al.: Human T-cell leukemia-lymphoma virus (HTLV) is in T but not B lymphocytes from a patient with cutaneous T-cell lymphoma. Proc Natl Acad Sci USA 79:5680, 1982

Haynes BF, Miller SE, Palker TJ, et al.: Identification of human T cell leukemia virus in a Japanese patient with adult T cell leukemia and cutaneous lymphomatous vasculitis. Proc Natl Acad Sci USA 80:2054, 1983

Popovic M, Sarin PS, Robert-Guroff M, et al.: Isolation and transmissin of human retrovirus (human T-cell leukemia virus). Science 219:856, 1983

Intracisternal A-type Particles

Kuff EL, Lueders KK, Scolnick EM: Nucleotide sequence relationship between intracisternal type A particles of *Mus musculus* and an endogenous retrovirus (M432) of *Mus cervicolor.* J Virol 28:66, 1978

Kuff EL, Feenstra A, Lueders K, et al.: Intracisternal A-particle genomes as movable elements in the mouse genome. Proc Natl Acad Sci USA 80:1992, 1983

Lueders KK, Kuff EL: Sequences associated with intracisternal A particles are reiterated in the mouse genome. Cell 12:963, 1977

Ono M, Cole MD, White AT, et al.: Sequence organizatin of cloned intracisternal A particle genes. Cell 21:465, 1980

Shen-Ong GLC, Cole MD: Differing populations of intracisternal A-particle genes in myeloma tumors and mouse subspecies. J Virol 42:411, 1982

VL30 Sequences

Giri OP, Hodgson CP, Elder PK, et al.: Discrete regions of sequence homology between cloned rodent VL30 genetic elements and AKV-related MuLV provirus genomes. Nucl Acid Res 11:305, 1983

Itin A, Rotman G, Keshet E: Conservation patterns of mouse "viruslike" (VL30) DNA sequences. Virology 127:374, 1983

copia* Sequences of *Drosophila

Hoffman-Falk H, Einat P, Shilo BZ, et al.: *Drosophila melanogaster* DNA clones homologous to vertebrate oncogenes: Evidence for a common ancestor to the src and abl cellular genes. Cell 32:589, 1983

Shiba T, Saigo K: Retrovirus-like particles containing RNA homologous to the transposable element *copia* in *Drosophila melanogaster.* Nature 302:119, 1983

CHAPTER 9

The Bacteriophages

In 1915 Twort published a note describing the infectious destruction of micrococcal colonies and offered three possible explanations for this phenomenon: (1) the destroyed colonies represented a stage in the bacterial life cycle that induced normal colonies to undergo a glassy transformation; (2) the lytic agent was an enzyme that caused both cell destruction and the production of more enzyme; and (3) the causative agent was a virus that grew in bacteria and destroyed them. All of these explanations could be reconciled with the original findings that the agent would not grow on any medium, passed through bacteria-proof filters, and was inactivated by heating to 60C for 1 hour. d'Hérelle, who discovered this phenomenon independently, soon demonstrated the particulate nature of what he called "bacteriophages." The elegant pioneering work of Burnet and of Schlesinger in the 1930s confirmed the viral nature of the Twort-d'Hérelle agents.

Early hopes of using the action of phage on susceptible bacteria as a means of preventing and treating infectious diseases were not fulfilled (Chap. 1). However, in the early 1940s, Delbrück and a group of investigators around him realized that the availability of viruses multiplying in cloned populations of rapidly growing host cells provided an ideal tool for gaining an insight into the mechanisms of biologic self-replication. Their expectation was amply borne out. The bacteriophage-bacterium system proved to be highly amenable to experimentation, and intensive investigation of it over the last four decades has provided many of the fundamental concepts concerning molecular genetics, nucleic acid replication, and the tran-

TABLE 9-1. CHARACTERISTICS OF SOME WELL-STUDIED BACTERIOPHAGES

		Particle Dimensions (nm)			Nucleic Acid			
Phage	Host	Head	Tail Length	Particle Structure	Type	Strandedness	Mol Wt $\times 10^6$	Structure
T1	*E. coli*	50	150	Hexagonal head, simple tail	DNA	DS	27	Linear
T2, T4, T6	*E. coli*	80 × 110	110	Prolate icosahedral head, complex tail with fibers	DNA	DS	112	Linear, contains glycosylated 5-hydroxymethylcytosine
T3, T7	*E. coli*	60	15	Hexagonal head, short tail	DNA	DS	25	Linear
T5	*E. coli*	65	170	Hexagonal head, simple tail	DNA	DS	80	Linear, one strand segmented
N4	*E. coli*	70	15	Hexagonal head, short tail	DNA	DS	40	Contains U
Lambda	*E. coli*	54	140	Hexagonal head, simple tail	DNA	DS	31	Linear, cohesive ends
P22	*S. typhimurium*	55	20	Hexagonal head, complex tail	DNA	DS	27	Linear, circularly permuted, terminally redundant
SPO1, SP82	*B. subtilis*	100	210	Hexagonal head, complex tail	DNA	DS	100	Linear, contains 5-hydroxymethyluracil
φ 29	*B. amyloliquefaciens*	30 × 40	30	Prolate icosahedral head with attached fibers, complex tail with collars and neck appendages	DNA	DS	11	Linear
PM2	*Pseudomonas BAL-31*	60	None	Hexagonal head, envelope contains lipid	DNA	DS	6	Circular
φX 174, S13, M12, G4	*E. coli*	27	None	Icosahedral	DNA	SS	1.6	Circular
fl, fd, M13 φ 6	*E. coli*	5–10 × 800	None	Filamentous	DNA	SS	1.3	Circular
	Pseudomonas phaseolica	65	None	Polyhedral head, envelope contains lipid	RNA	DS	9.5	3 linear segments (2.2, 2.8 and 4.5 × 10^6)
MS2, f2, fr,Qβ	*E. coli*	24	None	Icosahedral	RNA	SS	1.2	Linear

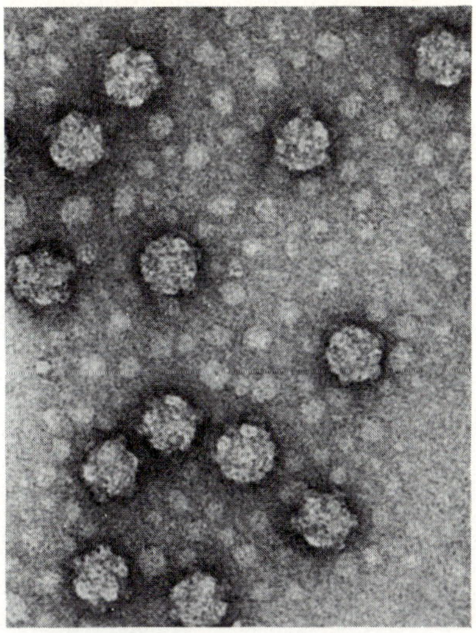

Figure 9-1. Bacteriophage ϕX 174. × 225,000. *(Electron micrograph by Dr. R.B. Luftig.)*

scription and translation of genetic information. These concepts are applicable not only to bacterial viruses but also to animal viruses and to cells in general. Thus, although bacteriophages were a failure as therapeutic agents, they have proved invaluable for the elucidation of the reactions most basic to life.

Structure of Bacteriophages

There are bacteriophages for every bacterial species. Very few have been investigated in detail, but intense concentration on a small number of them has permitted rapid progress. Many of the well-studied phages are active on *Escherichia coli* or on *Bacillus* or *Pseudomonas* species (Table 9-1).

Structure of Phage Capsids

The structure of bacteriophages is governed by the same principles as are described in Chapter 2. Some of the smaller phages, such as ϕX 174 and MS2, have icosahedral capsids (Fig. 9-1); others, such as phage fl, are filamentous and possess helical symmetry (Fig. 9-2). Larger phages generally consist of a head that comprises the phage genome enclosed within a single capsid shell that is usually hexagonal and may or may not be elongated, and a tail that serves both as the cell attachment organ and as a tube through which phage DNA passes into the host cell. The complexity of this tail varies greatly from phage to phage, but in most phages it conforms to one of three morphologic patterns. In the first, exemplified by coliphages T3 and T7, the tail is very short (Fig. 9-3). In the second, exemplified by coliphages T1 and lambda, the tail is long but rather simple in construction. It consists essentially of a noncontractile flexible tube that may or may not possess a knob or one or several spikes or fibers at its distal end (Fig. 9-4). The third morphologic tail pattern, exhibited by the coliphages T2, T4, and T6, the so-called T-even phages, is staggeringly complex (Fig. 9-5). These tails consist of a hollow core that is attached at one end to the head and bears at its distal end a hexagonal base plate to which are attached six pins and six long tail fibers bent in the middle. A thin collar with several (possibly six) whiskers is attached to the core close to the head, and it is surrounded for most of its length by a sheath composed of 24 rings of helically arranged capsomers. These tails, which consist of more than 20 different protein species, serve as syringes by means of which phage DNA is injected into the cell (p. 164).

Very few phages are enveloped. Among them are the *Pseudomonas* phages PM2 (Fig. 9-6) and ϕ6.

Structure of Phage Nucleic Acids

Bacteriophage genomes take several forms (Table 9-1). Most of them consist of single, linear, double-stranded

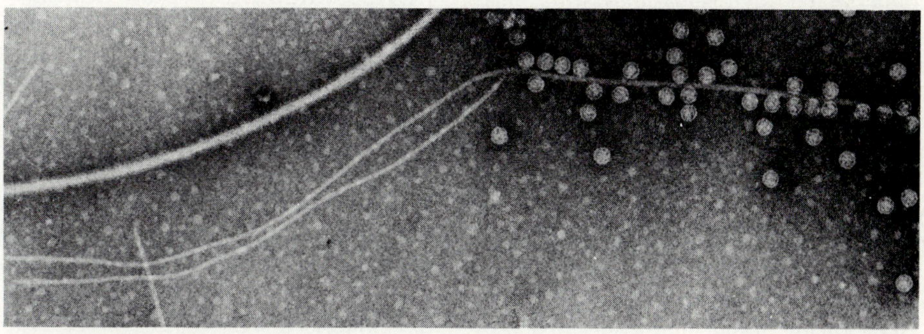

Figure 9-2. An F-pilus with two types of male-specific phage attached: icosahedral RNA-containing MS2, and filamentous DNA-containing fl. The former are attached along the entire length of the F-pilus; the latter are adsorbed by their ends to the tip of the pilus. *(From Caro and Schnos: Proc Natl Acad Sci USA 56:128, 1968.)*

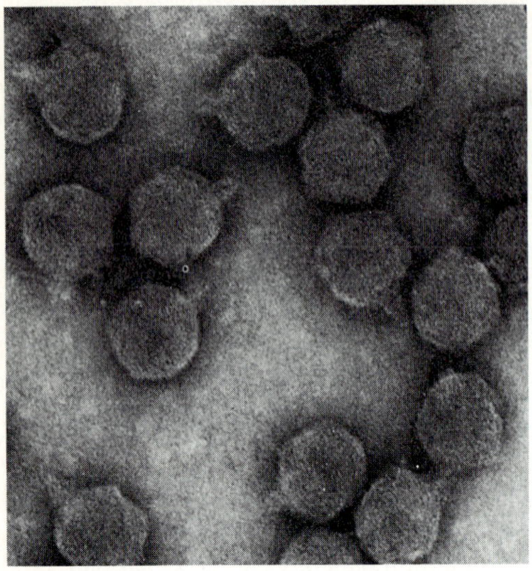

Figure 9-3. Bacteriophage T7. × 225,000. *(Electron micrograph by Dr. R.B. Luftig.)*

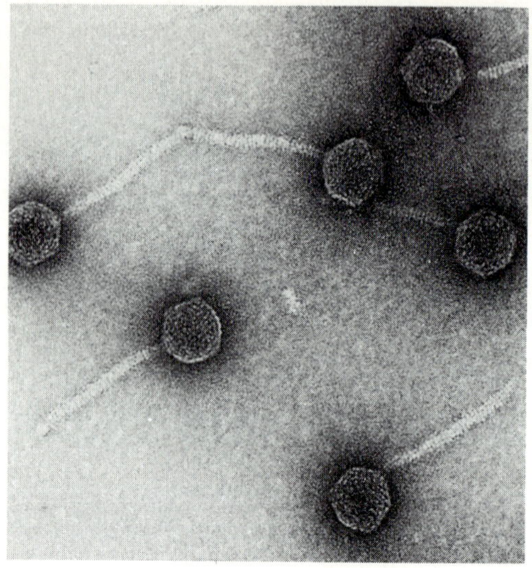

Figure 9-4. Bacteriophage lambda. × 135,000. *(Electron micrograph by Dr. R.B. Luftig.)*

DNA molecules that vary in molecular weight from about 1 million to more than 100 million. Some of them, in particular those of the T-even phages, exist in a form that is both circularly permuted and terminally redundant. In them the nucleotide sequence of some genomes is A, B, C, D, . . . W, X, Y, Z, A, B; of others B, C, D, . . . W, X, Y, Z, A, B, C; of others still C, D, . . . W, X, Y, Z, A, B, C, D; and so on. In other words, all contain the same sequences, but the terminal sequences differ in individual genomes and some nucleotides are reiterated at the ends of the genomes. This is because their replication proceeds via replicative intermediates that consist of many genomes linked covalently end-to-end, which are then cut at random so as to yield molecules of the same size (p. 170). The reason for the terminal redundancy is to avoid loss of the gene that would otherwise be cut at each end.

Other phage genomes, such as that of PM2, consist of circular double-stranded DNA; others, such as those of phages ϕX 174, G4, and fd, consist of single-stranded circular DNA with plus polarity, and still others are linear single-stranded nonpermuted RNA molecules with plus polarity, analogous to poliovirus RNA. There is also a phage of *Pseudomonas phaseolica*, ϕ6, that contains double-stranded RNA. Like the double-stranded RNA-containing genomes of animal viruses, ϕ6 RNA is segmented. It consists of three unique segments whose molecular weights are 2.2, 2.9, and 4.8 million.

Phage nucleic acids are infectious, just as are the nucleic acids of animal viruses. The bacterial cell wall, however, presents a more formidable barrier to the entry of nucleic acids than is presented by the plasma membrane of animal cells, and infection by naked phage nucleic acids, termed transfection, can only be demonstrated under special circumstances. Transfection of whole bacterial cells is rare. Cells of *Bacillus subtilis* that are competent for transformation can be transfected, and so can cells of *E. coli* treated with Ca^{2+} (only with lambda DNA).

The most readily transfectible bacterial forms are spheroplasts, and frozen-thawed cells that can be transfected not only with small single-stranded phage RNAs and DNAs but also with large double-stranded phage DNAs.

Unusual Nucleic Acid Bases. Whereas the genomes of animal viruses contain only the normal nucleic acid bases, adenine, guanine, cytosine, and uracil or thymine, phage genomes sometimes contain unusual or substituted bases. For example, the DNA of the T-even bacteriophages contains not cytosine but 5-hydroxymethylcytosine and glycosylated 5′-hydroxymethylcytosine; the DNA of certain *B. subtilis* phages contain not thymine but uracil, 5-hydroxymethyluracil, glycosylated and phosphorylated 5-(4′, 5′-dihydroxypentyl) uracil, or α-glutamyl thymine; and in the DNA of a *Pseudomonas acidovorus* phage, thymine is partially replaced by 5-(4′-aminobutylaminomethyl) uracil, also known as α-putrescinylthymine.

Glycosylation and Methylation. The bases of bacteriophage DNA are often glycosylated and/or methylated in highly characteristic patterns. Both 5-hydroxymethylcytosine and 5-hydroxymethyluracil are often glycosylated by phage-coded enzymes, that is, they are linked to either one or two glucose residues via α or β bonds. In the T-even phages the situation is as shown in Table 9-2. In addition, a small proportion of the cytosine and adenine residues in phage DNAs is generally methylated by host-specified enzymes.

The presence of modified bases alters the properties of phage DNAs in two major ways. First, both glycosylation and, especially, methylation confer resistance to degradation by nucleases. Bacteria guard themselves against foreign DNAs by degrading them with highly specific restriction endonucleases, and in order to prevent their own DNA from being destroyed, they cause methyl

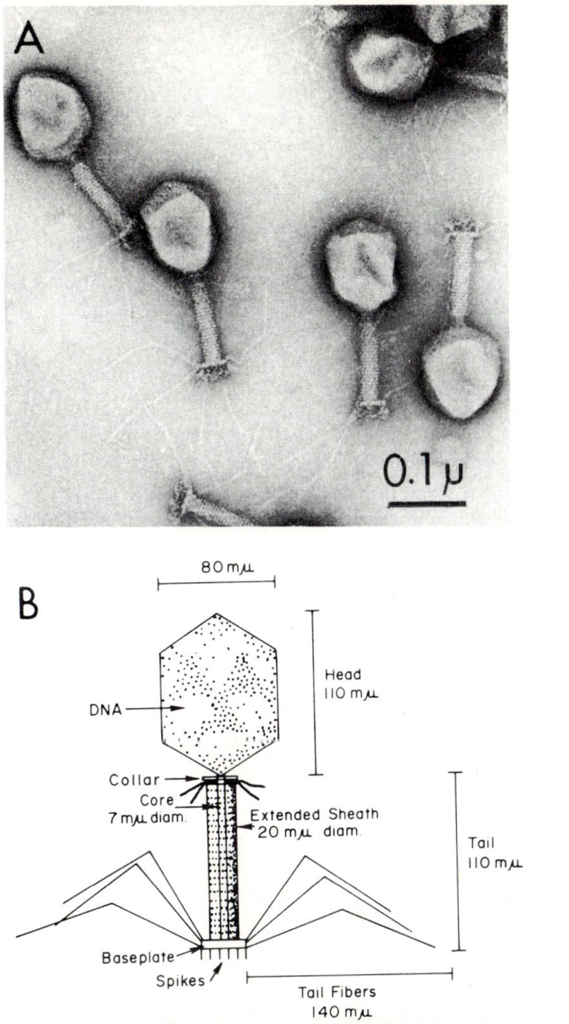

Figure 9-5. **A.** Bacteriophage T4. × 100,000. **B.** Model of phage T4. *(Electron micrograph by Dr. R.B. Luftig.)*

groups to be attached to their own DNA in specific locations. Since phage nucleic acids also become methylated, highly specific restriction patterns, known as "host-induced modifications," exist among bacteriophages. For example, the DNA of a phage grown in host A will be methylated by that host's enzymes in such a manner that it will be resistant to that host's restriction endonucleases, but most of the DNA of this phage will be degraded by the restriction endonucleases of other bacteria. However, any DNA molecules that escape degradation in such hosts can replicate, and their progeny will then be modified by the methylating enzymes of the new hosts, acquiring new specificities in the process.

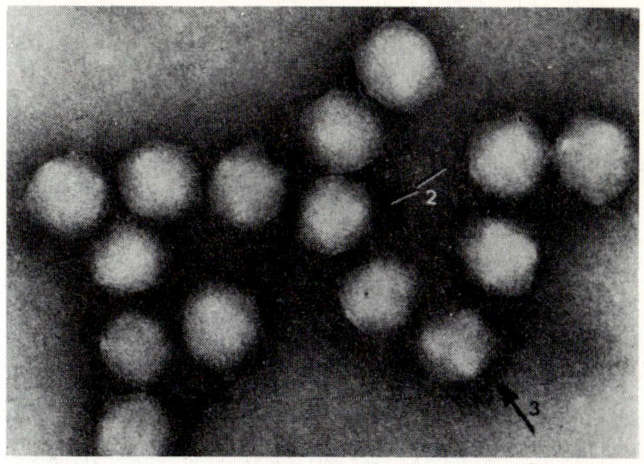

Figure 9-6. The enveloped phage PM2 fixed with glutaraldehyde and negatively stained with phosphotungstate. The numbered arrows indicate axes of two-fold and three-fold symmetry. × 120,000. *(From Silbert et al.: Virology 39:666, 1969.)*

Second, modification of the apolar character of pyrimidine 5′-methyl substituents alters the stability of the DNA double helix. In general, uncharged and negatively charged substituents decrease helix stability, and positively charged substituents increase it (by neutralizing some of the phosphate negative charges). Such modified bases could further protect DNAs from host and phage nucleases, serve as signals for transcription and replication, and facilitate packaging of DNAs on the one hand, and their injection into cells on the other (see below). However, although modified bases are clearly advantageous under certain specific sets of conditions, their presence has not conferred sufficient survival advantage during evolution for them to become used widely in nature.

Physiology of Lytic Phage Infection

Like animal viruses, some bacteriophages lyse their hosts, while others integrate their genomes into the host genome. The former are known as virulent phages, the latter

TABLE 9-2. EXTENT OF GLYCOSYLATION OF 5-HYDROXYMETHYLCYTOSINE IN THE DNA OF T-EVEN PHAGES*

Phage	Not Gylcosylated	α-Glucosyl	β-Glucosyl	β-1 : 6-Glucosyl-α-Glucosyl
T2	25	70	0	5
T4	0	70	30	0
T6	25	3	0	72

From Lehman: J Biol Chem 235:3254, 1960.
*Figures represent percentages.

as temperate or lysogenic phages. We will consider first the lytic phage one-step multiplication cycle, which is formally analogous to that of animal viruses (Chap. 4) but proceeds much more rapidly. For example, whereas the length of the latent period (the interval between infection and release of progeny virus) is at least 4 hours for poliovirus and 12 hours for vaccinia virus, the latent period is 13 minutes for phages T1, T7, and ϕX 174, and 21 to 25 minutes for the T-even phages and MS2.

Adsorption

The initial step of the phage multiplication cycle illustrates with particular clarity the existence of virus-specific receptors on host cells. Phages are usually highly specific for a limited number of bacterial host strains. The basis of this specificity resides in the complementarity of the molecular configurations on phage attachment organs on the one hand, and on receptor molecules on the bacterial surface on the other. The nature of the phage attachment organ varies from phage to phage: small icosahedral phages, such as ϕX 174 and MS2, have multiple attachment sites; filamentous phages, such as f1, adsorb with their ends (Fig. 9-2); tailed phages adsorb with the knobs, spikes, or fibers that are located at the tips of their tails. Phage receptors on the bacterial surface are sometimes on lipopolysaccharide, at other times on lipoprotein, and sometimes on F pili, which causes the phages that adsorb to them, typically single-stranded DNA-containing and RNA-containing phages, to be male-specific (Fig. 9-2).

Mutations in bacteria that destroy the complementarity of the phage-receptor interaction result in resistance. Phage populations usually contain mutants that are themselves altered in such a way as to restore the necessary complementarity. These are known as "host-range mutants" and can grow in the mutated bacteria.

Bacteria capable of adsorbing the same phage are often antigenically related. This observation has found diagnostic application in the practice of phage typing. In this method the sensitivity/resistance patterns of bacterial strains to a series of bacteriophages are determined. Since these patterns are both readily determined and highly characteristic, they are useful tests for identification. For example, some phages of *Salmonella typhi* are specific for strains possessing the Vi antigen, which is characteristic of virulent strains, and these phages are used for the identification of virulent strains of typhoid bacilli. Several other phage-typing systems exist, the best known being that for staphylococci.

Injection and Uncoating

The events immediately following phage adsorption are involved with the injection of phage nucleic acid into the cell. These events provide an excellent illustration of the general principle that uncoating of viral genomes involves the physical separation of genome and capsid. This was first shown in 1952 by Hershey and Chase in an experiment that represents one of the milestones of virology. They infected bacteria with phage T2 labeled in the protein with the radioisotope ^{35}S. Following an incubation period of several minutes, the mixture of phage and bacteria was sheared by blending in a Waring blender. After blending, only a small amount of radioactive label was associated with the bacteria. When this experiment was repeated with phage in which the DNA had been labeled with the radioisotope ^{32}P, the converse was true, that is, the radioactive label was now associated with the cells. This experiment was correctly interpreted as signifying that the DNA had passed into the interior of the cell, while the protein coat had remained attached to the outer cell surface from which it could be dislodged by shearing forces. Since the bacteria from which phage coats were removed by shearing yielded normal phage progeny, this experiment clearly showed that viral DNA itself contained all the information necessary for phage multiplication.

The actual infection process has been best studied for the T-even phages. Following adsorption by means of the tail fiber-receptor interaction, the six tail pins make contact with the host surface and firmly anchor the phage tail plate to it. The conformation of the tail plate (an extremely complex structure consisting of at least 14 different protein species) then changes. The reason for this change is apparently the fact that several of the tail plate components are enzymes. The six wedges that constitute the major portion of the base plate possess dihydrofolate reductase activity, and the central tail plug possesses both thymidylate synthetase and folyl polyglutamate cleaving activity. It is thought that the configuration of these components changes as a result of their interaction with substrates that leak from cells in response to infection. These conformational changes apparently trigger a change in the manner in which the protein subunits of the tail sheath are arranged, as a result of which the sheath contracts, thereby driving the tail core about 12 nm into the bacterial cell (Fig. 9-7). The phage DNA then passes through the tail core into the bacterial cell (Fig. 9-8). The holes created in the cell membrane by the phage tail cores are normally quickly sealed by cell wall material newly synthesized under the control of a phage gene called "spackle." Clearly, it would not be to the advantage of the phage to permit these holes to remain, since cell contents would leak out through them. In fact, if the multiplicity of infection is too high, excessive leakage does occur, resulting in a phenomenon known as "lysis from without," and the multiplication cycle is aborted.

As pointed out previously, most phages do not possess tails with contractile sheaths, and still others possess no tails at all. Nevertheless, here also the phage protein coat remains on the outside, and only the nucleic acid is introduced into the cell.

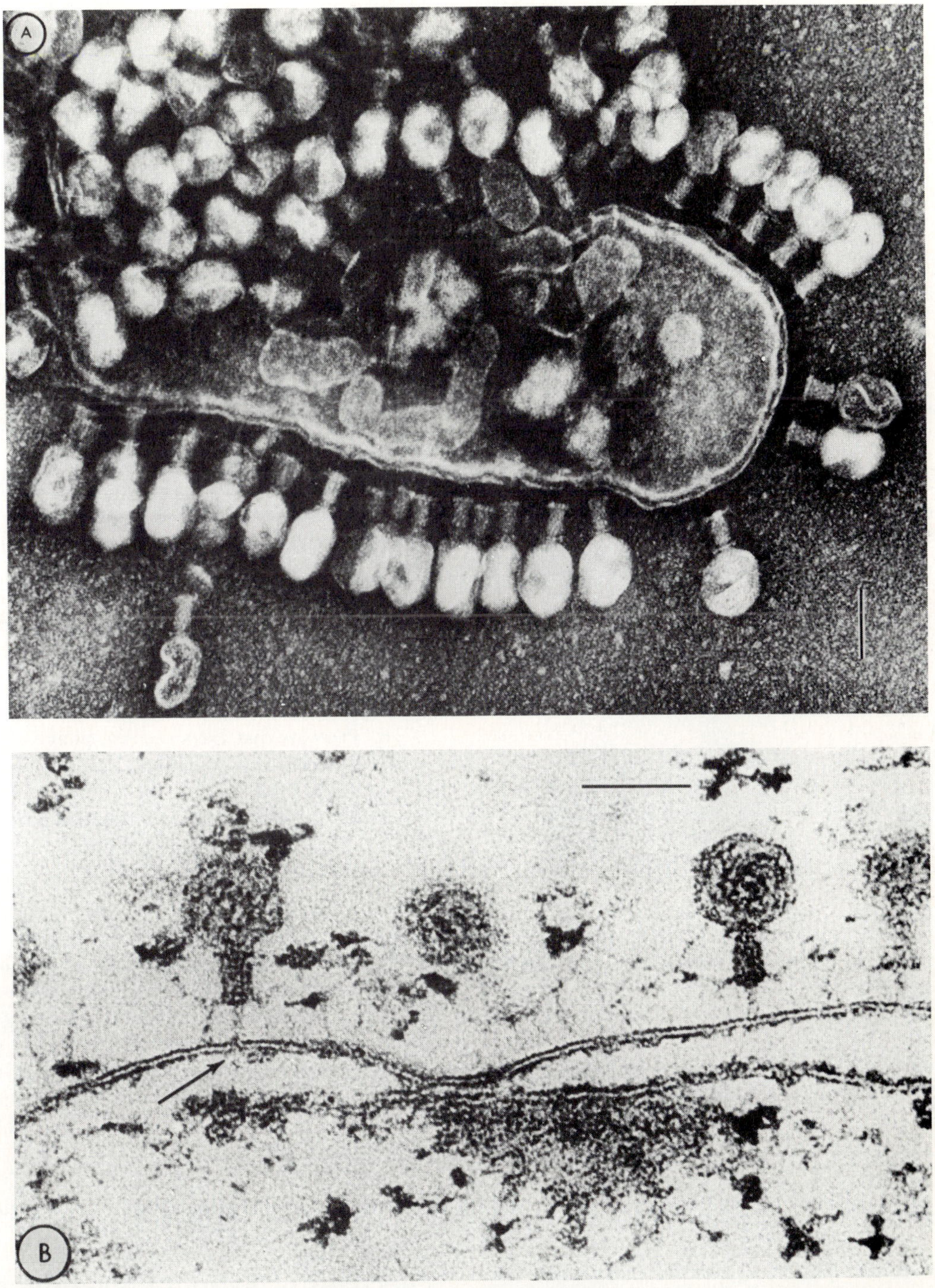

Figure 9-7. Bacteriophage T4 adsorbed to *Escherichia coli.* **A.** The phages' sheaths are contracted, and their base plates are 30 to 40 nm from the cell wall. **B.** The phages visible in this section are seen to be attached to the cell wall by the tail fibers. The cell wall appears as two continuous electron-dense lines separated by an electron-lucent space. The arrow indicates where the tail core of an adsorbed phage may have penetrated the cell wall. *(From Simon and Anderson: Virology 32:279, 1967.)*

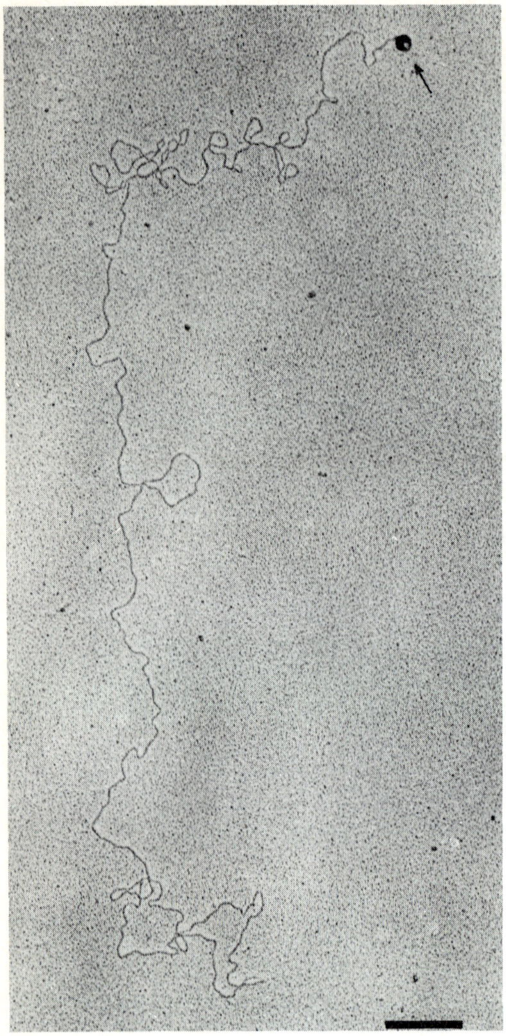

Figure 9-8. A T7 phage particle ejecting its DNA after being treated with formamide. Almost the entire DNA molecule (12 μm long) has been ejected. The bar represents 0.3 μm. *(Courtesy of Dr. Kaoru Saigo.)*

Multiplication Cycle of Phages Containing Double-stranded DNA

Nature of Information Encoded in Phage Genome

During the phage multiplication cycle, the genetic information encoded in the viral genome expresses itself according to an exquisitely refined transcription program that has been studied intensively along the lines discussed in Chapter 4. In fact, many of the techniques and methods that are now being applied to the analysis of the multiplication cycles of animal viruses were first designed and developed for studying the multiplication of bacteriophages. These techniques include, first and foremost, the extensive use of conditional lethal mutants, both temperature-sensitive and missense, such as amber (Chap. 6). Thousands of phage mutants have by now been isolated and characterized with respect to the function in which they are defective. For example, there are mutants that fail to synthesize early proteins, mutants that fail to replicate phage DNA, mutants that fail to form mature phage particles, and so on. Over 100 such functions, each corresponding to a specific gene, have so far been discovered for bacteriophage T4, which is probably about one half of the total number of T4 genes. For smaller, less complicated phages, this proportion is considerably higher.

Most of the known T4 genes have been mapped. All lie on a circular linkage map, a finding that, together with the fact that T4 DNA is a linear molecule, indicates that it is circularly permuted (Fig. 9-9). Similar maps have been prepared for several other phages, notably T3 and T7, lambda and P22, SP01 and SP82, and the small phages that contain single-stranded nucleic acid.

The proteins specified by the genes of the large complex phages, such as the T-even phages, have a variety of functions. Most of them can be grouped into eight classes:

1. Proteins that repair the bacterial cell membrane early in infection
2. Enzymes that degrade host DNA
3. Enzymes that synthesize nucleic acid precursors
4. Proteins that function in phage DNA replication
5. Proteins that program transcription of the phage genome
6. Proteins that are structural phage components
7. Proteins that function catalytically in phage morphogenesis
8. Enzymes that degrade the bacterial cell wall and cell membrane during the late stages of the multiplication cycle

In addition, the T-even phages code for eight species of transfer RNA, the genes for which are clustered in a small region of the phage genome where they may form a single transcription unit or operon. Mutants lacking these genes can multiply, but their burst size, or yield, is smaller than that of wild-type phage. This suggests that the phage-coded transfer RNAs supplement the reading capacity of those codons that are used more commonly by the virus than by the host, thereby ensuring optimal rates of phage protein synthesis.

We will now consider each of the eight categories of proteins and examine their role in phage multiplication.

Functions of Various Categories of Phage Gene Products

Proteins that Repair Bacterial Cell Membrane Early in Infection

Infection causes the bacterial cell membrane to become leaky, so that cellular contents begin to escape; but within several minutes sealing occurs, and the preinfection integ-

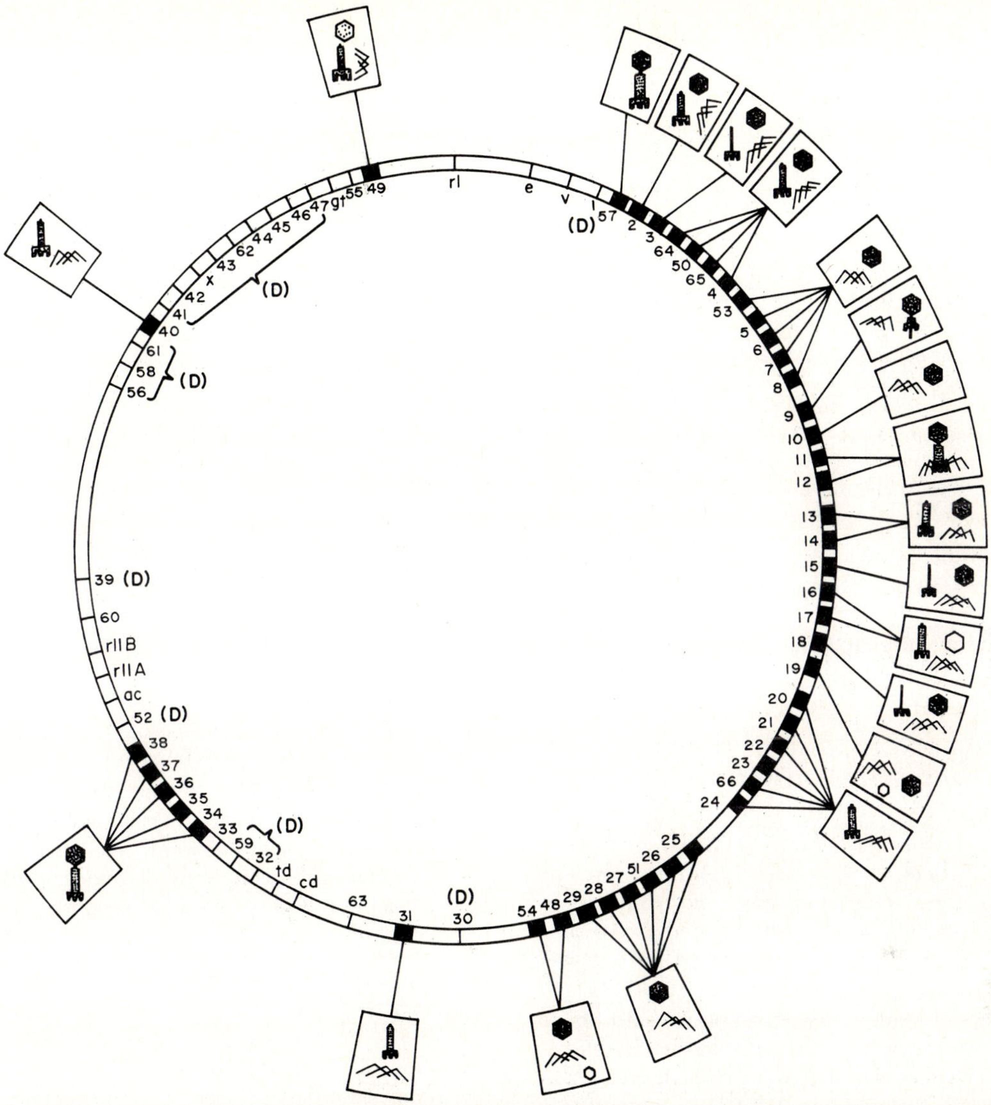

Figure 9-9. Simplified genetic map of T4. The solid segments indicate late genes with morphogenetic functions, while the short bars represent early genes with enzymatic or regulatory functions. Genes with functions in DNA replication are identified by (D). The boxes indicate viral components, such as heads, tails, and tail fibers, that are present in extracts of cells infected with conditional lethal mutants under restrictive conditions. *(Adapted from Edgar and Wood: Proc Natl Acad Sci USA 55:498, 1966.)*

rity of the membrane is restored. The precise mechanism by which this is achieved is not clear, but it is known that at least five phage-coded proteins are synthesized very early during the infection cycle and incorporated into the cell membrane.

Enzymes that Degrade Host DNA

Among the earliest effects of phage T4 infection is the breakdown of host DNA (Fig. 9-10), which has several consequences. First, it provides a source of nucleic acid precursors, which may be limiting under certain conditions. More important, transcription of host-specified messenger RNAs ceases abruptly. Since most bacterial messenger RNAs are short-lived, this not only leads to the sudden cessation of host-specified protein synthesis but also quickly provides ribosomes for the translation of phage-specified messenger RNA. The following is a graphic example of the consequences of the cessation of host protein synthesis. If a culture of *E. coli* grown in glucose-containing medium and infected with T4 is transferred to medium containing lactose, phage infection is aborted. The reason is that lactose utilization requires the induction of the synthesis of certain proteins, among them a perme-

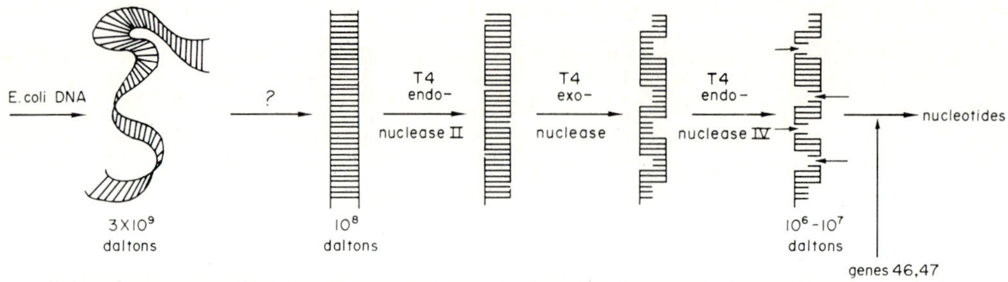

Figure 9-10. A tentative scheme to account for the degradation of *E. coli* DNA after infection with phage T4. *E. coli* DNA is first degraded to fragments about one-tenth its size, which are then nicked by endonuclease II. The nicks are then widened by an exonuclease, and the single-stranded stretches so produced are cut by endonuclease IV. The products are duplex DNA molecules that are more than 100 times smaller than the original *E. coli* genome. Since fragments of this size accumulate in cells infected with phage mutants carrying lesions in genes 46 and 47 but not in cells infected with wild-type phage, these genes presumably code for enzymes that function in their further degradation. *(Adapted from Warner et al.: J Virol 5:700, 1970.)*

ase and the enzyme β-galactosidase. T4 infection halts host protein synthesis and therefore prevents these enzymes from being synthesized. Thus, lactose cannot be metabolized, energy production is prevented, and no phage progeny can be formed.

Enzymes the Synthesize Nucleic Acid Precursors

Numerous enzymes function in the synthesis of nucleic acid precursors, particularly when the phage DNA contains both unusual bases and substituted bases. For example, in the case of T4, which contains glycosylated 5-hydroxymethylcytosine instead of cytosine, the following enzymes are required: (1) enzymes that destroy deoxycytidine triphosphate (so that cytosine is not incorporated into phage DNA), (2) an enzyme that hydroxymethylates deoxycytidylic acid, and (3) enzymes that glycosylate 5-hydroxymethylcytosine residues in polymerized DNA. In addition, numerous enzymes, among them enzymes that function in the synthesis of the other three deoxyribonucleoside triphosphates, are specified by the T-even genome. They are not absolutely essential but increase the yield of progeny phage.

Proteins that Function in Phage DNA Replication

The replication mechanism of double-stranded phage DNA is exceedingly complex, and although enormous effort has been devoted to its elucidation, no clear picture has yet emerged. The following facts are pertinent:

1. Phage DNA replicates by a semiconservative mechanism.
2. During the early stages of the replication of some phage DNAs, extensive recombination occurs. This results in the dispersal of the parental genome among numerous progeny genomes.
3. Phage DNA most probably replicates while associated with membrane in some as yet unspecified manner.
4. The replication of some double-stranded DNA genomes, notably those of the T-even phages, is accompanied by extensive recombination that leads to the formation of giant molecules that consist of up to 100 repeats of the phage genome.
5. Progeny phage genomes are cut from this intermediate in headful units that consist of circularly permuted and terminally redundant genomes (see above).

Among the enzymes known to function in the replication of T4 DNA are a DNA-unwinding protein (coded by gene 32), DNA polymerase (coded by gene 43), a polynucleotide ligase (coded by gene 30), several DNA-binding proteins of unknown function (for example, the proteins encoded by genes 44, 62, and 45), and several nicking enzymes (nucleases).

Proteins that Function in Transcription Programming

Phage genomes, like all other genomes, express themselves via messenger RNA. In fact, it is worth noting that messenger RNA was discovered in phage-infected cells. In 1956 Volkin and Astrachan noted that the base composition of newly synthesized RNA in T2-infected *E. coli* resembled that of T2 DNA rather than that of host DNA, and in 1959 Brenner, Jacob, and Meselson firmly established the concept of messenger RNA by showing that this RNA combines with ribosomes and is responsible for the synthesis of phage proteins.

Phage-specified proteins, like those specified by animal virus genomes (Chap. 4), are synthesized in a strictly ordered sequence. The necessity for this is obvious; for example, enzymes breaking down host DNA should be synthesized first, and viral structural proteins should be synthesized last. There are two ways of achieving programmed protein synthesis: (1) the entire viral genome is transcribed continuously and translation is programmed, or (2) transcription is programmed and messenger RNAs are translated as they are formed. Although the former mechanism may apply to a few species of messenger RNA, it is primarily transcription that is programmed in phage-infected and animal virus-infected cells. This is shown most readily by hybridization experiments of the following type. At various times after infection, cells are incubated for brief periods, e.g., for 2 minutes, with RNA precursors labeled with some radioisotope. On extraction, such cells yield labeled messenger RNA populations synthesized from 0 to 2, 2 to 4, 4 to 6, and so on, minutes after infection. These messenger RNA populations are then allowed to hybridize with denatured phage DNA in the presence of excess unlabeled messenger RNA extracted from cells at various stages of infection. If the labeled and unlabeled RNA populations are identical, the large excess of unlabeled RNA will, by competition, prevent the labeled RNA from hybridizing. If the two populations are different, the presence of unlabeled RNA will have no effect on the ability of labeled RNA to hybridize to DNA.

Another type of analysis that can be carried out is to hybridize the messenger RNA molecules that are formed at various times after infection to the series of fragments that are generated when phage DNA is digested with restriction endonucleases. As described in Chapter 4, such fragments can be ordered to provide restriction endonuclease fragment maps. With this technique, it can readily be demonstrated that different regions of the phage genome are transcribed at different stages of the multiplication cycle. The situation here is quite analogous to that described in Chapter 4 concerning the sequential expression of viral genetic information during the multiplication of the double-stranded DNA-containing poxviruses and herpesviruses. There are "immediate early" T4 genes, "early" genes, several classes of "middle" genes, and finally the truly "late" genes that code for most of the T4 structural proteins.

How is such a complex transcription program managed? The complete answer is not yet evident, but one of the factors of critical importance is certainly the specificity of the transcribing enzymes. Since phages do not contain RNA polymerases, the first phage genes are always transcribed by the host RNA polymerase. The *E. coli* RNA polymerase is a complex enzyme that consists of four subunits—two α subunits, one β subunit and one β' subunit—and has associated with it a protein molecule, the σ factor, which controls its specificity. The sequences of the phage genome that are transcribed by this enzyme are specified by the presence of initiation and termination signals that it can recognize and are usually not large. The messenger RNAs transcribed by it are known as early or immediate early RNAs (in the case of very complex programs).

The remainder of the transcription program is managed by proteins specified by early phage messenger RNAs. There are two principal means by which this is accomplished. The first, employed by the simpler phages, such as T7, involves the synthesis of a new RNA polymerase, the specificity of which is such that it transcribes its homologous DNA more efficiently than host DNA. The second means, employed by the more complex phages, such as T4, involves the synthesis of a series of proteins that modify the host RNA polymerase in a series of successive steps. These steps are as follows. Within 30 seconds, one of the α subunits is ADP-ribosylated and the σ factor is partially phosphorylated. During the next 5 minutes both the β and the β' subunits are altered in some as yet unspecified manner that changes their antigenicity and tryptic peptide maps, and between 5 and 10 minutes later, the β' subunit is further modified, as evidenced by an alteration in its electrophoretic mobility. Finally, after 10 minutes, three phage-coded proteins, the proteins encoded by genes 55, 33, and 45, become associated with the modified enzyme. If the ability to recognize and react with promoters and transcription termination signals of each of these modified RNA polymerase species is different, these modifications could readily effect transcription programs such as those described above.

Structural Phage Components

The messenger RNAs that code for the proteins described so far are, with few exceptions, transcribed only from parental DNA. Those that code for the proteins to be described now are usually transcribed only from progeny DNA. These proteins are known as the "late" proteins, and the quantitatively most important late proteins are the structural components of progeny phage particles (compare Chap. 4). Tailed phage particles are complex structures composed of a large number of protein species; for example, T4 contains at least 30 protein species, and even simple phages, such as T7 and lambda, contain 10 to 15 different species.

Proteins that Function Catalytically in Morphogenesis

Phage genomes usually code for several proteins that function in a catalytic capacity during morphogenesis. For example, in addition to the 30-odd structural protein species, T4 DNA codes for at least 17 additional proteins that are also essential for the formation of mature phage particles. Their nature and the precise manner in which they function is largely unknown (but see below for the scaffolding protein). The genes for tail proteins are clustered into three sets in the T4 genome (Fig. 9-9): one for proteins of which only very few copies are needed, one for proteins of which intermediate numbers of copies are needed, and one for proteins of which very many copies per cell are needed. The genetic apparatus for tail formation is thus very highly refined. The situation seems to be similar for several other phages.

Enzymes Necessary for Progeny Phage Liberation: Cell Lysis

Most virulent phages are liberated from their hosts by a mechanism that differs fundamentally from any employed by animal viruses (Chap. 4): the bacterial cell suddenly lyses, thereby liberating the entire progeny. This is known as cell lysis, and, in the case of the T-even phages, is the result of the function of two late phage-coded proteins. One is a lipase encoded by the *t* gene, which attacks the cell membrane, thereby halting metabolic processes; the other is the enzyme lysozyme, encoded by the *e* gene, which then hydrolyzes the cell wall.

Phage Morphogenesis

Phage morphogenesis has been investigated most intensively for coliphages T4, T3, and T7, and lambda, and for the *Salmonella* phage P22. The most successful approach has been to study the products of infection of a large number of conditional lethal mutants, both temperature-sensitive and amber, under restrictive conditions. Cells infected with structural or catalytic gene mutants under restrictive conditions accumulate not mature phage particles but phage components, such as immature and mature proheads, mature heads, tail fibers, tail cores, tail sheaths, partially assembled tails, and so on. As a result, it has been possible to link defects in both structural and catalytic proteins to specific genes whose location on the genetic map of the phage DNA could be identified.

Phage morphogenesis often involves the processing of capsid proteins by means of proteolytic cleavage (during T4 and P2 head assembly, as well as during T5 and lambda tail assembly). Possible reasons why viral capsid proteins are synthesized in the form of precursors are discussed in Chapter 4.

As for the study of the morphogenetic pathway itself, one of the most useful approaches has been to examine the ability of extracts of cells infected with phage mutants to complement each other. In other words, pairs of such extracts are mixed, and one determines whether infectious phage particles are formed from the components present in each. By such means, the scheme for T4 assembly shown in Figure 9-11 has been worked out. Heads, tails, and tail fibers are assembled independently of each other and then combine to form complete virus particles. Heads begin as complex core-containing immature proheads that are assembled on the cytoplasmic membrane of the bacterial cell. They are then proteolytically processed to proheads, which are released from the membrane and filled with DNA, a process that requires the function of several gene products.

Detailed insight into the mechanism by which DNA is

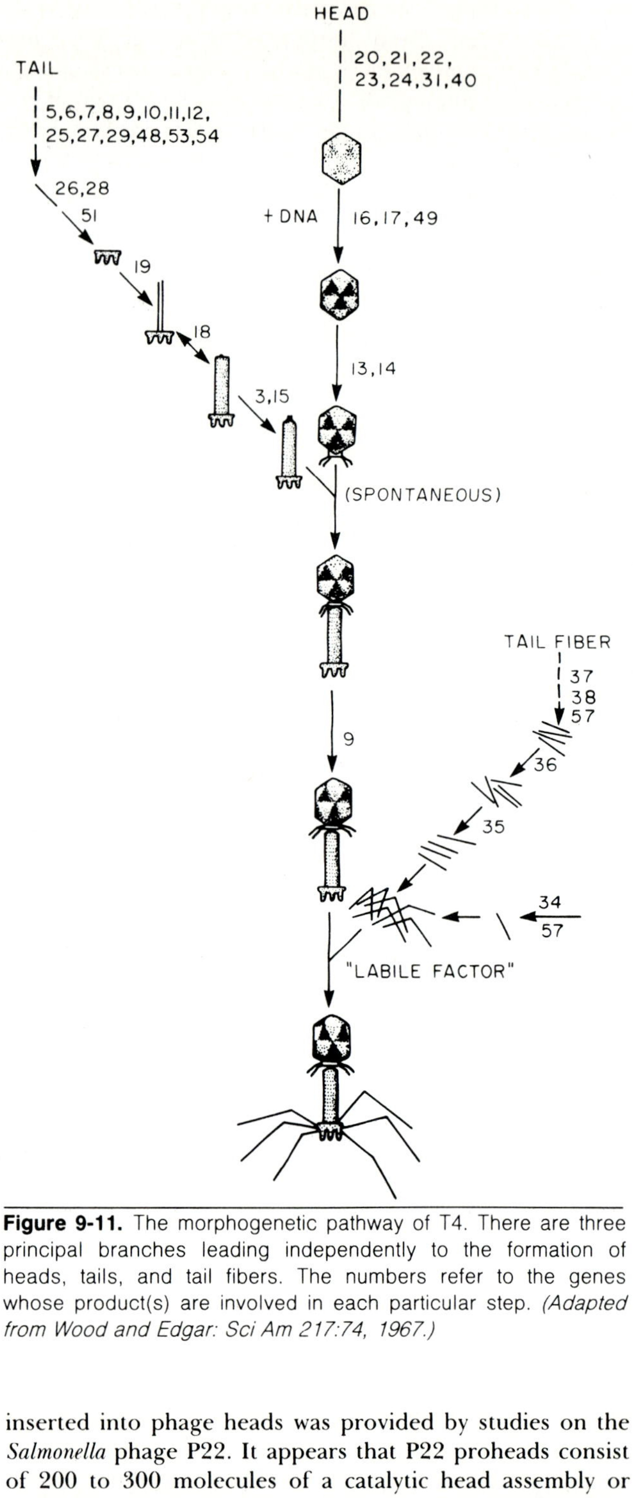

Figure 9-11. The morphogenetic pathway of T4. There are three principal branches leading independently to the formation of heads, tails, and tail fibers. The numbers refer to the genes whose product(s) are involved in each particular step. *(Adapted from Wood and Edgar: Sci Am 217:74, 1967.)*

inserted into phage heads was provided by studies on the *Salmonella* phage P22. It appears that P22 proheads consist of 200 to 300 molecules of a catalytic head assembly or scaffolding protein around which the actual phage head components are assembled. During DNA packaging the scaffolding protein exits and is replaced by DNA. Possibly the exit of the scaffolding protein exposes charged sites that serve to collapse the DNA. The actual amount of DNA that is inserted into the phage head is determined by the so-called headful cutting mechanism, that is, the DNA, in the form of long multimers, is inserted until the head is full, and the DNA is then cut by special endonucleases.

As for tail assembly, this is an extremely complex process that requires the functioning of at least 25 genes (including the genes encoding the tail structural components). One of the proteins involved in tail assembly is a fibrous core component that may act as a ruler that specifies the length of the T4 tail.

Multiplication Cycle of Phages Containing Single-stranded DNA

Several *E. coli* phages contain not double-stranded but single-stranded DNA (Table 9-1). The most completely studied of these phages is φX 174, whose genome is a plus-stranded single-stranded DNA molecule 5375 nucleotides long (mol wt 1.7×10^6), which was sequenced in 1976. It contains 10 genes that have been mapped (Table 9-3). The φX 174 genome was the first shown to contain overlapping genes, both in the same and in different reading frames, and genes within genes. Three of the proteins specified by φX 174 DNA are structural proteins, four are involved in DNA synthesis, one causes cell lysis, and the function of one is not clear.

The main problems posed by the discovery of these phages were (1) how does single-stranded DNA replicate and still obey the rules of base pairing, and (2) since messenger RNAs are transcribed from double-stranded DNA, how can single-stranded DNA serve as their template? These questions were answered when it was found that upon entering the host cell, single-stranded DNA is converted to a double-stranded replicative form.

A scheme describing the mode of replication of φX 174 DNA is presented in Figure 9-12. Although most of the steps depicted are no doubt oversimplified, the scheme's key elements have been demonstrated experimentally. The parental DNA (V) first attaches to a host cell membrane component (M), and a complementary strand is synthesized so as to yield a supercoiled circular double-stranded replicative form, known as RF1. This is then nicked by an endonuclease to yield RF2, a relaxed circular molecule (step 2). In step 3 the V strand is elongated using the C strand as template, and a new C strand is synthesized, with the elongated portion of the V strand serving as its template. This process is a modification of the rolling circle mode of DNA replication. In step 4 this intermediate is split into a membrane-attached RF1 identical to the original one and a free RF1. The original RF1 then repeats steps 2 to 4, forming new RFs, while the free RF1 has two options. If membrane sites are available, it can attach to them (step 5) and then also generate progeny RFs, or it may be converted to RF2 (step 6), on which the V strand is again elongated (step 7). This intermediate is then split to yield another RF2 (possibly via RF1) and a V strand, which is encapsidated (step 8). The net result is that double-stranded RF molecules first replicate and then serve as templates for the synthesis of large numbers of single-stranded progeny DNA molecules. It is worth noting that infectious φX 174 DNA has been synthesized in vitro with purified enzymes. It was the first functioning DNA genome to be synthesized outside a living cell.

TABLE 9-3. GENES AND GENE FUNCTIONS OF THE SINGLE-STRANDED DNA-CONTAINING BACTERIOPHAGE φX 174

Gene Designation	Molecular Weight of Protein Product	Function
A	56,000	RF replication, ss DNA synthesis
*A**	35,000	DNA synthesis
B	14,000	SS DNA synthesis
C	7,000	SS DNA synthesis
D	17,000	SS DNA synthesis
E	10,000	Lysis
J	4,000	Structural
F	46,000	Major capsid protein
G	19,000	Spike (vertex) protein
H	36,000	Spike (vertex) protein

Adapted from Denhardt: In Fraenkel-Conrat and Wagner (eds): Comprehensive Virology, vol. 7, p 1, 1977. New York, Plenum.
The coding regions for the A* protein and A protein overlap; the coding region for the A* protein is the righthand (C terminal) three fifths of the *A* gene in the same reading frame. The coding region for the B protein is entirely within that of the A/A* protein(s) in a different reading frame. Similarly, the coding region of the E protein is entirely within that of the D protein in a different reading frame. The gene order, starting from the junction of the *A* and the *H* gene, is *A(A*) (B)-C-D(E)-J-F-G-H.*

The enzymology of φX 174 DNA replication is extraordinarily complex. It requires at least 12 *E. coli* proteins, including DNA polymerase III, DNA polymerase I, ss DNA binding protein, DNA ligase, DNA gyrase, the products of genes dnaC and dnaB as well as of several others involved in priming, and the φX 174 A protein, which is the only protein encoded by φX 174 DNA that is directly involved in its replication (the functions of the A* protein and of the B, C, and D proteins not being known with certainty).

Messenger RNAs are transcribed from membrane-bound RFs. Among the proteins into which they are translated are the structural phage components, one species of which attaches to the loose end of progeny V strands that arise in step 7, thereby initiating encapsidation.

The mutiplication cycle of the filamentous phages f1, fd, and M13 differs somewhat from that of φX 174. Whereas nascent φX 174 DNA is immediately encapsidated, forming progeny that accumulates within the cell and is eventually liberated when cells lyse, large amounts of free viral DNA accumulate intracellularly in the case of the filamentous phages. These molecules are then encapsidated at the cell membrane, and virus particles are released without cell lysis in a process that is in part analogous to that by which enveloped animal viruses are released from their host cells.

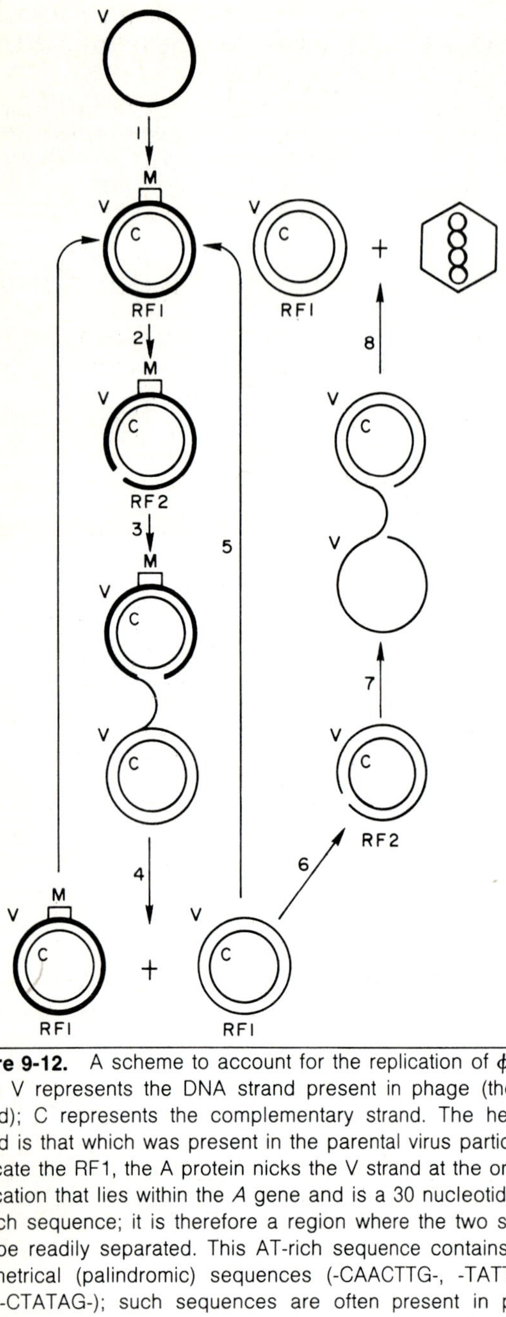

Figure 9-12. A scheme to account for the replication of ϕX 174 DNA. V represents the DNA strand present in phage (the plus strand); C represents the complementary strand. The heavy V strand is that which was present in the parental virus particle. To replicate the RF1, the A protein nicks the V strand at the origin of replication that lies within the *A* gene and is a 30 nucleotide-long AT-rich sequence; it is therefore a region where the two strands can be readily separated. This AT-rich sequence contains three symmetrical (palindromic) sequences (-CAACTTG-, -TATTATA-, and -CTATAG-); such sequences are often present in protein binding sites. The A protein becomes covalently attached to the 5′ end of the nicked strand and then initiates DNA synthesis in a rolling circle mode. It also linearizes and circularizes the displaced plus strand after each round of replication.

Multiplication Cycle of Phages Containing Single-stranded RNA

Single-stranded RNA-containing phages are small icosahedral viruses that resemble picornaviruses. Like them, their capsids consist of 180 protein molecules, but whereas there are 60 molecules each of three different protein species present in picornaviruses, all 180 protein molecules are identical in the case of the RNA phages. In addition, each phage particle contains one molecule of an additional protein, the maturation or A protein, which is necessary both for proper assembly and for ability to adsorb. The RNA of these phages has a molecular weight of just over 1 million, which is less than one-half the size of the picornavirus genome.

Most of the known RNA phages are coliphages. They fall into three or four serologic groups. Most of the well-studied RNA phages (f2, fr, MS2, R17, and so on) belong to one group, while one, Qβ, belongs to another. All RNA phages are male-specific because their receptor sites are on F-pili.

Study of the multiplication cycle of these phages has provided important clues for investigations of animal viruses that contain RNA. In addition, their extraordinary simplicity—they are the simplest viruses known—has made them fascinating objects for the elucidation of fundamental biologic processes.

The genomes of RNA phages comprise only three genes. These are, from the 5′-terminus of the RNA, the genes for the A protein, the coat protein, and the RNA polymerase. The latter protein is actually only one of four proteins that together make up the functional RNA polymerase, the others being three bacterial proteins that are normally located on ribosomes, namely, factor i, elongation factor Tu, and elongation factor Ts. The precise function of these host-coded components of the viral RNA polymerase is not known, but it has been suggested that they somehow control specificity and affinity for initiation sites and that they are essential for maintaining the enzyme complex in its active conformation.

The genomes of RNA phages possess plus polarity and start functioning as messenger RNA very soon after they enter cells. After coding for the RNA polymerase, they replicate by a mechanism similar to that described for poliovirus RNA (Fig. 4-28). This involves, first, the formation of complementary minus strands and then their successive transcription into progeny plus strands. Coat protein then begins to be synthesized in large amounts together with some A protein. As soon as their concentrations are sufficiently high, encapsidation of RNA commences and mature progeny phage accumulates (Fig. 9-13). These events are quite analogous to those that occur during the picornavirus multiplication cycle (Chap. 4).

Programming of RNA Phage Multiplication Cycle

The multiplication cycle of RNA phages, like that of other viruses, is programmed, with the various reactions necessary for morphopoiesis taking place in a regularly progressing sequence. Yet, the genome of RNA phage is too small to encode proteins with a purely regulatory function. How then does it happen that coat protein, which is present in virus particles in 180-fold excess over A protein, is in fact

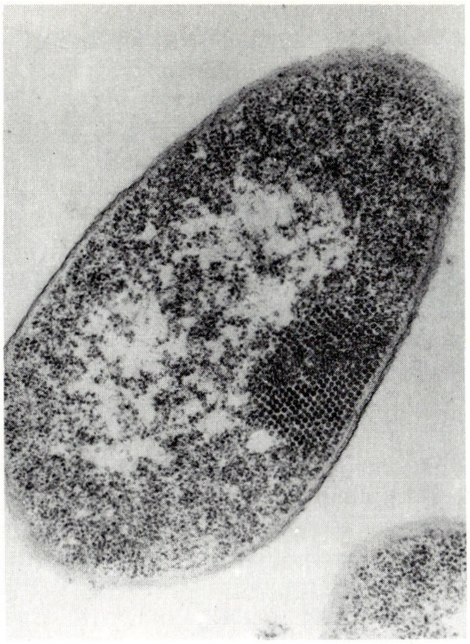

Figure 9-13. An *E. coli* cell 50 minutes after infection with MS2. Note the paracrystalline virus particle array. The virus is slightly larger than the ribosomes which are present throughout the cell. This cell is about to lyse. × 37,500. *(Courtesy of Dr. M. Van Montagu.)*

synthesized in vastly greater amounts than A protein? What mechanism causes the RNA polymerase to be synthesized early during the infection cycle, when it is needed, and not throughout the cycle? And since parental RNA genomes must be both translated and transcribed, what mechanism prevents collisions between ribosomes, which traverse messenger RNA from the 5'- to the 3'-terminus, and RNA polymerase molecules, which traverse templates in the opposite direction?

The genomes of RNA phages are polycistronic messenger RNAs. There are three ribosome attachment sites, one at the start of each cistron. Like other RNAs, they possess a pronounced secondary structure that is specified by base pairing between complementary nucleotide sequences. There is a marked difference in how accessible ribosome-binding sites at the 5'-termini of the three genes are to ribosomes. In normal phage RNA, the most accessible ribosome binding site is at the beginning of the cistron that codes for the coat protein, which would therefore be formed in the greatest amount. However, attachment of ribosomes there renders the site at the beginning of the polymerase cistron also accessible to ribosomes, so that during the initial stages of infection both coat protein and polymerase are formed freely. Coat protein itself, however, can bind to the ribosome-binding sites at the beginning of the A protein and polymerase cistrons, thereby preventing ribosome attachment, so that as coat protein accumulates, it gradually inhibits translation of these two cistrons more and more strongly. The net result is that the A protein cistron is translated only infrequently throughout most of the infection cycle, and the polymerase cistron is translated frequently during the early stages but only very infrequently during the later stages of the infection cycle.

The collision problem is solved in the following manner. When a polymerase molecule attaches to the 3'-terminus of the RNA strand, it also binds to the coat protein cistron ribosome-binding site, thereby preventing further ribosome attachment. When ribosomes have cleared from the region between these two points, the polymerase can progress along the RNA strand unimpeded.

It is clear therefore that, although it is very simple and small, the RNA phage genome regulates a sophisticated transcription and translation program. This is because several of the proteins that it encodes possess dual functions.

Lysogeny

Not all phage infections result in lysis of the host cell. There are some phages that, upon entering a sensitive cell, either elicit a lytic response, that is, a typical multiplication cycle controlled by a transcription program that involves expression of the entire phage genome, or a second type of response in which all phage genes except one are completely repressed and in which the phage genome is either inserted into the host genome or exists in the bacterial cell in free plasmid-like form. The phage genome, the prophage, behaves from then on like any other portion of the bacterial chromosome, and the bacteria that harbor prophage appear perfectly normal. Occasionally, however, the integrated prophage is excised from bacterial DNA, and phage multiplication and cell lysis ensue. This phenomenon is therefore known as "lysogeny." Bacteria that harbor such prophages are known as lysogens, and phages capable of eliciting the lysogenic pathway are known as lysogenic, or temperate, phages.

When it was discovered that some animal viruses could enter into a similar relationship with their hosts (Chap. 8), the analogy between them and temperate phages was quickly recognized. Although there are differences in the manner in which tumor viruses and temperate phages interact with their host cells, the concepts that evolved from studies of temperate phages have profoundly influenced our thinking concerning tumor viruses.

Prophage

The frequency of lysogenization varies both with the phage-host system and with the multiplicity of infection. It is greater the higher the multiplicity. This suggests that each phage genome has a finite probability of lysogenization. The number of any particular species of prophage per lysogen is generally the same as the number of bacterial genomes, which suggests that the prophage attachment site is restricted to a particular locus on the bacterial chromosome. That a unique location generally exists can be demonstrated by genetic studies, such as the interrupted mating technique. However, occasionally there is more than one attachment site for the same prophage, and all may be occupied simultaneously. Superinfection may result in the integration of two prophages at the same site, inserted either into one another or adjacent to each other. Further, bacterial chromosomes generally contain prophage attachment sites for several different unrelated prophages, and all of these may be occupied at the same time. Finally, one temperate phage, phage mu, has no specific integration site but can insert its genome anywhere in the bacterial chromosome. However, it is not essential that the prophage be integrated. If prophage cannot integrate (because of mutations, for example, in the attachment site or in the enzyme system responsible for integration), it can exist and be carried in the lysogen in the form of supercoiled circular plasmid-like molecules.

Concept of Immunity

Under normal conditions prophage is stable. Termination of the lysogenic state occurs spontaneously with low frequency (of the order of 10^{-5}). The phage genome is then excised from the host chromosome (see below), and a normal lytic multiplication cycle ensues. Cultures of lysogenic bacteria therefore contain low titers of infectious virus, but they are not lysed by it: they are immune. This is not because the phage cannot adsorb and inject its DNA but because the injected DNA cannot express itself and replicate. The reason for this is that one of the prophage genes codes for a repressor that prevents transcription of all other phage genes, both those on prophage and those on superinfecting phage genomes. Immunity is highly specific; bacteria lysogenic for one phage are only immune to it and to closely related phages. It is ability to effect immunity, that is, possession of a repressor gene, that is the essential attribute of a lysogenic phage, not ability to integrate its DNA into that of the host cell.

Nature of Phage Lambda

The best known of the many temperate bacteriophages is the coliphage lambda, probably the most intensively studied of all viruses. The exquisite and intricate mechanisms that control its interaction with the host and its multiplication represent the system par excellence with which to study biologic control. We will, therefore, discuss the mechanisms that operate in lysogeny in terms of the lambda system.

Phage lambda possesses a hexagonal head and a simple noncontractile tail with one terminal tail fiber; it comprises about 10 protein species. Its DNA, which contains no unusual bases, is linear and has a molecular weight of 31×10^6, representing about 50 genes. Figure 9-14 shows a simplified genetic map of lambda. About 20 genes code for its structural proteins and for proteins that function in its morphogenesis. These genes, which include genes *A* to *J*, are in the left arm of the DNA, which contains 55 percent guanine plus cytosine. Some 30 other genes have been identified as regulating in one way or another the interaction of the lambda genome with that of the host cell and its transcription and translation. These genes are located in the right arm of the DNA, which contains 46 percent guanine plus cytosine. Not all genes are transcribed from the same DNA strand. As shown in Figure 9-14, some genes are transcribed from one strand, while others are transcribed in the opposite direction from the other strand.

Events Leading to Lysogeny: Integration

When lambda DNA enters the cell, it cyclizes and forms covalently closed circles. Within a brief critical period of time the decision is then made as to whether a lytic multiplication cycle is to be initiated or whether the phage genome is to be repressed. The decision is influenced principally by how rapidly several viral gene products reach critical concentrations and begin to function.

The critical genes and control elements are illustrated in Figure 9-15, which is an enlargement of one portion of the lambda genetic map. The key element is the operator O_R, a sequence located at map position 78.5. It is about 50 nucleotides long and contains three 9 bp long sequences to which *E. coli* DNA-dependent RNA polymerase and two types of phage lambda-coded repressor proteins can bind. At the very beginning of infection, only RNA polymerase binds there and transcribes both genes that flank O_R, one from one strand and the second from the other. The gene on the left is the *cI* gene that encodes the lambda repressor, a 236 amino acid long protein (mol wt 26,000) with two domains, an N-terminal domain that rec-

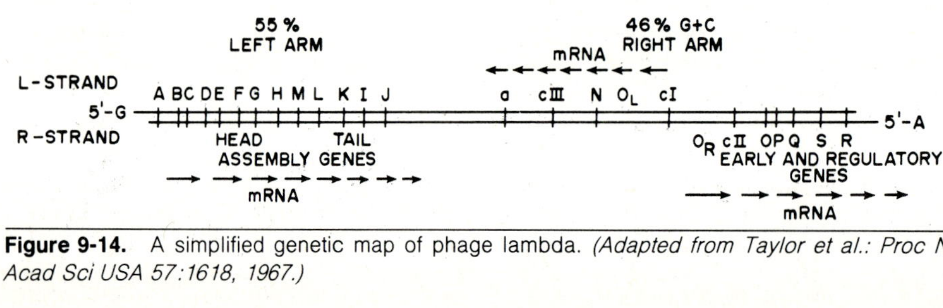

Figure 9-14. A simplified genetic map of phage lambda. *(Adapted from Taylor et al.: Proc Natl Acad Sci USA 57:1618, 1967.)*

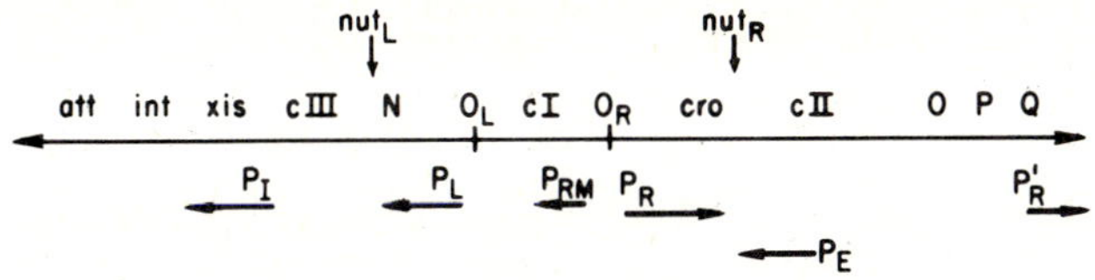

Figure 9-15. Portion of the lambda genetic map centered around operator O_R. It illustrates the various genes and control elements that determine whether the lytic or lysogenic pathway will be followed. For details, see text.

ognizes operator sites and a C-terminal domain that provides contacts for dimerization, dimers being the form in which it binds to O_R. The gene on the right is the *cro* gene, which encodes the *cro* repressor, a 66 amino acid long protein (mol wt 8000), the dimeric form of which also binds to O_R. The nature of lambda infection depends on whether more *cI* or more *cro* gene product is synthesized. If more *cro* repressor is made, it binds to O_R, preventing lambda repressor from binding there, and prevents the synthesis of the *cII* and *cIII* gene products that greatly increase lambda repressor synthesis (see below). In essence, it greatly reduces lambda repressor synthesis. As a result, a second operator, O_L, is not blocked by lambda repressor, and RNA polymerase binds there and proceeds to transcribe gene N. Expression of this gene is essential for the transcription of most of the lambda genome. The reason is that the early lambda genes, except *cI* and *cro,* contain transcriptional terminators, short sequences that cause RNA polymerase to cease transcription. The N gene product, a very basic protein 107 amino acids long (mol wt 12,000), is an antiterminator. It prevents, via a very complex mechanism that involves at least five host proteins, termination of transcription by attaching to so-called *nut* sites (*N* protein *ut*ilization sites) which are located just upstream from these terminators. If *N* gene product is bound to *nut* sites, RNA polymerase reads through the transcriptional terminators into adjacent genes, and in particular into gene *O,* the product of which is essential for lambda DNA replication, and into gene *Q,* the product of which is an antiterminator for lambda late genes. As a result, a normal lytic lambda multiplication cycle ensues, just like that described above for T4.

If, on the other hand, more *cI* product, that is, lambda repressor, is made than *cro* repressor, then the lambda repressor binds very tightly to operator O_R. This turns off transcription from promoter P_R (and therefore prevents synthesis of *cro* repressor) and turns on transcription from promoter P_{RM}. In fact, transcription from P_{RM} is much more efficient if O_R is occupied by lambda repressor than if it is not occupied. Lambda repressor is thus a positive regulator of its own synthesis.

The interaction of lambda repressor and *cro* repressor with the operator O_R thus forms an exquisitely sensitive, efficient, and sophisticated molecular switch capable of switching between two physiologic states in response to a transient signal. It represents the most intensively studied and best understood interaction between protein and nucleic acid.

In addition to lambda repressor positively controlling its own synthesis, two other early proteins augment *cI* transcription. These are the proteins encoded by genes *cII* and *cIII,* both of which promote transcription from P_E, a promoter that appears to lie within gene *cII,* from which transcription of *cI* can be initiated. Not only that, but the *cII* protein also positively regulates transcription, from promoter P_I, of the *int* gene, which codes for the integrase, the enzyme necessary for the integration of lambda DNA into that of the host cell. Thus, if lambda repressor is synthesized in excess over *cro* repressor, it binds to O_R and promotes its own transcription from P_{RM}, and the *cII* and *cIII* proteins additionally stimulate its transcription from P_E. All this causes a rapid buildup of lambda repressor. The *cII* protein also causes the formation of large amounts of integrase, and then, no more *cII, cIII,* and integrase proteins being required, the lambda repressor rapidly and with extraordinary efficiency binds to both O_R and O_L, thus blocking all transcription of the lambda genome except that of gene *cI.* That is, it prevents the synthesis of all lambda proteins except its own.

Once a cell contains sufficient lambda suppressor and also adequate amounts of the *int* gene product, the lambda genome is integrated into the host genome by a mechanism that is illustrated schematically in Figure 9-16. The phage DNA region aa′ between genes *J* and *cIII* aligns itself with region bb′, the prophage attachment site on the bacterial chromosome, which is situated between the galactose and biotin genes. Enzyme(s) encoded by the phage *int* system then make scissions in all four nucleotide strands, the phage DNA is inserted by means of double crossing over, and covalent bonds are then reformed. The lambda genome is now integrated. If the aa′ and bb′ regions do not match, usually because of a deletion, the phage genome cannot become integrated. It then multiplies in the host cell as an episome. In either event, the only lambda gene that is transcribed is gene *cI.*

Release from Repression: Induction

The termination of the lysogenic state, or induction, requires both release from repression and excision of the phage DNA from the host DNA. The cellular signal for release from repression is inhibition of host DNA synthesis, such as starvation of thymine-requiring mutants of thymine, treatment with inhibitors of DNA replication, such as mitomycin C, or irradiation with ultraviolet (UV) light. All these treatments initiate a multifunctional cellular response termed the SOS pathway, which causes the cellular *recA* protein, a protein that normally functions in genetic recombination, to be activated as a protease. This protease then cleaves the lambda repressor between amino acids 111 and 112, thereby inactivating it. As a result, RNA polymerase can again bind to operators O_L and O_R and initiates transcription there. As a result enzymes specified by the *int* and *xis* phage genes are synthesized, and these enzymes excise the phage DNA from the host DNA. Excision proceeds essentially via reversal of the integration

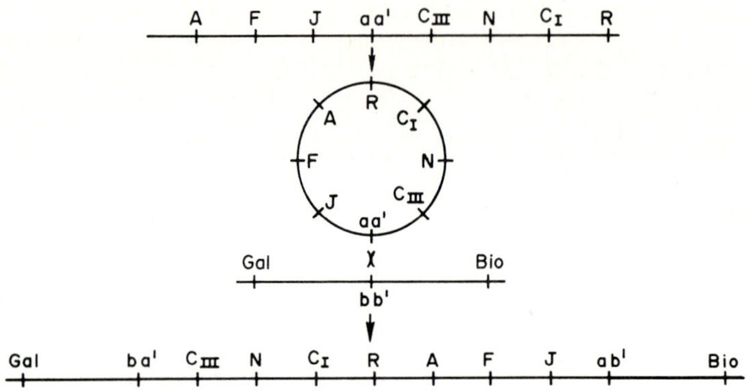

Figure 9-16. The Campbell model for prophage integration. After circularization of lambda DNA by joining of cohesive ends, reciprocal recombination between phage aa' and bacterial bb' recognition sites provides for linear insertion of the viral DNA into that of the host. *(Adapted from Echols and Joyner: In Fraenkel-Conrat (ed): Molecular Basis of Virology, 1968. New York, Reinhold Book Corp.)*

process and yields a circular phage DNA molecule that, active lambda repressor no longer being present, replicates in the normal manner characteristic of virulent lambda infection. Under appropriate conditions, treatment with mitomycin C or UV irradiation induces all cells in cultures of lysogenic bacteria at the same time, with lysis and progeny phage liberation occurring some 20 minutes later.

The juxtaposition of bacterial and phage genes in the chromosome of the lysogen sometimes leads to excision of some bacterial DNA together with phage DNA. This provides an opportunity for the transfer of bacterial genetic material from one bacterium to another via phage; this is known as transduction.

Significance of Lysogeny

Every bacterium may well carry one or more prophages. There are numerous defective or cryptic prophages, that is, prophages that lack the complete set of information necessary for phage multiplication, so that even when induced and therefore excised, no infectious phage particles are formed. Bacteria harboring such prophages are analogous in some respects to cells transformed by defective SV40 (Chap. 7). Even if they possess complete genomes, lysogenic phage cannot be detected unless there are available nonimmune bacterial indicator strains that lack prophage attachment sites and that can be infected by the lytic pathway.

Lysogenic Phage Conversion

Although in most cases the phenotype of bacteria that carry prophage is indistinguishable from that of bacteria that do not, there are several interesting examples where there is a clear difference. These bacteria exhibit the phenomenon known as lysogenic conversion.

One case of lysogenic conversion involves the phage-mediated conversion of the somatic O antigen of *Salmonella.* This antigen forms part of the lipopolysaccharide structure of the cell wall and is composed of highly esterified lipid (lipid A) linked to a polysaccharide core to which are attached side chains consisting of repeating sequences of a variety of sugars. The antigenic specificity resides in the sugars and can be modified by altering their nature.

A wide variety of temperature phages of *Salmonella* can modify the antigenic properties of the somatic O antigen. For example, the O antigen of *Salmonella anatum* normally has the antigenic formula 3,10 (based on its response pattern to various antisera) and carries terminal O-acetyl-D-galactosyl groups linked by means of α-1:6 linkages to D-mannosyl residues. When lysogenized by the temperature phage ϵ^{15}, antigenic specificity 10 is lost, and specificity 15 is acquired. This is due to loss of the O-acetyl group and replacement of the α-1:6 bond by a β-1:6 bond. Cells lysogenized by phage ϵ^{15} can themselves be lysogenized by phage ϵ^{34}, which causes a further change in antigenic specificity, this time due to the addition of D-glucosyl residues by means of β-1:4 linkages. There are numerous other examples.

There is no doubt that the chemical alterations in *Salmonella* polysaccharides are phage-induced, since ϵ^{15} causes repression or inhibition of the α-1:6-galactosyl transferase and acetylase and encodes a β-1:6-galactosyl transferase. These converting functions are, however, not essential to the phage, since mutants defective in them grow well. On the other hand, it is significant that ϵ^{15} cannot adsorb to cells with antigenic specificity 3,15, that is, cells carrying ϵ^{15} cannot be infected by it. It is likely that the significance of this type of lysogenic conversion lies in the specification of host range patterns, perhaps to augment phage immunity systems.

A second example of lysogenic conversion concerns *Corynebacterium diphtheriae.* Toxigenic strains carry the prophage β, and nontoxigenic strains can be made toxigenic by lysogenization. It is clear that the structural gene for toxin is located on the phage genome, since phage mutants coding for defective toxin have been isolated. However, it is not clear what advantage the phage gains by coding for a protein with the remarkable biologic and enzymatic properties of the toxin. Most probably, the advantage relates not to the phage but to the bacterial lysogen. In other words, corynebacteria that can synthesize toxin most probably have a survival advantage over those that cannot do so.

A third example involves *Clostridium botulinum* types C and D, which produce toxin only when demonstrably infected with (and yielding) phages CE β and DE β, respectively. However, with types C and D, the relation between host cell and phage may not be true lysogeny, since infected *C. botulinum* becomes nontoxigenic (and nonvirogenic) when treated with antiserum to phage.

FURTHER READING

Books and Reviews

DOUBLE-STRANDED DNA-CONTAINING PHAGES

Anderson TF: Reflections on phage genetics. Annu Rev Genet 15:405, 1981

Cairns J, Stent GS, Watson JD: Phage and the origins of molecular biology. New York, Cold Spring Harbor Laboratory, 1966

Casjens S, King J: Virus assembly. Annu Rev Biochem 44:555, 1975

Earnshaw WC, Casjens SR: DNA packaging by the double-stranded DNA bacteriophages. Cell 21:319, 1980

Eiserling FA: Bacteriophage structure. In Fraenkel-Conrat H, Wagner RR (eds): Comprehensive Virology. New York, Plenum, 1979, vol 13, p 543

Hausmann R: Bacteriophage T7 genetics. Curr Top Microbiol Immunol 75:77, 1976

Koerner JF, Snustad DP: Shutoff of host macromolecular synthesis after T-even bacteriophage infection. Microbiol Rev 43:199, 1979

Kruger DH, Schroeder C: Bacteriophage T3 and bacteriophage T7 virus-host cell interactions. Microbiol Rev 45:9, 1981

Mathews CK: Reproduction of large virulent bacteriophages. In Fraenkel-Conrat H, Wagner RR (eds): Comprehensive Virology. New York, Plenum, 1977, vol 8, p 179

Murialdo H, Becker A: Head morphogenesis of double-stranded DNA containing bacteriophages. Microbiol Rev 42:529, 1978

Reanney DC, Ackermann H: Comparative biology and evolution of bacteriophages. Adv Virus Res 27:206, 1982

Wagner ES, Auer B, Schweiger M: *Escherichia coli* virus T1: Genetic controls during virus infection. Curr Top Microbiol Immunol 102:131, 1983

Warren RAJ: Modified bases in bacteriophage DNAs. Annu Rev Microbiol 34:137, 1980

Wood WB, King J: Genetic control of complex bacteriophage assembly. In Fraenkel-Conrat H, Wagner RR (eds): Comprehensive Virology. New York, Plenum, 1979, vol 13, p 581

PHAGE LAMBDA: LYSOGENY

Calendar R, Geisseloder J, Sunshine MG, et al.: The P2-P4 transactivation system. In Fraenkel-Conrat H, Wagner RR (eds): Comprehensive Virology. New York, Plenum, 1977, vol 8, p 329

Campbell A: Defective bacteriophages and incomplete prophages. In Fraenkel-Conrat H, Wagner RR (eds): Comprehensive Virology. New York, Plenum, 1977, vol 8, p 259

Echols H, Murialdo H: A genetic map of lambda. Microbiol Rev 42:577, 1978

Gottesman S: Lambda site-specific recombination: The att site. Cell 25:585, 1981

Greenblatt J: Regulation of transcription termination by the N gene protein of bacteriophage lambda. Cell 24:8, 1981

Herskowitz I, Hagen D: The lysis-lysogeny decision of lambda: Explicit programming and responsiveness. Annu Rev Genet 14:402, 1980

Johnson AD, Poteete AR, Lauer G, et al.: Lambda repressor and cro—components of an efficient molecular switch. Nature 294:217, 1981

Nash HA: Integration and excision of bacteriophage lambda: The mechanism of conservative site-specific recombination. Annu Rev Genet 15:143, 1981

Scott JR: Immunity and repression in bacteriophage P1 and P7. Curr Top Microbiol Immunol 90:49, 1980

Shimatake H, Rosenberg M: Purified lambda regulatory protein cII positively activates promoters for lysogenic development. Nature 292:128, 1981

Ward DF, Gottesman ME: Suppression of transcription termination by phage lambda. Science 216:946, 1982

Weisberg RA, Gottesman S, Gottesman ME: Bacteriophage lambda: The lysogenic pathway. In Fraenkel-Conrat H, Wagner RR (eds): Comprehensive Virology. New York, Plenum, 1977, vol 8, p 197

SINGLE-STRANDED RNA AND DNA-CONTAINING PHAGES

Denhardt DT, Dressler D, Ray DS (eds): The Single-stranded DNA Phages. New York, Cold Spring Harbor Laboratory, 1978

Fiers W: Structure and function of RNA bacteriophages. In Fraenkel-Conrat H, Wagner RR (eds): Comprehensive Virology. New York, Plenum, 1979, vol 13, p 69

Ray DS: Replication of filamentous bacteriophages. In Fraenkel-Conrat H, Wagner RR (eds): Comprehensive Virology. New York, Plenum, 1977, vol 8, p 105

Zinder ND: Portraits of viruses: RNA phage. Intervirology 13:257, 1980

Selected Papers

THE LYTIC PHAGE MULTIPLICATION CYCLE

Black LW, Silverman DJ: Model for DNA packaging into bacteriophage T4 heads. J Virol 28:643, 1978

Brennan SM, Chelm BK, Romeo JM, et al.: A transcriptional map of the bacteriophage SP01 genome: II. The major early transcription units. Virology 111:604, 1981

Coombs DH, Eiserling FA: Studies on the structure, protein composition and assembly of the neck of bacteriophage T4. J Mol Biol 116:375, 1977

Crowther RA, Lenk EV, Kirkuchi Y, et al.: Molecular reorganization in the hexagon to star transition of the base plate of T4. J Mol Biol 116:489, 1977

Fuller MT, King J: Purification of the coat and scaffolding proteins from procapsids of bacteriophage P22. Virology 112:529, 1981

von Gabain A, Bujard H: Interaction of *Escherichia coli* RNA polymerase with promoters of several coliphage and plasmid DNAs. Proc Natl Acad Sci USA 76:189, 1979

Heintz N, Shub DA: Transcriptional regulation of bacteriophage SP01 protein synthesis in vivo and in vitro. J Virol 42:951, 1982

Kozloff LM, Lute M, Crosby LK: Bacteriophage T4 virion baseplate thymidylate synthetase and dihydrofolate reductase. J Virol 23:637, 1977

Majumder HK, Bishayee S, Chakraborty PR, et al.: Ribonuclease

III cleavage of bacteriophage T3 RNA polymerase transcripts to late T3 mRNAs. Proc Natl Acad Sci USA 74:4891, 1977

Matsuo-Kato H, Fujisawa H, Minagawa T: Structure and assembly of bacteriophage T3 tails. Virology 109:157, 1981

McCorquodale DJ, Chen CW, Joseph MK, et al.: Modification of RNA polymerase from *Escherichi coli* by pre-early gene products of bacteriophage T5. J Virol 40:958, 1981

Milhausen MJ, Whiteley HR: In vitro synthesis of a peptide which modifies the transcriptional specificity of *Bacillus subtilis* RNA polymerase. Biochem Biophys Res Commun 99:900, 1981

Minagawa T, Murakami A, Ryo Y, et al.: Structural features of very fast sedimenting DNA formed by gene 49 defective T4. Virology 126:183, 1983

Nordstrom B, Randahl H, Slaby I, et al.: Characterization of bacteriophage T7 DNA polymerase purified to homogeneity by antithioredoxin immunoadsorbent chromatography. J Biol Chem 256:3112, 1981

Spiegelman GB, Whiteley HR: Bacteriophage SP82 induced modifications of *Bacillus subtilis* RNA polymerase result in the recognition of additional RNA synthesis initiation site on phage DNA. Biochem Biophys Res Commun 81:1058, 1978

Talkington C, Pero J: Restriction fragment analysis of the temporal program of bacteriophage SP01 transcription and its control by phage-modified RNA polymerases. Virology 83:365, 1977

PHAGE LAMBDA: LYSOGENY

Ho Y-S, Lewis M, Rosenberg M: Purification and properties of a transcriptional activator: The cII protein of phage lambda. J Biol Chem 257:9128, 1982

Hochschild A, Irwin N, Ptashne M: Repressor structure and the mechanism of positive control. Cell 32:319, 1983

Hoyt MA, Knight DM, Das A, et al.: Control of phage lambda development by stability and synthesis of cII protein: role of the viral cIII and host hfla, himA and himD genes. Cell 31:565, 1982

Kikuchi Y, Nash HA: The bacteriophage lambda int gene product. J Biol Chem 253:7149, 1978

Sanger F, Coulson AR, Hong GF, et al.: Nucleotide sequence of bacteriophage lambda DNA. J Mol Biol 162:729, 1982

Sauer RT, Ross MJ, Ptashne M: Cleavage of the lambda and P22 repressors by recA protein. J Biol Chem 257:4458, 1982

Shaw JE, Jones BB, Pearson ML: Identification of the N gene protein of bacteriophage lambda. Proc Natl Acad Sci USA 72:2225, 1978

Takeda Y, Folkmanis A, Echols H: Cro regulatory protein specified by bacteriophage lambda: Structure, DNA-binding and repression of RNA synthesis. J Biol Chem 252:6177, 1977

SINGLE-STRANDED NUCLEIC ACID-CONTAINING PHAGES

Arai K-I, Kornberg A: Mechanism of dnaB protein action. IV. General priming of DNA replication by dnaB protein and primase compared with RNA polymerase. J Biol Chem 256:5267, 1981

Grant RA, Lin T-C, Konigsberg W, et al.: Structure of the filamentous bacteriophage f1. J Biol Chem 256:539, 1981

Meyer TF, Geider K: Enzymatic synthesis of bacteriophage fd viral DNA. Nature 296:828, 1982

Sanger F, Coulson AR, Friedmann T, et al.: The nucleotide sequence of bacteriophage ϕX174. J Mol Biol 125:225, 1978

Shlomai J, Polder L, Arai K-I, et al.: Replication of ϕX174 DNA with purified enzymes. I. Conversion of viral DNA to a supercoiled, biologically active duplex. J Biol Chem 256:5233, 1981

DIPHTHERIA TOXIN PRODUCTION

Uchida T, Kanei C, Yoneda M: Mutations in corynephage β that affect the yield of diphtheria toxin. Virology 77:876, 1977

SECTION II

CLINICAL VIROLOGY

CHAPTER 10

Host-Virus Interactions

As available knowledge has increased, discussion of virus infections in humans has become increasingly detailed and concepts of virus–host interaction have been expanded. Initially, only acute self-limited illnesses, such as a respiratory tract infection or measles, were included. The number of viruses identified that cause specific illnesses with a short course and attendant morbidity and mortality has greatly increased with the availability of cell cultures.

A second virus–host interaction is that of teratogenesis. Viral agents, such as rubella and cytomegalovirus (CMV), are well appreciated causes of intrauterine infection. The consequences of such infection are dependent upon such factors as the time of infection, the agent causing the infection, and the response of the host. One virus may cause alterations in organogenesis, as is the case with rubella virus, or another, such as CMV, may cause destruction of poorly differentiated tissue. The immature fetus does not mimic the adult immune response to infection, and thus it has been shown with rubella and CMV that infectious viruses may replicate and be present for months or years. The effects of virus replication may be compounded by the additional consequences of the host's response to the virus, for example, circulating immune complexes are demonstrable in infants with congenital CMV.

Virus latency and recurrent infection with the same agent are well documented in the case of the herpes group of viruses. Herpes simplex virus is notorious for its ability to cause intermittent overt infection and has been demonstrated to be latent in neural tissue. CMV may be intermittently excreted by the infected individual, and when appropriate studies have been done, such as restriction endonuclease analysis, it appears that the infecting virus is a single strain of virus. Similarly, it has long been appreciated that varicella virus infection induces a primary generalized illness and, in subsequent years, a localized infection in the form of zoster with the same virus. Epstein–Barr virus, the etiologic agent of infectious mononucleosis, would certainly appear to cause latent infection of circulating lymphocytes and perhaps of other cells. The herpes group of viruses exemplifies a type of virus–host interaction where an initial infection is followed by an indeterminate period of time when no demonstrable signs of infection are present and subsequent recurrent active infection occurs.

At the present time it is apparent that some human viruses may cause persistent infection of the host. The most salient example of this is hepatitis B virus, which may be present in large quantities for years. The results of this persistent infection can be asymtomatic infection or symptomatic aggressive liver disease, with the possible outcomes of cirrhosis and hepatocellular carcinoma linked to this infection. The central nervous system infections with enteroviruses occurring in patients with agammaglobulinemia are a second example of persistent infection but one that is dependent on an abnormal host response. Virus may be readily detectable for years in the central nervous system, and the clinical manifestations are progressive and ultimately fatal. Serologic studies indicate that human papovaviruses (BK and JC) asymptomatically infect the majority of persons by adulthood, yet disease becomes apparent only with immunosuppression. Relentlessly progressive central nervous system disease, such as Kuru or Jacob–Creutzfeldt disease, is due to transmissible agents called chronic infectious neuropathic agents, or CHINA viruses. These agents have not been visualized or isolated.

A final example of the spectrum of illness is oncogenesis. It now seems quite certain that several human viruses are linked to the ability to form tumors in people. Hepatitis B virus is associated with hepatocellular carcinoma. Epstein–Barr virus has been associated with Burkitt's lymphoma and a polyclonal malignant lymphoma, as well as nasopharyngeal carcinoma. Finally, the recently recognized human leukemia viruses must be considered in any discussion relating viruses to human malignancy. Thus, in general terms, our appreciation of the virus–host interaction has extended across the spectrum from acute, temporally limited illness through persistent infection to latency and recurrent infection, as well as teratogenesis and oncogenesis.

The virus–host interaction is likely to differ for viral agents of different groups. The age of the infected individual can influence the outcome of the host–virus interaction by virtue of variations in the immune response. Many other specific features of the virus–host interaction will determine which tissues of the host are infected and, therefore, where the detectable effects of infection will be.

Invasion of Host

The virus must first gain access to the host, and most often this is via mucous membranes of the respiratory, gastrointestinal, or genitourinary tracts. Aerosolization of virus affords entry into respiratory tract, whereas direct inoculation of virus occurs with sexual transmission and fecal–oral spread. Less frequently, the virus may gain entry through the skin or by direct inoculation into the bloodstream, as occurs with insect vectors or transplacental transmission of agents. Intact skin poses obvious problems for viral entry with the layers of keratinized nonmetabolizing cells. Mucous membrane surfaces are bathed in an array of secretions, including saliva and mucus, and these materials contain both nonspecific and specific defenses against invasion by viral pathogens.

Adherence of the virus to the host cells is essential to invasion of the cell. This is mediated by specific receptors of the virion and host. For polioviruses, the neuronal affinity is mediated by specific receptors, as is the species susceptibility. The specific cell receptors are known to be coded for by human chromosome 19. The specific viral receptor is unknown.

The ability of viruses to survive transit through the gastrointestinal tract may be partially dependent upon their acid stability, as with the enteroviruses. A protease resistant outer capsid protein (μlC) enables reovirus type 1 to survive transit through the gastrointestinal tract, adsorb to M epithelial cells, and subsequently replicate. There are mucoproteins in host secretions containing sialic acid that may be the receptor recognized by several viruses of the myxo/paramyxovirus families. There may be competition by the mucoproteins for the virus, which would diminish its infectivity by preventing contact with cells.

Influential features of the outcome of the virus–host contact include many factors that are not completely understood. The age of the host is clearly important when such agents as herpes simplex virus, rotavirus, hepatitis B virus, and adenoviruses are considered. In the case of herpes simplex virus, an overwhelming disseminated infection may occur in the unfortunate newborn infant who acquires infection during delivery. In the absence of immunocompromise this is an almost unheard of event in older individuals. In the case of rotaviruses, asymptomatic excretion of virus appears to be the rule in the newborn nursery when such infection is documented. On the other hand, these viruses are the leading cause of diarrhea in infants between the ages of 6 months and 18 months. Although hepatitis B virus can infect and ultimately cause serious disease in any age individual, it is far more likely to become established as a persistently infecting agent if an infant acquires this virus in the newborn period. It has been estimated that 90 percent of infants who contact this virus in the perinatal period become chronic carriers of hepatitis B virus. This is clearly not the case for older children or adults who acquire infection with this agent. Adenoviruses can cause a severe and overwhelming pneumonia in infants, and this is very unusual in older individuals unless immunosuppression or immunodeficiency exists.

Another such factor influencing the outcome of the infection is the nutritional status of the host. Elaborate studies have been done to define the changes in the host's immune status with malnutrition. The complex changes in immune function that are secondary to protein calorie malnutrition contribute to the severity of the infection.

Multiplication in Host Cell Tissues

Virus replication must occur when the virus gains access to the host if infection is to occur. Assuming the virus gains access to the relatively few permissive cells, other features of the environment in the host can limit virus replication. The paramyxoviruses have a surface fusion protein that is essential for induction of infection and is responsible for cell-to-cell spread of virus. This protein must be cleaved by a host cell protease for the virus to be infectious. Thus, the tissue tropism may be determined by the presence of an appropriate host cell protease capable of cleaving the target protein.

As virus replication must occur intracellularly, viruses gain access to both the professional phagocytes and host cells that do not normally phagocytize. Their intracellular replication may provide a protected environment, as they are clearly inaccessible to such elements of the host immune system as antibody. In certain instances, for example, lymphocytic choriomeningitis in animals, it is easy to demonstrate that the virus actually infects the effector cells of the immune system. This too will have a distinct effect on the outcome of the infection if virus can continue its replication within these cells and alter their function or destroy them.

As intracellular pathogens, viruses may spread by lysing the host cell, in which case the virus will spread via the extracellular environment and ultimately be accessible to all elements in the host immune system. Enteroviruses are examples of agents that are generally thought to lyse cells. Secondly, viruses may spread from cell to cell, as do those viruses having a fusion protein responsible for the joining of cellular membranes. Measles virus is a good example of an agent that can spread by fusion of adjacent cell membranes. Intact infectious virus is also released to the extracellular environment by budding from the host cell. Finally, some viruses may be passed directly from the parent cell to progeny cells without being liberated.

Children with immunodeficiencies have provided insight into the normal host–virus interaction. Several children with combined humoral and cellular immunodeficiencies have been observed to have chronic pulmonary infection with a parainfluenza virus because they are not able to eradicate viruses from their respiratory tract. The deficient cellular immunity seems more important, as children with only antibody deficiency have not had prolonged respiratory tract infection with these viruses. These cellular immunodeficient children have also been observed to have virus detectable in tissues other than the respiratory tract. It is not yet clear whether these viruses are mutants whose cleavage requirements have been altered or whether this is simply related to the persistent infection and the inability to prevent virus dissemination. The paramyxoviruses are only one group of agents that are known to cause difficulty in these children. The herpes agents and measles virus produce lethal infections. These children have also been demonstrated to have noncultivatable adenoviruses and/or rotaviruses present in the gastrointestinal tract for prolonged periods of time with active gastrointestinal disease.

It is possible to speculate that those viruses that insert viral proteins into host cell membrane by fusion during cell entry or cause de novo expression of viral antigens on the cell surface prior to formation of intact infectious virus might conceivably be rapidly eliminated if host defense mechanisms, antibody, complement, and sensitized lymphocytes, can destroy the cell in which the virus is replicating. It is also possible that the infection will actually be temporarily amplified if the infected cell is identified and lysed by the host defense mechanisms at a time when infectious progeny are contained within the cytoplasm.

Antibody

The host sees the virus as multiple antigens. Whether this is as multiple determinants on a single protein and/or as multiple proteins, the host develops numerous specific responses to these antigens. Generally speaking, neutralization of the virus involves the interaction of antibody with surface protein(s). In the case of reoviruses the sigma 1 capsid protein stimulates the production of antibody that is capable of neutralizing the virus. The sigma 3 protein, an outer capsid antigen, also stimulates antibody that is capable of neutralizing the virus. The use of monoclonal antibodies has allowed more intricate dissection of the interaction of such proteins with specific determinants of the virus. Thus, with polioviruses, at least two different antigenic sites on a single protein (VP1) have been shown to be capable of neutralizing the virus. Neutralization of infectivity may not of itself indicate destruction of virus. The interaction of virus and antibody occurs rapidly, and one antibody molecule can neutralize one virus particle. Presumably, the entire capsid of the virus is altered conformationally, or additional combining sites are obscured. Initial combination of antibody with the virus results in loss of infectivity, but release of antibody from the virus particle restores infectivity. When antibody–virus mixtures are prepared in vitro, there is almost always a small unneutralizable fraction of virus as a result of virus–antibody complexes, with subsequent dissociation of infectious virus from antibody. The presence of these complexes can be demonstrated by neutralization of all residual infectivity by anti-immunoglobulin serum.

There is general agreement that the most significant role of antibody is to prevent reinfections, although antibody may contribute to the termination of primary infection by limiting the spread of extracellular virus. These generalizations may also be applicable to virus replication in the cells of mucous membranes, although when the primary site of replication is the mucosa, IgA antibody becomes more important than IgG antibody.

Much of what we know about the host–virus interaction is a result of the unfortunate natural occurrence of immunodeficient patients. These patients, who are unable to synthesize antibodies normally, provide useful data through the observation of their interaction with viruses. Such patients generally receive replacement globulin, which provides them only with humoral IgG. Nevertheless, even before this human deficiency was recognized, many of the common viral infections did not appear to be a major problem for these patients. They were able to cope normally with vaccinia immunization and such illnesses as varicella and measles. They have not had recognized problems with such viruses as RSV, influenza, herpes simplex, or CMV. On the other hand, inability to limit replication of viruses in the central nervous system is now recognized to be a consequence of humoral antibody deficiency. Enteroviruses may replicate specifically in neuronal cells, as the polioviruses do, or generally in central nervous system tissue, as other enteroviruses seem to do. These unfortunate patients sustain persistent and chronic infections with these viruses in this sequestered location, and antibody therefore is important in the termination of these infections.

Virus–antibody complexes may circulate and be responsible for pathology within the host. Infants congenitally infected with CMV have been shown to have circulating complexes of virus and antibody. Such complexes have been shown to be deposited in the kidney. Similarly, patients with hepatitis B infection have also been shown to have circulating immune complexes and have had resultant pathology, such as arthritis and glomerulonephritis, as a result of these circulating complexes. In the experimental animal, perhaps the most extensively studied system is that of lymphocytic choriomeningitis (LCM). In utero and neonatal infection of mice with this virus produces an initially asymptomatic infection. Persistent lifetime viremia is established, and the blood contains virus–antibody complexes. Study of the animal has demonstrated that antibody to each of the polypeptides of the virus is present, yet virus is not cleared from the animal. In fact, the infectious virus that circulates is protected by being bound to antibody. These complexes may lead to glomerulonephritis, choroiditis, and vasculitis, with virus subsequently multiplying in the tissues where the complexes are deposited. It is not clear in this animal model why cytotoxic T cells are not detectable. However, some fascinating observations have been made, demonstrating that initially the viral antigens are expressed on the surface of infected cells as well as in the cytoplasm. Sequentially, the surface antigen diminishes, which may be related to the capping and subsequent stripping of the antigen from the cell by antibody. The viral nucleoprotein in the cytoplasm persists, but the cell is then no longer susceptible to specific lysis, as there are no expressed viral antigens on its surface. Simultaneously, in both in vivo and in vitro infection, defective interfering LCM virus is present. It has been demonstrated that defective virus can block infection with wild-type LCM virus. Details of these interactions are not clearly delineated, but in this model the host can be immunologically intact and yet the virus is able to escape immune surveillance and successfully establish persistent infection.

The concept that these persistently infected cells manage to survive despite intracellular virus replication is important. Some functions of the cells may be lost. For example, infection of the pituitary has resulted in absence or diminution of growth hormone because of the presence of LCM virus. There are no hallmarks of tissue destruction or inflammation in this setting, and by light microscopy the tissue morphology appears normal. With the use of appropriate antisera, however, viral nucleoprotein can be demonstrated within the cytoplasm of the cells. This infection would go undetected without knowledge of the infectious agent and use of specific antisera.

Complement

The alteration of the cell membrane by such enveloped viruses as measles or respiratory syncytial virus is apparent, with the resulting fusion of cell membranes producing multinucleated giant cells. Thus, with adsorption of the virus to the cell, the cell membrane is altered and viral proteins can be inserted in the host cell membrane without de novo synthesis of viral antigens. The presence of complement may initiate lysis of either cell free virus or virally infected cells in the presence of antibody. The expression of viral antigens on the cell surface has been more carefully described for enveloped viruses, but this is also true for reovirus (nonenveloped)-infected cells, which are replicating virus. For some of the other viruses, the expression of their proteins on the cell surface has yet to be delineated. Thus, in the presence of complement, antibody may result in lysis of the infected cell and/or the virus particle.

Adverse Consequences of Altered Virus–Host Interactions

Atypical measles is an example of an adverse effect that may be precipitated by the combination of virus infection and host response. The atypical measles syndrome occurred in persons who had received inactivated measles virus vaccine and subsequently, some months to years later, contacted wild-type measles virus. It has been learned that the formalin-inactivated measles virus vaccine had lost the fusion, or F, protein. Therefore, the vaccine recipients never formed antibody to the F protein but did form antibody to the hemagglutinin and all other proteins of measles virus. Introduction of wild-type virus into such a host permitted its replication and its cell-to-cell spread. An anamnestic response in antibody occurred with recognition of the expressed hemagglutinin, as well as a cell-mediated immune response to the other viral proteins. Virus replication and cell-to-cell spread could not be eliminated until antibody to the fusion protein formed. It is also possible that infected cells expressing antigen could exhibit capping and liberate antigen–antibody complexes. Thus, a different result of infection with measles virus was produced by the antecedent immunization with an incomplete antigen. It is assumed that the unusual manifestations of illness, including the prominent pulmonary disease, a vasculitic type rash, arthritis, and hepatic dysfunction, are more likely a result of the host response to the virally infected cells than a result of virus replication alone, since these manifestations differ from those of natural measles.

Cell-mediated Immunity

Antigens are processed by macrophages and T cells. Clearly, macrophages phagocytize virus particles and, in some instances, destroy the virus. In other instances, the virus may replicate and destroy the macrophage. Sensitized T cells have been demonstrated to an array of human viruses. Such cells must recognize more than the viral antigens, that is, they must share the H2 antigens with the target cells. Interactions of various subgroups of T cells are complex. If the sensitized lymphocyte can eliminate the infected cell prior to the production of infectious progeny, the infection may be aborted.

Again, using measles virus as an example, this virus has been isolated from circulating lymphocytes by cocultivation of these cells in vitro. It is not yet known whether the inability to produce infectious virus in lymphocytes is related to absence of a host cell protease capable of cleaving the fusion protein. Experimentally, infection of lymphocytes can occur in vitro without any demonstrable expression of antigens on the cell surface or in the cytoplasm until a mitogenic stimulus is applied for the cells. The infected lymphocytes appeared morphologically normal but did not function normally as effectors in antibody-dependent cell-mediated cytotoxicity assays. Thus, this is another potential example of infected cells having an altered specific function but otherwise appearing normal. The phenomenon of loss of intradermal sensitivity to tuberculin protein has long been recognized with acute measles infection. Is this because effector cells are now infected with measles virus and have lost their effector functions?

Finally, it has been suggested that inflammation might nonspecifically destroy contiguous infected cells. All of the contributing features to the inflammatory response, such as the lymphokines, including migration inhibition factor and interferon, may contribute nonspecifically to the control of infection. Further details of the host response to infection are given in the following chapters.

FURTHER READING

Buchmeier MJ, Welsh RM, Dutkof J: The virology and immunobiology of LCMV infection. Adv Immun 30:275, 1980

Choppin PW, Richardson CD, Merz DC: The functions and inhibition of the membrane glycoproteins of paramyxoviruses and myxoviruses and the role of the measles virus M protein in subacute sclerosing panencephalitis. J Infect Dis 143:352, 1981

Fishaut M, Tubergen D, McIntosh K: Cellular response to respiratory viruses, with particular reference to children with disorders of cell-mediated immunity. J Pediatr 96:179, 1980

Fraenkel-Conrat H, Wagner RR (eds): Virus–host interactions. Comprehensive Virology. New York, Plenum, 1979, vol 15

Oldstone MBA: Immunopathology of persistent viral infections. Hosp Pract 17:61, 1982

Zinkernagel RM: Major transplantation antigens in host responses to infection. Hosp Pract 13:83, 1978

CHAPTER 11

Diagnostic Virology

Specific diagnosis of virus infection is useful to the practicing physician by delineating an etiologic agent for the observed illness. This information may alter unnecessary antimicrobial therapy, allow earlier discharge from the hospital, provide a more accurate prognosis, or generate informative research data. Additionally, some diagnoses may prevent nosocomial transmission or alert the physician to possible transmission in the community. New viruses or unique manifestations of old viruses may be identified. Finally, a specific diagnosis may allow appropriate use of prophylactic agents or vaccines.

The time required for viral diagnosis by standard inoculation of tissue culture, embryonated egg, or animals often exceeds the duration of the illness in question. Increasingly rapid diagnosis will provide far more information for the responsible physician. Antigen detection rather than isolation of virus will ultimately replace the classic, more cumbersome isolation techniques. Development of specific antiviral drugs will produce a need for more rapid specific diagnosis if the drug is to be administered effectively.

Viral diagnostic facilities vary greatly, and the clinician must determine what specific resources are available in his or her hospital or community. The facilities of the municipal or state health departments are accessible without direct patient costs, and through these laboratories referral of clinical materials can be made to the Centers for Disease Control in Atlanta, Georgia. In addition, laboratories within community hospitals and associated with medical schools are accessible in some areas. More recently, commercial laboratories have incorporated some viral diagnostic skills into their available procedures. Generally, these utilize serologic diagnosis or consist of commercially available kits containing reagents for detection of a few specific antigens, e.g., HBsAg or rotavirus.

There are viral illnesses where the accurate diagnosis is of extreme importance to the patient, the patient's family, or his or her community. The correct diagnosis of an initial case of paralytic poliomyelitis can allow effective immunization to be instituted in a susceptible community, thereby preventing a sizable outbreak of disease. This requires isolation, identification, and typing of the virus in the laboratory. When rubella infection is suspected in the first trimester of pregnancy, the currently available accurate serologic means of diagnosis are mandatory to confirm the diagnosis prior to any consideration of pregnancy interruption. The serologic assessment of rubella immunity should become an integral part of the female premarital examination and is required by law in many states, since attenuated rubella vaccine offers a means of establishing immunity in susceptible women prior to pregnancy. Introduction of varicella into the hospital setting of high-risk patients is a frequent problem. Ascertainment of the susceptibility of exposed persons and protection of those at high risk with prophylactic zoster immune globulin requires laboratory definition of the serologic status of many persons.

Finally, within the framework of any program responsible for training physicians, it is important that these physicians become familiar with viral illnesses, institute appropriate control measures when necessary, and provide appropriate prophylaxis for others when this is available. Laboratory documentation of viral illness confirming the clinical impression or, in some cases, providing an unsuspected diagnosis will improve the judgment of these physicians providing patient care in the years to come.

Treatment of Specimens

A basic understanding of the laboratory procedures is necessary in order to utilize optimally the available virus laboratory facilities. Whenever a specimen is submitted, adequate information must accompany the request. This information is essential, as specimens are often processed in the laboratory according to their source and the physician's provisional diagnosis. Commonly needed information includes patient identification and age, the clinical diagnosis, the referring physician, the source of the specimens, and the date they were obtained. In addition, it is often helpful to know whether the patient has recently received viral vaccines. The responsible laboratory processing these materials should be consulted whenever questions arise, as they will be able to specify the optimal handling of the materials.

Patient materials are cultured for the presence of viruses to detect a specific etiologic agent. Tissue culture systems are usually more readily available, less cumbersome, and less expensive than embryonated eggs or animals. The cells utilized are dictated in part by the facilities available in the particular laboratory and by the suspected type of infection. It is usually advisable to collect the specimens as early as possible in the course of a clinical illness. Since viral agents are not affected by antimicrobial agents, cultures may be obtained even if therapy for potential bacterial pathogens has previously been initiated. Such mate-

TABLE 11-1. SUGGESTED SPECIMENS TO BE SUBMITTED FOR VIRAL DIAGNOSIS

Clinical Illness	Suspected Virus	Clinical Specimens	Postmortem Materials	Notes
Respiratory		N-P secretions	Lung, trachea, blood	Immunofluorescence requires intact cells in secretions, immunocompromised patients may have virus in tissue other than respiratory tract
Pharyngitis, croup, bronchiolitis, pneumonia	Influenza, parainfluenza, respiratory syncytial virus, reovirus, adenovirus		Stool, eye	
Gastrointestinal	Rotavirus, adenovirus, Norwalk-like, miscellaneous others	Stool	Intestinal contents	Examination by EM or testing for antigen more productive than attempted cell culture isolation, if parotitis present, culture throat and urine
Diarrhea				
CNS		CSF, throat, stool	Brain, liver, intestinal contents	No routine serology available for enteroviruses except polioviruses; many enteroviral syndromes are without symptoms
Meningitis/encephalitis	Enteroviruses, mumps, herpes simplex virus, togaviruses			
		Brain tissue, blood, brain	Brain tissue, other viscera	Togaviruses present in CNS tissue and blood; serologic diagnosis more practical
Gingivostomatitis		Vesicle fluid, throat swab or mouth wash, vaginal swab		
Keratoconjunctivitis				
Genital vesicular lesions				
Vesicular lesions of lip				
Eczema vaccinatum	Herpes simplex			
Chickenpox				
Zoster	Varicella			
Mononucleosis	EBV CMV	Buffy coat, urine, throat swab	Lung, kidney, salivary gland	Serologic assessment of antibodies to EBV include IgM, IgG, anti-VCA, EBNA, EA
Hepatitis	HBV HAV NANB	Serum, liver, stool	Liver, blood	Serologic assessment allows detection of HBV antigens and antibodies (HBsAg, HBeAg, αHBsAg, αHBeAg, αHBeAg); IgM anti-HAV provides estimate of recent infection
Measles	Measles	Respiratory secretions, blood, urine	Brain, lung	
SSPE		CSF	Brain, lung	CSF antibodies for measles virus
Intrauterine or perinatal infection	CMV	Buffy coat, urine	Liver, kidney, intestinal contents	
	Rubella	Throat, urine, blood,		
	Enteroviruses	Throat, stool, blood, CSF		
	Herpes simplex virus	Throat, stool, blood, CSF		

rials are obtained from the same site(s) as specimens for bacterial cultures (Table 11-1). Respiratory tract secretions, stool, urine, cerebrospinal fluid, pleural fluid, pericardial fluid, blood, bone marrow, vesicle fluid, and skin scrapings may be utilized in attempted virus isolations. Tissue specimens from biopsies or postmortem examinations are suitable for attempted virus isolation if fresh or frozen but not in formalin.

The principles adhered to in the collection of bacterial specimens are applicable to specimens submitted for virus culture. Containers must be clean and sterile and handled accordingly. The more stable viral agents include vaccinia, the enteroviruses, and the adenoviruses. As it is rarely possible to know the particular etiologic agent until the virus is isolated, all specimens should be treated as though the agent is potentially labile. Many viruses tend to be unstable at an acid pH or at temperatures above 4C. All patient specimens should be transported as rapidly as possible to the laboratory. If a delay of even 1 hour occurs, the material should be refrigerated at 4C or transported on ice. Freezing materials at −20C for brief periods of time may inactivate many of the more labile enveloped viruses, and keeping specimens at 4C is preferred. Delays of several days prior to inoculation usually necessitate freezing of the specimens, preferably at −70C.

In addition to their heat and acid lability, many viruses do not withstand drying. Swabs of mucosal surfaces, skin scrapings, and tissues are placed in a transport medium, which provides stability with a protein source such as 0.5 percent gelatin or antibody-free serum and a buffered salt solution essential to preserve infective virus. Several such media are commercially available or easily made. Veal infusion broth or Stuart's transport medium is employed by bacteriology laboratories. A 1 percent solution of skimmed milk in distilled water, Hanks' balanced salt solution with 10 percent fetal calf serum, or 0.5 percent bovine albumin or minimal essential medium and 40 percent sucrose have been used successfully. All of these media have antibiotics (e.g., penicillin, 50 units/ml, amphotericin, 1 μg/ml; streptomycin, 5 μg/ml) added to prevent overgrowth by resident host bacterial flora and to decrease exogenous contamination of the specimen.

Identification of Virus

Isolation of an agent from a patient, especially from a mucosal surface, does not alway prove an etiologic relationship to his illness. For this reason, patients being thoroughly evaluated for viral disease should have both acute and convalescent sera drawn for antibody determinations. The acute specimen of blood is obtained from the patient as early as possible in the illness, and the convalescent specimen is drawn 2 to 3 weeks later. The serum is separated and kept at refrigerator or freezer temperature. Whole blood should not be frozen, as the erythrocytes lyse and the subsequent assay of hemolyzed serum is difficult and inaccurate.

The traditional techniques to assay viral antibodies include complement fixation (CF), hemagglutination inhibition (HI), and neutralization of the viral cytopathic effect. The commonly accepted serologic confirmation of acute infection is a four-fold or greater rise in antibody titer when serial two-fold dilutions of serum are employed in these traditional test procedures. Complement fixation offers a relatively rapid, efficient way of screening sera for a number of viral antibodies. It is particularly useful in determining that recent infection has occurred. As a general rule, the antibodies thus detected are group-specific and not type-specific. For example, adenovirus antibody can be distinguished from poliovirus antibody, but antibody to type 1 adenovirus cannot be distinguished from any other adenovirus CF antibody. Complement-fixation antibodies usually decline more rapidly than do specific neutralizing antibodies, so that their absence does not necessarily denote susceptibility.

Hemagglutination-inhibition studies are limited by the fact that not all viruses possess a hemagglutinin. Agents with recognized hemagglutinins are influenza, mumps, measles, the parainfluenzae, rubella, vaccinia, variola, the arboviruses, reoviruses, and some of the adenoviruses and echoviruses. The limitations of the test itself are primarily technical, as it is often difficult to eliminate nonspecific inhibitors of hemagglutination from the serum being tested. The HI antibodies are type-specific, and the method is quite sensitive, correlating well with the antibodies observed in the neutralization test.

Neutralizing antibodies are highly specific for virus type, appear early in the course of illness, and persist for a long time thereafter. The determination of neutralizing antibody requires the growth of an agent in a cell culture or an animal system. The serum in question is incubated with the suspected etiologic agent and is then placed into the appropriate culture system. The results are commonly unavailable for at least a week, as the appearance of the cytopathic effects in the cell culture or illness in the animal determines the length of time necessary for the performance of the test.

Technologic innovations are changing traditional serologic methods. Enzyme-linked immunosorbent assay (ELISA) tests, radioimmunoassays (RIAs), and quantitative immunofluorescence determinations are reporting results with numerical values that have no obvious correlation with traditional values that are reported as the reciprocal of two-fold dilutions. Each test brings with it a new set of values, each of which must be compared to acceptable standards. Each method demands individual interpretation. Currently, such serologic procedures are coming into general use. Many laboratories are dependent upon the manufacturers' standards and are not aware of the limitations of the pre-licensure testing or of the variability of the procedure itself and cannot relate the information obtained to older methods. Thus, there are many predictable changes occurring in laboratory serology, and there is already attendant confusion concerning interpretation of the data. The utilization of these methods will increase the availability of tests, and ultimately will increase the sensitivity and efficiency of testing.

Regardless of the method employed, serologic demonstration of an antibody response may provide evidence of infection in the absence of virus isolation from cultures. Unfortunately, documentation of infection is delayed because of the need to assess convalescent serum for antibodies and is limited by the multiplicity of viruses infecting humans. Serology may also be used to assay the immune status of an individual following previous infection or vaccination.

Antigen Detection

In recent years the development and application of new technology has begun to be applied to detection of viral antigen in clinical materials. The site of virus multiplication, the complex composition of patient specimens, and the differences in amount of virus present influence the usefulness of these techniques. Far better serologic reagents, such as monoclonal antibodies, have the potential of increasing the sensitivity and specificity of antigen detection. Methods, such as immunoprecipitation and countercurrent immunoelectrophoresis, have been utilized for specific viruses, such as varicella and hepatitis. These tests have provided more rapid recognition of the viral antigens than cell culture isolation of virus and have made tests available on a larger scale but have been superseded by more sensitive methods such as ELISAs or RIAs. No other human virus has been as easily demonstrable in serum as HBV and its antigens because of the quantity that is present.

ELISAs are being increasingly applied to the detection of viral antigens. Reagents are less costly than radiolabeled materials, and expensive equipment is not a necessity. ELISAs are designed with a specific enzyme linked to antibody. The enzyme (e.g., alkaline phosphatase) can produce a color change when provided with the right substrate (e.g., *p*-nitrophenyl phosphate). The visible color change is appreciated with the eye and can be easily quantitated by a spectrophotometer. In practice, antigen is adsorbed to a surface (microtiter plate, metal beads, and so on), and the test serum is added. Any specific antibody will attach to antigen. Enzyme-labeled antiglobulin is then added and attaches to the bound antigen–antibody complex. After exhaustive washing, addition of the substrate results in the visible color change. If no specific antibody is present, the enzyme-labeled antiglobulin will not adhere to the plate, and no hydrolysis of substrate can occur.

Immunofluorescence has been utilized for rapid viral diagnosis of respiratory tract infections, vesicular exanthems, and examination of tissues. Respiratory epithelial cells obtained from nasal secretions may be examined by indirect immunofluorescence for the presence of many of the common respiratory viruses. A large successful experience with diagnosis of respiratory syncytial virus, parainfluenza, influenza, and adenovirus infections has been accumulated in European laboratories. Meticulous preparation of materials is required, and antisera, which are not generally available, must be both sensitive and specific. The basic techniques can be standardized but still require an experienced person to interpret the results. The method offers possible etiologic diagnosis within one working day, which is a distinct advantage to the clinician. Standardization of reagents and increased availability will render immunofluorescence a more broadly available method.

Experimental detection of viral nucleic acids and proteins has reached a level of sensitivity and practicality that has begun to permit investigators to apply the technology to clinical materials. Immobilization of the DNA, RNA, or protein on nitrocellulose paper precedes the use of an enzyme or radiolabeled probe that specifically binds to the nucleic acid or protein and is detected by the reaction product or autoradiography. Epstein–Barr virus and cytomegalovirus DNA have been reproducibly demonstrated in peripheral lymphocytes by placing lymphocytes on nitrocellulose paper and performing in situ hybridization with appropriately labeled probes.

The sensitivity and specificity make this approach to detection of a known virus attractive. The obvious disadvantage is the multiplicity of agents infecting humans and the need for multiple specific probes. Clearly, the physician's knowledge of the clinical illness and epidemiology must be utilized when a patient is having materials submitted for analysis. Ideally, definition of group-reactive antigen or nucleoprotein would occur initially, so that, for example, definition of an influenza virus versus a parainfluenza virus would precede subsequent, more specific identification. In many instances, the rapid detection of an etiologic virus without type specificity would provide extremely useful information. To identify influenza A viral antigens in secretions provides the physician with the opportunity to use antiviral therapy for the patient, prophylaxis of contacts at risk, and administration of vaccine in the setting of an outbreak among high-risk persons. Knowing the specific serotype would not add appreciably to the initial decisions.

Electron Microscopic Examination

The electron microscope has been utilized recently to assist in viral diagnosis. Negative staining by heavy metal salts allows electron microscope visualization and morphologic characterization of the virus group. Examination of materials from vesicular lesions by experienced personnel can readily distinguish a viral agent of the herpes group from one of the poxvirus group. Identification of the etiologic agent of hepatitis B was accomplished by electron microscope visualization of the virus. Another example of the use of the electron microscope has been the detection of previously unrecognizable virus particles in stool specimens. Ten percent suspensions of stool examined directly will reveal the presence of virus at a concentration of 10^5 particles/g of stool. These observations have led to the identification of agents, such as rotaviruses and Norwalk-like agents, now considered causative in acute gastrointestinal disease. The human rotaviruses are not yet easily grown in any cell culture system, so antigen detection by electron microscopy or ELISA is the most practical diagnostic method at the present time. Other refinements of methodology have broadened the diagnostic applications of the electron microscope. The use of specific antiserum causes adherence of virions to antibody and results in clumps of virus particles. This clumping permits detection of smaller numbers of virus particles. Such immune electron microscopy provides direct visualization of the antigen–antibody reaction. Although such work is primarily investigational at the present time, new insights into gastrointestinal disease have come from work with the electron microscope. The future will see electron microscope diagnosis supplanted by more practical methods.

Tissue Pathology

Any laboratory where tissue pathology is done can examine tissues by microscopy, which may facilitate a viral diagnosis. Histologic examination of pertinent clinical specimens with hematoxylin and eosin or Giemsa stains may disclose pathognomonic features of virus infection, such as inclusion bodies of multinucleate giant cells. If specific antisera are available, immunofluorescence may also be used.

Measles infection, either that of natural disease or of attenuated virus, may produce multinucleate giant cells in the urine, as well as intranuclear and intracytoplasmic inclusions. Such findings have also been described in the sputum or throat scrapings of patients with giant cell pneumonia or in malnourished patients with measles. Rubella, mumps, Coxsackie A virus, and variola have been reported to produce eosinophilic cytoplasmic inclusions in the cells of the urine sediment. Agents, such as cytomegalovirus and herpes simplex, have been observed to produce intranuclear inclusions in cells in the urine. Such positive findings in the urine, sputum, or tissues will point toward the probability of virus infection, but without culturing the virus, the laboratory cannot identify the specific agent involved. The absence of such findings does not exclude viral disease, and it is very important to recognize that many agents (for example, the enteroviruses) do not cause specific hallmarks of virus infection.

Cutaneous lesions, such as vesicles, macules, or pustules, can also be examined for the presence of multinucleate giant cells and inclusion-bearing cells. Materials obtained from such lesions can be examined easily and quickly. The vesicle is sponged with alcohol (if no virus cultures are being taken from the lesion), and the roof of the vesicle is reflected. The fluid is blotted, the base of the lesion is scraped, avoiding gross bleeding when possible, and the cellular material is spread on a glass slide and air dried. It can be fixed with methyl alcohol and stained with Wright or Giemsa stain. Giant cells are readily apparent, and inclusions may be seen with carefully made preparations. The presence of such giant cells will exclude vaccinia and variola from the differential diagnosis but will not distinguish between herpes simplex and varicella-zoster. Similarly, the diagnosis of herpes simplex infection of the female genital tract can be approached by obtaining a swab of the cervix and examining by Papanicolaou stain for giant cells and/or intranuclear inclusions. Again, immunofluorescence may provide specific etiologic information in some of these situations.

The information provided in this brief discussion can be applied in the diagnosis of the virus infections discussed in the subsequent clinical virology chapters.

FURTHER READING

Gardner PS, McQuillin J: Rapid Virus Diagnosis. Application of Immunofluorescence. London, Butterworth, 1974

Hsiung GD: Diagnostic Virology, 3rd ed. New Haven, Yale University Press, 1982

Lennette EH, Schmidt NJ: Diagnostic Procedures for Viral, Rickettsial and Chlamydial infections, 5th ed. Washington, D.C., Am Public Health Assoc, 1979

McIntosh K, Wilfert C, Chernesky M, et al.: Summary of a workshop on new and useful techniques in rapid viral diagnosis. J Infect Dis 142:793, 1980

Rapid Laboratory Techniques for the Diagnosis of Viral Infections. Report of a WHO scientific group. Tech Rep Series 661. Geneva, WHO, 1981

Yolken RH: Enzyme immunoassays for the detection of infectious antigens in body fluids: Current limitations and future prospects. Rev Infect Dis 4:35, 1982

CHAPTER 12

Poxviruses

The family Poxviridae includes 20 or more mammalian viruses in five genera, a group of bird viruses (genus *Avipoxvirus*), and nearly two dozen insect species (*Entomopoxvirus*). They are large, brick-shaped, enveloped, containing double-stranded DNA, two lateral bodies, and a central core or nucleoid. They possess a common internal nucleoprotein antigen and share the clinical manifestation of vesicular skin lesions in the susceptible host. Until recently, smallpox (variola), an *Orthopoxvirus*, received most attention because of its responsibility for epidemic disease throughout the world for many centuries. With smallpox eradication in 1977, poxvirus research and surveillance programs have been emphasized to investigate the relationships of other mammalian poxviruses and to explore the possiblity of mutations with reemergence of variola.

Smallpox (Variola)

Smallpox is a member of the genus *Orthopoxvirus*, which includes also vaccinia, monkeypox, buffalopox, camelpox, cowpox, rabbitpox, and mousepox (ectromelia). There is only one serotype, which has apparently persisted for many years. The disease was recognized as a major health problem for at least 3000 years. Early epidemics may have been confined to the Orient, Middle East, and Africa until spread into Europe by the Arab expeditions of the sixth century. Early 16th century Spanish conquistadors introduced smallpox to the Western Hemisphere with transmission to Aztec natives. It spread throughout the Americas. Early American colonists were familiar with the illness. A noteworthy epidemic in 1721 involved 5889 of Boston's 12,000 inhabitants. The publication in 1798 by Edward Jenner of his work with cowpox heralded the beginning of a new era in the prevention of smallpox. Despite widespread acceptance of vaccination and its use with increasing frequency throughout Europe and the United States, another century passed before major epidemics were eliminated in these nations. By 1967 there were still 33 countries, mainly in Asia and Africa, where smallpox remained endemic, claiming millions of victims annually. The World Health Organization (WHO) program for eradication was initiated that year and culminated in success, with the last naturally occurring case detected in Somalia in October 1977.

Epidemiology

Humans were the only known natural host of smallpox virus, but nonhuman primates have been successfully infected in the laboratory. Transmission of virus occurred directly from person to person. The major source of infectious material was respiratory tract secretions with droplet spread. The virus was able to persist for lengthy periods in the protein and cellular debris of the sloughed scabs, but they were of minor importance in transmission. Susceptible members of a patient's household were the most likely to become infected. Another group with a high rate of spread were unimmunized hospital personnel caring for a patient with the illness. Although respiratory tract shedding of small amounts of virus preceded the appearance of the exanthem (Fig. 12-1), the patient was most infectious with the onset of rash for 7 to 14 days.

Widespread use of smallpox vaccine was responsible for striking alterations in the geographic patterns of the disease. The last recorded case in the United States was an importation in 1949, but there had been 48,000 patients in 1930. The WHO eradication program began in 1967, when 62 nations still harbored the disease. By 1974 only 8 countries reported cases, and it was endemic in only 4 (India, Pakistan, Bangladesh, and Ethiopia). The last-known naturally acquired case was recorded in the town of Merka, Somalia, on 26 October 1977. Because there is no evidence that smallpox virus persists in the human host and there is no animal reservoir, it is likely that deep-freezes in four laboratories (U.S., U.S.S.R., South Africa, and England) now hold the only variola virus remaining in the world.

Clinical Illness

Three main forms of disease were seen in unvaccinated patients. Classic smallpox (variola major) was a severe, biphasic, febrile illness with a mortality rate of 20 to 50 percent. Variola minor (alastrim) had <1 percent mortality, while an intermediate form of smallpox ranged from 10 to 15 percent mortality rate. An initial prodromal phase was characterized by abrupt onset of high fever, chills, headache, backache, and malaise for 2 to 4 days. The patient was toxic and obtunded or delirious. This was followed by a sudden, dramatic improvement as temperature fell and respiratory symptoms developed. At this time rash began, often starting on the face and arms but progressing to involve the trunk and lower extremities. Simultaneously, an enanthem appeared with painful ulcers of the buccal, pharyngeal, and bronchial mucosa. The rash started as macules, which within a few hours had become papules. Over the next several days the lesions vesiculated and then, between the seventh and ninth days evolved into frank pustules. Fever rose again, and the patient became severely ill with constitutional symptoms as well as intensely painful local lesions. By the tenth day the pustules started to rupture and then to crust, with sloughing of the scabs over the next 5 to 10 days, leaving scars in the areas of previous involvement.

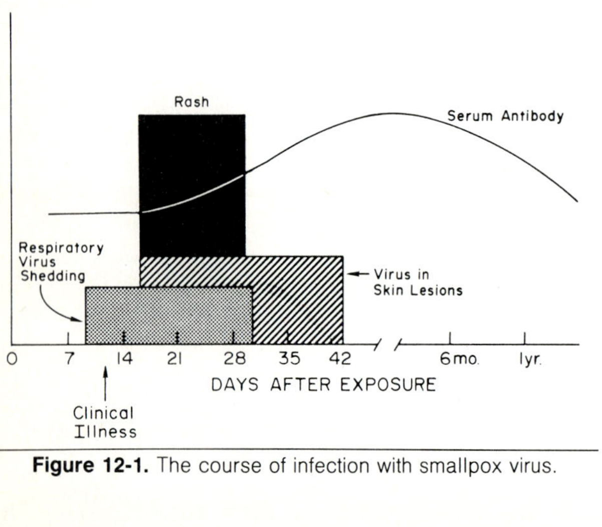

Figure 12-1. The course of infection with smallpox virus.

There was considerable individual variation in the clinical picture, and the rash ranged from discrete to confluent lesions. A small number of patients underwent severe hemorrhagic smallpox, with a rapid, fulminant course, including hemorrhages of the skin and mucous membranes in the absence of the usual eruption. This form of the disease was almost always fatal. In contrast, a very mild, modified illness occurred in partially immune individuals. Because patients did not feel ill and remained ambulatory, they were a source of virus spread throughout the community.

Variola minor had a prolonged incubation period of 15 to 20 days, a mild prodromal phase, a discrete, rapidly evolving eruption, moderate constitutional symptoms, and a mortality rate of less than 1 percent.

Complications included pneumonia, keratitis with corneal damage, encephalitis, and peripheral neuritis. Most common were secondary bacterial infections of the skin and respiratory tract, with cellulitis, furunculosis, impetigo, and pneumonia. Bacteremia resulted in metastatic foci, including pyogenic arthritis and osteomyelitis. No specific effective antiviral chemotherapy was available, but the oral administration of methisazone (methylisatin-beta-thiosemicarbazone) very early in the incubation period diminished the attack rate in susceptible contacts. Supportive therapy with fluids, electrolyte replacement, nutritional supplementation, and antibiotic treatment of secondary bacterial complications was of importance.

Pathology and Pathogenesis

After its entry via the upper respiratory tract, smallpox virus spread to regional lymphatics and nodes, from which a primary viremia then emanated. Dissemination was widespread, with involvement of all tissues, especially epithelial cells. Lesions began in the areas surrounding infected endothelial cells of small vessels. The skin lesions evolved as foci of mononuclear cell infiltration and edema, progressing to swollen epithelial cells within which acidophilic inclusions (Guarnieri bodies) appeared in the cytoplasm. Epithelial cell necrosis and accumulations of interstitial fluid resulted in vesicle formation. A similar evolution took place in mucous membranes, where rapid unroofing of the vesicle surface initiated ulcerative lesions. Focal necrotic lesions also developed in spleen, testis, liver, lung, and other organs. Virus released from these multiple sites of replication produced a secondary viremia coinciding with the eruptive phase of the disease.

Those patients at the extremes of life, the young infant and the aged, had more severe disease and were more likely to die as a result. Prognosis correlated well with the severity of the prodromal phase and the type of rash. Striking toxemia and prostration in the first days of illness heralded a poor outcome. The hemorrhagic rash presaged an 80 percent or higher mortality; confluent exanthem, 50 percent; discrete lesions, less than 10 percent.

Immunity

An attack of smallpox confers active immunity of lifetime duration. Prior to the discovery of vaccination, variolation was widely practiced as a means of inducing active immunity. A mild form of illness ensued, which in most instances produced enduring immunity. However, occasional recipients developed severe smallpox from variolation, and there were deaths in 1 to 2 percent.

The introduction of vaccination in 1798 began one of the fascinating sagas of medical history. With abundant controversy, vaccination gradually achieved a widespread role as the principal prophylactic method for smallpox prevention. It was not until the WHO program began in 1967 that the final stages in disease eradication provided the culmination in 1977 of Jenner's observations 181 years earlier.

Following natural infection or immunization, virus-specific antibodies appear in the patient's serum. These will fix complement, inhibit hemagglutination, neutralize viral infectivity, and/or inhibit agar gel precipitation (AGP).

Diagnosis

When smallpox was a common disease, diagnosis was often established on the basis of (1) a clinically compatible illness, (2) a known recent exposure in an endemic area, and (3) the absence of a history of vaccination or a visible vaccination scar. When the infection had become a rarity, laboratory confirmation of any suspected case was absolutely essential because of the public health implications. A number of available techniques (Table 12-1) offer rapid and reliable laboratory diagnosis.* In actual practice those laboratories most familiar with smallpox virus employed four tests: electron microscopy (EM), AGP, and viral propagation in cell cultures and on the chorioallantoic membrane (CAM). Electron microscopic identification of a poxvirus may be accomplished within an hour; AGP requires only 1 to 4 hours. Rapid diagnosis is, therefore, possible with the skill of those working regularly with various poxviruses.

Because chickenpox (varicella), disseminated herpes hominis, vaccinia, and some noninfectious exanthemata may mimic smallpox, it is not surprising that many false alarms have been avoided or aborted by use of the techniques listed. Monkeypox, although indistinguishable by EM and AGP, produces distinct CAM lesions that can be identified by pock morphology. Vaccinia and variola are similarly distinguished by varying pock characteristics and growth in cell culture systems. In the 4 years from January 1978 to March 1982, 176 smallpox suspects have been investigated in 60 different countries. Aside from 2 laboratory-acquired smallpox cases in 1978 in Birmingham, England, all have been disproven.

*Any suspicious patient or specimen material should be discussed promptly with the Centers for Disease Control, Atlanta, Georgia, telephone number (404) 633-3311, Biohazards Control Officer.

TABLE 12-1. LABORATORY METHODS FOR POXVIRUS DIAGNOSIS

A. Direct visualization of poxvirus
   1. Electron microscopy (EM)
B. Visualization of elementary bodies
   1. Light microscopy of stained smears
C. Identification of viral antigens
   1. Agar gel precipitation (AGP)
   2. Fluorescent antibody (FA)
   3. Complement fixation (CF)
D. Isolation of virus
   1. In ovo on chorioallantoic membrane (CAM)
   2. In cell cultures
      a. Primary rhesus kidney cells
      b. Infant foreskin fibroblasts (FS-32)
      c. Vero cells
E. Serologic confirmation
   1. Specific antibody rise (four-fold) in paired sera
      a. Complement fixation (CF)
      b. Virus neutralization (VN)
      c. Agar gel precipitation (AGP)
      d. Hemagglutination inhibition (HI)

Prevention

The appropriate use of vaccination has prevented smallpox. Vaccinia virus confers protective immunity against variola for a lengthy period of time, albeit less enduring than the active immunization produced by the disease itself. Past field experience with studies of vaccine prophylaxis under conditions of natural exposure demonstrated a 99 percent efficacy for 1 year, 95 percent for 3 years, 85 percent for 10 years, and 50 percent for 20 years. Previously vaccinated individuals, whose immunity had waned, tended to have a much milder illness and a mortality rate far lower than that of unvaccinated patients. This ameliorating effect persisted as long as 20 years.

Vaccinia

Jenner introduced vaccination to the public with a paper published in 1798 based on his studies begun in 1796. It is not possible to establish with certainty today what virus he actually employed or what has happened to it over the ensuing nearly two centuries of multiple human and animal passages. Jenner believed his strain was horsepox (grease) which had been passed in cows before transfer to humans. Laboratory markers show that current vaccinia strains differ from cowpox as well as from other orthopoxviruses. Some investigators suggest that it is a recombinant of cowpox and smallpox.

Until 1971 it was recommended that all infants in the United States receive smallpox vaccination as a routine component of the childhood immunization schedule. The absence of endemic smallpox, the absence of disease importations since 1949, and the recognition of certain common and other rare complications of vaccination led public health and pediatric authorities to discontinue this practice after 1971–1972. Until that time nearly four million primary vaccinations and eight million revaccinations had been performed annually. With careful surveillance of vaccine complications, it was possible to exclude certain candidates who were at increased risk of these problems. Patients with exfoliative dermatitis (especially eczema) were likely to develop diffuse vaccinial lesions over the involved skin. This followed accidental vaccination of patients themselves or exposure to household or other close contacts who had an active vaccinial lesion. Individuals with immunodeficiency or those being treated with immune-suppressive therapy, particularly those with compromised T cell function, were more apt to develop progressive vaccinia. It was not possible to predict the rare patient who might develop encephalitis in the 10 to 14 days after inoculation, but there seemed to be an increased risk correlated with increasing age at the time of primary vaccination. Autoinoculation was relatively common among infants who scratched the site of their primary lesion and then introduced the virus elsewhere on their uninvolved skin. This was not a source of any serious problems unless the secondary site was the eye, where keratitis was a possible outcome. Local bacterial infections with pyogenic skin flora, especially staphylococci or streptococci, occasionally precipitated a cellulitis at the lesion site.

Molluscum Contagiosum

This infection of humans is caused by a poxvirus that does not replicate in any current in vitro cell culture systems but can be visualized by electron microscopy of affected cells from papillomatous skin lesions. It may be related to another poxvirus, the Yaba monkey tumor agent. The lesions are easily distinguished by their umbilicated appearance produced by central degeneration and by the formation of satellite nodules at the periphery of the parent lesion. They are 2 to 5 mm long, pink, white, or yellow, shiny, and rounded. On pathologic examination, the epidermis shows ballooning degeneration, acanthosis, hyperplasia, and the presence of large acidophilic inclusions (molluscum bodies) in superficial epithelial cells. The incubation period varies widely from 14 to 50 days.

In children the lesions are commonly on the face, trunk, or limbs. Adults often acquire their infection by sexual transmission and develop genital lesions. Most patients have fewer than 20 individual papules, but some immunocompromised individuals may have hundreds of lesions. Although spontaneous resolution usually occurs, this may require 6 to 36 months, so that surgical removal, cryotherapy, or other physical methods have been employed to accelerate clearing.

Orf

This old Saxon term refers to the infection of humans with the parapoxvirus of contagious pustular dermatitis (scabby mouth) of sheep and goats. In lambs the disease is characterized by the development of watery papillomatous lesions on the cornea, lips, and mouth, which usually resolve in 4 to 6 weeks without consequence. In humans, vesicles usually develop at the site of abrasions on the hand or face, which may evolve into hyperplastic nodular masses accompanied by regional lymphadenopathy. Ordinarily, lesions require no treatment. Since parapoxviruses and orthopoxviruses are only very distantly related immunologically, vaccination provides no protection. Orf is an occupational disease associated with handling of sheep, particularly in shearers.

Milker's Nodules (Pseudocowpox)

This condition is also caused by a *Parapoxvirus* (paravaccinia). It is a cutaneous disease of the udders of cow that may be transmitted to humans by contact. Lesions appear 1 to 2 weeks after contact and are similar to those produced by contagious pustular dermatitis. Recovery is complete in 4 to 8 weeks. Reinfection may occur, indicating that immunity does not last long.

Cowpox

Cowpox, an *Orthopoxvirus,* produces a vesicular eruption on the udders of cattle from which it may be transmitted to humans. Usually the illness in humans is a limited vesicular eruption of the skin, although rarely the disease develops into a widespread eruption with systemic symptoms.

Currently, reports of human cowpox are exceedingly rare, and doubts exist whether the cow is indeed the true reservoir host of this virus. Spontaneous cowpox virus infections have been detected in humans with no prior contact with cows and in some large felines (tigers) in Russian, Swedish, and English zoos. A similar, closely related virus was isolated from gerbils in the Turkmen Republic of U.S.S.R., suggesting that rodents in western Europe may be the true natural reservoir of cowpox.

Monkeypox

From 1970 through 1982, more than 70 laboratory-confirmed cases of human infection with this *Orthopoxvirus* have been reported, mainly in the tropical rain forest areas of West and Central Africa. The responsible agent had initially been recovered in the 1950s and 1960s from monkeys who became ill in captive laboratory colonies. Human illness closely resembles smallpox and, therefore, is critically important in surveillance for any recrudescence of variola infections. Monkeys are suspected to be the reservoir of this apparent zoonosis, but the epidemiology remains unclear. Antibodies specific to monkeypox virus have been detected in sera of wild monkeys trapped in West Africa. One human case has been reported in an infant bitten 12 days earlier by a chimpanzee.

Of 63 cases reported by WHO field teams, most were children under 15 years of age with no history of prior smallpox vaccination. There were 8 deaths. Although secondary spread from human to human appears unusual, 6 of 139 unvaccinated close contacts of the initial patients developed rash 7 to 20 days after exposure.

FURTHER READING

Arita I, Cromyko A: Surveillance of orthopoxvirus infections, and associated research, in the period after smallpox eradication. Bull WHO 60:367, 1982

Benenson AS: Smallpox. In Evans AS (ed): Viral Infections of Humans, 2nd ed. New York, Plenum, 1982, chap 22, pp 541–568

Dales S, Pogo BGT: Biology of poxviruses. In Kingsbury DW, Zur Hausen D (eds): Virology Monographs. New York, Springer-Verlag, 1981, vol 18

Fenner F: A successful eradication campaign. Global eradication of smallpox. Rev Infect Dis 4:916, 1982

Mutombo MW, Arita I, Jezek Z: Human monkeypox transmitted by a chimpanzee in a tropical rain-forest area of Zaire. Lancet 1:735, 1983

Ricketts TF, Byles JB: The diagnosis of smallpox (Reprinted from the 1908 London edition). US Dept of HEW, Bureau of Disease, Prevention and Environmental Control, Division of Foreign Quarantine, 1966, vols I and II

World Health Organization: Declaration of global eradication of smallpox. Weekly Epidemiol Rev 55:148, 1980

CHAPTER 13

Herpesviruses

The group of human herpesviruses includes herpes simplex virus (HSV) types 1 and 2, varicella-zoster virus (VZV), cytomegalovirus (CMV), and Epstein–Barr virus (EBV). These large, enveloped DNA viruses are responsible for a broad spectrum of clinical illness and share the unique characteristic of becoming latent in the body after a primary infection and having the potential for subsequent reactivation after varying periods of time. This persistence in the body has raised concern about potential oncogenicity, and, indeed, HSV and EBV have been associated with human cancer, and CMV has been shown to have transforming properties. Most people have antibodies to these viruses as adults, and although most of the clinical diseases are only temporarily annoying, life-threatening infections can occur.

Herpes Simplex Virus

Infections caused by herpes simplex virus have troubled us throughout history. Diseases resembling herpes were described in biblical times with the term "herpes" (from the Greek work, ερπειν, to creep) first appearing around 100 AD in descriptions of herpes labialis. Genital herpes infection was described by the physician to the king of France in 1736.

In 1912 Gruter and Lowenstein first transmitted HSV infection by using material from herpes keratitis and labialis to infect rabbit corneae. Since that time, advances in viral technology have led to the development of in vitro models of infection, recognition of the two types of HSV, increasing understanding of the mechanisms of latency and reactivation, and development of the first successful antiviral agents for use against HSV.

Epidemiology

Herpes simplex viruses are found worldwide, with humans as the only natural reservoir. Since the virus cannot remain infectious for long outside the body, direct contact with infected secretions is the mode of spread. Generally, HSV type 1 is transmitted in oral secretions, while HSV type 2 is transmitted genitally. Asymptomatic excreters can transmit infection, although that amount of virus is less than that seen in active lesions and presumably less infectious. Serologic studies indicate that lower socioeconomic status is associated with greater rates of seropositivity, which is thought to be related to closer living conditions with increased chance for spread. Primary infection with HSV-1 often occurs very early in life, and by adulthood, 30 to 100 percent of populations, depending on socioeconomic status, will have antibodies. In contrast, HSV-2 antibodies do not appear until puberty, and the acquisition rate is highest from 14 to 29 years, reflecting the venereal transmission of this virus. A sharp increase in the number of recognized cases has been noted recently in the United States, making genital herpes infection one of the most common venereal diseases seen today. Other modes of infection include autoinoculation to another body site and transmission from mother to infant via an infected birth canal at the time of delivery.

Recurrent infections can occur following primary infection with either HSV-1 or HSV-2. Recurrent disease is not usually as severe as primary disease, and most recurrences are due to reactivation of endogenous virus rather than to reinfection.

Pathogenesis

Herpes simplex virus enters the body through skin and mucous membranes. Most primary infections go unrecognized or are subclinical. When studied histologically, a local lytic infection of the parabasal and intermediate epithelial cells is noted, with an accompanying local mononuclear inflammatory response. Together, these make up the characteristic vesicle of HSV infection. Multinucleated cells and occasional typical Cowdry type A intranuclear inclusions are seen, along with ballooning degeneration of the cells and chromatin margination. During primary infection, involvement of the lymphatics and regional lymph nodes is common, and viremia with further dissemination can occur in patients who do not have an intact immune system.

HSV becomes latent following a primary infection by traveling up the sensory nerves to the corresponding sensory ganglia. Human autopsy studies have demonstrated the presence of latent virus in sacral, trigeminal, and vagal ganglia. The site of latency is felt to be within the neuron where viral DNA has been detected, but the exact physical nature of latent HSV is still not known. The signal for reactivation is also still a mystery, but various stimuli, such as fever, stress, sunlight, and local trauma, may be recognized by individuals as precipitating factors. Following reactivation, the virus presumably travels back down the sensory nerve pathway and again establishes infection on the skin or mucous membranes. Antibody titer is not usually affected, and lesions may or may not be clinically evident.

Both humoral and cell-mediated immune mechanisms contribute to limitation of virus spread, but the severe forms of disseminated HSV infection are more often seen in patients with depressed cell-mediated immunity. Viremia disseminates the virus in severe cases, resulting in infection that can involve the liver, lungs, kidneys, and central nervous system. Infants and malnourished or immunosuppressed patients are at highest risk for this often lethal complication.

Clinical Illness

Neonate

Herpes simplex virus infection of the newborn can be a devastating and often fatal disease, with an estimated incidence of between 1 in 3000 and 1 in 30,000 live births. Although cases of true intrauterine infection have been described, most infants seem to be infected via passage through the mother's infected birth canal or via retrograde spread of maternal genital infection shortly before birth. Since most genital herpes is due to HSV-2, most babies are also infected with this virus type. If HSV-1 is transmitted, it causes an identical disease picture. In a natural history study of neonatal HSV occurring in 56 mother–infant pairs, Whitley et al. found that 70 percent of the mothers had asymptomatic infection at the time of delivery, and nearly 50 percent of the births occurred prematurely.

Disease becomes apparent in infants from birth to 4 weeks of age, depending on the time of infection. Disseminated congenital infection is manifest at birth or soon after by seizures, irritability, jaundice, hepatosplenomegaly, bleeding disorders, chorioretinitis, pneumonitis, and skin vesicles. Progressive deterioration, with respiratory distress, circulatory collapse, and coma, often follows, and death occurs in up to 70 percent of untreated infants. Neonatal infections acquired during labor and delivery are clinically manifest around the end of the first week of life. Skin vesicles alone were the presenting sign in 70 percent of the neonates studied, but continued progression to involvement of other sites occurred in a further 70 percent of these infants. About 20 percent of infants, however, never developed skin vesicles, and viral isolation from other sites was required for diagnosis.

Disease that remains localized to the skin, eye, or mouth carries a better prognosis (mortality 30 percent) compared with localized central nervous system or disseminated disease (mortality 50 percent and 80 percent, respectively), which make up more than three quarters of all cases. Vidarabine therapy has markedly decreased the mortality of this disease, but few treated survivors of the localized central nervous system and disseminated forms of infections are neurologically normal at 1 year of age.

Oropharynx

Most primary HSV infections of the mouth are clinically inapparent. Those that are symptomatic most often present in early childhood (ages 1 to 6) as gingivostomatitis. This disease occurs year-round and begins with fever, drooling, and a sore mouth following an incubation period of 2 to 12 days. Initial pharyngeal erythema and edema progresses to vesiculation involving the pharyngeal and oral mucosa and gum tissue. Ulceration occurs quickly and may be accompanied by gingival bleeding. Lesions primarily involve the buccal mucosa, tongue, soft palate, and lips, in contrast to herpangina, caused by Coxsackie A virus, which primarily affects the posterior oropharynx. Tender submandibular and cervical adenopathy is common. Fever, pain, and toxicity may last several days, and secondary dehydration may occasionally become a problem. The illness lasts 1 to 2 weeks, and recovery is complete. Young adults may have a different presentation of their primary oral HSV-1 infection, with involvement of tonsils and the posterior pharnyx. This must be distinguished from other common causes of pharyngotonsillitis. This picture may also be seen in 10 percent of patients with primary genital HSV infections, presumably due to orogenital contact.

Herpes labialis (fever blister) is the most common disease caused by HSV, affecting 20 to 40 percent of the population. In contrast to the intraoral location of primary gingivostomatitis, recurrences usually occur at the vermilion border of the outer lip. A prodrome of pain, burning, tingling, or itching often precedes the clinical development of vesicles, which usually appear at the same location with each recurrence. Pain and viral titer decrease rapidly after 24 hours, and complete healing occurs within 7 to 10 days.

Eye

HSV infections involving the eye are usually due to type 1 virus. The disease is most often unilateral and can present as follicular conjunctivitis or blepharitis with associated preauricular adenopathy. Corneal involvement, in the form of dendritic lesions or punctate opacities on the epithelium, occurs in some patients. In the absence of stromal involvement, the eye heals without scarring in 1 to 3 weeks, but delayed healing, aggravated by the host's immune response, is sometimes seen if the infection spreads more deeply into the stroma and may be associated with opaque scars that require surgical therapy.

Recurrent eye disease occurs within 2 years in 25 to 50 percent of patients who experience recognized primary infection. Dendritic keratitis is the most common form and is easily diagnosed using fluorescein staining. Amebic ulcers (named for their shape) occasionally occur, especially in those patients treated with topical steroids, and can be a destructive and chronic problem. Unilateral keratoconjunctivitis and blepharitis may also be seen as manifestations of recurrent disease.

Genitalia

Primary genital infection with HSV may go unnoticed by the patient or run a distressing clinical course that can involve many body sites. The incubation period is 2 to 7 days. HSV-2 causes 70 to 90 percent of these infections. The 10 to 30 percent associated with HSV-1 usually result from oral–genital contact. Patients who present with symptoms have multiple painful vesicular or ulcerated lesions, vaginal or urethral discharge from the associated cervicitis or urethritis, and local itching. Tender inguinal adenopathy is common, and about 40 percent of patients will have associated systemic findings, including fever, malaise, myalgias, or photophobia. Dysuria and urinary retention secondary to urethral involvement may be seen, and some patients have an accompanying sacral radiculomyelitis that can be associated with neuralgia and urinary retention. Viral meningitis has been documented in 4 to 8 percent of cases, implying that viremia has occurred, and is accompanied by CSF pleocytosis. Cerebrospinal fluid culture for HSV is positive in this situation, in contrast to encephalitis due to HSV, where virus isolation from cerebrospinal fluid is distinctly unusual. The symptoms of primary genital disease last for 2 weeks, and healing of the lesions is usually complete at the end of 3 weeks. This disease has been seen in young children, and as with other sexually transmitted diseases presenting at a young age, the possibility of child abuse should be kept in mind.

Recurrent genital HSV disease is clinically much milder than its primary form. Approximately 70 percent of patients experience prodromal symptoms that are followed by the development of a small group of vesicles that may coalesce to form one or two ulcers. Pain and itching, if present, can last 3 to 4 days but are much milder than with primary infection. Lesions are usually healed in 7 to 10 days. In a study of 137 patients with a first symptomatic episode and 87 patients with recurrent disease, Corey et al. noted that only 14 percent of HSV-1 infections versus 60 percent of HSV-2 infections recurred during mean follow-up of 221 days. The probability of recurrence was directly related to the presence and titer of neutralizing antibody to HSV-2 in convalescent serum. Symptomatic patients with recurrent genital disease have five to eight recurrences per year, but cervical and urethral shedding of virus can occur without disease, so the true recurrence rate is unknown. The majority of recurrences are due to reactivation of endogenous virus, but reinfection with a different strain can occur.

The most important complication of this disease is the emotional stress that patients experience in dealing with a chronic illness that affects their sexual relationships. Women have the added burden of being at increased risk for abnormalities in cervical cytology and need to be monitored during pregnancy to avoid exposing their infants to herpes infection at the time of birth.

Perianal Area

Primary HSV disease of the anus and perianal area is being recognized with increasing frequency, particularly in male homosexuals. Vesicles and ulcers can be seen in the perianal and anal area and are associated with pain, itching, discharge, and tenesmus. Bilateral inguinal adenopathy is common, and systemic symptoms similar to those seen in primary genital infection have been noted.

Skin

Primary HSV infection of the skin occurs following a break in the integrity of this important host defense, and several well-recognized syndromes have been described. Young children with eczema can develop a rare but potentially fatal disease known as "eczema herpeticum." The term "Kaposi's varicelliform eruption" has also been used for this disease, but its use should be avoided since it implies a different etiologic agent. High fever and irritability are followed by the development of crops of vesicles that may continue to appear over the course of a week. Fever and toxicity subside after 7 to 10 days, and lesions are usually healed by the end of the third week unless bacterial superinfection complicates the process.

Primary infection of the finger, "herpetic whitlow," causes intense pain and itching, usually involving just one digit. Vesicles form deep under the skin and the accompanying axillary adenopathy and neuralgias can be impressive. Medical and dental personnel are at risk due to occupational exposure while examining infected patients, but this infection also occurs in the general population. Virus is readily communicated from these lesions, and medical personnel should cease all patient care while the disease is active. Lesions heal in 2 to 3 weeks and should not be incised, since bacterial superinfection is a frequent complication of this unnecessary procedure.

Superficial skin abrasions can also become infected with HSV. In wrestlers, this presentation has come to be known as "herpes gladiatorum." Burn patients are susceptible to developing HSV infections involving damaged skin areas.

Brain

Herpes simplex infection of the brain is considered to be the most common cause of fatal sporadic encephalitis occurring in the United States, and although still relatively uncommon (with an estimated incidence of 1 case/million/year), it carries a mortality rate of up to 70 percent in untreated cases. Outside of the neonatal period, disease is almost always caused by HSV-1 and can affect persons of any age. Herpes encephalitis can occur as a primary infection, but many patients have a history of prior HSV infection with detectable antibody titers in acute-phase serum. Only 8/92 encephalitis patients studied by Whitley et al. had HSV isolated from a peripheral site in addition to the brain isolate. Restriction endonuclease patterns were identical for five of the pairs but different in three. The reason for such rare involvement of the brain in HSV infections, which are otherwise so common in the general population, is still unclear.

The clinical illness can begin suddenly or after a flulike illness. Fever, headache and stiff neck, and behavioral changes are common, and most patients will have focal neurologic signs. Findings in the cerebrospinal fluid are quite variable, but elevated protein, pleocytosis, and erythrocytosis, can all be seen. Most cases will eventually demonstrate localized abnormalities by electroencephalography, technetium brain scanning, or computerized axial tomography of the head, but these changes may take days to become detectable. Localization to the temporal lobe is characteristic, but other areas of brain involvement have also been described, and the process can even be patchy and diffuse. Since isolation of HSV from cerebrospinal fluid is rare and noninvasive techniques may not be helpful early in the disease process, brain biopsy is still generally recommended for appropriate histologic and culture diagnosis. Untreated, the disease can run a very rapid course, progressing from lethargy to coma and death. The mortality in biopsy-proven untreated cases is 60 to 80 percent, and more than 90 percent of survivors have significant neurologic sequelae.

Immunocompromised Host

Severe herpes simplex infections can complicate the course of patients with a variety of immunocompromised states. Patients who are HSV seropositive before receiving bone marrow, cardiac, or renal transplants have a reactivation rate of 35 to 85 percent. Many reactivation episodes are asymptomatic, but severe and/or chronic disease may cause significant morbidity in this population, and patients have died from HSV pneumonia. HSV reactivation in patients receiving immunosuppressive therapy for malignancy correlates with suppression of cell-mediated immunity. Similarly, patients with congenital or acquired immunodeficiency syndromes affecting cell-mediated immunity may have severe, persistent infection. Patients with severe combined immunodeficiency, nucleoside phosphorylase deficiency, common variable immunodeficiency, and the newly described acquired immune deficiency syndrome (AIDS), primarily affecting young homosexual males, fall into this category.

Oncogenic Potential

HSV-2 has been associated with squamous cell carcinoma of the cervix, although inconsistencies exist in the data used to support this contention. Evidence centers around the following findings: (1) HSV can transform cells in vitro, (2) antibodies to HSV-2 are found more frequently and in higher titer in patients with cervical carcinoma than in controls, and (3) HSV-2 DNA and mRNA have been detected in some cancer cells. Conflicting results have been reported by different laboratories and may reflect different definition of patient and control groups, different serologic techniques and reagents, and possibly different geographic factors. At this time one can say that there is an association between HSV-2 and cervical carcinoma, but it remains to be proven that a cause-and-effect relationship exists.

Diagnosis

Patients presenting with fever, localized vesicular rash (especially one that involves mucous membranes), and constitutional symptoms should be suspected of having primary HSV infection. Clinical recognition of recurrent disease is made easier if the patient can give a history of previous similar eruptions. Confirmation of the diagnosis, especially in the face of severe illness where antiviral therapy is considered, is most reliably made by virus isolation. Infection of embryonated eggs or experimental animals has become unnecessary in light of the advances made in tissue culture techniques. Several primary cell lines, including rabbit kidney, human amnion, and human embryonic kidney, can be used to cultivate HSV, in addition to continuous human diploid and monkey kidney cell strains. Because of its rapid growth, cytopathic effect due to HSV can be seen in 24 to 48 hours if a large enough inoculum is used. Specimens for culture should be obtained from fresh vesicular lesions, which contain the highest titer of virus, and inoculated onto tissue cultures as soon as possible.

A more rapid bedside procedure, known as the Tzanck preparation, is made by scraping the base of a suspected skin lesion, fixing the specimen with ethanol, and staining with Wright or Giemsa stain. Examination under the microscope will reveal multinucleated giant cells indicative of HSV or varicella-zoster infection. The Papanicolaou stain may also be used to demonstrate intranuclear inclusions, but both of these techniques are less sensitive than is actual virus isolation. Paired acute and convalescent sera may show a rise in neutralizing or complement-fixing antibodies in primary infection but are unreliable in diagnosing recurrent disease. Immunofluorescence has been used to rapidly detect HSV antigen in brain and other tissue specimens but is not as sensitive as tissue culture in detecting small amounts of HSV. Electron microscopy has also been used for rapid diagnosis but suffers from the same insensitivity problem and is unable to differentiate among the herpes group viruses, since thay are morphologically similar.

Treatment

The development of effective antiviral therapy for the treatment of HSV infections has been one of the most important breakthroughs in medical virology. Although supportive care is still an important part of the management of all HSV infections, several antiviral agents have been shown to effectively treat various syndromes associated with this virus.

Idoxuridine

Idoxuridine (5-iodo-2′-deoxyuridine, IUDR) was the first agent shown to be efficacious against HSV. Developed in 1959, this deoxythymidine analog inhibits thymidine kinase and is incorporated into viral and cellular DNA. Its associated myelosuppressive effect makes it too toxic for systemic use, and its primary usefulness has thus been in the topical treatment of dendritic herpes keratitis. Development of in vitro resistance can be easily demonstrated, and lack of clinical response has been noted in several studies. Some patients develop allergic responses to application of the solution. Controlled clinical studies determined that use of idoxuridine is harmful in the treatment of encephalitis due to HSV, and its efficacy in the treatment of skin infections has not been well supported.

Vidarabine

This purine analog was first shown to have anti-HSV activity in 1964 after having been developed as an anticancer agent. Also known as ara-A and adenine arabinoside, the compound is phosphorylated within the cell and, in its triphosphate form, acts as a preferential noncompetitive inhibitor of viral DNA polymerase over host DNA polymerase. It is used topically to treat HSV keratitis and is effective against some IUDR-resistant isolates. Vidarabine has much lower toxicity than IUDR, which enables it to be administered systemically. Multicenter studies using the intravenous form of the drug have demonstrated that it clearly reduces mortality and favorably affects morbidity in patients who have HSV encephalitis or disseminated neonatal HSV infection, although many survivors are still left with significant neurologic sequelae. As with IUDR, there is no benefit from topical application to oral or genital lesions.

Trifluridine

Trifluridine (trifluorothymidine, TFT), is another deoxythymidine analog. First synthesized in 1962 as an anticancer agent, this agent is useful topically in the treatment of herpes keratitis. Its antiviral activity is thought to be a result of direct incorporation into viral DNA. Myelosuppression occurs following systemic administration, and therefore its use is also limited to topical therapy of HSV keratitis. Trifluorothymidine has better efficacy against stromal disease than either IUDR or vidarabine, and it can effectively treat disease caused by some viruses that are resistant to those agents.

Acyclovir

The latest antiherpes agent licensed for use is acyclovir (acycloguanosine, ACV), a deoxyguanosine analog first reported as an antiherpes agent in 1977 by Schaeffer and Elion. Its major advantage is a selective action on HSV-infected cells and consequent low toxicity for normal uninfected host cells. The compound itself is relatively inert, but HSV thymidine kinase, present in infected cells, preferentially phosphorylates acyclovir to its monophosphate form. Cellular thymidine kinase has a much lower affinity for the drug, so this step does not occur to any great extent in uninfected cells. Further phosphorylation to the triphosphate form is accomplished by cellular enzymes, and acyclovir-triphosphate then can act as an inhibitor of, and substrate for, the HSV DNA polymerase and effectively stop viral replication. When topical acyclovir is used for treatment of primary genital infection due to HSV, duration of viral shedding and time to crusting are shorter than in placebo-treated patient with primary disease, but only duration of viral shedding was shortened in patients with recurrent disease. The intravenous form, when used in the treatment of severe genital herpes infections and HSV disease in the compromised host, has an even more dramatic effect on the clinical and virologic course of the disease. An oral preparation is still being clinically tested but has suppressed symptomatic recurrences in immunosuppressed patients who were given the drug for up to 65 days.

Prevention

Avoidance of infection is currently the mainstay of prophylaxis attempts. Neonates and children with extensive areas of eczema should avoid contact with persons having active HSV lesions. Patients with genital HSV infection should abstain from close sexual contact during the time that active lesions are present. Cesarean section is recommended for mothers in labor who have genital lesions, or are known to be virus-positive, if the membranes have not been ruptured for more than 4 hours.

In terms of more specific prevention, prophylactic administration of acyclovir to seropositive bone marrow transplant recipients has been shown to prevent acute reactivation of HSV, although some patients did develop mild disease after cessation of the drug. Attempts at vaccine development have been discouraging to date and raise a number of questions concerning possible teratogenicity, oncogenicity, and effects on latency and recurrent disease. It must be remembered that patients with latent virus that recurs already have detectable antibodies in their serum, which, therefore, can hardly be called protective.

Varicella-Zoster Virus

Infection with varicella-zoster virus (VZV) is an experience most people have before reaching adulthood. Primary infection produces the disease, varicella (or chickenpox), a common childhood disease that is considered a normal part of growing up. Adults and those individuals who are immunosuppressed form a small group at risk of developing a much more serious illness that can be fatal. Individuals who have had prior varicella infection may later develop zoster, which is the illness produced by reactivation of latent VZV.

The distinction between chickenpox and smallpox was first made in 1802 by Heberden. Von Bohan, in 1892, was the first to propose that varicella and zoster were the same infectious agent after observing cases of chickenpox that occurred in close family contacts of zoster patients. The theory that zoster is a manifestation of reactivation of latent varicella virus was expressed by Garland in 1943. Propagation of the virus in tissue culture was accomplished by Weller and co-workers in 1952. This was followed by investigations that show that virus isolates from chickenpox and zoster patients are identical immunologically and morphologically and that the molecular weight of their DNA and restriction endonuclease patterns are the same.

Epidemiology

The only natural hosts for VZV are humans, although an animal model of experimental infection in guinea pigs has been described and may be useful in studying pathogenesis and effect of therapy. Outbreaks of varicella occur worldwide, primarily in late winter and early spring, with transmission occurring by close personal contact. It is assumed that virus is present in the respiratory tract of infected patients, since transmission of disease from an infected person prior to development of a rash has been noted, and epidemiologic studies document high communicability primarily by aerosolized virus. The incubation period is 10 to 23 days, and studies of household outbreaks indicate that 88 percent of the susceptibles will develop disease within 2 weeks of exposure and 96 percent within 1 month. Vesicular fluid from skin lesions contains easily detectable, significant amounts of virus, particularly during the first 3 days of rash, and close contact with this material is also a potential mode of transmission. Susceptible children exposed to a household member with zoster can also develop chickenpox, but the attack rate is much lower.

A much rarer form of transmission can occur during pregnancy. If a woman develops varicella during the first trimester, she may have as much as a 1 in 14 chance of transmitting the infection to the fetus. A spectrum of clinical findings has been described in these infants with congenital varicella syndrome. This is in contrast to those fetuses infected later in pregnancy, who are normal at birth but have zoster as their first manifestation of VZV disease postnatally.

In contrast with varicella, zoster occurs year-round and is generally believed to be the result of activation of latent VZV. It can affect patients of any age but occurs with increased frequency after the fourth decade and in immunosuppressed populations. There is no clear evidence to support the view that zoster can develop as a consequence of exposure to a patient with varicella or zoster. A population study reported by Ragozzino et al. has also disputed the notion that patients with zoster have an increased risk of developing cancer.

Pathogenesis

Because of the lack of good animal models, our understanding of the pathogenesis of VZV infection is based on clinical observations. After first contact with the virus, perhaps via the respiratory tract, a secondary site of replication is probably established within the body. Peripheral blood cell-associated viremia has been documented during the incubation period and during active infection in immunosuppressed children but not in normal children. Presumably the virus spreads via the bloodstream to the skin. Sequential histologic sections taken during the course of varicella infection demonstrate the presence of eosinophilic intranuclear inclusions in endothelial cells that surround small blood vessels in the corium, followed by spread to other cells and the formation of multinucleated cells. The fluid that accumulates between the prickle cell layer and outer epidermis forms the vesicle characteristic of the VZV rash. The lesion evolves as polymorphonuclear leukocytes invade the corium and appear in the vesicular fluid, which then becomes cloudy. Scab formation follows reabsorption of this fluid, and eventually the epidermis desquamates.

The sequence of events involved in the establishment of ganglionic infection is unknown. During active zoster infection, the skin pathology is the same as for varicella, although the lesions are generally confined to a single dermatome. Within the dorsal spinal ganglion corresponding to the distribution of the lesions, intense inflammation can be detected, with hemorrhagic necrosis of nerve cells and destruction of portions of the ganglion. Observation of virus particles in ganglion and perineural cells also adds credence to the theory that VZV becomes latent in the dorsal spinal ganglia following varicella infection and can be activated to travel down sensory nerves and establish infection of the skin. In contrast to HSV, however, the isolation of VZV during this proposed latent state has not been accomplished. It is possible that VZV reactivates periodically, as suggested by a longitudinal serologic study, but is aborted before causing the full constellation of signs recognized as zoster. Support for this concept comes from the occurence of the pain syndrome typical of zoster that is reported by some patients who never develop skin lesions.

Intact cellular immunity is important in preventing reactivation. Thus, immunosuppression due to malignancy, chemotherapy, or both is associated with an increased rate of reactivation. In vitro lymphocyte stimulation responses to VZV antigen wane with advancing age and may contribute to the propensity for VZV reactivation in older individuals.

Clinical Illness

Varicella

Following the incubation period of 10 to 23 days (mean 14.3 days), uncomplicated infection becomes manifest as a vesicular eruption beginning on the scalp and trunk and spreading to the extremities. Children may have an associated fever of 38 to 39C for 2 to 3 days, which parallels the severity of the rash, but they generally feel fairly well during the illness. Macules quickly evolve to papules and superficial vesicles 2 to 3 mm in diameter, appearing in crops that are characteristically in different stages of development. The pruritis that accompanies the vesicle stage can be distressing to both the child and the parents. Mucous membrane lesions can appear in the mouth, conjunctivae, rectum, and vagina, but because of their location, they rupture easily and appear as ulcers. Lesions can continue to appear for up to 1 week and tend to cluster in areas of irritation. Total lesion counts vary considerably from a few to many hundreds, with older children and secondary cases tending to have more lesions. The vesicles differ from smallpox in their superficial nature, the distribution, and the simultaneous existence of different lesion stages.

Varicella in adolescents and adults is generally more severe, and may be preceded by a 1 to 2 day prodrome of fever, malaise, anorexia, and headache. Fever tends to be higher and the rash more profuse than in young children. Primary viral pneumonia, uncommon in children, has been documented in 14 percent of military recruits studied with varicella but was accompanied by clinical signs in only 4 percent. Nonetheless, fatal cases of varicella pneumonia in adults have been described.

Immunosuppressed patients who develop varicella may go on to suffer from progressive varicella, with continued lesion formation into the second week of illness and temperature elevations up to 40 to 41C. Lesions may be more deep-seated than usual, and visceral spread in the form of pneumonia, meningoencephalitis, and hepatitis can be seen. This form of illness occurs in approximately 30 percent of children with leukemia and carries a mortality rate of 20 percent. The overall mortality in children with leukemia who develop varicella is 7 percent.

There are several well-described complications of varicella in normal children, although it should be emphasized that uncomplicated disease with complete recovery is the rule. Acute cerebellitis is the most common neurologic manifestation of varicella and usually occurs at the end of the first week of rash, although it occasionally precedes lesion development. Fulminant encephalitis, occurring in less than 1 of every 1000 cases, has been noted to occur shortly after varicella lesions appear. Some of these cases are now felt to be examples of Reye's syndrome, which has been epidemiologically associated with varicella infection. Less common neurologic manifestations include aseptic meningitis, Guillain–Barré syndrome, and myelitis. Bleeding disorders, such as Henoch–Schönlein purpura and purpura fulminans, may occur 1 to 2 weeks into the illness. Secondary skin infections are usually due to staphylococci or streptococci and, prior to antibiotic availability, served as foci for systemic infection.

Congenital and Neonatal Varicella

Women who have varicella during the first trimester may transmit the infection to their infants. The spectrum of manifestations of the congenital varicella syndrome includes cicatricial lesions of an extremity in a dermatomal distribution, growth retardation, microphthalmia, cataracts, chorioretinitis, deafness, and cortical atrophy of the brain.

If primary maternal varicella infection occurs within 4 days prior to or after delivery, the attack rate of infection for the infant is about 20 percent. Mortality in these infants, however, is about 35 percent because they cannot control viral replication like an older child. Transmission of maternal IgG antibody across the placenta will partially protect the newborn infant, who will then develop only mild infection.

Zoster

Radicular pain is often the first manifestation of zoster, particularly in adults. The rash appears morphologically similar to varicella, but its unilateral distribution covers only one to three dermatomes. New lesions may appear for several days, and occasionally a few may be found outside the original dermatomes. Thoracic dermatome involvement is most common. Involvement of the ophthalmic division of the fifth cranial nerve becomes a particular problem in elderly populations, where it occurs more frequently than in the young. Complications such as iritis, conjunctivitis, keratitis, and ocular muscle paralysis can occur. Other reported complications include Bell's palsy and the Ramsay Hunt syndrome.

Patients receiving radiation therapy or organ transplants and those with malignancies, especially Hodgkin's disease and chronic lymphocytic leukemia, have a higher incidence of zoster. From 24 to 50 percent of the immunosuppressed population develop disseminated zoster, which is heralded by the onset of new lesions in a generalized distribution beginning about 1 week after the localized lesions appear. Visceral involvement in the form of hepatitis, pneumonitis, and occasionally encephalitis occurs in 10 to 20 percent, and the mortality rate in this population is 0 to 3 percent. Postherpetic neuralgia is a frequent and quite disabling sequela of zoster in both normal and immunosuppressed patients and may last for months following lesion healing. Studies addressing this problem have defined the term in such a variety of ways that the exact incidence of this complication is unknown. It occurs more after age 60 and can be severe enough to prevent sleep.

Diagnosis

Typical cases of varicella and zoster can usually be diagnosed on clinical grounds. An exposure history to chickenpox is often possible to elicit in patients suspected of having varicella, but patients with zoster, particularly the elderly, may not be able to remember having chickenpox in the past. Herpes simplex can occasionally present in a zosteriform distribution, and disseminated disease due to either HSV or VZV may be difficult to differentiate. In these cases, culture of vesicular fluid will correctly identify the causative agent. Human diploid fibroblasts support the growth of VZV, and isolation is best accomplished if lesions are cultured within 3 days of onset. The lability of the virus requires that samples be kept at 4C and transported promptly to the laboratory or inoculated directly onto the cell culture. Viremia may be detectable by culture of white blood cells in patients with progressive varicella or disseminated zoster. Detection of VZV antigen in vesicle fluid is also possible using counterimmunoelectrophoresis (CIE).

Acute and convalescent serum will show a rise in titer of antibody to VZV if further confirmation is needed. The complement-fixation (CF) test is adequate for this purpose but not sensitive enough to pick up low levels of antibody for determination of susceptibility. Some of the more sensitive, but not yet generally available, serologic tests include fluorescent antibody to membrane antigen (FAMA), immune adherence hemagglutination antibody (IAHA), enzyme-linked immunosorbent assay (ELISA), radioimmunoassay (RIA), immunoperoxidase antibody (IPA), and complement-enhancing neutralizing antibody.

Treatment

Uncomplicated varicella is a benign disease that requires only supportive care. Drying lotions, such as calamine, can reduce pruritis, and effects of scratching can be minimized by cutting the fingernails. The use of aspirin in varicella should be avoided because it has been epidemiologically associated with an increased risk of developing Reye's syndrome.

Several agents have been tried in the treatment of varicella in immunosuppressed patients, although none have yet been approved for this indication. High-dose interferon diminished the duration of new lesion formation and reduced the incidence of serious dissemination compared to placebo in a study of children with cancer. Vidarabine (ara-A) has also been shown to decrease new lesion formation, mean daily lesion counts, and duration of fever, and it prevented visceral disease when given within 3 days of onset. A collaborative study of the effect of acyclovir on chickenpox in immunosuppressed children indicated that administration of this antiviral agent also prevented visceral dissemination when given early in the course of the disease.

Treatment of zoster in normal patients is mainly limited to control of the accompanying pain. Steroids given early in the course have been shown to significantly reduce postherpetic neuralgia. A placebo-controlled trial of intravenous acyclovir found that the rate of healing was significantly increased and the period of pain was shortened by this agent.

Studies of immunosuppressed patients with zoster have shown that high-dose interferon decreased the time of new lesion formation, the incidence of dissemination, postherpetic neuralgia, and visceral complications. Vidarabine therapy also has been shown to decrease dissemination, visceral complications, and rate of cutaneous dissemination. The duration of post-herpetic neuralgia was diminished although the frequency of this complication was the same as that seen in the placebo group. Therapy with acyclovir has produced similar results.

Prevention

Since uncomplicated varicella is usually a mild illness, attempts at preventing it are not thought to be worthwhile. The focus has been in preventing infection with VZV in the immunocompromised patients who can suffer more significant morbidity and occasional mortality from this virus. Children incubating varicella should not be electively admitted to the hospital, where contact with immunocompromised patients may result in transmission of disease. If hospitalization is unavoidable, patients with varicella and zoster should be kept in strict isolation.

Passive immunization has been shown to be effective in modifying or preventing illness. Initial studies of immune serum globulin (ISG) showed that the severity of disease could be diminished if administration occurred within 72 hours of exposure. Testing with the high-titered, convalescent, IgG fraction of plasma from recuperating zoster patients, known as "zoster immune globulin" (ZIG), prevented disease in healthy children and modified illness in susceptible immunosuppressed patients. ZIG has effectively prevented severe varicella in the susceptible newborn whose mother developed varicella within 4 days of delivery. Outdated, high-titer normal donor plasma has been used to make varicella-zoster immune globulin (VZIG) and is available for use in high-risk cases. It should be administered within 72 hours of exposure or delivery for optimal benefit.

Experimental live attenuated VZV vaccine has been developed in Japan, which results in no morbidity in serosusceptible normal children and adults. It is immunogenic, and antibodies can be detected for as long as 2 years. When this vaccine is given to immunosuppressed children, a few will have mild rash and will rarely transmit virus to susceptible household contacts. Protective neutralizing antibody levels develop and predictably persist in those who develop rash. A proportion of these patients lose detectable antibodies with time. Thus far, these children have been protected from severe varicella, but reinfection, as manifested by antibody rise after exposure, is fairly common. Longitudinal studies with the vaccine are in progress.

Cytomegalovirus

This member of the group of herpesviruses is another ubiquitous agent and is responsible for a broad spectrum of disease affecting humans in many different clinical settings. While the great majority of cytomegalovirus (CMV) infections are inapparent, this virus is now known to be the most common cause of congenital viral infection, an etiologic agent of the mononucleosis syndrome, and a feared pathogen in post bone marrow transplant patients.

The first description of probable congenital CMV disease was published by Rippert in 1904. In examining sections of kidney from a stillborn child, he noted large protozoan-like cells. In 1907, Lowenstein described intranuclear and intracytoplastic inclusions in the parotid glands of infants, and over the next 25 years, further case reports of apparent cytomegalic inclusion disease appeared in the literature. Isolation of murine cytomegalovirus was accomplished by Smith in 1954 and followed by the independent isolation of human CMV by Smith, Rowe, and Weller. Since that time, the development of serologic tests has further enabled investigators to define the importance of this virus as a cause of human infection.

Epidemiology

Serologic studies using the complement-fixation (CF) test have shown that the prevalence of CMV antibodies in adults is 40 to 100 percent depending on socioeconomic conditions. CMV is found worldwide and has no seasonal predilection. Age at CMV antibody acquisition is dependent on the mode of transmission. Population studies have shown that serologic conversion rates increase in early childhood, with a peak at 1 to 2 years. A second slow increase in the seroconversion rate occurs in adults from 16 to 50 years, although detection of virus shedding is not as common after the age of 30 years.

Several methods of CMV transmission have been described and result in different manifestations of infection. Intrauterine infection occurs in 0.05 to 2 percent of all live births, as documented by infant viruria shortly after birth. The neonatal infection rate following primary CMV in mothers during pregnancy is high, and 23 percent of infants born to women with seroconversion during pregnancy have stigmata of congenital CMV infection at birth. Numerically, more babies with intrauterine infection are born to seropositive mothers with secondary or reactivation infection. These infants are less likely to be symptomatic at birth than those infected during primary infection.

Perinatal CMV infection of an infant is much more common than intrauterine infection, occurring in 3 to 10 percent of babies born in various populations. In contrast to intrauterine CMV, viruria is not detectable until 4 to 8 weeks of age. Several prospective studies of pregnant women have documented an increased rate of cervical CMV excretion during the latter stages of pregnancy. Infants born to mothers who excrete virus in the third trimester or postpartum have a higher infection rate than those born to non-CMV excreters, suggesting that infection during the birth process probably occurs. Some immune mothers have also been shown to excrete CMV into breast milk. Infants who are breastfed by these mothers have a higher infection rate than their bottle-fed counterparts. A recent day-care center study has suggested that toddlers in this setting may acquire CMV infection from children who orally excrete the virus. CMV was recovered from toys mouthed by children known to be oral excreters, and the infection rate was highest in the 1 to 2 year age group, corresponding to the age where the oral excretion rate and oral contact between children was highest.

Several pieces of evidence point to venereal transmission as another mode of CMV acquisition. The virus has been isolated from semen and secretions from the female genitourinary tract. Multiple sex partners are associated with higher cervical infection rates in women, and homosexual males have a higher urinary CMV isolation rate and seropositivity rate than do heterosexual males. Cases of CMV mononucleosis transmitted by sexual contact have been reported.

Blood transfusions have also been implicated as a source of CMV. A postperfusion syndrome of fever, splenomegaly, and atypical lymphocytosis was noted in patients following extracorporeal cardiopulmonary bypass surgery for open heart surgery and linked to CMV. Susceptible infants of seronegative mothers who receive blood from seropositive donors are also at high risk and can develop severe and sometimes fatal infection. Most posttransfusion infections outside of the neonatal period are asymptomatic. The risk of infection is about 3 percent per unit transfused and greatest if donors are seropositive and recipients seronegative. CMV can infect peripheral blood leukocytes, but isolation of virus from donor blood has not been successful.

CMV infection occurs in most patients about 2 months (range 1 to 4 months) following bone marrow or renal transplantation. There is some evidence that the donor kidney may be a source of primary CMV following renal transplantation, although isolation of the virus from this organ has not been possible. Cytotoxic drug regimens, which are part of the care of transplant patients, have been associated with development of virus shedding in seropositive patients, presumably on the basis of depression of cell-mediated immunity. The use of antithymocyte globulin, cyclosporin A, and cyclophosphamide has been particularly associated with an increased incidence of viremia and CMV illness. Graft-vs.-host (GVH) reactions in bone marrow transplant recipients are also associated with a higher incidence of CMV infection. Patients with malignancy and undergoing chemotherapy form another high-risk group.

Pathogenesis

Primary infection, as mentioned above, can be acquired through the bloodstream or through presumed oral, venereal, and respiratory routes. Epithelial cells in the oropharnyx may serve as a primary focus, with spread to lymphoid tissue and leukocytes finally producing viremia. Patients with CMV mononucleosis often have virus isolated from peripheral leukocytes for up to 3 weeks following infection, and persistence for as long as 3 months has been documented.

The typical cytopathology seen with CMV infection is the presence of large giant cells with intranuclear inclusions. These inclusions have been shown to contain virions and specific viral antigens. In young children the salivary glands, particularly the parotid, are a site of localization, but this has not been demonstrated in older children and adults. Virus shedding occurs over prolonged periods of time from throat, breast milk, feces, semen, and cervix in spite of the presence of antibody to CMV. After active shedding ceases, the virus presumably enters into a latent state, possibly in the leukocytes, and can be reactivated on a periodic basis under a number of different conditions.

Clinical Illness

Congenital Cytomegalic Inclusion Disease

Twenty percent of all infants with congenital CMV infection are symptomatic at birth and may manifest hepatosplenomegaly, jaundice, petechiae, microcephaly, chorioretinitis, and cerebral calcifications. Lethargy, respiratory distress, and seizures can occur shortly after birth, often followed by death in days to a few weeks. This severe form of disease is found in 25 percent of symptomatic infants (5 percent of all infants born with congenital infection). The other 75 percent of the symptomatic infants (15 percent of the total born with congenital infection) manifest psychomotor retardation, hepatomegaly, or deafness. The remaining 80 percent, detected by viruria within 1 week after birth, are clinically asymptomatic at birth, but over time, 5 to 20 percent of this group may manifest evidence of central nervous system involvement, such as sensorineural hearing loss and school failure problems.

Perinatal CMV

The vast majority of infants who acquire CMV in the perinatal period are asymptomatic. Pneumonitis and manifestations of the mononucleosis syndrome may be seen occasionally, with onset during the first 3 months of life, but subtle long-term CNS sequelae have not yet been detected. Infection in the neonatal period via blood transfusion, however, can be serious and sometimes fatal.

CMV Mononucleosis

This syndrome may occur in children but is most commonly seen in adults. Fever is the dominant symptom, accompanied by an absolute lymphocytosis with atypical lymphocytes that are detectable within 1 to 2 weeks of onset of fever. Unlike EBV-induced mononucleosis, tonsillopharyngitis, splenomegaly, and lymphadenopathy are uncommon. Mildly elevated liver function tests are present but usually not associated with severe hepatitis or jaundice. Prospective studies of mononucleosis patients have documented that CMV infection is responsible for about 45 percent of heterophil-negative cases. The clinical picture of posttransfusion CMV mononucleosis, which occurs 3 to 4 weeks after transfusion, is the same as that described for spontaneous CMV mononucleosis. Associated findings that are occasionally observed include interstitial pneumonitis, hepatitis (with or without granulomas), meningoencephalitis, Guillain–Barré syndrome, myocarditis, hemolytic anemia, and thrombocytopenia.

CMV in Immunocompromised Patients

Primary and reactivation CMV infections are commonly manifest about 2 months posttransplantation, affecting nearly all renal transplant recipients and half of the bone marrow recipients. Most of these renal patients (50 to 60 percent) have asymptomatic infection with CMV, 40 to 50 percent will have a self-limited nonspecific syndrome, and 2 to 3 percent develop disseminated disease and death. CMV can cause renal disease, with diminished renal function. This should be carefully distinguished from rejection because immunosuppressive therapy should be decreased, not increased. Symptomatic CMV infection is more likely to occur in primarily infected patients than in those who are initially seropositive. Interstitial pneumonitis can be a rapidly fatal process in transplant recipients. In bone marrow transplant recipients, the incidence of CMV pneumonia is about 20 percent, and mortality is more than 80 percent.

Patients with leukemia or lymphoma, especially children, are at high risk for acquiring CMV infection. The rate of seroconversion has been related to the number of chemotherapeutic agents used. Clinical syndromes in this population include pneumonia, fever and rash, gastrointestinal involvement, and myocarditis. In both the posttransplant and malignancy groups, CMV has frequently been isolated with other agents. Its role as a copathogen in the recently described acquired immune deficiency syndrome (AIDS) is also currently under study.

Diagnosis

The manifestations of CMV disease are not distinctive enough to make a clinical diagnosis without laboratory confirmation. Isolation of the virus is the most specific means of making a diagnosis, and cytopathic effect can be detected as early as 3 to 4 days postinoculation with a large inoculum, although sometimes 1 to 2 weeks are required. Histologic examination of lung biopsy tissue will often reveal the presence of cytomegalic cells, primarily in the alveolar and bronchial epithelium, in patients with CMV pneumonitis.

Complement-fixing antibodies can be detected in immunosuppressed patients undergoing clinical CMV infection but are not sensitive enough to reliably diagnose perinatal and cervical infection. Serologic tests with increased sensitivity include indirect fluorescent antibody (IFA) and anticomplement immunofluorescent (ACIF) tests.

Treatment

Significantly less progress has been made in the development of effective therapy for CMV infections than for either HSV or VZV. Many antiviral agents have been tested on the more severe forms of disease, but none has yet been found to be clinically useful. Human leukocyte interferon has been used to treat congenital CMV and infection in renal and bone marrow transplant recipients. There was no clinical benefit for any patients except for a delay of virus excretion in the renal transplant group. Initial treatment and prophylaxis studies of recombinant α-$_2$ interferon in bone marrow transplant recipients demonstrated that it did not prevent CMV infection or clinically benefit the patients. Therapy with cytosine arabinoside (ara-C), vidarabine (ara-A), idoxuridine (IUDR), and acyclovir (ACV), including combination studies of vidarabine or acyclovir with human leukocyte interferon, has been unsuccessful to date.

Prevention

Efforts at vaccine development have been targeted at preventing the most serious forms of CMV illness—primary infection in the immunosuppressed and congenital CMV infection, which is the cause of severe neurologic sequelae in more than 5000 children born each year in the United States. Since reactivation occurs in the presence of specific antibody, the theoretical effect of vaccine on already seropositive patients should be nil. Concern exists over questions of potential oncogenicity and effect of vaccine on the latent state and reactivation potential of CMV, but development has continued and human trials are currently in progress.

Two vaccine strains have been studied, the AD169 and Towne 125 strains. Both have been shown to be immunogenic as defined by seroconversion, although titers diminish over time, and there has been no evidence of persistent infection. Vaccination with Towne 125, however, failed to protect seronegative renal transplant recipients who received kidneys from seropositive donors. Further studies are currently underway.

Epstein–Barr Virus

Epstein–Barr virus (EBV), like its fellow members of the human herpesvirus group, is a common cause of infection worldwide. Infection in early childhood is largely asymptomatic, but adolescents and young adults often develop the disease, infectious mononucleosis. Patients undergoing posttransplant immunosuppression or those with various congenital immunodeficiency syndromes may develop more severe disease, and reports of the development of fatal polyclonal lymphomas associated with the presence of EBV genome and antigens in tumor tissue are increasing. EBV has now been firmly associated with African Burkitt lymphoma and nasopharyngeal carcinoma.

Although EBV is the most recently recognized member of the human herpesviruses, clinical descriptions of infectious mononucleosis date back to 1889, when Emil Pfeiffer reported the characteristic findings of Drüsenfieber, (glandular) fever, including fever, adenopathy, sore throat, and occasional hepatosplenomegaly. In 1920, Sprunt and Evans named the disease and described the characteristic mononuclear leukocytosis. Three years later, Downey and McKinley definitively described the morphologic appearance of atypical lymphocytes in infectious mononucleosis. Paul and Bunnell discovered the heterophil antibody in 1932, which, with Davidsohn's addition of guinea pig kidney and beef red blood cell absorption, enabled clinicians to make a serologic diagnosis.

In 1958 Burkitt described a malignant tumor involving the jaw and abdomen that occurred in children of central and western Africa. Because the distribution of the tumor seemed to be affected by climate, a search for an infectious agent carried by an anthropod vector was begun. Culture of the tumor cells was accomplished by Epstein and Barr in 1964, and electron microscopy of these cells revealed the presence of viral particles typical of the herpes group. Henle and Henle developed an indirect immunofluorescent antibody test for EBV antibody in 1966 that helped to define epidemiologically the importance of this virus. When their technician developed infectious mononucleosis in 1968 after working with Burkitt tumor tissue, serial examination of her serum showed the development of EBV antibodies, her lymphocytes were able to be grown in tissue culture, and EBV antigen was detected in the lymphocytes. The link with EBV and infectious mononucleosis has been subsequently confirmed.

Epidemiology

Seroepidemiologic studies indicate that EBV infections occur in all populations, with age of acquisition determined by socioeconomic factors. Seroconversion has been documented shortly after birth in New Guinea, Polynesia, and Ghana, where poor hygiene and low socioeconomic conditions predominate, while the more industrialized populations, such as England, Sweden, and the United States, tend to delay their encounter with this virus until adolescence and adulthood. Increasing use of day-care centers may change this pattern, however, as seen with CMV. EBV antibodies can be found in 90 to 95 percent of most adult populations.

When primary EBV exposure occurs early in childhood, infection most often goes unrecognized. Seroconversion has been documented following nonspecific febrile illness, upper respiratory infection, pharyngotonsillitis, rash, lymphadenopathy, hepatosplenomegaly, and pneumonia. Sometimes infectious mononucleosis-like illness occurs in young children, but this presentation becomes much more common in college-age populations, where 28 to 74 percent of students with documented seroconversion have associated mononucleosis. Throat washings from acutely ill patients yield EBV, and excretion may continue intermittently for months after all signs of illness have disappeared. Cultures of throat washings from 10 to 20 percent of healthy seropositive adults who have no history of mononucleosis yield low titers of EBV, indicating that intermittent excretion occurs even after clinically inapparent infection. This helps to explain why only 6 percent of patients with mononucleosis can report exposure to another case of mononucleosis. EBV has been isolated from saliva, parotid gland secretions, and B lymphocytes but not from other sources of transmissions, such as feces, urine, or the genital tract. Intimate oral contact is thus felt to be the primary mode of transmission. Infection via blood transfusions and bone marrow has been reported but occurs much less frequently than CMV-induced posttransfusion mononucleosis. The virus does not seem to be very contagious, since follow-up studies of susceptible college roommates of mononucleosis patients found that the risk of infection was no greater than in the general population. A family study of EBV transmission in households following diagnosis of a child with infectious mononucleosis found evidence of spread in 20 percent, with an incubation period of 4 to 6 weeks.

Pathogenesis

Since saliva seems to be the probable mode of transmission, it is thought that the virus attaches to cells in the oropharynx, perhaps in the parotid glands, where it is able to replicate. Bloodstream invasion occurs at some point, with the ensuing infection of B lymphocytes and dissemination through the lymphoreticular systems. During acute clinical disease, 0.005 to 0.5 percent of circulating mononuclear cells have been found to contain EBV. The polyclonal activation of B cells by EBV is accompanied by production of antigens that are expressed by the cell. Actively proliferating T cells belonging to the B suppressor/cytotoxic subset then appear, accounting for most of the atypical lymphocytes seen on peripheral smears taken from patients with infectious mononucleosis.

Histologic examination of the enlarged lymph nodes accompanying mononucleosis reveals enlarged, active lymphoid follicles and germinal centers but an intact reticular framework. The spleen can be enlarged two to three times its normal size, and blast cells are seen throughout the red pulp. Tonsils, lung, liver, heart, kidneys, adrenals, skin, and central nervous system can also be involved with focal mononuclear infiltrates. The host's antibody response to EBV infection forms the basis of laboratory diagnosis.

EBV remains latent in the blood, lymphoid tissue, and throat of individuals who have been infected and is reactivated, as detected by intermittent oral shedding, by as yet undefined mechanisms. The importance of cellular immune mechanisms has been suggested by a higher prevalence of EBV excretion in patients with malignancy and those receiving immunosuppressive therapy.

Clinical Illness

Infectious Mononucleosis

Infectious mononucleosis is the most commonly recognized manifestation of EBV infection. This is a disease primarily seen in adolescents and young adults, although cases may occasionally be seen in young children and the elderly, and the spectrum of illness is very broad. Onset of disease can be abrupt or heralded by a prodrome of chills, sweats, anorexia, or malaise. The classic clinical triad of sore throat, which can be extremely severe, fever, and lymphadenopathy is often accompanied by hepatosplenomegaly. Fever may be as high as 40C and usually resolves in 1 to 2 weeks. Tonsillopharyngitis is accompanied by thick exudate in about half of the patients, and palatal petechiae can occasionally be seen. The lymphadenopathy occurs in over 90 percent of patients and is usually symmetrical, involving the posterior cervical chain. Anterior cervical, submandibular, axillary, and inguinal node involvement can also be present. Adenopathy usually subsides in days to weeks depending on the severity of the illness. Splenomegaly is maximal in the second week and is detectable in half of the patients with mononucleosis if it is looked for regularly during the course of illness. Hepatomegaly occurs in 10 to 15 percent of patients, with associated mild elevations in hepatic cellular enzymes, but only 5 percent of patients will develop jaundice. Various forms of skin rash may also be seen in 5 percent of patients. If, for some other reason, individuals are given ampicillin during the course of their illness, more than 90 percent will develop a pruritic maculopapular eruption. Although the exact mechanism is not known, this usually does not imply an allergic response to penicillin.

The vast majority of patients will recover uneventfully, but occasional individuals may exhibit complications. Splenic rupture, heralded by abdominal pain, most commonly occurs in the second or third week of illness. This dramatic but rare complication is often preceded by trauma and has fostered recommendations against contact sports and vigorous palpation of the spleen during the first weeks of illness. Neurologic complications occur in less than 1 percent of patients and can present as encephalitis, meningitis, Guillain–Barré syndrome, myelitis, Reye's syndrome, and cranial nerve palsies. Autoimmune hemolytic anemia is noted in 0.5 to 3 percent of patients, with hemolysis becoming apparent after the second week of illness. Thrombocytopenia is common but only rarely severe. Pericarditis and myocarditis have been reported, and serologic evidence of acute EBV infection has been found in children with pneumonia, some of whom had evidence of infection with other pathogens. Persistent infection with EBV producing illness lasting longer than 1 year has been described in several patients presenting with nonspecific malaise, fever, and weight loss.

EBV in Immunosuppressed Patients

Severe and sometimes fatal infection with EBV has been described in several groups of patients with underlying immunodeficiencies. The X-linked recessive lymphoproliferative syndrome (XLP) has been described in several kindreds and is associated with an extreme susceptibility to serious EBV infection. Fatal EBV disease occurs in 40 to 50 percent, 15 to 30 percent have acquired variable immunodeficiency, and 40 percent develop lymphoreticular malignancies. A functional T cell defect and deficiency of natural killer (NK) cell activity have been demonstrated. A non-X-linked form has been described in a family where three siblings developed severe infectious mononucleosis associated with diminished NK cell activity. Renal transplant recipients have occasionally been reported to develop polymorphic diffuse B cell hyperplasias and polymorphic B cell lymphomas. EBV genome has been detected in tumor cells of patients with serologic evidence of primary or reactivated EBV infection.

Burkitt's Lymphoma and Nasopharyngeal Carcinoma

Several lines of evidence point to the association of EBV to African Burkitt's lymphoma and nasopharyngeal carcinoma. EBV genome has been detected in the tumors, tumor cells express EBV-associated nuclear antigen (EBNA), and patients have high titers to EBV antibodies. Salivary IgA antibody to EBV viral capsid antigen is currently being used as a screening tool to detect early nasopharyngeal carcinoma in China, where the frequency of this tumor is very high.

Diagnosis

Because infection with EBV produces such a broad range of clinical illness, the diagnosis is usually based on laboratory findings. The hematologic picture is often the first clue, with 70 percent of patients having an absolute lymphocytosis at presentation. Atypical lymphocytes are not specific for EBV infection, but at the height of lymphocytosis, they account for about 30 percent of the differential count. Some patients may have none while others have up to 90 percent of their total lymphocyte count made up of these large cells with lobulated nuclei and vacuolated, basophilic cytoplasm. Neutropenia and thrombocytopenia are common.

Heterophil antibodies are present in 90 percent of adult cases at some point during the illness, usually peaking at 2 to 3 weeks. Children in the 2 to 5 year group develop detectable heterophil antibodies when they present with classic infectious mononucleosis, but since this is an unusual manifestation of disease in this age group, the majority of children will not have a positive test.

Immunofluorescent tests for EBV-specific antibodies are used in heterophil-negative and atypical cases to confirm EBV infections. Antibodies to viral capsid antigen (VCA) arise early and are detectable in virtually all patients. IgG VCA persists for life, while IgM VCA lasts only 4 to 8 weeks, making it a more specific indicator of acute infection. There are two types of antibody to early antigen (EA). Anti-D diffusely stains both the nuclei and cytoplasm of infected cells and is detected in 70 percent of patients with infectious mononucleosis. It persists for 3 to 6 months following infection and is also detected in patients with nasopharyngeal carcinoma. Anti-R stains only aggregates in the cytoplasm and is seen in atypical, protracted cases of mononucleosis and in patients with African Burkitt's lymphoma. Antibodies to Epstein–Barr nuclear antigen (EBNA) appear 3 to 4 weeks after infection and persist for life, as do antibodies to soluble complement-fixing antigen (anti-S) and neutralizing antibodies. Isolation of EBV is not routinely available because of the need for specific laboratory methods involving cultivation of lymphocytes and antigen detection. Throat washings and lymphocytes yield virus in 80 to 90 percent of patients with infectious mononucleosis in an experimental laboratory. EBV antigen detection in lymphocytes will become more practical as labeled specific antibodies or probes become available.

Treatment

Infectious mononucleosis is generally a self-limited disease, and treatment is limited to supportive measures. Bed rest during the acute stage is advocated, and contact sports should be avoided for the first 2 to 3 weeks. Fever and sore throat can usually be relieved by aspirin or acetaminophen. Patients with severe disease manifest by impending airway obstruction, hemolytic anemia, thrombocytopenia, and progressive neurologic involvement may be treated with corticosteroids, but this is not felt to be necessary in mild cases. The use of steroids has been shown to decrease the duration of fever, and response is usually prompt.

EBV is inhibited in vitro by vidarabine, phosphonoacetic acid, and acyclovir. Clinical trials of acyclovir for use in the treatment of infectious mononucleosis, the X-linked recessive lymphoproliferative syndrome, and posttransplant EBV-associated lymphomas are currently in progress.

Prevention

Patients with infectious mononucleosis need not be isolated, since intimate contact is necessary for disease transmission. Immunization has been considered, but the problem of potential oncogenicity will be difficult to overcome unless purified polypeptides with immunogenic properties can be developed.

FURTHER READING

HERPES SIMPLEX VIRUS

Allen WP, Rapp F: Concept review of genital herpes vaccines. J Infect Dis 145:413, 1982

Arvin AM, Pollard RB, Rasmussen LE, et al.: Cellular and humoral immunity in the pathogenesis of recurrent herpes viral infections in patients with lymphoma. J Clin Invest 65:869, 1980

Bastian FO, Rabson AS, Yu CL, et al.: Herpesvirus hominis: Isolation from human trigeminal ganglion. Science 178:306, 1972

Binder PA: Herpes simplex keratitis. Surv Ophthalmol 21:313, 1977

Cook ML, Bastone B, Stevens JG: Evidence that neurons harbor latent herpes simplex virus. Infect Immun 9:946, 1974

Corey L: The diagnosis and treatment of genital herpes. JAMA 248:1041, 1982

Corey L, Nahmias AJ, Guinan ME, et al.: A trial of topical acyclovir in genital herpes simplex virus infections. N Engl J Med 306:1313, 1982

Hanshaw JB, Dudgeon JA: Herpes simplex infection of the fetus and newborn. In Major Problems in Clinical Pediatrics. Viral Diseases of the Fetus and Newborn, Philadelphia, Saunders, 1978, vol. 17

Nahmias AJ, Roizman B: Infection with herpes simplex viruses 1 and 2. N Engl J Med 289:667, 719, 781, 1973

Nahmias AJ, Dowdle WR, Schinazi RF (eds): The Human Herpes Viruses: An Interdisciplinary Perspective. New York, Elsevier, 1981

NIAID Collaborative Antiviral Study: Adenine arabinoside—therapy of biopsy-proven herpes simplex encephalitis. N Engl J Med 297:289, 1977

Nilsen AE, Aasen T, Halsos AM, et al.: Efficacy of oral acyclovir in the treatment of initial and recurrent genital herpes. Lancet 2:571, 1982

Openshaw H, Puga A, Notkins AL: Herpes simplex virus infection in sensory ganglia: Immune control, latency and reactivation. Fed Proc 38:2660, 1979

Rawls WE, Garfield CH, Seth P, et al.: Serological and epidemiologic considerations of the role of herpes simplex virus type 2 in cervical cancer. Cancer Res 36:829, 1976

Reeves WC, Corey L, Adams HG, et al.: Risk of recurrence after first episodes of genital herpes. N Engl J Med 305:315, 1981

Saral R, Burns WH, Laskin OL, et al.: Acyclovir prophylaxis of herpes simplex virus infections: A randomized double-blind, controlled trial in bone marrow transplant recipients. N Engl J Med 305:63, 1981

Spruance SL, Overall JC, Kern ER, et al.: The natural history of recurrent herpes simplex labialis: Implications for antiviral therapy. N Engl J Med 297:69, 1977

Stevens JG: Latent herpes simplex virus and the nervous system. Curr Top Microbiol Immunol 70:31, 1975

Whitley RJ, Nahmias AJ, Soong S-J, et al.: Vidarabine therapy of neonatal herpes simplex virus infection. Pediatrics 66:495, 1980

Whitley RJ, Nahmias AJ, Visintine AM, et al.: The natural history of herpes simplex virus infection of mother and newborn. Pediatrics 66:489, 1980

Whitley RJ, Soong S-J, Hirsch MS, et al.: Herpes simplex encephalitis: Vidarabine therapy and diagnostic problems. N Engl J Med 304:313, 1981

VARICELLA-ZOSTER VIRUS

Arbeter AM, Starr SE, Wiebel RE, et al.: Live attenuated varicella vaccine: Immunization of healthy children with the OKA strain. J Pediatr 100:886, 1982

Arvin AM, Kushner JH, Feldman S, et al.: Human leukocyte interferon for the treatment of varicella in children with cancer. N Engl J Med 306:761, 1982

Bastian FO, Rabson AS, Yee CL, et al.: Herpesvirus varicellae: Isolated from human dorsal root ganglia. Arch Pathol 97:331, 1974

Burgoon CF, Burgoon JS, Baldridge GD: Natural history of herpes zoster. JAMA 164:265, 1975

Burke BL, Steele RW, Beard OW: Immune responses to varicella zoster in the aged. Arch Intern Med 142:291, 1982

Brunell PA: Zoster in infancy: Failure to maintain virus latency following intrauterine infection. J Pediatr 98:71, 1981

Brunell PA, Ross A, Miller LH, et al.: Prevention of varicella by varicella zoster immune globulin. N Engl J Med 280:1191, 1969

Brunell PA, Shehab Z, Geiser C, et al.: Administration of live varicella vaccine to children with leukaemia. Lancet 2:1069, 1982

Eaglstein WH, Katz R, Brown JA: The effects of early corticosteroid therapy on the skin eruption and pain of herpes zoster. JAMA 211:1681, 1970

Feldman S, Hughes WT, Daniel CB: Varicella in children with cancer—seventy-seven cases. Pediatrics 56:388, 1975

Feldman S, Hughes WT, Kim HY: Herpes zoster in children with cancer. Am J Dis Child 126:178, 1973

Gordon JE: Chickenpox: An epidemiologic review. Am J Med Sci 244:362, 1962

Merigan TC, Rand KH, Pollard RB, et al.: Human leukocyte interferon for the treatment of herpes zoster in patients with cancer. N Engl J Med 298:981, 1978

Orenstein WA, Heymann DL, Ellis RJ, et al.: Prophylaxis of varicella in high-risk children: Dose-response effect of zoster immune globulin. J Pediatr 98:368, 1981

Peterslund NA, Seyer-Hansen K, Ipsen J, et al.: Acyclovir in herpes zoster. Lancet 2:827, 1981

Ragozzino MW, Melton JL, Kurland LT, et al.: Risk of cancer after herpes zoster: A population-based study. N Engl J Med 307:393, 1982

Steele RW, Myers MG, Vincent MM: Transfer factor for the prevention of varicella zoster infection in childhood leukemia. N Engl J Med 303:355, 1980

Takahashi M, Otsuka T, Okuno Y, et al.: Live vaccine used to prevent the spread of varicella in children in hospital. Lancet 2:1288, 1974

Weller TH: Serial propagation in vitro of agents producing inclusion bodies deriving from varicella and herpes zoster. Proc Soc Exp Biol Med 83:340, 1953

Whitley RJ, Chien LT, Dolin R, et al.: Adenine arabinoside therapy of herpes zoster in the immunosuppressed. N Engl J Med 294:1193, 1976

Whitley RJ, Hilty M, Haynes R, et al.: Vidarabine therapy of varicella in immunosuppressed patients. J Pediatr 101:125, 1982

Whitley RJ, Soong S-J, Dolin R, et al.: Early vidarabine therapy to control the complications of herpes zoster in immunosuppressed patients. N Engl J Med 307:971, 1982

CYTOMEGALOVIRUS

Drew WL, Mintz L, Miner RC, et al.: Prevalence of cytomegalovirus infection in homosexual men. J Infect Dis 143:188, 1981

Evans AS (ed): The risk factors of cytomegalovirus infection transmitted by blood transfusion. Yale J Biol Med 49:3, 1976

Fiala M, Payne JE, Berne TV: Epidemiology of cytomegalovirus infections after transplantation and immunosuppression. J Infect Dis 132:421, 1975

Hanshaw JB: Congenital cytomegalovirus infection: A fifteen-year perspective. J Infect Dis 123:555, 1971

Hanshaw JB, Scheiner AP, Moxley AW, et al.: School failure and deafness after "silent" congenital cytomegalovirus infection. N Engl J Med 295:468, 1976

Ho M (ed): Cytomegalovirus, Biology and Infection. New York, Plenum, 1982

Huang E-S, Alford CA, Reynolds DW, et al.: Molecular epidemiology of cytomegalovirus infections in women and their infants. N Engl J Med 303:958, 1980

Lang DJ, Kummer JF: Cytomegalovirus in semen: Observations in selected populations. J Infect Dis 132:472, 1975

Meyers JD, McGuffin RW, Bryson YJ, et al.: Treatment of cytomegalovirus pneumonia after marrow transplant with combined vidarabine and human leukocyte interferon. J Infect Dis 146:80, 1982

Meyers JD, Spencer HC, Watts JC, et al.: Cytomegalovirus pneumonia after human marrow transplantation. Ann Intern Med 82:181, 1975

Pass RF, August AM, Dworsky M, et al.: Cytomegalovirus infection in a day-care center. N Engl J Med 307:477, 1982

Pass RF, Stagno S, Myers GS, et al.: Outcome of symptomatic congenital cytomegalovirus infection: Results of long-term longitudinal follow-up. Pediatrics 66:758, 1980

Pass RF, Whitley RJ, Diethelm AG, et al.: Cytomegalovirus infection in patients with renal transplants: Potentiation by antithymocyte globulin and an incompatible graft. J Infect Dis 142:9, 1980

Schopfer K, Lauber E, Krech U: Congenital cytomegalovirus infection in newborn infants of mothers infected before pregnancy. Arch Dis Child 53:536, 1978

Stagno S, Pass RF, Dworsky MF, et al.: Congenital cytomegalovirus infection: The relative importance of primary and recurrent maternal infection. N Engl J Med 306:945, 1982

Stagno S, Reynolds DW, Huang E-S, et al.: Congenital cytomegalovirus infection: Occurrence in an immune population. N Engl J Med 296:1254, 1977

Stagno S, Reynolds DW, Pass RF, et al.: Breast milk and the risk of cytomegalovirus infection. N Engl J Med 302:1073, 1980

Stagno S, Reynolds D, Tsiantos A, et al.: Comparative serial virologic and serologic studies of symptomatic and subclinical congenitally and natally acquired cytomegalovirus infection. J Infect Dis 132:568, 1975

Starr SE, Glazer JD, Friedman HM, et al.: Specific cellular and humoral immunity after immunization with live Towne strain cytomegalovirus vaccine. J Infect Dis 143:585, 1981

Suwansirikul S, Rao N, Ho M, et al.: Clinical manifestations of primary and secondary CMV infection after renal transplantation. Arch Intern Med 137:1026, 1977

Yeager AS, Grumet FC, Hafleigh EB, et al.: Prevention of transfusion-acquired cytomegalovirus infections in newborn infants. J Pediatr 98:281, 1981

EPSTEIN–BARR VIRUS

Cheeseman SH, Henle W, Rubin RH, et al.: Epstein–Barr virus infection in renal transplant recipients: Effects of antithymocyte globulin and interferon. Ann Intern Med 93:39, 1980

Epstein MA, Achong BG (ed): The Epstein–Barr Virus. New York, Springer-Verlag, 1979

Epstein MA, Achong BG, Barr YM: Virus particles in cultured lymphoblasts from Burkitt's lymphoma. Lancet 1:702, 1964

Fleisher G, Lennette ET, Henle G, et al.: Incidence of heterophil antibody responses in children with infectious mononucleosis. J Pediatr 94:723, 1979

Fleisher GR, Pasquariello PS, Warren WS, et al.: Intrafamilial transmission of Epstein–Barr virus infections. J Pediatr 98:16, 1981

Gerber P, Nonoyama M, Lucas S, et al.: Oral excretion of Epstein–Barr virus by healthy subjects and patients with infectious mononucleosis. Lancet 2:988, 1972

Grose C, Henle W, Henle G, et al.: Primary Epstein–Barr virus infections in acute neurologic disease. N Engl J Med 292:392, 1975

Hallee TJ, Evans AS, Niederman JC, et al.: Infectious mononucleosis at the United States Military Academy: A prospective study of a single class over 4 years. Yale J Biol Med 47:182, 1974

Hanto DW, Frizzera G, Gajl-Peczalska KJ, et al.: Epstein–Barr virus-induced B cell lymphoma after renal transplantation: Acyclovir therapy and transition from polyclonal to monoclonal B cell proliferation. N Engl J Med 306:913, 1982

Hanto DW, Frizzera G, Purtilo DT, et al.: Clinical spectrum of lymphoproliferative disorders in renal transplant recipients and evidence for the role of Epstein–Barr virus. Cancer Res 41:4253, 1981

Heath CW, Brodsky AL, Potolsky AI: Infectious mononucleosis in a general population. Am J Epidemiol 95:46, 1972

Henle W, Henle G, Hewetson J, et al.: Failure to detect heterophile antigens in Epstein–Barr virus infected cells and to demonstrate interaction of heterophile antibodies with Epstein–Barr virus. Clin Exp Immunol 17:281, 1974

Henle W, Henle G, Ho HC, et al.: Antibodies to Epstein–Barr virus in nasopharyngeal carcinoma, other head and neck neoplasms and control groups. J Natl Cancer Inst 44:225, 1970

Kieff E, Dambaugh T, Heller M, et al.: The biology and chemistry of Epstein–Barr virus. J Infect Dis 146:506, 1982

Porter DD, Wimberly I, Benyesh-Melnick M: Prevalence of antibodies to EB virus and other herpesviruses. JAMA 208:1675, 1969

Purtilo DT, Bhawan J, Hutt LM, et al.: Epstein–Barr virus infections in the X-linked recessive lymphoproliferative syndrome. Lancet 1:798, 1978

Purtilo DT, Cassel CK, Yang JPS, et al.: X-linked recessive progressive combined variable immunodeficiency (Duncan's disease). Lancet 1:935, 1975

Robinson J, Brown N, Andiman W, et al.: Diffuse polyclonal B cell lymphoma during primary infection with Epstein–Barr virus. N Engl J Med 302:1293, 1980

Sawyer RN, Evans AS, Niederman JC, et al.: Prospective studies of a group of Yale University freshmen. 1. Occurrence of infectious mononucleosis. J Infect Dis 123:263, 1971

Svedmyr E, Jondal M: Cytotoxic effector cells specific for B cell lines transformed by Epstein–Barr virus are present in patients with infectious mononucleosis. Proc Natl Acad Sci USA 72:1622, 1975

Tosato G, Magrath I, Koski I, et al.: Activation of suppressor T cells during Epstein–Barr-virus-induced infectious mononucleosis. N Engl J Med 301:1133, 1979

Zur Hausen H, Schulte-Holthausen H, Klein G, et al.: EBV DNA in biopsies of Burkitt's tumors and anaplastic carcinomas of the nasopharynx. Nature 228:1056, 1970

CHAPTER 14

Adenoviruses and Adenovirus-associated Viruses

Adenoviruses

Adenoviruses were first isolated in the winter of 1952–1953 by two groups of investigators. Rowe and his colleagues at the National Institutes of Health cultured adenoids surgically removed from young children and isolated an agent from 33 of 53 adenoids that caused cytopathic effects in the epithelial cells. During the same winter, an epidemic of acute respiratory illness occurred in military recruits at Fort Leonard Wood, Missouri. Although many of the infections were caused by type A influenza, approximately 20 percent of the patients did not have myxovirus infection. The throat washings from one of these patients contained a virus that caused similar cytopathic effects in tissue culture and was related by complement-fixation and neutralization tests to the agent described by Rowe and co-workers. The recovery of these prototype adenovirus strains illustrates their ability to cause epidemic and endemic respiratory illness and also to establish latent or persistent infections in normal hosts. The adenoviruses were named as a group in 1956 by Enders et al. to serve as a reminder of the source of the original prototype strain of adenoviruses and also to designate the prominent involvement of lymphoid tissue in these infections.

Classification

There are at present 34 recognized serotypes of human adenoviruses and 5 candidate serotypes. The 34 human adenoviruses are subdivided by their biophysical, biochemical, biologic, and immunologic characteristics into 5 subgroups (A,B,C,D,E), as indicated in Table 2-4. The biophysical and biologic characterizations of these viruses and the clinical syndromes caused by the subgroups are remarkably parallel. Subgroup A adenoviruses (types 12, 18, and 31) are regularly isolated from the feces of apparently healthy humans, and the incidence of antibody to them is high. This group of adenoviruses is associated with the induction of tumors in hamsters. Subgroup B adenoviruses (types 3, 7, 11, 14, 16, 21, and 34) are most frequently isolated from the throat washings of patients during epidemics of acute respiratory illness and may be associated with severe pneumonia. This group of adenoviruses is not associated with latency. Subgroup C adenoviruses (types 1, 2, 5, and 6) are most commonly isolated from the respiratory tract and gastrointestinal tract of children with mild upper respiratory infections; they are also isolated from long-term cultures of adenoid or tonsillar tissue. Apparently, subgroup C adenoviruses are able to establish latent or masked infections in lymphoid tissue, which persist for extended periods of time. Subgroup D adenoviruses (types 8, 9, 10, 13, 15, 17, 18, 19, 20, 22, 23, 24, 25, 26, 27, 28, 29, 30, 32, and 33) are most often associated with the clinical entities of conjunctivitis and pharyngoconjunctival fever. They are not usually associated with the development of latent infections. Antibodies to these serotypes are also less commonly detected in seroepidemiologic surveys of the population. The only subgroup E adenovirus is adenovirus type 4, which has been associated with severe respiratory disease in both sporadic and epidemic form and with pharyngoconjunctival fever.

Several other adenoviruses have been isolated from patients with clinically significant illness over the past years. They are classified as new serotypes on the basis of unique serum neutralization tests and restriction endonuclease analysis of their genomes. Adenovirus 35 was first isolated in 1972 from the lung and kidney tissues of an immunosuppressed patient who died from interstitial pneumonia following kidney transplant. It has since been frequently identified in immunosuppressed patients with a variety of clinical illnesses and occasionally from nonimmunocompromised patients. Adenovirus 36 was isolated in February 1978 in a stool specimen from a 6-year-old child with enteritis. Adenovirus 37 was first identified in May 1976 in an eye swab from a patient with epidemic catarrhal conjunctivitis. It has also been associated with pharyngoconjunctival fever, and conjunctivitis and urethritis. Adenovirus 38 is the first of the adenoviruses to be termed "noncultivatable," "fastidious," or "enteric." Studies in the United States, England, and the Scandinavian countries have associated this adenovirus with approximately 5 to 15 percent of infantile gastroenteritis. Adenovirus 39 was recently isolated from a stool specimen obtained from a 2-year-old South American child hospitalized with severe respiratory illness.

Clinical Associations

Adenoviruses show a predilection for infection of conjunctival, respiratory, and intestinal epithelium, in addition to regional lymphoid tissue. Incubation periods have been 1 to 2 weeks where discernible. Latent infections, clinically asymptomatic infections, and prolonged viral shedding following clinical illness (particularly of the intestine) have all been described.

Respiratory Illness

Adenoviruses of subgroups B and C cause acute respiratory illness. Subgroup B viruses, particularly serotypes 3, 7, and 14, cause epidemics of respiratory disease in addition to sporadic cases of illness, while subgroup C serotypes 1, 2, 5, and 6 cause sporadic mild respiratory illness of infants and children and can also establish latent infections in tonsillar tissue. Characteristically, the patient with adenoviral respiratory infection is febrile, with pharyngitis, cervical adenitis, and conjunctivitis. Coryza and cough are also frequently present. Atypical pneumonia may occur, and adenoviruses have been recovered from the lungs of fatal cases of pneumonia. A pertussis-like syndrome has been associated with adenovirus infection. Gastrointestinal symptoms can be prominent, and occasionally adenovirus-induced lymphoid hyperplasia in the gastrointestinal tract can serve as a focus, promoting intussusception.

Adenoviruses are responsible for a significant proportion of serious, acute, lower respiratory tract infections in children. Adenovirus infection may occur at any time of the year, but large outbreaks of pharyngoconjunctival fever tend to occur in the summer and are associated with swimming pools. Prolonged excretion of virus, both from the pharynx and from the intestinal tract, may follow illness. Therefore, fecal to oral spread and respiratory droplet transmission contribute to the spread of virus in the community.

Outbreaks of severe pulmonary disease due to adenovirus types 3, 7, and 21 have been well documented in children as well as in adults in closed populations. Affected children are generally young infants or toddlers less than 3 years old. Longitudinal studies of these children show that a significant proportion will develop evidence of chronic pulmonary disease. Adenovirus types 3, 4, 7, 14, and 21 have also been associated with epidemics of febrile respiratory illness in closed populations, particularly among military recruits. Syndromes include an influenza-like illness, febrile pharyngitis, and atypical pneumonia. The conjunctival mucosa is frequently involved, and there are occasionally gastrointestinal symptoms.

Conjunctivitis

Epidemic keratoconjunctivitis is most commonly caused by adenovirus type 8. Several recent outbreaks due to both adenovirus type 19 and the candidate serotype adenovirus 37 have been described. The disease is characterized by the acute onset of tearing, erythema, suffusion, lymphoid follicles beneath the conjunctiva, and preauricular adenopathy. As the conjunctivitis begins to subside after 1 to 2 weeks, discrete corneal infiltrates appear. The latter may persist for 1 to 2 years.

Gastroenteritis

Adenoviruses can often be cultured from the stools of children with and without symptomatic diarrhea or gastroenteritis. Early epidemiologic studies show that adenoviruses types 1 through 31 are not related to gastrointestinal disease. Several large epidemiologic studies have used electron microscopy to screen the stools of children admitted to the hospital with diarrhea for the presence of virus particles. These studies, which established the rotaviruses and a group of 27 nm viruses related to the prototype Norwalk agent as etiologic agents for acute infectious gastroenteritis in children, also showed that some children had adenovirus-like particles present in their stools. In approximately half the children with gastroenteritis and adenovirus particles detectable in stools by transmission electron microscopy, no adenovirus could be isolated in tissue culture. These noncultivatable, enteric adenoviruses form a unique serotype of adenoviruses, candidate serotype 38, which may be responsible for between 5 and 15 percent of endemic diarrhea in young children (Chapter 17).

Cystitis

Adenovirus 11 infection is a cause of acute hemorrhagic cystitis in children. In a study of hermorrhagic cystitis conducted in Sendai, Japan, and Chicago, Illinois, 51 percent of the Japanese children and 23 percent of the American children had adenoviruria during their illness. Shedding of virus in the urine was associated with rising levels of neutralizing type-specific antibody during convalescence and the detection of adenovirus antigens in exfoliated bladder cells by immunofluorescence, supporting the association of adenovirus infection with hemorrhagic cystitis. Hemorrhagic cystitis due to adenovirus 11 has also been reported in several renal transplant recipients. Adenovirus 21 has been infrequently associated with hemorrhagic cystitis in children.

Clinically, hemorrhagic cystitis due to adenoviruses is an acute self-limited disease lasting 4 or 5 days in the typical American population. Males are affected more commonly than females. Gross hematuria, frequency, and dysuria are common. Enuresis, fever, and suprapubic pain are infrequent symptoms.

Other Clinical Adenovirus Infections

Several other syndromes and illnesses have rarely been associated with adenovirus infection. Among them are myocarditis, hepatitis, renal disease, arthritis, acute and subacute meningoencephalitis, and general exanthems. Many of the higher adenovirus serotypes have been recovered from persons with inapparent infections, and their significance in disease is uncertain. Several of the newly defined adenovirus serotypes, particularly candidate adenovirus 35, have been isolated from immunosuppressed patients and may cause life-threatening infections, primarily interstitial pneumonitis. These infections may represent reactivation of latent virus in a manner analogous to cytomegalovirus infection in this population.

Epidemiology

Human adenoviruses spread from person to person with no other known reservoir. Serologic evidence of infection with one or more subgroup C serotypes is common by age 5. Approximately 5 to 10 percent of civilian respiratory disease appears to be due to adenovirus infection. Occasional outbreaks of subgroup D conjunctival infection have been linked to swimming pools, but most have no such association.

The method of acquisition of adenovirus appears to be important in determining disease. Attempts to artificially induce conjunctivitis in volunteers are unsuccessful unless the conjunctival surface is mildly irritated by swabbing. Dusty environments, chlorinated swimming pool water, and optical instruments, such as tonometers, can all provide the necessary conjunctival irritation and, in some cases, transmit the virus as well.

Nasopharyngeal inoculation of volunteers with adenovirus and ingestion of the virus usually results in asymptomatic infection or mild, afebrile illness. However, inhalation of adenovirus aerosols into the lower respiratory tract has resulted in the full range of clinical syndromes. It is thus suggested that the epidemic adenovirus disease seen in army recruits is the result of airborne spread, facilitated by close contact within a large group of susceptibles. The fecal shedding of virus may facilitate transmission by the fecal to oral route, thus contributing to the spread of infection, particularly between young children or where personal hygiene and sanitation are poor.

Diagnosis

The differential diagnosis of the clinical syndromes caused by adenoviruses includes infections with bacteria, chlamydia, *Mycoplasma pneumoniae,* and several other viruses. The differentiation between streptococcal and adenovirus pharyngitis and a culture for streptococci should be obtained whenever possible. The atypical pneumonia caused by adenoviruses cannot be clinically distinguished from that caused by mycoplasma, and as many as one in five persons with adenovirus atypical pneumonia have modest elevations in cold agglutinins.

Adenoviruses can be recovered in cell culture from respiratory secretions, throat swabs, urine, feces, blood, and biopsy or autopsy tissue of infected persons. Cell culture isolation remains the most sensitive means of detecting these viruses except for the fastidious enteric adenoviruses. The specimen is inoculated into susceptible cells of human origin. Human embryonic kidney (HEK) cells are the most sensitive, but continuous human cell lines, such as HeLa, Hep-2, or KB cells can also be used. Typical adenovirus cytopathic effects (cpe) are grape-like clusters of rounded, refractile cells that have intranuclear inclusions when stained with hematoxylin and eosin. Cpe may be seen in 2 to 7 days but can require several weeks; the rapidity of appearance of cpe depends on virus concentration, serotype, and host tissue. Identification of the agent as an adenovirus can be accomplished using antiserum to detect the hexon group antigen by fluorescent-antibody (FA) or complement-fixation (CF) tests. A monoclonal antibody specific for adenovirus hexon protein has recently been described. Although adenoviruses can be subgrouped according to their hemagglutination reaction with rhesus and rat blood cells, identification of serotype is usually accomplished by neutralization tests. Adenoviruses or adenoviral antigens have also been detected in clinical specimens using electron microscopy, enzyme-linked immunoabsorbent assays (ELISAs), and radioimmunoassays. These methods of adenoviral antigen detection are of primary importance in the diagnosis of adenoviral enteric disease in which virus isolation cannot be accomplished.

Because adenoviruses can be recovered from healthy persons, increases in antibody titer between acute and convalescent sera should be sought to document recent acute infection. This may be done using a complement-fixation test for the group-reactive adenovirus hexon antigen or specific neutralization or hemagglutination-inhibition tests employing type-specific antisera.

Treatment

Treatment of adenovirus infections is symptomatic and supportive. Secondary bacterial infection is not common. Interferon has been used for treatment of adenoviral keratoconjunctivitis. Although there appears to be little modification of the course of established conjunctivitis, interferon does seem to protect against severe manifestations of disease in the contralateral eye in those cases presenting with only one eye involved.

Prevention

Immunity following adenovirus infection is serotype-specific and appears to be long lasting. Because of the problem that adenovirus infections pose in military recruit camps, vaccines have been developed and tested in these populations. Experience with subcutaneous inoculation of an inactivated polyvalent vaccine containing types 3, 4, and 7 indicated that such vaccines could control infection.

More recently, infectious adenovirus vaccines of types 4, 7, and 21 have been developed for oral administration. The virus is encased in an enteric-coated capsule and is released in the intestine, where it causes an asymptomatic, nontransmissible infection. Good protection has been provided by these vaccines. However, the rate of seroconversion to adenovirus 7 and 21 decreases when several vaccine types are given simultaneously.

Currently, efforts are being directed toward the exploration of additional forms of immunoprophylaxis, including new modes of vaccine administration and the development of purified subunit vaccines. The development of new vaccines, particularly those that do not require administration of whole virus, is desirable, since adenoviruses may establish persistent infection and are capable of both including tumors in lower animals and causing transformation of cells in vitro.

Adeno-associated Viruses

The adeno-associated viruses (AAV) are small DNA viruses of the parvovirus family. AAV were first observed by electron microscopy as small particles in adenovirus preparations. They were thought to represent either precursor or breakdown products of the adenovirus virions. It was later determined that they represented a second virus that was biologically and structurally different from adenovirus. Four serotypes of AAV have been identified. AAV-1 was isolated from adenovirus preparations that had been cultured in both human and monkey cells, AAV-2 and AAV-3 were isolated from human cell lines and considered to be human serotypes, and AAV-4 has only been isolated from African green monkey cells. Since the initial demonstration of AAV, serotypes of bovine, avian, equine, and canine origin have been discovered. The host range of AAVs is not as limited as that of their helper adenoviruses: avian AAVs can productively infect man using a human adenovirus helper, and herpes simplex viruses type 1 and type 2 can provide the necessary helper functions for AAV replication.

Several seroepidemiologic studies have shown that AAV infection is common in the general population. Antibodies are generally acquired between 6 months and 2 years of age, and 50 to 80 percent of persons tested can be shown to have serologic evidence of AAV infection. AAV cryptically infects human and primate cells in vivo, and latent infection of human cells with AAV has been documented. No overt clinical syndromes have been associated with the AAV infection.

Coinfection or previous infection of cells with AAV may modify the ability of some DNA viruses to transform those cells or induce tumor formation in animal models. The ability of adenovirus 12 to induce tumors in hamsters is decreased from 44 to 18 percent by AAV infection. Perinatal transplacental infection of mice with AAV protects these mice against a lethal postnatal adenovirus infection. In a study of patients with either cervical carcinoma or carcinoma of the prostate, neoplasms for which an etiologic role for herpes simplex virus has been discussed, the incidence of antibodies to AAV 2 and AAV 3 was lower than in a comparable group of patients without carcinoma who were matched for sex and age. The suggestion implicit in these studies is that patients with AAV infection may be at decreased risk of developing either cervical or prostatic carcinomas when later exposed to herpes simplex virus. These data are provocative and not proven. Any role of AAV in human disease remains to be established.

FURTHER READING

Books and Reviews

ADENOVIRUSES

Chanock RM: Impact of adenoviruses in human disease. Prev Med 3:466, 1974

Spencer MJ, Cherry JD: Adenoviral infections. In Fergen RD, Cherry JD (eds): Textbook of Pediatric Infectious Diseases. Philadelphia, Saunders, 1981

Tullo AB: Clinical and epidemiological features of adenovirus keratoconjunctivitis. Trans Ophthalmol Soc UK 100:263, 1980

ADENO-ASSOCIATED VIRUSES

Berns KI, Hauswirth WW: Adeno-associated viruses. Adv Virus Res 25:407, 1979

Selected Papers

ADENOVIRUSES

Brandt CD, Kim HW, Vargosko AJ, et al.: Infections in 18,000 infants and children in a controlled study of respiratory tract disease. I. Adenovirus pathogenicity in relation to serologic type and illness syndrome. Am J Epidemiol 90:484, 1969

D'Angelo LJ, Hierholzer JC, Kennlyside RA, et al.: Pharyngoconjunctival fever caused by adenovirus type 4: Report of a swimming pool-related outbreak with recovery of virus from pool water. J Infect Dis 140:42, 1979

Faden H, Gallagher M: Disseminated infection due to adenovirus type 4. Clin Pediatr 19:427, 1980

Fox JP, Hall CE, Cooney MK: The Seattle virus watch. Am J Epidemiol 105:362, 1977

Harnett GB, Bucens MR, Clay SJ, Saker BM: Acute haemorrhagic cystitis caused by adenovirus type 11. Med J Aust 1: 565, 1982

Hierholzer JC, Sprague JB: Five-year analysis of adenovirus and antibody levels in an industrial community following an outbreak of keratoconjunctivitis. Am J Epidemiol 110:132, 1979

James AG, Lang WR, Liang AY, et al.: Adenovirus type 21 bronchopneumonia in infants and young children. J Pediatr 95:530, 1979

Ladisch S, Lovejoy FH, Hierholzer JC, et al.: Extrapulmonary manifestations of adenovirus type 7 pneumonia simulating Reye syndrome and the possible role of an adenovirus toxin. J Pediatr 95:348, 1979

Mackey JK, Green M, Wold WSM, et al.: Analysis of human cancer DNA for DNA sequences of human adenovirus type 4. J Natl Cancer Inst 62:23, 1979

Mufson MA, Belshe RB: A review of adenoviruses in the etiology of acute hemorrhagic cystitis. J Urol 115:191, 1976

Nicolas JC, Ingrand BF, Bricout F: A one-year virological survey of acute intussusception in childhood. J Med Virol 9:267, 1982

Sundmacher R, Wigand R, Cantell K: The value of exogenous interferon in adenovirus keratoconjunctivitis: Preliminary results. Graefe's Arch Clin Exp Ophthalmol 218:139, 1982

Takafuji ET, Gaydos JC, Allen RG, et al.: Simultaneous administration of live, enteric-coated adenovirus types 4, 7 and 21 vaccines: Safety and immunogenicity. J Infect Dis 140:48, 1979

Wenman WM, Pagtakhan RD, Reed MH, et al.: Adenovirus bronchiolitis in Manitoba. Chest 81:605, 1982

Zahradnik JM, Spencer MJ, Porter DD: Adenovirus infection in the immuno-compromised patient. Am J Med 68:725, 1980

ADENO-ASSOCIATED VIRUSES

Blacklow NR, Hoggan MD, Kapikian AZ, et al.: Epidemiology of adenovirus-associated virus infection in a nursery population. Am J Epidemiol 88:368, 1968

Buller RML, Janik JE, Sebring ED, et al.: Herpes simplex virus type 1 and 2 completely help adenovirus-associated virus replication. J Virol 40:241, 1981

Lipps BV, Mayor HD: Defective parvoviruses acquired via the transplacental route protect mice against lethal adenovirus infection. Infect Immun 37:200, 1982

Maza M, Carter BJ: Inhibition of adenovirus oncogenicity in hamsters by adeno-associated virus DNA. J Natl Cancer Inst 67:1323, 1981

Rosenbaum MJ, Edwards EA, Pierce WE, et al.: Serologic surveillance for adeno-associated satellite virus antibody in military recruits. J Immunol 106:711, 1971

Yates VJ, Dawson GJ, Pronovost AD: Serologic evidence of avian adeno-associated virus infection in an unselected human population and among poultry workers. Am J Epidemiol 113:542, 1981

CHAPTER 15

Human Papovaviruses

Papillomaviruses

Papillomaviruses are the etiologic agents causing warts in humans and papillomas in rabbits, dogs, and livestock. The inability to propagate human papillomaviruses in cell culture systems has impeded their classification and characterization based on biologic properties. Papillomaviruses have now been assigned to several different groups based on patterns of restriction endonuclease digestion of their DNA, DNA homology, and serologic cross-reactivity. A classification of human papillomaviruses is provided in Table 2-4. Each type of human papillomavirus (HPV) is associated with the production of a single variety of wart. A single clinical type of wart, however, may be caused by several HPV types.

Epidemiology and Clinical Associations

The papillomaviruses associated with common warts (common, plantar, or flat warts) are usually found in children and young adults. Natural transmission of these viruses is presumed to be through contact and minor abrasions. There are no specific predisposing factors for the development of common warts, although more extensive warty disease may be seen in individuals with primary immune deficiencies and patients treated with immunosuppressive therapy. These warts usually are caused by HPV types 1, 2, 3, and 4. HPV types 1, 2, and 3 are commonly isolated from warts of patients age 5 to 15, while HPV-4 warts occur predominantly in patients age 20 to 25. Serologic studies show corresponding serotype-specific antibody rises in these age groups. HPV-7 infection is also associated with the development of common warts. It is seen only in the warts found in meat handlers. The natural history of these lesions is spontaneous regression.

The warts and macular lesions associated with epidermodysplasia verruciformis may be seen throughout the lifetime of infected individuals. The natural route of transmission for the three HPV serotypes associated with these lesions (HPV-5, 8, and 9) is not known. Epidermodysplasia verruciformis is a familial disease that may be linked to an autosomal recessive gene. It is usually associated with depressed cell-mediated immunity, which may contribute to the lifetime persistence of disseminated wart lesions. Malignant conversion of some of the warty lesions, particularly those associated with HPV-5, is observed in approximately 25 percent of the affected patients. Those warts that undergo malignant transformation usually occur on sun-exposed areas.

Condylomata acuminata are genital warts caused by HPV-6. They generally occur in young adults, and their transmission is mainly venereal. Sexual promiscuity and changes in hormone balance (for example, in pregnancy) may be predisposing factors for their development. Condylomata acuminata may regress spontaneously but are subject to recurrence and may give rise to extensive lesions. Malignant conversion of these anogenital warts has been observed in rare instances in lesions of the vulva, penis, and anus. Laryngeal papillomas form another group of HPV-caused lesions. The juvenile type of laryngeal papillomatosis is generally found in children under 5 years of age. The HPV-6 genome has been demonstrated in some of these lesions, suggesting that the development of these papillomas follows transmission of virus at birth from mothers with condylomata acuminata to their children. Laryngeal papillomas are also seen in adults, and a small percentage of these lesions can also be shown to contain the HPV-6 genome. Laryngeal papillomas show frequent and rapid recurrence after excision, but their malignant conversion is only rarely observed. Reported transformation has usually been seen after radiation therapy of the lesions. In the absence of radiation therapy, malignant transformation may be associated with heavy smoking. A new type of human papillomavirus, HPV-11, has recently been reported to be another etiologic agent of laryngeal papillomatosis.

Epidermal infection with human papillomaviruses is associated with the development of serotype-specific antibodies and cell-mediated immunity. Both IgM and IgG humoral antibodies appear in wart patients. Detection of IgG antibodies and cell-mediated immunity correlate with resolution of the warts. The number of warty lesions and the persistence of those HPV infections is inversely related to the presence of IgG antibody. Thus, those patients without any antibodies to HPV are more likely to have a greater number of warts that persist for a longer period of time. Those patients who possess HPV-specific IgM but have not developed HPV-specific IgG have intermediate numbers of warts and intermediate healing times.

Human Papillomaviruses in Cancer

Most human papillomaviruses, including the etiologic agents of common, plantar, and flat warts, are entirely benign and are not associated with subsequent development of carcinomas. However, as indicated previously, several HPVs have recently been implicated in the malignant transformation of special groups of warty lesions to squamous cell carcinomas. HPV-6 is related to juvenile laryngeal papillomatosis and the malignant transformation of condylomata acuminata. Recently, Ostrow and his colleagues have identified HPV-5-specific nucleotide sequences in the squamous cell carcinomas evolving from the chronic wart disease, epidermodysplasia verruciformis. Not only was HPV-5 DNA present in the warty lesions of these patients, but the viral genome could also be detected in a subcutaneous metastatic tumor from one of these patients. This latter observation eliminated the possibility that the HPV-5 DNA present in the malignant tumors in these patients resulted from cross-contamination from an adjacent benign wart containing HPV-5 genome but does not establish the virus as the etiologic agent of the carcinoma.

An additional papillomavirus-associated clinical entity that may be linked to malignancy has been reported recently. It is described as both noncondylomatous cervical wart viral infection and subclinical papillomavirus infection. Lesions are associated with atypia on Papanicolaou smears and appear as abnormal mucosa with vascular surface contour and pigment changes similar to cervical intraepithelial neoplasia under colposcopy. Tissue sections from cervical biopsies taken from these lesions show pathologic changes that are similar to, but distinct from, those of cervical intraepithelial neoplasia. HPV-specific antigens have been detected in 50 percent of these dysplastic cervical lesions using a cross-reactive genus-specific antiserum. This association of HPV infection with cervical dysplasia is of particular interest, since cervical dysplasia is epidemiologically associated with carcinoma in situ and invasive cervical carcinoma. The role that HPV infection plays in cervical intraepithelial neoplasia is not yet known.

Several points may be made regarding the relationship between papillomaviruses and carcinomas. The oncogenic potential of any given papillomavirus type is unique. Therefore, the viruses of common warts probably have low oncogenic potential, while HPV-5 and HPV-6 are more strongly related to the development of malignancies. The role of cocarcinogens may be crucial to potentiating papillomavirus-induced malignant transformation. This is particularly evident in epidermodysplasia verruciformis, where malignant transformation of warty lesions occurs only in those areas exposed to UV light. Additionally, the malignant transformation associated with HPV-6 in laryngeal papillomatosis appears to occur only after radiation therapy to the lesions. The immunocompetence of the host also effects the transformation of viral papillomas. Defects in immunity in patients with epidermodysplasia verruciformis or immunosuppression (such as in renal transplant patients) are associated with both an increased number of warts and an increased incidence of cutaneous carcinomas. The state of the papillomavirus genome in the malignant transformed cell is unknown at this time.

Polyomaviruses

Classification

In 1971 two human polyomaviruses were isolated. Each was designated by the initials of the person from whom it was obtained. BKV was isolated by Gardner et al. from the urine of a patient receiving immunosuppressive therapy following kidney transplant. This urine contained transitional epithelial cells with enlarged inclusion-bearing nuclei. Electron microscopic examination of the exfoliated cells showed the presence of intranuclear virus-like particles of the size and structure typical of polyomaviruses. The virus hemagglutinates human type O and guinea pig red blood cells. In serologic tests, BKV reacts slightly with antisera specific for SV40 but not with antisera against polyomavirus or human papillomaviruses. JCV was isolated by Padgett et al. from brain tissue obtained at autopsy from a person with progressive multifocal leukoencephalopathy (PML). JCV also hemagglutinates human and guinea pig erythrocytes. Weak reactions are detected between JCV and antisera against SV40.

Other viruses serologically indistinguishable from BKV and JCV have been recovered from a wide variety of patients. Although these viruses are isolated with the highest frequency from patients immunocompromised either by virtue of inherent defects in immunity or by immunosuppression due to pregnancy or suppressive medication, they can also be isolated at a low frequency from apparently normal individuals. All JCV-related viruses tested appear to be identical to prototype JCV. Most BKV-related viruses are very similar to the prototype BKV, although some differences may be seen with DNA reassociation techniques and restriction endonuclease mapping.

Epidemiology

Several epidemiologic studies of human polyomaviruses have shown that these infections are widespread in many parts of the world. Infection with these viruses is a common occurrence during childhood, with BKV and JCV infections occurring independently. Approximately 80 percent of children age 5 to 9 can be found to have antibodies to BKV present in their serum. Antibody to JCV may be acquired somewhat later in life. Padgett and Walker found that 65 percent of children in Wisconsin were JCV-seropositive by 10 to 14 years of age. In another study, 50 percent of the children had antibodies to JCV by the age of 3 years. Seventy to one hundred percent of adults are seropositive for antibodies to both JCV and BKV. There is probably no animal reservoir for these viruses.

The high incidence of infection with these viruses implies that they are transmitted easily. However, almost nothing is known about the route of transmission. The viruses have, with rare exception, been recovered only from the urine. It may be, however, that a respiratory route of viral transmission is the source of most primary BKV and JCV in infections.

Several recent studies have addressed the possibilities of congenital infections with human polyomaviruses. For example, in a serologic study of pregnant women in the United States, four-fold or greater polyomavirus antibody rises during pregnancy occurred. These antibody titer changes were all consistent with virus reactivation. Virus-specific IgM was detected in the serum of mothers after BKV reactivation but not after JCV reactivation. No evidence of congenital transmission of either JCV or BKV has been found in either English or American studies, although some Japanese studies have turned up some positive evidence.

A high percentage of adults have antibodies to BKV and JCV detectable decades after their primary childhood infection. Many patients have significant levels of antibody against BKV prior to immunosuppression and nevertheless show four-fold or greater rises of titer thereafter. In some persons this increase has been correlated with the appearance of IgM antibodies in the serum. These data suggest that there is lifelong persistence of virus with reactivation of virus subsequent to immunosuppression.

Clinical Association

Primary Infection

A mild respiratory illness has been recorded in children at the time of appearance of antibodies to BKV. Goudsmit et al. retrospectively investigated sera from 177 children admitted to hospital for acute respiratory disease. Sera from 7 of these children showed seroconversion suggestive of primary infection with BKV. All children with BKV infection had upper respiratory tract infections, and BKV was associated with 8 percent of all upper respiratory tract infections in this series. Tonsillar tissue from children with recurrent attacks of acute respiratory disease has been found to contain BKV DNA by hybridization with cloned genomic DNA of prototype BKV, but no infectious virus could be isolated from these tonsils.

Primary infection with JCV has not been documented. The lack of data regarding primary JCV infections may be related to difficulty in obtaining primary fetal glial cells for virus isolation. In addition, the slightly older age of children when infected may make primary JCV disease less severe and preclude patients seeking medical attention.

Urinary Tract Infection

BKV was first isolated from the urine of an immunosuppressed patient who had received a kidney and ureter transplant 3 months previously. Virus-containing cells were shed from the lumen of a stenosed donor ureter. Subsequently, Coleman et al. documented the excretion of large quantities of polyomavirus-infected cells in the urine of renal transplant patients who had been given large doses of cortisol steroids for possible rejection episodes. The transplanted ureters of these patients proved to be stenosed and ulcerated, and the urothelium contained cells with large inclusion bodies containing polyomavirus particles. Hogan et al. studied infection of JCV and BKV in 61 immunosuppressed renal transplant patients. Polyomavirus excretion was detected in the urine of 12 of 61 patients (20 percent), 11 of whom excreted JCV, while 9 excreted BKV. Serologic data suggested that most JCV infections were primary, while most BKV infections resulted from virus reactivation. Urinary tract excretion of polyomavirus is associated with drug-dependent diabetes mellitus, arterial occlusive disease, and urethral stricture with loss of renal function.

Progressive Multifocal Leukoencephalopathy

The one disease closely linked to human polyomaviruses is progressive multifocal leukoencephalopathy (PML). PML is an uncommon, generally fatal, demyelinating disease that occurs in patients with altered immunocompetence. It occurs most frequently as a complication in patients with chronic lymphocytic leukemia or Hodgkin's disease but may also be seen in patients who are immunosuppressed following renal transplantation or with inherited immunodeficiency syndromes.

PML is caused by infection of oligodendrocytes by polyomavirus (most commonly JCV). Several cases of PML have been associated with an SV40-like virus designated as SV40-PML. Pathologic lesions of PML occur in both the gray and white matter and may be distributed throughout the neuraxis. These lesions are classically small discrete areas of demyelination that may become confluent. Cytologically, the outstanding features are unusual astrocytes with bizarre chromatin patterns and atypical oligodendroglia with enlarged, ill-defined inclusions. As a result of the infection of the oligodendrocytes, demyelination occurs. Presumably, this oligodendroglial degeneration is secondary to activation of previously latent JCV by immunosuppression.

Although PML is now recognized as a viral disease, diagnosis of this illness still rests on finding the characteristically altered oligodendroglia in biopsied brain tissue. Studies of serum antibody levels are not helpful because of the high background level of antibody in the general population and because affected patients often have impaired immune responses. Neither specific JCV antibodies nor other proteins characteristic of demyelinating disease have been found in the cerebrospinal fluid. In a recently reported case of PML in a male homosexual with T cell insufficiency, oligoclonal bands were documented.

There is no known treatment for PML. Human leukocyte interferon has been used for prophylaxis of BKV and JCV infections in renal transplant patients with success.

Oncogenicity of Human Polyomaviruses

The human polyomaviruses, BKV and JCV, are oncogenic in neonatal hamsters. Tables 15-1 and 15-2 document the types of tumors that are induced by BKV and JCV, respectively, in these laboratory animals. Malignant, histologically distinct brain tumors developed in two of four adult owl monkeys inoculated with JCV intercerebrally, subcutaneously, and intravenously simultaneously. Four owl monkeys inoculated similarly with BKV and four inoculated with SV40 did not develop tumors after 3 years.

TABLE 15-1. TYPES OF TUMORS INDUCED BY BK VIRUS IN HAMSTERS

Osteosarcoma
Fibrosarcoma
Undifferentiated and poorly differentiated sarcoma
Ependymoma
Choroid plexus papilloma
Reticulum cell sarcoma
Insulinoma

TABLE 15-2. TYPES OF TUMORS INDUCED BY JC VIRUS IN HAMSTERS

Medulloblastoma
Undifferentiated neuroectodermal tumor
Glioblastoma
Ependymoma
Pineocytoma
Meningioma
Neuroblastoma
Leiomyosarcoma
Hemangioma

Attempts have been made to associate BKV and JCV infection with human tumors, using both serologic and DNA hybridization techniques on hundreds of patients and tumors. All results have been uniformly negative. No data, therefore, exist linking BKV or JCV to human carcinomas.

SV40 is tumorigenic in laboratory animals. It produces subclinical infections indicated by serum antibody prevalence and virus isolation in humans. SV40-contaminated poliovirus vaccine was administered to millions of people in the early 1960s. Although it has been reported that SV40-like antigens are present in the tumors of patients with meningiomas and other brain tumors, there is no evidence that cancer trends have been affected by poliovirus vaccine containing SV40. Mortimer et al. recently reported on the 17- to 19-year follow-up of newborns exposed to SV40-contaminated poliovirus vaccine in the first 3 days of life and found no excess risk of cancer of any sort.

FURTHER READING

Books and Reviews

Adler A, Safai B: Immunity in wart resolution. J Am Acad Dermatol 1:305, 1979

Bender ME, Pass F: Papillomaviruses and cutaneous malignancy. Int J Dermatol 20:468, 1981

Briggman RA, Wheeler CE: Immunology of human warts. J Am Acad Dermatol 1:297, 1979

Dvoretzky I, Lowy DR: Infections by human papillomavirus (warts). Am J Dermatopathy 4:85, 1982

Howley PM: The human papillomaviruses. Arch Pathol Lab Med 106:429, 1982

Mantyjarvi RA: New oncogenic human papovaviruses. Med Biol 57:29, 1979

Orth G, Jablonska S, Breitburd F, et al.: The human papillomaviruses. Bull Cancer 65:151, 1978

Padgett BL, Walker DL: Natural history of human polyomavirus infections. In Stevens JG (ed): Persistent Viruses. New York, Academic Press, 1978, p 751

Shah K, Nathanson N: Human exposure to SV-40: Review and comment. Am J Epidemiol 103:1, 1976

Von Krogh G: Warts: Immunologic factors and prognostic significance. Int J Dermatol 18:195, 1979

Selected Papers

Coleman DV, et al.: A prospective study of human polyomavirus infection in pregnancy. J Infect Dis 142:1, 1980

Daniel R, Shah K, Madden D, et al.: Serological investigation of the possibility of congenital transmission of papovavirus JC. Infect Immun 33:319, 1981

Dei R, Marmo F, Corte D, et al.: Age-related changes in the prevalence of precipitating antibodies to BK virus in infants and children. J Med Microbiol 15:285, 1982

Gardner DV, Field AM, Coleman DV, et al.: New human papovavirus (BK) isolated from urine after renal transplantation. Lancet 1:1253, 1971

Goudsmit J, Baak ML, Slaterus KW, et al.: Human papovavirus isolated from urine of a child with acute tonsillitis. Br Med J 283:1363, 1981

Goudsmit J, Wertheim-van Dillen P, van Strien A, et al.: The role of BK virus in acute respiratory disease and the presence of BKV DNA in tonsils. J Med Virol 10:91, 1982

Grossi MP, et al.: Lack of association between BK virus and ependymomas, malignant tumors of pancreatic islets, osteosarcomas and other human tumors. Intervirology 15:10, 1981

Heritage J, Chesters PM, McCancer DJ: The persistence of papovavirus BK DNA sequences in normal human renal tissue. J Med Virol 8:143, 1981

Hogan TF, Borden EC, McBain JA, et al.: Human polyomavirus infections with JC virus and BK virus in renal transplant patients. Ann Intern Med 92:373, 1980

Miller JR, et al.: Progressive multifocal leukoencephalopathy in a male homosexual with T-cell immune deficiency. N Engl J Med 307:1436, 1982

Mortimer EA, Lepow ML, Gold E, et al.: Long-term follow-up of persons inadvertently inoculated with SV40 as neonates. Med Intell 305:1517, 1981

Mounts P, Shah KV, Kashima H: Viral etiology of juvenile- and adult-onset squamous papilloma of the larynx. Proc Natl Acad Sci USA 79:5425, 1982

Orth G, et al.: Identification of papillomavirus in butchers' warts. J Invest Dermatol 76:97, 1981

Ostrow RS, Bender M, Niimura M, et al.: Human papillomavirus DNA in cutaneous primary metastasized squamous cell carcinomas from patients with epidermodysplasia verruciformis. Proc Natl Acad Sci USA 70:1634, 1982

Padgett BL, Walker DL, ZuRhein GM, et al.: Cultivation of papova-like virus from human brain with progressive multifocal leucoencephalopathy. Lancet 1:1257, 1971

Pfister H, zur Hausen H: Seroepidemiological studies of human papilloma virus (HPV-1) infections. Int J Cancer 21:161, 1978

Reid R, Stanhope CR, Herschman BR, et al.: Genital warts and cervical cancer. I. Evidence of an association between subclinical papillomavirus infection and cervical malignancy. Cancer 50:377, 1982

Reid R, Laverty CR, Coppleson M, et al.: Noncondylomatous cervical wart virus infection. Obstet Gynecol 55:476, 1980

Shah K, Daniel R, Madden D, et al.: Serological investigation of BK papovavirus infection in pregnant women and their offspring. Infect Immun 30:29, 1980

Shokri-Tabibzadeh S, Koss L, Molnar J, et al.: Association of human papillomavirus with neoplastic processes in the genital tract of four women with impaired immunity. Gynecol Oncol 12:S129, 1981

Tabuchi K, Kirsch WM, Low M, et al.: Screening of human brain tumors for SV40-related T antigen. Int J Cancer 21:12, 1978

Zang KD, May G: Expression of SV40-related T antigen in cell cultures of human meningiomas. Naturwissenschaften 66:59, 1979

CHAPTER 16

The Enteroviruses

The *Enterovirus* genus of the Picornaviridae family contains six major groups: polioviruses, echoviruses, Coxsackie viruses group A and group B, the new enterovirus serotypes 68, 69, 70, and 71, and hepatitis A viruses. All of these viruses infect and multiply in the gastrointestinal tract. There are three distinct poliovirus serotypes, 23 Coxsackie A serotypes, 6 Coxsackie B serotypes, 31 echovirus serotypes, 4 viruses designated as enteroviruses 68–71, and 1 serotype of hepatitis A.

Enteroviruses are 30 nm particles composed of a single-stranded RNA genome with a protein coat of icosahedral symmetry. The viruses are indistinguishable morphologically, stable at pH 3, and resist inactivation by ether. Assignment of a virus to one of these groups is based on biophysical properties, differences in growth and tissue culture systems, pathogenicity for various strains of laboratory animals, and serologic reactivity.

The RNA of enteroviruses is a positive single strand and, therefore, by definition, serves as the messenger RNA for the replication cycle of the virus. All enteroviruses code for four proteins (VP1, VP2, VP3, VP4), derived by cleavage of a precursor polyprotein, that constitute the capsid of the virus. Experiments with members of each of these groups suggest that the four capsid proteins contain the antigens that determine the serotype of the virus strain. Recent work suggests that VP2 induces specific neutralizing antibodies for several echoviruses and Coxsackie B viruses. Group-reactive antigenic determinants are found in all of the capsid proteins for Coxsackie B viruses. In contrast, it would appear that antibody to VP1 of the polioviruses is neutralizing and, therefore, defines serotype specificity. However, antibodies to other capsid polypeptides seem to contribute to neutralization. More than one capsid protein may be required to form the antigenic determinant that elicits the formation of serotype-specific antibodies.

History

Sporadic cases of paralytic disease are as old as recorded history. A famous Egyptian stele from the period 1580 to 1350 BC depicts a priest with a flail atrophic lower limb, typical of paralytic polio. Sir Walter Scott underwent an illness in 1772 that was one of the earliest and certainly the most renowned case of polio described in the British Isles. Acute paralytic illness in children was first described by Underwood in his textbook in 1789, while the name "anterior poliomyelitis" is attributed to Kussmaul in the late nineteenth century. The term "poliomyelitis" was derived from the Greek for gray marrow of the spinal cord and the Latin (*itis*) for inflammation. The location of the involved cells in the anterior horns of the spinal cord contributed the designation "anterior." Outbreaks of illness were regularly identified in the nineteenth and twentieth centuries by the observation of paralysis among young children. The first isolations of poliovirus were achieved in 1908 by the inoculation of central nervous system tissue into susceptible monkeys via the intracerebral route. In 1949, Enders, Robbins, and Weller reported their classic experiments on the cultivation of poliovirus in tissue cultures of nonneural human cells.

The histories of the other enteroviruses are relatively recent. In 1948, Dalldorf and Sickles isolated a filterable agent from a stool of a patient from Coxsackie, New York, who had paralytic illness. Subsequently, a large group of antigenically related agents has been characterized and designated Coxsackie (A and B) viruses. The echoviruses were also isolated initially from human fecal specimens, frequently from patients without overt disease, and their name represents an acronym (*e*nteric, *c*ytopathic, *h*uman, *o*rphan). With increasing clinical study, they have been associated with a wide variety of illness, so that most no longer are "orphans." As distinct antigenic serotypes were identified, they were assigned sequential numbers. Since 1969, new enterovirus types have been assigned enterovirus type numbers rather than being subclassified as Coxsackie viruses or echoviruses, hence, the designation enteroviruses 68 through 71. Finally, hepatitis A virus now appears to be a member of the picornavirus family.

Epidemiology

The epidemiology of all human enteroviruses is quite similar. The pattern is most clearly defined for the polioviruses because paralytic disease has been so readily identifiable. As early as 1916, the clinical epidemiologic features were defined on the basis of an outbreak that occurred that year in New York City. These principles were: (1) Poliomyelitis is, in nature, exclusively a human infection, transmitted from person to person without the necessary intervention of a lower animal or insect host. (2) The infection is far more prevalent than is apparent from the incidence of clinically recognized cases, since a large majority of persons infected become carriers without clinical manifestations. It is probable that during an epidemic, such as that in New York City, a very considerable proportion of the population became infected, adults as well as children. (3) The most important agencies in disseminating infection are the unrecognized carriers and perhaps mild, abortive cases ordinarily escaping recognition. It is fairly certain that frank paralytic cases are a relatively minor factor in the spread of infection. (4) An epidemic of 1 to 3 recognized cases per 1000, or even less, immunizes the general population to such an extent that the epidemic declines spontaneously due to the depletion of susceptible persons.

Enteroviruses have a worldwide distribution, with increased prevalence during the warm months of the year in temperate climates. Within the United States, some variation in geographic distribution of infections may be due to importation of viruses, for example, from Latin America. Epidemics occur between May and October in the United States and other areas of the north temperate zone. The seasonal prevalence of these viruses is shown in Figure 16-1. Sporadic infections due to these viruses can occur at any time throughout the year.

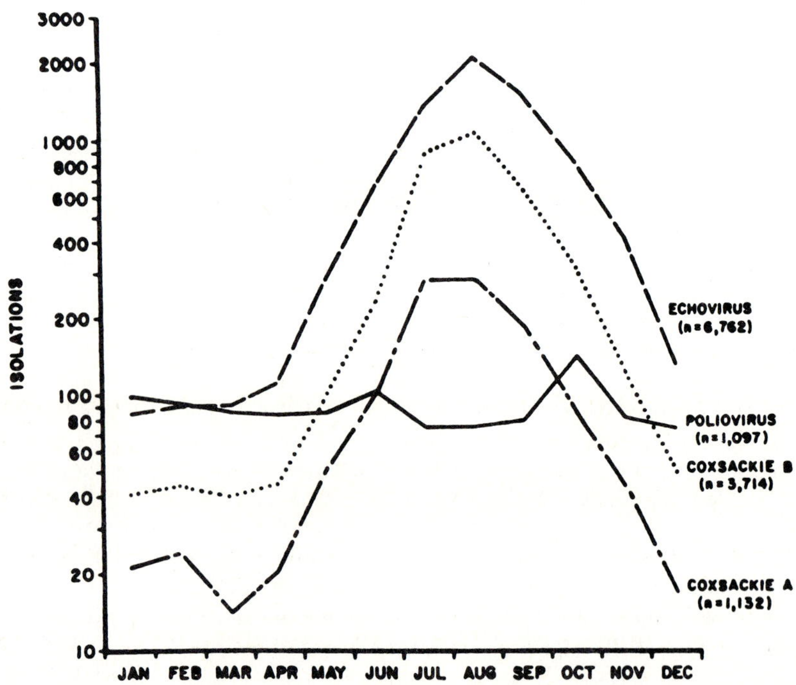

Figure 16-1. Seasonal prevalence of human enterovirus infections, United States, 1970–1979. *(From CDC Enterovirus Surveillance Summary 1970–1979. Issued November 1981, p 6. U.S. Dept. HHS, PHS.)*

The seroepidemiology of enterovirus infections, including polio and hepatitis A viruses, demonstrates an increased transmission of infection at a young age among persons of lower socioeconomic status. Crowding creates intimate living conditions, and it may also be associated with poor hygiene, which enhances the fecal to oral transmission of these agents.

Enterovirus illness and laboratory isolation of enteroviruses is most commonly reported from children in the 1- to 4-year age group. It is not clear whether such data reflect an enhanced concern over any illness at that age, whether the infections occur more frequently in infants, or whether they are more likely to be overt rather than occult. Nevertheless, when specific outbreaks occur within a community, a broad age spectrum of persons may be infected.

A 2- to 5-year periodicity has been observed with Coxsackie B infection, suggesting that a limited number of serotypes contributes to this pattern. These agents are also able to cause outbreaks of disease when a newly susceptible population is present in the community. When a specific virus circulates frequently, younger infants are more likely to be susceptible and develop disease. Perhaps the numerous serotypes of echoviruses have a broader range of age-related attack rates, since a given serotype circulates through a community sporadically. It is unlikely that any individual would encounter all serotypes of enteroviruses in childhood.

The clinical epidemiology of these infections suggests that respiratory excretion of virus is not as important a means of spread as is fecal to oral transmission. Intimate human contact is important in transmission of virus, and communicability within households is greatest between children. Diapered infants appear to be more efficient disseminators of infection than do other individuals. In the current era of day-care centers and nursery schools, it has already been shown that hepatitis A virus is transmitted in this setting and, if present, is transmitted to virtually all children in the nursery. It is likely that outbreaks of infection due to other enteroviruses are also occurring in these facilities.

Community outbreaks of enterovirus infection can spread to hospital nurseries. A newborn who acquires virus from the mother or from nursery personnel may spread it throughout the nursery. The viruses can be introduced into intensive care units by patients or personnel. Recognition of such infections imposes a need to institute isolation precautions, such as cohorting of infants and personnel, to minimize spread of infection.

Clinical Illness

The broad spectrum of clinical disease produced by the enteroviruses overlaps among groups. A listing of the various syndromes is included in Table 16-1. The more common manifestations associated with infection are discussed briefly.

TABLE 16-1. CLINICAL MANIFESTATIONS OF ENTEROVIRUS INFECTIONS

	Viruses Implicated			
		Coxsackie		
Clinical Syndrome	Polio	A	B	Echo
Asymptomatic infection	X	X	X	X
Nonspecific febrile illness	X	X	X	X
Respiratory disease		X	X	X
Exanthems		X	X	X
Enanthems		X		
Pleurodynia			X	
Orchitis			X	
Myocarditis			X	
Pericarditis			X	X
Aseptic meningitis and meningoencephalitis	X	X	X	X
Disseminated neonatal infection			X	X
Transitory muscle paresis	X	X	X	X
Paralytic disease	X	X	X	X

Febrile Illness

The great majority of infections with enteroviruses produce no specific clinical hallmarks. Although the portal of entry is the gastrointestinal tract, they are not frequently responsible for gastroenteritis. In young children, undifferentiated febrile illness, nonspecific malaise, and myalgias are frequently associated with enterovirus infections. There is nothing unique about this type of clinical presentation. A recent prospective study of newborn infants in Rochester, New York, demonstrated that during a typical enterovirus season, as many as 13 percent of infants acquired infection with these viruses during the first month of life. Although 80 percent of these patients were asymptomatic, most of the symptomatic infants were admitted to the hospital because they were suspected of having bacterial sepsis. These observations allow an estimate of the frequency of enterovirus infection of very young infants. It is an impressive 7 infections per 1000 live births, which occur in the first month of life during the months of seasonal prevalence of these agents. It has come to be appreciated that enterovirus infection is as common as other neonatal infections of widespread clinical concern.

Congenital and Neonatal Infections

Transplacental and neonatal transmission have been demonstrated with Coxsackie B viruses, resulting in a serious disseminated disease that may include hepatitis, myocarditis, meningoencephalitis, and adrenal cortical involvement. Infants infected in the newborn period with echoviruses have died with disseminated disease, with the predominant feature of the infection being hepatic necrosis. Serologic studies have suggested that maternal antibody protects the infant from severe disease, although they may acquire infection, as documented by virus excretion. When poliovirus infections were common, examples of transmission from infected mother to fetus were apparent by the birth of a paralyzed infant.

Respiratory Disease

Mild upper respiratory tract illness has been associated with several of the Coxsackie and echoviruses. Very few cases of pneumonia have been attributed to Coxsackie virus infection.

Exanthems and Enanthems

Various enteroviruses (particularly echoviruses 9 and 16, and Coxsackie A9, A16, and B5) have been associated with large outbreaks of febrile rash disease. Younger children are more likely to develop exanthems, which vary widely in their characteristics. Small vesicular lesions have been described on the hands and feet in association with ulcers of the buccal mucosa (hand–foot–mouth disease), particularly with Coxsackie A16. Macular and maculopapular eruptions indistinguishable from rubella have been observed with a number of the Coxsackie and echoviruses. Petechiae have accompanied some rashes, especially with echovirus 9. The presence of virus has been demonstrated in the skin lesions themselves. Some of the syndromes include an associated enanthem. Herpangina, one of these, is most commonly associated with Coxsackie A infections. Ulcerative lesions of the mucosa appear on the posterior pharynx and soft palate. The associated discomfort, fever, and sore throat are prominent. Because many different serotypes of the echo and Coxsackie groups can cause identical clinical pictures, virus isolation is necessary to identify the specific etiologic agents.

Pleurodynia (Bornholm Disease)

This is a febrile illness with extreme myalgia, pleuritic chest pain, and headache. Most often it has been associated with Coxsackie B viruses, but other agents have occasionally been recovered from patients.

Orchitis

Although viral orchitis most often is due to mumps, it has accompanied infections with the Coxsackie B viruses.

Myocarditis and Pericarditis

Isolated myocarditis and/or pericarditis in older children and adults has been shown to result from Coxsackie B or echovirus infections. The spectrum has ranged from benign, self-limited pericarditis to severe, chronic, fatal myocardial disease.

Viral Meningitis and Meningoencephalitis

Many of the enteroviruses have been isolated from the cerebrospinal fluid (CSF) of patients suffering from aseptic meningitis and/or encephalitis. These illnesses are characterized by varying degrees of fever, headache, nuchal rigidity, malaise, and altered central nervous system function. The most severely affected patients may be obtunded or comatose. The least involved patients may complain only of mild headache and/or stiff neck. A CSF pleocytosis is detected, with usually less than 500 cells per microliter. Early in the disease, these cells are likely to be predominantly polymorphonuclear leukocytes, but after 24 to 48 hours of illness, mononuclear cells are the majority. The CSF protein may be normal or mildly elevated, but the glucose is normal. Most patients with enteroviral meningitis recover so that pathologic descriptions are based on only a few cases. There is inflammation of the meninges with perivascular inflammatory cell infiltration. The most acute processes are likely to have a predominance of polymorphonuclear cells, whereas mononuclear cells become predominant after a relatively few days. The prognosis for patients with enteroviral central nervous system infections is better than that for similar pyogenic infections. Although most of the youngest infants appear to recover completely, several longitudinal studies of such patients have demonstrated that neurologic deficits, particularly in receptive language function, are demonstrable in babies sustaining such infection during the first several months of life.

Paralytic Disease

Poliovirus infection, especially with types 1 and 3, was responsible for almost all the paralytic disease associated with the enteroviruses. Occasional cases of transient paralysis and muscle weakness have been noted with these viruses, particularly the Coxsackie B agents. With classic paralytic polio, there is a 2 to 6 day incubation period with an initial nonspecific febrile illness. This probably coincides with early replication of virus in the pharynx and gastrointestinal tract. With the subsequent hematogenous spread of virus, central nervous system involvement may result in meningitis and anterior horn cell infection. From 1 to 4 percent of susceptible patients infected with polioviruses develop central nervous system involvement. The spectrum of paralytic disease is enormously variable and may involve only an isolated muscle group or extensive paralysis of all extremities. Characteristically, the picture is one of asymmetrical distribution, the lower extremities more frequently involved than the upper. Large muscle groups are more often affected rather than the small muscles of the hands and feet. Involvement of cervical and thoracic segments of the spinal cord may result in paralysis of the muscles of respiration. Infection of cells in the medulla and the cranial nerve nuclei results in bulbar polio with compromise of the respiratory and vasomotor centers. With the return of the patient's temperature to normal, the progress of paralysis ceases, and the subsequent weeks and months reveal a varying spectrum of recovery ranging from full return of function to significant residual paralysis. Atrophy of involved muscles becomes apparent after 4 to 8 weeks. Recovery may be exceedingly slow, and its full extent cannot be judged for 6 to 18 months.

Pathology

Most Coxsackie and echovirus infections are transient and nonfatal, therefore limited histologic information is available. The pathogenic changes of poliovirus in the central nervous system are most prominent in the spinal cord, medulla, pons, and midbrain. After initial cytoplasmic alterations in the Nissl substance of the motor neurons, nuclear changes develop next, and pericellular infiltrates of polymorphonuclear and mononuclear cells accumulate. The final stage is destruction, with neuronophagocytosis and dropping out of the necrotic cells.

Fatal newborn infection with enteroviruses has shown nonspecific but extensive damage of the infected tissues. The echovirus infections are associated with hepatic necrosis and evidence of disseminated intravascular coagulation in multiple organs. If the patient has lived long enough, the liver may then show cirrhosis, as opposed to the acute process.

Immunity

Enteroviruses gain entry into the host via the mouth. The virus establishes infection in the oral pharynx and portions of the gastrointestinal tract, where multiplication subsequently occurs. Virus then gains access to adjacent lymph nodes and the bloodstream. The incubation period of enterovirus infection is usually from 1 to 5 days (Fig. 16-2). Invasion of other tissues, such as the meninges or the myocardium, typically occurs from 7 to 10 days after initial exposure to the virus, resulting in the classic biphasic illness such as occurs with poliovirus infection.

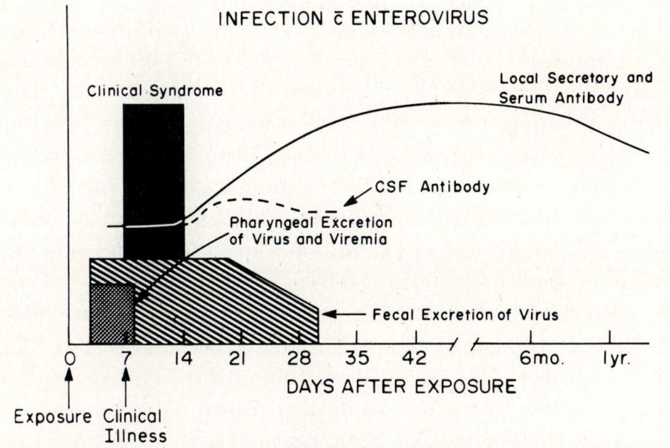

Figure 16-2. The course of typical enterovirus infection.

Enteroviruses induce secretory and humoral antibody responses. The humoral responses are initially predominantly IgM antibodies, followed by IgA and IgG antibodies that persist for months to years. Coproantibodies, primarily IgA, have been studied as a response to administration of poliovirus vaccines or to natural infection, e.g., by echovirus type 6. Local secretory immunoglobulin A production occurs at the site of contact of virus with lymphoid cells. The antibody formation and virus excretion for typical enterovirus infections are depicted in Figure 16-2. Development of type-specific antibody provides lifelong protection against clinical illness due to the same agent. Local reinfection of the gastrointestinal tract may recur, but this is accompanied by only an abbreviated period of virus replication without clinical illness.

In experimental poliovirus infection, specific IgG antibody-producing cells and measurable antibodies can be demonstrated in areas of the central nervous system where virus is replicating. Local central nervous system antibody production is independent of systemic humoral antibody production. Although specific central nervous system enterovirus antibodies are probably produced primarily within the central nervous system, some passive transfer of serum antibody to the CSF may occur as permeability is increased by inflammation. In viral meningitis, only minimal elevation of CSF globulin has been documented. Evidence for the extreme importance of central nervous system antibody is deduced from agammaglobulinemic patients who are unable to eliminate enteroviruses from the central nervous system. Administration of extraordinarily large quantities of parenteral globulin or plasma with specific antibody is necessary to passively achieve measurable antibody levels in the CSF.

Cellular immunity against enterovirus infection is not well defined. Circulating peripheral white blood cells have been a source of virus isolation during acute illness. Recognition of virus by lymphocytes occurs in experimental models employing Coxsackie viruses. The abnormal response of some children with immunodeficiency disease to infection with attenuated polioviruses may offer further insights to immune processes normally stimulated by enterovirus infection.

Diagnosis

The clinical illnesses in some instances may permit a presumptive diagnosis of enterovirus infection. However, as shown in Table 16-1, the spectrum of illness is wide. The time of the year may be an indication, with a predilection for summer and early autumn circulation of enteroviruses occurring in the temperate zones. Specimens for virus isolation should be obtained early in the course of illness. The CSF of patients with viral meningitis and/or meningoencephalitis has been a rich source of enteroviruses, except for the three polio types. Materials, such as pleural and pericardial fluid, should also be cultured when available.

Specific etiologic diagnosis of enteroviral disease is presently dependent upon demonstration of the enterovirus by cell culture techniques. Unfortunately, most of the Coxsackie A viruses grow poorly in cell cultures, and newborn mice provide a more reliable system for detection of these agents. The distinction between Coxsackie groups A and B has classically depended on the pathologic lesions produced in mice. Group A viruses cause generalized myositis and flaccid paralysis. Group B viruses cause focal myositis and typical lesions in the infrascapular fat pad and brain. Various primate and human cell culture systems will support replication of most of the enteroviruses, with cytopathic effects revealing their presence. The specimens submitted most often for attempted virus isolations are nasopharangeal swabs and stool specimens. An enterovirus may be excreted in fecal material for several weeks after the onset of clinical illness. Recovery of an enterovirus from the throat or stool of the patient does not in itself establish this as the etiologic agent of the illness observed. The temporal association of illness, virus recovery, and an antibody rise specific to that agent provide firmer evidence of a causative relationship.

A potentially useful and more practical approach to diagnosis would be the demonstration of viral antigen in clinical specimens, especially CSF. It would be ideal if antigen could be detected by a method capable of providing a specific diagnosis within hours. Although there are only scanty data concerning the quantitation of enterovirus present in various sites, it would appear that an efficient diagnostic test for the detection of virus/antigen in the CSF or blood should be capable of detecting as little as 1 to 100 tissue culture infectious doses of virus. Diagnostic assays, such as the enzyme-linked immunosorbent assay (ELISA) tests, presently available for antigen detection do not achieve this level of sensitivity. On the other hand, excretion of these viruses in stool is more likely to produce 10^3 to 10^7 tissue culture infectious doses of virus. The existing assays are capable of detecting this quantity of virus. Thus, at the present time virus isolation remains the most sensitive and specific means of diagnosing enterovirus infections. It is anticipated that future tests for antigen detection and body fluids will be more sensitive.

Acute and convalescent serum samples obtained from 7 to 21 days apart will help to define quantitative changes in antibody titers. Complement fixation, virus neutralization, immunoprecipitation, and, in a few instances, hemagglutination inhibition are the available techniques for assaying enterovirus antibodies. Neutralizing antibodies are type-specific, whereas complement fixation demonstrates group-reactive antibodies. In the course of a lifetime, humans sustain multiple infections, occult or overt, with a variety of enteroviruses. A specific infection elicits the production of antibody specific to that virus type but also may prompt an anamnestic response demonstrated by an increase in group-reactive antibody and by parallel rises in antibodies to serotypes of some of the other enteroviruses previously encountered. The concomitant serologic rises in antibody titer create some problems with serologic surveys, rendering the complement-fixation test inadequate to define a specific infection. The isolation of a specific virus provides the opportunity for assessment of the patient's antibody against his or her own viral agent. In the absence of the recovery of a virus, one faces the problem of seeking specific antibody rises against the whole genus of *Enterovirus*. Thus the complexity of serology makes the serologic diagnosis of these infections impractical.

Prevention

Because there currently is no specific treatment for enterovirus infections, efforts have focused on means of prevention. The multiple antigenic types and the usually benign, self-limited course of most echovirus and Coxsackie virus infections have resulted in little stimulus for the development of vaccines. The story of the poliovirus vaccines, however, has been one of the most exciting and rewarding sagas in the history of microbiology. Prior to the work of Enders and colleagues with successful tissue culture techniques for growth of the polioviruses, there had been several ill-fated vaccines prepared from emulsions of spinal cord removed from monkeys infected with wild-type poliovirus. These preparations were treated with formalin or other inactivating agents. Trials of such vaccines in 1935 proved unsuccessful and unacceptable.

Enders' tissue culture techniques lent themselves to the propagation in vitro of sufficient amounts of relatively pure poliovirus, so that controlled formaldehyde inactivation could be used to produce noninfectious virus that retained its antigenicity. Salk and his colleagues pursued this line of research and by 1954 were able to embark on a field trial that established the efficacy of an inactivated poliovirus vaccine in the prevention of paralytic disease. This was a trivalent preparation incorporating the three poliovirus types. After an initial series of two or three injections spaced several weeks to months apart, followed by a booster 6 to 12 months later, there was demonstrable serum antibody to all three polio serotypes. The vaccine was widely used in the United States during the 5 years from 1956 through 1960. The results were dramatic. Previous years had seen from 10,000 to 20,000 cases of paralytic disease reported annually. With the widespread use of Salk vaccine, this rapidly dropped to 2000 to 3000 cases annually, as increasingly large numbers of susceptible individuals were immunized (Fig. 16-3).

By the early 1960s, a second vaccine was available. Strains of poliovirus that Sabin had selected and studied in his laboratory were proven attenuated for monkey and humans. Their ingestion resulted in intestinal infection and virus excretion, so that humoral and gastrointestinal tract immunity developed without any illness. Because these could be administered more readily, by the oral route, and

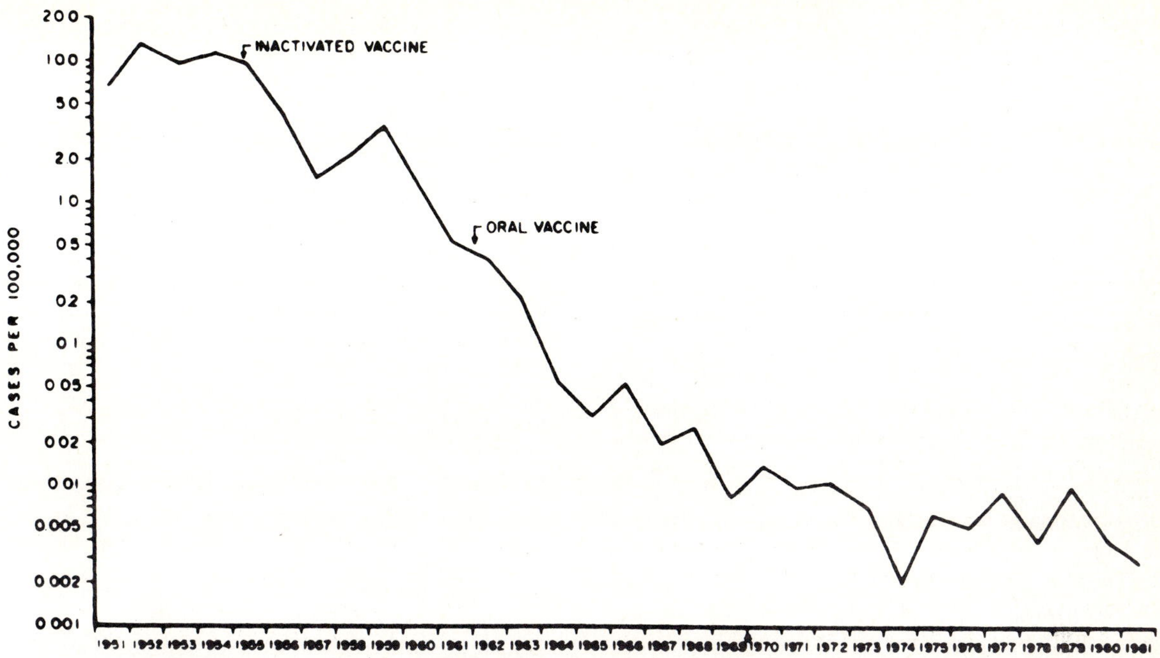

Figure 16-3. Reported paralytic poliomyelitis attack rates, United States, 1951–1981. *(From CDC Poliomyelitis Surveillance Summary 1980–1981. Issued December 1982, p 9. U.S. Dept. HHS, PHS.)*

because their multiplication in the gastrointestinal tract more closely mimicked natural infection, they offered certain selected advantages, which led to their replacing the injectable Salk vaccine. Over the first 5 years of the 1960s, more than 400 million doses of oral vaccine were distributed in the United States. At the same time, trials also were successfully conducted in European nations, Japan, and other countries. The use of oral vaccine in this country was accompanied by a further decrease in the annual reported polio cases (Fig. 16-3), so that beginning in 1966 fewer than 100 have occurred each year. Between 1969 and 1981 with continued use of the oral vaccines, 203 cases of paralytic disease were reported in the United States. In less than 20 years, a disease that had claimed thousands of victims annually and had been the source of indescribable community anxiety was reduced to a rarity!

In the complex processes of vaccine development, commercial production, and widespread utilization, a number of unexpected events took place that merit consideration. After the highly successful field trials of 1954, commercial manufacture of the Salk type vaccine was licensed. Within a few weeks of its use, paralytic disease was observed in April through June 1955 among children in California and Idaho who had received some of the first lots of commercial vaccine manufactured by the Cutter Laboratories. By the time this had been fully investigated and resolved, it was learned that there were 204 cases of vaccine-associated disease. Seventy-nine were among children who had received the vaccine, 105 were among their family contacts, 20 were in community contacts. Nearly three quarters of the cases were paralytic, and there were 11 deaths. The agent isolated from these patients was type 1 poliovirus. Laboratory tests on vaccine distributed by Cutter Laboratories revealed viable virulent type 1 poliovirus in 7 of 17 lots. Revisions of the federal regulations governing the steps in vaccine manufacture were promptly promulgated and implemented to prevent recurrence of such a tragic episode.

Manufacturers faced further difficulties in maintaining the fine balance between the complete elimination of the infectious live virus from the production process and the retention of effective antigenicity of the inactivated components. A number of lots of vaccine subsequently proved to be poorly antigenic for type 3 poliovirus. As a result, when community polio outbreaks occurred among well-immunized groups, there were breakthroughs with paralytic disease, especially due to type 3 virus, in previously immunized subjects. Such an outbreak was studied in 1959 in Massachusetts, where an analysis of polio cases revealed that 47 percent (62 of 137) of the patients had previously received three or more inoculations of inactivated vaccine.

Enthusiasm for attenuated oral vaccine was enhanced by the aforementioned unfortunate episodes involving inactivated vaccine. A final unanticipated discovery in 1960 was the detection of a simian virus, SV-40, as a contaminant of the monkey kidney cell cultures utilized in the preparation of both inactivated and oral attenuated vaccines. Once again, a revision of standards for preparing and testing the tissue cultures was necessary to exclude this previously unrecognized agent. In the United States, inactivated vaccine has been used sparingly in the past 15 years. Almost all immunization has been conducted with the oral attenuated product. A number of European countries, especially those in Scandinavia, have adhered to the use of inactivated vaccine. With successful production of fully potent antigens, their record of achievement in the control of polio has been parallel to that of this country.

The marked decrease in paralytic disease due to wild polioviruses has disclosed a small but significant number of oral vaccine recipients who have developed paralytic illness in temporal association to the ingestion of vaccine. In addition to these few cases among recipients of vaccines, there have also been paralytic episodes reported among susceptible family or community contacts of the vaccine recipients. These have been few in number and are difficult to characterize with complete clarity. A small portion of these patients have been found to be immunodeficient children, particularly those with congenital hypogammaglobulinemia. One concern has always been that the attenuated strains of virus might prove genetically unstable in human intestinal passage, so that increased neurovirulence might result from widespread dissemination. This has not been demonstrated. Monovalent oral polio vaccine (MOPV) was used extensively until 1964, when it was supplanted by trivalent vaccine (TOPV). With MOPV the risk of vaccine-associated illness in recipients was estimated to have been 0.19 per million doses distributed. With TOPV an overall figure of risk to recipients and their contacts has been calculated at 0.28 per million or 1 case per 3.6 million doses.

The achievements with poliovirus vaccination have been impressive in the United States, Canada, most of Europe, Australia, and some Asian and African nations. Polio remains an endemic disease in many tropical lands. It is premature, therefore, to relax the use of poliovirus vaccination in those parts of the world where the disease has been nearly eradicated. The possibility of the inadvertent introduction of virulent virus is omnipresent. A number of such episodes have occurred already on the Texas–Mexico border. Although polio immunization is now confined principally to infants and children, it is recommended that adult Americans traveling abroad to endemic areas receive polio vaccine prior to departure. Armed Forces recruits are routinely administered oral poliovirus vaccine. Its major use remains that for infants and children in the first 18 months of life.

FURTHER READING

Beatrice S, Katze MG, Zajac BA, et al.: Induction of neutralizing antibodies by the Coxsackie virus B3 virion polypeptide VP2. Virology 104:426, 1980

Centers for Disease Control Enterovirus Surveillance. Summary 1970–1979. Issued November 1981. USDHHS, PHS

Hughes JR, Wilfert CM, Moore M: Echovirus 14 infection associated with fatal neonal hepatic necrosis. Am J Dis Children 123:61, 1972

Kibrick S, Benirschke K: Severe generalized disease (encephalohepatomyocarditis) occurring in the newborn period and due to infection with Coxsackie virus, group B. Pediatrics 22:857, 1958

Melnick JL, Rennick V: Infectivity titers of enterovirus as found in human stools. J Med Virol 5:205, 1980

Modlin JF: Fatal echovirus 11 disease in premature neonates. Pediatrics 66:775, 1980

Modlin JF, Polk BF, Horton P, et al.: Perinatal echovirus infection: Risk of transmission during a community outbreak. N Engl J Med 305:368, 1981

Morbidity and Mortality Weekly Report. Annual Summary 1980. 30[54]:25, 103, 1982

Morens DM: Enteroviral disease in early infancy. J Pediatr 92:374, 1978

Nathanson N, Langmuir AD: The Cutter incident, I, II, II. Am J Hyg 78:16, 1963

Nightengale EO: Recommendations for a national policy on poliomyelitis vaccination. N Engl J Med 297:249, 1977

Ogra PL: Distribution of echovirus antibody in serum, nasopharynx, rectum and spinal fluid after natural infection with echovirus type 6. Infect Immun 2:150, 1977

Ogra PL, Ogra S, Al-nakeeb S, et al.: Local antibody response to experimental poliovirus infection in the central nervous system of rhesus monkeys. Infect Immun 8:931, 1973

Paul JR: A History of Poliomyelitis. New Haven, Conn., Yale University Press, 1971

CHAPTER 17

Viruses in Gastrointestinal Tract Infection

Acute infectious diarrheal illness is recognized as one of the leading causes of morbidity and mortality in developing nations. Even in developed countries, infectious gastroenteritis is cited as second only to respiratory infections as a cause of morbidity in childhood. Viral agents recognized during the past decade have been shown to be responsible for a large proportion of the diarrhea for which an etiologic agent can be defined. Acute viral gastroenteritis affects all age groups of people and may occur in either sporadic or epidemic form. Most such illnesses are self-limited, and in normal hosts recovery is complete. If severe dehydration occurs, morbidity and even mortality may be substantial.

Infection of the gastrointestinal tract with agents, such as the enteroviruses, is usually an asymptomatic infection. However, the initial virus replication may be followed by viremia, with spread of virus to other target organs and symptoms related to the infection of the additional tissues. Contrary to early suggestions, enteroviruses do not appear to be responsible for any significant proportion of gastrointestinal tract disease. It is also necessary to note briefly that several nondiarrheal diseases of the gastrointestinal tract have a postulated viral etiology. Intussusception occurs most commonly in children under the age of 2 years, and mesenteric lymph node enlargement in the area of the terminal ileum has been observed at the time of surgery. Since lymphoid hyperplasia may ocur in association with virus infection and adenoviruses have been isolated from children with intussusception, they are one of the etiologic agents suggested for this entity. Coxsackie B viruses have been epidemiologically associated with diabetes mellitus, and several case reports have associated Coxsackie B4 with the development of diabetes mellitus. Experimentally, other viruses have been shown to infect pancreatic beta cells, and reovirus type 3 and murine encephalomyocarditis virus can produce a diabetes-like syndrome in inbred strains of mice. It must be emphasized that intussusception and diabetes mellitus have not been proven to be of viral etiology. It may be that virus infection represents only one of several contributing factors to the development of subsequent disease.

The viral agents discussed in detail in this chapter are those that seem to be associated with clinical symptoms related to virus replication within the gastrointestinal tract.

Rotaviruses

In 1943 an outbreak of diarrhea occurring in infants was reported by Light and Hodes. They isolated a filterable agent from stool specimens that caused diarrhea in calves. They established the incubation period and reproduced diarrhea with serial passage of the agent. The pathology of the bowel, the development of immunity to the agent, and passive protection by the administration of immune serum were described. At the time there was no confirmation of the viral etiology of the diarrhea as no agent could be detected in available cell culture systems. It was not until 1973 when virus particles were visualized in a duodenal biopsy by electron microscopy that the etiologic agent was finally defined as a rotavirus. In the past decade, rotaviruses have come to be appreciated as the single most common agent causing epidemic diarrhea in infants from 6 to 24 months of age. Rotaviruses are known to cause diarrhea in foals, lambs, piglets, rabbits, deer, monkeys, and other species. Experimental infection of animals other than the species of origin occurs with most rotaviruses.

Rotaviruses constitute one genus of the family Reoviridae. The rotavirus genome consists of 11 segments

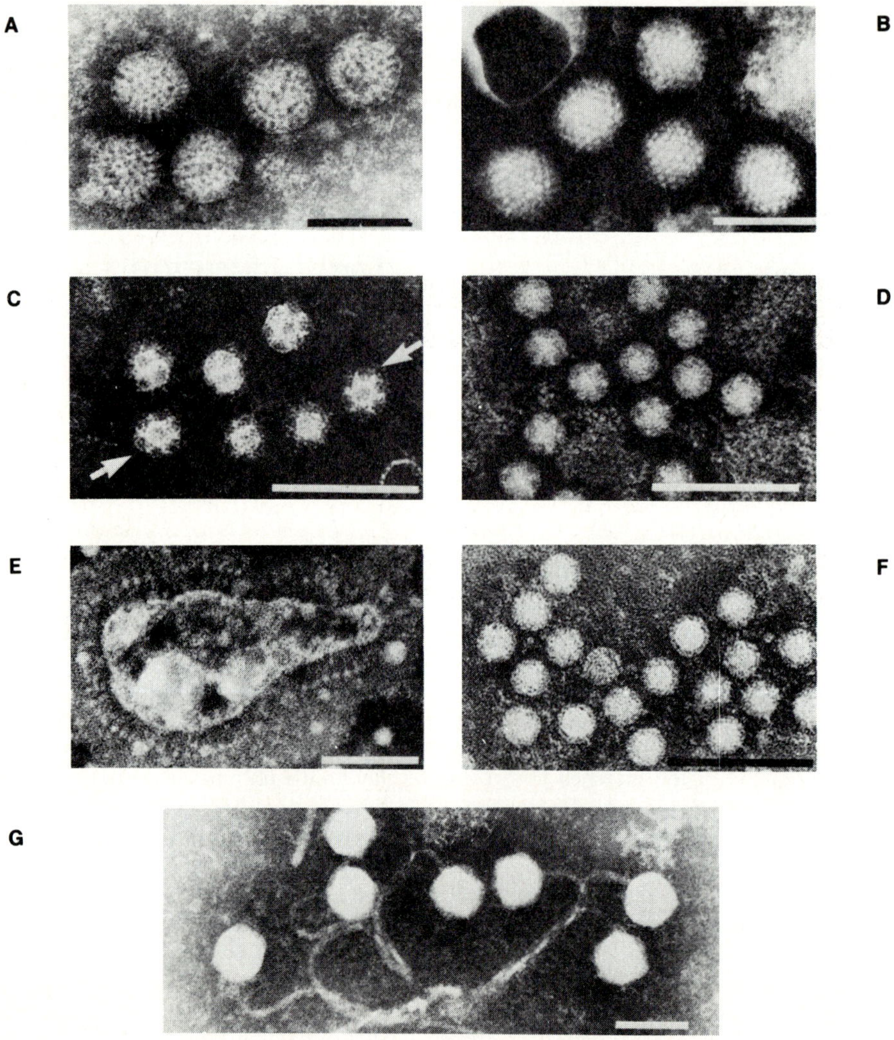

Figure 17-1. Viruses in feces from patients with gastroenteritis, negatively stained with 2 percent potassium phosphotungstate at pH 6.5. Bars present 100 nm. **A**. Rotaviruses. **B**. Adenoviruses. **C**. Calciviruses—two particles (arrowed) exhibit the characteristic morphology of a six-pointed star. **D**. Astroviruses—some particles show a five- or six-pointed star on the surface. **E**. Coronavirus—pleomorphic particle with large surface projections. **F**. Small round viruses (SRV)—particles with no obvious morphology and a diameter of 27 to 30 nm. **G**. Bacteriophages—these particles have hexagonal heads with long flexible tails attached to pieces of bacterial debris. *(Courtesy of H.A. Davies.)*

of double-stranded RNA, and rotavirus particles possess a double shell of outer and inner capsids (Fig. 17-1). The inability of these viruses to grow in the usual cell cultures has slowed research on them. It is the fourth gene that restricts ability of human rotaviruses to grow in cell culture, and if this gene is supplied by a bovine rotavirus (all animal rotaviruses *can* grow in cultured cells), the reassortant is able to grow. Gene *9* codes for the neutralizing antigen and gene *6* for the major internal structural protein responsible for type specificity. The fact that a high percentage of the strains can be typed indicates that the number of distinct serotypes may be limited. Additional information is of critical importance in defining the antigens responsible for inducing immunity and the feasibility of developing protective immunogens.

Epidemiology and Clinical Illness

Sporadic diarrhea occurring predominantly in infants and young children is associated with rotavirus infection. In fact, rotaviruses appear to be responsible for at least one half of the cases of infantile diarrhea that require hospitalization. Peak prevalence of rotavirus infection occurs during the cooler months of the year in temperate climates, but in tropical areas cases are identified throughout the year. Serum antibodies are usually acquired between the ages of 6 and 24 months. Transmission of rotavirus from person to person occurs via the fecal to oral route. The incubation period is 2 to 5 days. Adults are often contacts of symptomatc children and have infections that may be asymptomatic or associated with clinical illness. Asymptomatic or very mild infections, but not severe disease, have been reported in newborn nurseries.

Acute infection due to rotaviruses is characterized by the rather abrupt onset of severe watery diarrhea that is not characteristically associated with blood or mucus in the stool. Fever and vomiting are often present at the onset of illness. Dehydration and metabolic acidosis are observed in children hospitalized with this infection. Those most severely infected and affected are between the ages of 6 and 24 months of age.

Virus is excreted in large amounts, with as many as 10^{11} virus particles per gram of feces. Virus is excreted in feces for approximately 8 days after onset of symptoms. Virus does not seem to be shed from the respiratory tract, but aerosolization of fecally contaminated material may result in inhalation or ingestion of infectious virus.

Rotavirus particles have been visualized by electron microscopy in intestinal epithelial cells, aspirated duodenal secretions, and feces of infected persons. Morphologically, shortening and blunting of the villi of the duodenum and small intestine accompany acute illness. Virus particles are visualized in the cytoplasm and bud into the cisternae of the endoplasmic reticulum of the enterocytes. Immunofluorescence studies have also demonstrated rotavirus antigens in the cytoplasm of the villus epithelial cells but not in the cells of the crypts or lamina propria. This suggests that the specificity of the virus particle is for the mature or differentiated enterocytes located on the villi. This destruction of mature enterocytes is associated with the decrease in one or more mucosal disaccharidases. The destroyed infected cells are replaced by immature cells, which results in a deficit in glucose-facilitated sodium transport. Diarrhea then results from decreased absorption secondary to the altered ion transport in immature cells. In contrast to the toxin-mediated diarrheas, there is no increase in intestinal secretion. Complete recovery has been documented by biopsy as early as 4 weeks after the episode of diarrhea.

Host Response

Specific antibody has been demonstrable in the stool and serum. Primary infection seems to produce an initial serum IgM response, followed by an IgG response. Adults with rotavirus infection manifest an anamnestic response with elevation of IgG antibodies. Some studies in volunteers suggest that protection from infection with rotaviruses correlates better with secretory IgA of the small intestine than with serum antibody. Persons may experience more than one infection with rotaviruses. It is not yet clear whether these are always different serotypes.

Specific antibody has been demonstrated in colostrum and milk for as long as 9 months of lactation. In nurseries where rotavirus infection has been endemic, breast-fed infants seem to acquire infection less often than do formula-fed infants. Those who are infected excrete less virus and are less symptomatic. Antibodies in human colostrum and milk are capable of neutralizing rotavirus in vitro. Weaning from breast milk in developing nations is temporally associated with the onset of a diarrhea/malnutrition cycle. Despite the fact that breast milk has been shown to have preventive activity against undifferentiated infantile diarrhea and, even more specifically, has been shown to contain antibodies against some of the causative agents, breastfeeding is declining in popularity in many parts of the world with the greatest incidence of diarrheal disease. Breast milk does provide both specific and nonspecific protection.

Diagnosis

Human rotaviruses are extremely fastidious, but recent progress has been made in the cell culture propagation of these agents. Human rotavirus strains have been efficiently propagated directly from clinical specimens into cell cultures. In particular MA 104 cells, which are a line derived from embryonic rhesus monkey kidney, have been successfully used. The specimen is pretreated with trypsin (10 μg/ml), and 1 μg/ml of trypsin is added to the maintenance medium. The ability to grow these viruses in cell culture will enhance the study of these agents.

The quantity of virus excreted in fecal specimens has enabled various antigen detection systems to identify virus in the stool. Electron microscopic examination of fecal extracts obtained during the acute stage of gastroenteritis, particularly when specific antiserum is used to agglutinate virus particles, is almost invariably positive. Enzyme-linked immunosorbent assay (ELISA) and radioimmunoassay techniques have also become available for the detection of rotavirus particles in stool. All known rotaviruses share a common antigen thought to be located in the inner capsid, which makes the immunologic detection of these viruses a practical reality. Indirect assays employ an unlabeled specific antibody and subsequent measurement of the antibody/antigen combination with an enzyme-labeled antiglobulin. ELISAs are as sensitive as elecron microscopy and are more practical, since commercially marketed reagent kits are now available for detection of rotavirus in stool.

Prevention and Therapy

Therapy of viral gastroenteritis is limited to supportive measures, since there are no effective antiviral agents available for specific treatment.

There can be no doubt that prevention of rotavirus illness would be a major contribution to reduction or morbidity from gastroenteritis. For immunization to be effective, immunity within the gastrointestinal tract is probably a necessity. Various approaches to immunization that are being considered include a live attenuated human rotavirus vaccine, an attenuated reassortant rotavirus vaccine, a vaccine made from an animal rotavirus strain if such a strain is able to infect humans without causing illness, cloning of the human rotavirus genome by DNA technology, and production of synthetic vaccines derived from the specific amino acid sequences responsible for induction of protective antibodies. Reassortants have already been created, and work with human rotaviruses in cell culture has facilitated the study of these agents. The task of defining protective antigens has made the feasibility of a vaccine an accessible goal.

Norwalk Group of Viruses

Agents Associated with Epidemic Viral Gastroenteritis

Epidemic gastroenteritis occurs in a form that produces an explosive, self-limited disease lasting for 24 to 48 hours, may be communitywide, and involves school-age children, family contacts, and adults. Such as outbreak of gastroenteritis occurred in Norwalk, Ohio, in 1969. Within a matter of 48 hours gastrointestinal illness developed in half of the students and teachers in an elementary school, with the secondary symptomatic attack rate affecting approximately one third of family contacts. A bacteria-free filtrate from a stool specimen produced gastroenteritis in several volunteers, and stools from the infected individuals could be serially passaged in additional volunteers, but no agent could be isolated in the usual cell culture systems. In 1972, immune electron microscopy with serum from a symptomatic patient demonstrated small, 27-nm-diameter particles in an infectious stool filtrate. Norwalk agent particles contain RNA and only a single protein species with a molecular weight of 59,000. Among mammalian viruses in this size range, the caliciviruses are the only ones that possess a single structual protein. The Norwalk agent is, therefore, probably a calicivirus (Fig. 17-1).

Epidemiology and Clinical Infection

Roughly one third of outbreaks of gastroenteritis can be attributed to a Norwalk-like agent. This is a surprisingly high number and suggests that the antigenically unique viruses of this group may be limited in number. The settings in which such outbreaks have occurred include schools, recreational camps, cruise ships, persons using contaminated water, nursing homes, and ingestion of inadequately cooked shellfish. Outbreaks have occurred at all times of the year, and antibody surveys suggest that the agent occurs worldwide. In most undeveloped nations, infection occurs at an early age. In the United States, antibody is uncommon during childhood and develops during late adolescence and early adulthood.

Norwalk agents are transmitted by the fecal to oral route, and volunteers who have shed virus had detectable virus in their stools during the first 72 hours after the onset of illness. Although respiratory symptoms are very unusual, the rapidity of spread suggests that some aerolization of virus may occur from fecal contamination of the environment.

Infection with these agents result in delayed gastric emptying, although the gastric mucosa is morphologically normal. Microscopic broadening and blunting of the villi in the jejunum is apparent. The mucosa remains histologically intact, but there is mononuclear cell infiltration. Virus has not yet been detected in involved mucosal cells by elecron microscopy.

The majority of patients who sustain these infections have nausea, vomiting, and abdominal cramps, and about one half of them have associated diarrhea. Some have fever and chills. The symptoms last from 12 to 24 hours, and the incubation period appears to be around 48 hours. Usually the stools are not bloody and do not have mucus or leukocytes. A transient lymphopenia has been observed in volunteers challenged with these agents.

Host Response

Immunity to these viruses is a puzzling feature of the infections that they cause. Challenge of volunteers produces disease in some persons and not in others. Repeat challenge with homologous virus within several months of the original infection will not produce clinical illness. Subsequent challenge 2 to 4½ years later produces disease in the same volunteers who had symptomatic illness with the first contact with the virus. Those individuals who were asymptomatic and did not acquire infection with the first contact do not do so with subsequent challenge. Those individuals who acquire clinical infection have demonstrable antibody that wanes and then have an anticipated boost with a subsequent challenge. Volunteers who fail to develop illness have no demonstrable antibody. Measurement of intestinal antibody also showed that those individuals who develop illness have higher mean antibody titers in jejunal fluid than those who failed to develop illness. Neither serum nor local intestinal antibody correlates with resistance to a Norwalk challenge. Thus, individuals who have demonstrable serum antibody are those who are at risk for symptoms induced by infection. These findings are not understood, but it is possible that some individuals are not susceptible to these viruses by reason of genetically determined factors. It is also possible that repetitive exposure to the virus is necessary to induce an antibody response.

Diagnosis and Therapy

Immune electron microscopy is the best available procedure for identifying members of this group of agents. Specific coating of particles with antibody needs to be observed if the immune response is being assessed.

The radioimmunoassay is more efficient than immune electron microscopy because it is able to detect soluble as well as particulate antigens. This test depends on the availability of appropriate high titered serum. In research laboratories radioimmunoassay has been used to assess serum antibody status.

The illnesses associated with the Norwalk group of agents are generally self-limited and mild. No specific therapy is available. Replacement fluid therapy is essential in management of such patients. The rather simplistic approach of good handwashing and effective hygiene is the best we have to offer to prevent the spread of these viruses.

Coronaviruses

Coronaviridae are pleomorphic, enveloped, single-stranded RNA-containing viruses with widely spaced 20 nm club-shaped surface projections (Fig. 17-1). This group of viruses has been well identified as etiologic agents of respiratory and intestinal disease in animals. In 1960 the first of these agents was isolated from a human with a cold. It grew in human tracheal organ culture and was morphologically similar to infectious bronchitis virus, an avian coronavirus. A second isolate, now the prototype strain of human coronavirus (229E), was isolated in human kidney cell culture in 1962.

Human coronaviruses were first etiologically associated with upper respiratory tract disease in adults and lower respiratory tract disease in hospitalized children. It has also been found that coronaviruses may be responsible for an exacerbation of the respiratory symptomatology in hospitalized asthmatic children. Coronavirus infections tend to occur in small outbreaks that take place during the late winter and early spring. Sporadic outbreaks in other seasons can also occur. Periods of high incidence with one specific serotype have been reported to occur in cycles of 2 to 3 years. Reinfection with coronaviruses is a frequent event, as shown by the presence of infection in persons with preexisting neutralizing antibodies.

It was predicted in the mid-1970s that an association of coronaviruses with enteric disease of humans would be identified because of the known involvement of these agents with enteric disease in animals. Electron microscopic examination of stools then revealed coronavirus-like particles in human feces. In fecal specimens it has been estimated that there are as many as 10^8 coronavirus particles per gram of feces. Many of these particles are defective, which suggests that maturation may be faulty within the gastrointestinal tract.

Of interest is an apparent difference in the epidemiology of these viruses. They seem to be less likely to be responsible for diarrhea within the first year of life and are more commonly visualized in the diarrheal stools of older children and young adults. Enteric coronaviruses can be excreted for as long as a year and a half, and in some of the persistent excretors chronic gastroenteritis is present. Prolonged viral excretion complicates conclusions concerning the epidemiology because asymptomatic individuals can be excreting virus. It has been documented that endemic diarrheal disease occurs in situations where poor hygiene exists, and acquisition of virus does coincide with development of gastroenteritis.

Work with the coronaviruses isolated from humans has been difficult because they grow best in organ cultures, and those from the respiratory tract appear to require the use of ciliated epithelium. They are labile under conditions of virus purification. Thus, detailed analyses of avian and other mammalian coronaviruses have proceeded at a much more rapid rate. The successful cultivation in vitro of several human strains is beginning to advance our knowledge of these viruses. Human coronaviruses possess four major structural proteins; the surface projections that are responsible for hemagglutination and complement fixation consist of two large glycoproteins. There are at least two antigenic groups of mammalian coronaviruses. Coronaviruses do not appear to bud from the plasma membrane of infected cells but bud into the cisternae of the endoplasmic reticulum and are found in large intracytoplasmic vesicles (Chap. 4).

Enteric Adenovirus

The fastidious enteric adenoviruses were first described by Flewett in 1975. These agents have been established as a significant pathogen of diarrheal illness in children. Preliminary characterization of agents isolated from geographically distinct outbreaks indicates that they are all representatives of the adenovirus 38 candidate serotype (Fig. 17-1). These agents do not grow in the usual cell culture systems, and thus far successful in vitro cultivation has been dependent upon the use of Graham 293 cells, a human embryonic kidney cell line containing some of the genome of adenovirus type 5. In these cells the cytopathic effects produced are typical of adenoviruses.

These agents most often appear to be responsible for acute diarrhea in infants less than 1 year of age. The onset of illness is manifest by diarrhea, and the young child may also have respiratory symptoms, including cough, rhinorrhea, or wheezing. Pneumonia and conjunctivities have also been seen in association with adenovirus gastroenteritis. The illness is usually mild to moderate in severity and may occur in any month of the year. The viruses are visualized in the feces of patients for a period of 4 days to 2 weeks.

The estimated frequency of adenoviruses as a cause of diarrhea varies. If the study period is selected when rotavirus disease is not occurring, adenoviruses are responsible for a larger proportion of illness, recorded to be as high as 50 percent. If a prospective study is managed over a several year period, 4 to 8 percent of all the diarrhea observed may be associated with these fastidious adenoviruses. Serologic studies of children suggest that approximately one half of children have antibodies at an early age.

The diagnosis of these agents is also dependent upon demonstration of the virus particles or antigen in stool. Initial recognition by electron microscopy has been followed by the development of ELISAs and radioimmunoassays.

Astroviruses

Astroviruses were described in 1975 after visualization in the stool of newborn infants. They are 28-nm particles shed in the stool in very large numbers. They are present in the stools of infants both with and without acute gastroenteritis. The star shape designates the agents as astrovirus particles (Fig. 17-1). Similar morphologic structures have been identified in feces from both adults and children and in diarrheal feces from lambs and calves. These agents infect monolayers of human embryonic kidney cells without producing cytopathic effects. The evidence that they cause disease is equivocal. Early serologic studies have demonstrated seroconversion in association with demonstrable infection and fecal excretion. However, feeding of these agents to adult volunteers resulted in poor transmission of disease but antibody rises in the majority of volunteers. It may be that most adults have previously met the agents and, therefore, are protected against disease.

In lambs, these agents infect the epithelial cells and the subepithelial macrophages of the villi of the small intestine. Atrophy of the villi is demonstrable. At least in animals it would appear that they are capable of causing gastroenteritis.

Other Putative Viruses

The interest in examining feces by electron microscopy has resulted in the description of numerous virus species. Some of them are clearly defined as etiologic agents of gastroenteritis, and others have yet to be assigned a definitive etiologic role. The relationship to each other or other morphologic species also remains to be determined. These as yet unidentified and unclassified types of particles are discussed below.

Small Round Viruses, Picorna-Parvovirus-like

This is a heterogeneous collection of small round viruses visualized in stools. The particles have a diameter of 27 to 30 nm, no detectable surface structure, and do not grow in vitro in routine cell culture systems (Fig. 17-1). They have been seen in stools from patients who have no clinical symptoms. More information is needed to establish their causative role in gastroenteritis.

Mini-Reovirus

These agents are 30 nm particles with a double capsid. They have been visualized in stools from children with diarrhea and in infants who have acquired diarrhea within hospital settings. Additional information is needed to establish their role as etiologic agents in gastroenteritis.

FURTHER READING

GENERAL

Tyrrell DAJ, Kapikian AZ: Virus Infections of the Gastrointestinal Tract. New York, Basel, Marcel Dekker, 1982

ROTAVIRUSES

Blacklow NR, Cukor G: Viral gastroenteritis. N Engl J Med 304:397, 1981

Steinhoff MC: Rotavirus: The first 5 years. J Pediatr 96:611, 1980

NORWALK-LIKE AGENTS

Adler I, Vicki R: Winter vomiting disease. J Infect Dis 119:668, 1969

Agus SG, Dolin R, Wyatt RG, et al.: Acute infectious nonbacterial gastroenteritis: Intestinal histopathology. Histologic and enzymatic alterations during illness produced by the Norwalk agent in man. Ann Intern Med 79:18, 1973

Blacklow MR, Cukor G, Bedigian MK, et al.: Immunoresponse and prevalence of antibody to Norwalk enteritis virus as determined by radioimmunoassay. J Clin Microbiol 10:903, 1979

Blacklow MR, Dolin R, Fedson DS, et al.: Acute infectious nonbacterial gastroenteritis: Etiology and pathogenesis. Ann Intern Med 76:993, 1972

Dolin R, Blacklow MR, DuPont H, et al.: Transmission of acute infectious nonbacterial gastroenteritis in two volunteers by oral administration of stool filtrates. J Infect Dis 123:307, 1971

Greenberg HB, Valvesuso J, Kalica AR, et al.: Proteins of Norwalk virus. J Virol 37:994, 1981

Schaffer FL: Calicivirus. In Fraenkel-Conrat H, Wagner RR (eds): Comprehensive Virology. New York, Plenum, 1978, vol 14, p 249

OTHER VIRUSES

Flewett PH, Davies H: Caliciviruses in man. Lancet 1:311, 1976

MacNaughton MR, Davies HA: Human enteric Corona viruses. Arch Virol 70:301, 1981

Madaley CR, Cosgrove BP: Viruses in infantile gastroenteritis. Lancet 2:124, 1975

Madaley CR, Cosgrove BP, Bell EJ, et al.: Stool viruses in babies in Glasgow. I. Hospital admissions with diarrhea. J Hyg 78:261, 1977

Kurtz JB, Lee TW, Pickering D: Astrovirus-associated gastroenteritis in a children's ward. J Clin Pathol 30:948, 1977

Kurtz JB, Lee TW, Craig JW, et al.: Astrovirus infection in volunteers. J Med Virol 3:221, 1979

Chiba S, Sakuma Y, Kogasaka R, et al.: Fecal shedding of virus in relation to the days of illness in infantile gastroenteritis due to calicivirus. J Infect Dis 142:247, 1980

Kapikian AZ, Wyatt RG, Greenberg HB, et al.: Approaches to immunization of infants and young children against gastroenteritis due to rotaviruses. Rev Infect Dis 2:459, 1980

CHAPTER 18

Influenza Viruses

Members of this group of ubiquitous myxoviruses produce epidemic illness so regularly that all readers of this chapter will have experienced several infections by them. They have been inconstant companions of human beings for at least as long as recorded history, and the broad age range of those afflicted, as well as the broad spectrum of illness observed, was well described in English texts as early as the 16th century, when it was called the "newe acquaintance." Because of the seasonality of influenza epidemics, it was thought initially to be a disease affected by celestial movement ("malattia influenza per le stelle"), and this belief permanently baptized both the viruses and the clinical illnesses that they produce. Although several major epidemics occurred during the early part of the 20th century, the viral etiology of this disease was not demonstrated until the 1930s, and an understanding of the antigenic variability of these viruses and thus the periodic occurrence of epidemic illness had to await the more advanced virologic techniques of the 1940s and 1950s.

Clinical Features

As with most viral diseases, influenza represents a very broad spectrum of severity of clinical illness, from the occasional asymptomatic infection to the more common, bothersome, and irritating grippe, to the often fatal primary influenza pneumonia. The reasons for this wide variation are poorly understood and may be partly, but not exclusively, related to the age, health, and antigenic background of the patient, the presence of preexisting abnormalities of the pulmonary parenchyma or vasculature, and possibly to the virulence of the virus itself. The tissue tropism for influenza virus and thus the pathogenesis of infection may be explained by a unique virus–host cell interaction. Hemagglutinin, one of the glycoprotein spikes present on the surface of the virus (Chap. 8), is responsible for adsorption of virus to the host cell. The host cell receptors not only must contain N-acetyl neuraminic acid residues but must also express proteases that cleave the hemagglutinin to render it infectious. There is significant homology in the cleavage region between the hemagglutinin of influenza A and B as well as the F protein of paramyxoviruses. This suggests that fusion of viral and cellular membranes may occur during penetration.

The significant histologic abnormalities induced by the virus are relatively uniform, beginning with virus replication in all superficial respiratory cells, destruction of the ciliated columnar epithelium, and subsequent denudation of the tracheobronchial tree. These anatomic changes invariably lead to impairment in respiratory function and physiology, even in patients without obvious clinical evidence of pulmonary involvement. Defects include diminished defusing capacity, diminished tracheobronchial clearance, increased bronchial reactivity (sensitivity to irritation), and variable degrees of small airway obstruction. The pharyngitis and tracheitis thus induced explain the severe throat and substernal pain, cough, and shortness of breath often seen during acute illness, as well as the paroxysms of cough that may be exacerbated by sudden exposure either to cold or environmental pollutants for weeks after the subsidence of clinical illness. Some of the functional pulmonary defects may require weeks or, occasionally, months to disappear. Furthermore, influenza virus infection not only ablates the normal removal of bacteria in the mucous blanket by destroying ciliated cells but also decreases T lymphocyte function and granulocyte chemotaxis. The tracheobronchial tree that has been denuded of its usual defense mechanisms is therefore more susceptible to invasion by bacteria. This occurs most commonly in patients with chronic bronchitis (where large numbers of bacteria may already be present in the lower respiratory tract), in aged individuals, and in others with poor cough reflexes and poor efficiency of expectoration, or in any patient in whom pulmonary mechanics or host defense mechanisms are already abnormal.

The usual clinical disease begins rather suddenly within 1 or 2 days after exposure to infected aerosol droplets (Fig. 18-1), most often in epidemic circumstances and primarily during the colder months of the year. A sudden rise in temperature, sometimes to 102F, though rarely higher in adults, is accompanied by rigors and myalgias and is then followed by the variable appearance of sore throat, nasal congestion and dryness, conjunctivitis, a nonproductive cough, and headache. Marked lassitude and moderate anorexia accompany these symptoms and are frequently so severe that even the most stalwart and ambitious individual must spend the first day or two of illness in bed. Physical examination will reveal generalized vasodilation of the dermal and mucosal surfaces of the head and neck, as well as edema and little to moderate discharge from the upper respiratory tract. On auscultation, the lungs are generally clear in individuals with otherwise healthy pulmonary function. Young children, however, are prone to develop laryngotracheobronchitis, bronchiolitis, gastrointestinal upset, febrile seizures, conjunctivitis, and the common sequela of otitis media. Laboratory studies will generally show a moderate lymphocytopenia, and blood gas analysis will often indicate a surprising level of hypoxia even in patients without physical or roentgenologic evidence of pulmonary involvement. Patchy diffuse infiltrates of small size can occasionally be noted on chest x-ray. However, these are usually evanescent and of little consequence but must be differentiated from the more severe forms of pneumonia seen during influenza epidemics and described below. Acute bronchitis, possibly bacterial, and exacerbations of chronic bronchitis are seen more commonly. The symptoms generally subside within several days, and the patient is able to return to normal daily functions shortly thereafter. However, a severe postviral aesthenia, as well as a depressed affect, may be quite striking and persist for several weeks or more after resolution of the illness. The etiology of this weakness and easy fatigability is unknown, and its perceived severity is often proportionate to the expectations of the patient, as is often the case with infectious mononucleosis occurring during adolescence.

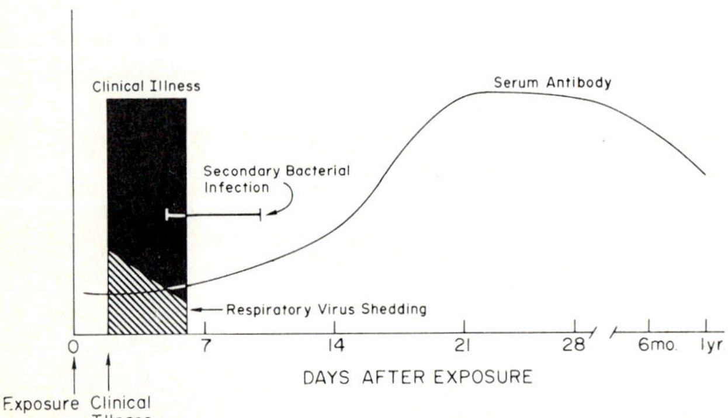

Figure 18-1. The course of influenza virus infection.

Pneumonias are the most common serious complications of influenza and can be divided into two fairly distinct types. The more common is that produced by secondary bacterial invasion. It occurs particularly in patients with preexisting lung disease and in elderly or debilitated individuals. It usually follows a brief quiescent period after the initial viral illness, at a time when the patient feels he is beginning to recover. The most common infecting organisms are pneumococci, *Haemophilus influenzae*, and staphylococci, although any species of bacteria can cause such an infection. The pneumonias themselves differ in no way from those caused by the same organisms under any other circumstance, and mortality is generally low (less than 20 percent). As with all bacterial pneumonias, nevertheless, the precise prognosis of the patient depends on the virulence and sensitivity to antibiotics of the infecting organism, the age and general health of the patient, the expertise of the physician, and the zeal and skill with which supportive care is given.

A second type of infection caused solely by the virus itself is much less common but considerably more lethal. The patient's clinical illness gives him no respite from the explosive onset of the grippe and continues inexorably through coughing, often in paroxysms, and marked shortness of breath, finally requiring admission to hospital. The sputum is scant, with little mucus, and is occasionally tinged with blood. Hypoxia is marked, and chest x-rays often reveal more than does physical examination. Initially there are small patches and streaks of hazy infiltration, usually extending from the hilum to involve one or several lobes. These infiltrates increase in size, distribution, and density each day in spite of increasing levels of respiratory support and the desperate use of antibiotics until near total opacification of both lung fields occurs, and the patient expires from extreme hypoxia. This sequence may evolve so rapidly that occasionally a patient may die suddenly after only a few days' or hours' symptoms, whereas patients with severely depressed cell-mediated immunity may rarely manifest a much more indolent course. On pathologic examination, the lungs appear firm and red, and the cut surfaces give the appearance of raw beef. Microscopic examination reveals no bacteria but rather severe interstitial edema and hemorrhage, as well as occlusion of alveoli with proteinaceous debris and blood. While this disease is seen most commonly in patients with mitral stenosis and, in some epidemics, in women during the last trimester of pregnancy, it may occasionally be seen in otherwise healthy individuals.

It should be emphasized that many more patients die as a result of influenza that can be accounted for solely by those succumbing from pneumonia. Total excess mortality (the difference between the observed and expected number of deaths in a given time period) is generally two to three times greater during influenza epidemics than mortality from pneumonias. This can be easily understood if one accepts that influenza infection causes major derangements in many of the body's homeostatic mechanisms, and a large number of patients with marginal cardiac, metabolic, neurologic, and renal function may succumb rapidly from their primary disease when overcome by the virus-induced stress of fever and hypoxia.

A number of other less common complications or sequelae of influenza have been observed at variable frequencies, and these include myositis, myocarditis, pericarditis, orbital cellulitis, aseptic meningitis, as well as a postinfectious neuritis impossible to distinguish from the Guillain–Barré syndrome. Elegant epidemiologic studies have strongly established that von Economo's encephalitis (encephalitis lethargica) and thus most postencephalitic parkinsonism were a result of H swine-like influenza, which was epidemic or sporadic between 1918 and the late 1920s. This illness has not been observed following infection with other strains of influenza, but an increased incidence of bacterial meningitis has occasionally been noted during some influenza epidemics, confirming experimental animal studies that demonstrated that influenza increases the susceptibility to meningococcal and *H. influenzae* infections by mechanisms that have not been fully elucidated.

Epidemiology

The interpersonal spread of influenza viruses is caused by the formation of virus-laden aerosol droplets when an infected patient sneezes or coughs. Individuals in the immediate vicinity inhale these particles, the larger ones being deposited in the nares and upper nasopharynx, the smaller ones reaching the lower tracheobronchial tree. If the virus is not neutralized, as for example by local IgA-specific antihemagglutinin antibody, initial replication occurs. Further replication, and thus clinical illness, is dependent on a host of factors, including local IgA, serum IgG, and possibly various effectors of cell-mediated immunity. The efficiency of aerosol spread is exceedingly high and is in direct proportion to the number of particles generated, the density of susceptibles, their physical and temporal contiguity to the aerosols, and the degree of stagnation of the ambient atmosphere. It is not surprising, therefore, to observe high attack rates (at times approaching 90 percent) in nursing homes, classrooms, barracks, ships, and aircraft, where these conditions are at their worst. Cigarette smoking increases the susceptibility to infection and is associated with more severe clinical illness. There is little evidence that other modes of contagion play a significant part in the spread of influenza, although the role of hand contact and certain fomites, such as nasal spray applicators and drinking glasses, remains to be investigated.

Young children of preschool or gradeschool age appear to be the most effective disseminators of this disease, probably as a direct result of their limited prior experience with influenza (and thus high attack rates), as well as their primitive concepts of hygiene when they are actively excreting virus. An explanation of the appearance of epidemic influenza in the winter in temperate zones has been assiduously sought, but few positive conclusions have been reached. It does not appear to be directly related to temperature, relative humidity, or the duration of sunlight exposure. Likewise, wetting or chilling of the susceptible, so prominent a factor in avian respiratory infections, also does not appear to influence the susceptibility to or virulence of human influenza infections. It must be remembered that influenza epidemics may occur at any time in the tropics, and there have been epidemics recorded in every month of the year in the United States. Our largest recorded epidemic occurred in the late summer and early fall of 1918.

An understanding of the periodicity of influenza epidemics and pandemics requires a basic knowledge of the ultrastructure of the virus, as delineated in Chapter 8, for the surface antigens of the virus and the antibodies they induce within a population determine the epidemiology of influenza. The lipid envelope of the virus is covered by a number of glycoprotein spikes made up primarily of hemagglutinin with a smaller number of separate neuraminidase spikes. Because neuraminidase cleaves neuraminic acid from glycoproteins or glycolipids, it permits elution of virus from cell receptors or glycoproteins in secretions. Thus neuraminidase facilitates cell-to-cell spread and may even remove neuraminic acid residues from hemagglutinin, facilitating its cleavage and activation. Antibody to hemagglutinin prevents infection, either in tissue culture or in people, whereas antibody to neuraminidase does not neutralize virus or prevent infection but does limit viral spread in tissue culture and, if antihemagglutinin antibody is absent, lessens the severity of clinical influenza. Changes in the amino acid sequences of these glycoproteins lead to changes in their antigenic identity. The mechanisms that engender these changes have been a matter of great speculation for many years. It is now known, however, that influenza viruses are genetically extremely unstable as a result of either recombination/reassortment, insertions, frequent point mutations, and/or an absence of "proofreading" enzymes found in most DNA viruses. All of these factors are further multiplied by the relatively high replication rate of influenza viruses.

Generally, when a new virus with a different hemagglutinin type appears, there is little antibody against it in the population at large. The first wave of the epidemic infects a substantial proportion (25 to 60 percent) of the population. The virus also has the opportunity to undergo spontaneous, albeit limited, mutation (antigenic drift), so that a separate wave occurring 1 to 5 years later infects many of the remaining antibody-negative individuals, as well as some of the individuals who were previously infected but whose antihemagglutinin antibody response was either initially low or had waned over the intervening years. This sequence continues until the vast majority of the population has developed protective levels of antibody. At that point, a new hemagglutinin type, which shares no obvious antigenic cross-reactivity with the first, begins the cycle once again.

The grouping of these major antigenic types is based on the ability to observe serologic cross-reactivity in hemagglutination- or neuraminidase-inhibition (HI or NI) tests. To date, there have been five major types of human influenza hemagglutinin identified (H swine, H0, H1, H2, and H3) and two major types of neuraminidase (N1 and N2). Antibody to one will not be protective against infection with the other. That a greater hierarchy occurs than can be detected by serologic HI assays, however, is demonstrated by the fact that one can note antigenic priming among members of the H swine, H0, and H1 group, and similar priming among the H2 and H3 groups. Such priming is observed when prior infection with one member of the group causes an accelerated antibody response when subsequent infection or immunization occurs with another member of the group. The immunologic relatedness of the H swine, H0, and H1 group is so strong, in fact, that they have all recently been placed in the same group, designated H1.

Serologic analysis of individuals who were alive during the epidemics occurring in the latter part of the 19th century and the early part of the 20th century have clarified and greatly expanded our understanding of the periodic recurrences of influenza epidemics. Epidemics of viruses bearing the H2 hemagglutinin occurred in 1889 to 1890, and these viruses were later replaced by viruses probably bearing the H3 antigen around 1900. The H swine antigen first appeared in 1918 and gave rise to one of the greatest epidemics in recorded history. Next to appear in the 1930s was the H0 antigen, and viruses carrying the H1 antigen became epidemic in 1946. The H2 antigen then reappeared in 1957, to be supplanted by the H3 antigen in 1968, a sequence similar to that noted in 1889 and 1900. After the abortive reappearance of viruses bearing the H swine antigen in 1976, the H1 antigen reappeared in Southeast China in mid-1977 and caused widespread epidemics with apparently low mortality throughout the world in 1977 and 1978. Since that time, both H1 and H3 viruses have circulated simultaneously in the world population, with outbreaks caused by H3 viruses generally associated with more significant morbidity. The coexistence of H1 and H3 antigens had not been regularly observed in the past and defies current epidemiologic explanation.

Many recent pandemics (1957, 1968, 1977) began in China. The reasons for this are not clear, although it has been hypothesized that the density of human and swine or duck populations in the area near Canton provides an opportunity for dual infections with viruses indigenous to each species. Subsequent recombination may produce numerous new viruses, some of which may be novel or more virulent or against which there is little protective antibody in the population. Credence was given to the possibility of increased interspecies virulence when the mass die-off of harbor seals on the New England coast in 1980 was found to have been caused by an influenza virus bearing avian markers. Although spread from China to the rest of the world may take several months or more, the inexplicable simultaneous appearance of a new influenza virus in several widely separated parts of the world is well documented and was observed even before the advent of rapid intercontinental travel. Epidemics tend to sweep rapidly through individual communities and rarely last more than a month from beginning to end. Mortality rates are difficult to quantitate, but are generally quite low, often being quoted as 0.01 to 0.1 percent for the population at large, although the case fatality rate is considerably higher in the very young and particularly the very old. No valid explanation has yet been brought forth to account for the high fatality rate, especially in patients in their third and fourth decades of life, observed in the 1918 H swine epidemic.

Influenza B viruses also undergo major and minor antigenic changes, though at lower frequencies and longer intervals. Epidemics caused by influenza B viruses have occasionally been associated with excess mortality, but the significance of major antigenic changes, as occurred for example in 1973, is more obvious in younger rather than older age groups. Children are more readily infected with this virus, are more obviously symptomatic once infected, and are more likely to suffer one of the most serious sequelae of infection by this virus, Reye's syndrome. The association of this disease, characterized by hepatocerebral fatty infiltration and degeneration, with influenza B and a few other virus infections, including influenza A, is extremely strong, and over 300 cases were noted in the United States during the brief influenza B epidemic of 1973–1974. The pathomechanisms of this disease remain to be elucidated, but epidemiologic studies have shown a considerably higher risk of this complication in those patients who received aspirin rather than acetaminophen as part of their treatment for clinical influenza. Although a direct cause-and-effect relationship has yet to be defined to the satisfaction of all concerned, it would seem most prudent to use acetaminophen rather than aspirin in children with influenza B infection, at least until the matter has been fully clarified.

Diagnosis

While the influenza viruses can produce a wide variety of clinical illnesses, it must also be remembered that a broad spectrum of infectious and noninfectious agents can produce clinical syndromes that are similar to those of influenza. Patients infected by other common respiratory pathogens (RSV, adenovirus, coronavirus, rhinovirus, parainfluenza viruses) will often state that they have "the flu." Although influenza is more easily diagnosed during epidemics, a pathognomonic complex of signs and symptoms does not exist, and there is little to distinguish it on clinical grounds from other illnesses that may also occur during these periods. Recent experience in the Caribbean, for example, has shown that even epidemic dengue is difficult to distinguish from influenza unless the patient has prominent respiratory signs and symptoms.

Rapid confirmation of the clinical impression of influenza can be obtained by examination of material obtained by swabbing the posterior pharynx. Viral antigen can be detected within nasopharyngeal cells by direct or indirect immunofluorescent stains directed at any of the viral antigens. Such tests, however, are not generally available and require excellent reagents and appropriate positive and negative controls, as well as experienced observers.

The virus may also be grown from nasopharyngeal swabs after inoculation into any of several substrates. One of the more convenient and effective is continuous Madin–Darby canine kidney (MDCK) cells. Other effective substrates are primary monkey kidney cells and the allantoic or amniotic cavity of 10-day-old embryonated hen's eggs. In most instances, little viral cytopathic effect is induced, and the presence of virus must be determined by immunofluorescence, hemadsorption, or hemagglutination. Plaques can be formed in MDCK cells if the overlay contains trypsin, but this is of little use in primary isolation. Viral culture of the blood is of no use, as viremia is exceedingly rare in influenza.

It is usually not practical, necessary, or even desirable to attempt virus isolation in most clinical situations. Nonetheless, programs of surveillance that include virologic culture of select populations, are highly necessary for the general well-being. Individuals involved in such programs serve as sentinels and permit the early awareness of epidemic influenza. These surveillance systems operate best when centralized, as through the Centers for Disease Control or the World Health Organization, and when they disseminate their information rapidly and effectively. Public health authorities may then make plans for immuno- or chemoprophylaxis.

Serologic confirmation of influenza infection is rarely required. If such a confirmation is deemed necessary for scientific investigational purposes, however, several facts should be borne in mind. Complement-fixation (CF) tests depend on the interaction between antibody and internal (nucleocapsid) proteins. Since these proteins are antigenically (if not chemically) identical for all viruses within a group (A, B, or C), positive CF tests can signify infection by a member of that group but cannot more specifically identify the virus. CF titers generally rise relatively rapidly (within 1 to 2 weeks), but their decline is somewhat variable, often in terms of several weeks to several months. In some patients, however, they may persist for longer periods of time, though usually at a rather low titer. A single postillness serum sample, therefore, cannot be considered absolutely diagnostic but does become more useful if the titer is elevated ($\geq 1:32$). Studies of postinfection CF titers are generally of more epidemiologic than clinical value.

A more precise method of determining acute influenza infection is the quantitation of HI antibodies simultaneously on a sample obtained before or at the beginning of illness and a second sample obtained 3 or more weeks later. A four-fold rise in antibody titer is considered diagnostic of influenza if the patient has not been recently vaccinated. Additionally, because this antibody is directed against the specific surface glycoprotein, the precise identity of the originally infecting organism can generally be determined with some precision.

Since most influenza infections are self-limited and recovery can be hastened only moderately by early amantadine therapy, the major goal in diagnosis is often to determine whether other diseases causing influenzal syndromes are present or whether pneumonia caused by bacterial superinfection has occurred. The criteria for establishing the latter diagnosis include sustained pyrexia, leukocytosis, evidence of pulmonary consolidation on physical or x-ray examination, and, most importantly, the presence of substantial numbers of granulocytes and bacteria in the sputum. It cannot be overemphasized that the ability to perform a proper gram stain of the sputum and examine it with accuracy is the sine qua non of a physician competent to treat all pneumonias, including those following influenza. The proper treatment and final clinical outcome of the patient will often be dependent on the physician's ability to distinguish granulocytes from epithelial cells (and thus to distinguish a sputum from spit) and to recognize properly stained bacteria.

Treatment

General supportive measures have been prescribed for centuries to alleviate the bothersome symptoms of common influenza. There is little evidence that any of these measures shortens the duration of illness or diminishes the frequency of complications. Antipyretics such as acetaminophen for fever, fluids for thirst, analgesics for muscle pains, and bed rest for lassitude all support the comfort of the patient. Topical and systemic decongestants relieve nasal obstruction, and antihistamines promote restful sleep.

Evidence is accumulating that amantadine, a symmetrical primary amine, is effective in the treatment of clinical disease caused by influenza A viruses. This effect must be carefully differentiated from its prophylactic effect, which will be discussed below. The interpretation and performance of studies on the therapeutic effectiveness of this synthetic inhibitor of viral uncoating are difficult because influenza is a fairly rapidly evolving and resolving illness, and only a few days of clinical disease are ordinarily observable after the patient has consulted with his physician and sought therapy. Earlier studies during the 1960s demonstrated that amantadine definitely lessened the number of days of pyrexia, but this effect appeared little different from that of aspirin. More recent studies, however, have shown that amantadine often diminishes the severity of most symptoms to a significant extent and hastens clinical recovery by 1 to 4 days if therapy is begun within 48 hours of the onset of symptoms. Although this improvement may appear to be of marginal benefit, any improvement will be welcomed by most patients. Amantadine also significantly reduces the titer and duration of viral excretion, which, while of little direct benefit to the patient may be very significant in terms of limiting the spread of disease. Most importantly, it has been demonstrated that the duration of altered pulmonary function (as measured by diminished frequency-dependent compliance), which may last for several weeks after clinical influenza, can be markedly shortened following amantadine therapy. The dose of amantadine is usually 100 mg by mouth twice a day. Side effects can occur with variable frequency and are more common in the elderly. The most common effects in young adults appear to be psychologic. Insomnia, excitement, and a poor attention span or difficulty in mental concentration may be seen in up to 10 percent of recipients. Some studies have shown that rimantadine, a close analog of amantadine, is associated with fewer adverse reactions. Other studies have shown that although amantadine does not induce adverse reactions that are more common or more severe than those associated with a commonly used antihistamine, the combination of the two agents markedly increases the frequency of these reactions. In older individuals, the drug can occasionally precipitate congestive heart failure, cause more severe mental changes, or be responsible for other less common adverse effects. Amantadine has also been administered by aerosol to the upper and lower tracheobronchial tract, but the advantages and practicality of this technique require further study.

Prevention

Because the therapy of influenza is limited, major attempts have been made to prevent this disease. That these efforts have not been successful in the past is confirmed by the large number of people who die during epidemics and even during interpandemic years. The etiology of this lack of success is primarily logistical and attitudinal (as was the case for smallpox) and not because effective prophylactic measures are not available. Early attempts at preventing the disease involved growing influenza viruses in the allantoic cavity of embryonated hens' eggs and inactivating the virus in this slurry with formaldehyde. These vaccines generally induced high levels of HI antibody, which were closely correlated with protection from infection. Serum HI antibodies of $\geq 1:32$ generally are associated with solid protection from infection, whereas lesser levels of antibody (1:8 and 1:16) are associated with either moderate protection from infection or attentuation of clinical disease. These early vaccines required large volumes of allantoic fluid for each vaccine dose and were associated with endotoxin-like reactions, consisting of fever, chills, lassitude, and myalgias, which the recipient often considered to be similar to (or worse than) the early phases of clinical influenza. The etiology of these reactions was not clear. It was thought that the large amount of nonviral (egg) protein present in the vaccines caused these reactions, although precise clinical investigations both in the 1940s and the 1970s did not support this hypothesis, and vaccines containing larger amounts of egg protein (such as the 17D yellow fever vaccine) do not induce such reactions. An equally valid hypothesis could be that the large amount of virus with its lipoprotein coat may cause these reactions. Vaccines produced in the late 1960s and early 1970s by density gradient centrifugation (Chap. 8), which eliminated most of the nonviral protein, were associated with fewer adverse reactions and equal immunogenicity, although very young individuals continued to experience at times severe and debilitating adverse reactions, including seizures. Disruption of the virus by a variety of detergents and solvents yielded vaccines that produced fewer adverse reactions and were equally immunogenic in primed populations. Single doses of such vaccines, however, are less immunogenic in individuals who have little or no prior antigenic experience with influenza. A second dose given a month or more later, however, ordinarily induces protective antibodies in over 85 percent of these recipients. The recent cloning of the hemagglutinin antigen by genetic engineering techniques is another step in the potential refinement of influenza vaccines.

Inactivated vaccines, nonetheless, are little used for a variety of reasons, the first being the memory of both the patients and doctors of older, more highly reactogenic vaccines. Second, these vaccines are effective only when the antigens in the vaccine are identical or closely related to the antigens of the epidemic virus. Since the preparation of these inactivated vaccines requires 6 to 9 months of lead time, a certain amount of guessing must occur each winter in an effort to establish which virus will be epidemic in the succeeding year. These prognostications are sometimes accurate. In addition, the immunity induced is not highly effective for much more than a year, so that annual vaccination must be given. Finally, the economics of vaccine production are difficult and marginal. Manufacturers must deal with an everchanging target, which only intermittently captures the attention of patients, public health authorities, and physicians. As a result, they tend to produce only the number of doses of vaccine they feel will be sold in the succeeding year. This has generally been in the range of 15 to 20 million doses annually in the United States. The practical problems of administering all of these doses at the optimal time (generally several weeks to a few months before the expected epidemic) can be easily imagined.

Because of these logistical problems, vaccine is currently recommended only for those who are at high risk of dying should they acquire influenza. They would include any patient with a chronic illness, particularly pulmonary, but also any chronic cardiac, metabolic, and neurologic disease, and the elderly (those over 65 years of age). Its use in vital community personnel, such as physicians, nurses, policemen, and firemen, was temporarily slowed by the occurrence of the Guillain–Barré syndrome in approximately 1 of 100,000 recipients of the A/New Jersey (swine) strain influenza vaccine. About 10 percent of these cases were fatal. Subsequent studies have shown that vaccines that do not contain the H swine antigen are not associated with Guillain–Barré syndrome, further emphasizing the unusual neuroreactivity of this virus as exemplified by the association of von Economo's encephalitis with natural infection only with this strain of influenza. It should be noted also that influenza vaccines, like other biologic response modifiers, transiently depress hepatic cytochrome *p*-450 enzymatic activity and thus diminish the rate of metabolism or degradation of certain drugs, such as theophyllin. This observation would have particular relevance to asthmatics receiving this drug and who are also a high-risk group requiring immunization.

As it is thought optimal by some to induce local (nasal and/or tracheobronchial) immunity to prevent respiratory disease, great enthusiasm has been generated over the past 3 decades in Eastern Europe and for the past 1 to 2 decades in the West for live influenza vaccines that may be applied topically in the nostrils. The viruses in these vaccines have been attenuated by a variety of means, including multiple egg passages, recombination with highly attenuated strains, cold adaptation, selection of temperature-sensitive mutants, or the selection of strains resistant to nonspecific inhibitors. Clinical studies with several of these types have shown that immunity can be induced at a level and duration roughly equivalent to that induced by inactivated vaccines. One advantage of these vaccines is that a much greater number of doses can be produced per embryonated egg. Fertilized eggs are often a limiting economic and supply factor in the production of influenza vaccines. A disadvantage of these vaccines, on the other hand, is that because they contain infectious virus, much more stringent testing in humans must be performed before their widespread general use in tens or hundreds of millions of recipients can be encouraged. When such testing is completed, the original epidemic strain for which the vaccine was designed has often disappeared from the population. Attempts to use nonhuman and in vitro models of immunogenicity and safety are being intensely investigated, but to date none has been sufficiently consistent and convincing to obviate or circumvent extensive and time-consuming clinical trials in humans.

Amantadine has also been shown to be effective in the prevention of influenza. Its efficacy is approximately that of inactivated vaccines. Its advantage is that its prophylactic activity is not as strain-specific as that of vaccines and therefore may be used when the virus epidemic in the population is different from that in the vaccine or when vaccines are not available. Its disadvantages are that it will induce a substantial number of side effects in patients who are otherwise healthy, and it must be taken regularly during the entire epidemic exposure season.

FURTHER READING

Barry DW, et al.: Comparative trial of influenza vaccine. I. Immunogenicity of whole virus and split product vaccine in man. Am J Epidemiol 104:34, 1976

Dolin R, Reichman RC, Madore HP, et al.: A controlled trial of amantadine and rimantadine in the prophylaxis of influenza A infection. N Engl J Med 307:580, 1982

Dowdle WR, Coleman MT, Gregg MB: Natural history of influenza type A in the United States, 1957–1972. Prog Med Virol 17:91, 1974

Hall WJ, Douglas RG, et al.: Pulmonary mechanics after uncomplicated influenza A infection. Am Rev Respir Dis 113:141, 1976

Jackson GG, Muldoon RL: Viruses causing common respiratory infections in man. V: Influenza A (Asian). J Infect Dis 131:308, 1975

Kark JD, Lebiush M, Rannon L: Cigarette smoking as a risk factor for epidemic A($H_I N_I$) influenza in young men. N Engl J Med 307:1042, 1982

Kavet J: A perspective on the significance of pandemic influenza. Am J Public Health 67:1063, 1977

Kilbourne ED: The Influenza Viruses and Influenza. New York, Academic Press, 1975

Linnemann CC, et al.: Reye's syndrome: Epidemiologic and viral studies, 1963–1974. Am J Epidemiol 101:517, 1975

Rogers DE, Louria DB, Kilbourne ED: The syndrome of fatal influenza virus pneumonia. Trans Assoc Am Physicians 71:260, 1959

Selby P (ed): Influenza: Virus, Vaccines and Strategy. New York, Academic Press, 1973

Stuart Harris CH, Schild GC: Influenza: The Viruses and the Disease. Littleton, Mass, Publishing Sciences Group, 1976

Webster RG, Laver WG, et al.: Molecular mechanisms of variation in influenza viruses. Nature 296:115, 1982

CHAPTER 19

Paramyxoviruses

Parainfluenza Virus

In the quarter of a century since their initial isolation, the epidemiology, clinical illnesses, and the host response to infection associated with these agents have been described, as well as some of the molecular events associated with replication. The pathogenesis of infection has been better understood with the advent of investigations by the molecular virologists. These paramyxoviruses have a nonsegmented single-stranded RNA genome with enveloped helical nucleocapsids. They have both hemagglutination and neuraminidase activity associated with one glycoprotein and cell fusion or red blood cell hemolytic activity attributed to a second membrane glycoprotein.

Clinical Illness

Parainfluenza virus type 1 has been the predominant agent associated with laryngotracheobronchitis (croup). This agent tends to occur in biennial epidemics that peak in the fall months. Children usually acquire infection between the ages of 6 months and 3 years. The vast majority of young adults have demonstrable serum antibodies against parainfluenza 1.

Parainfluenza type 2 is also associated with acute laryngotracheobronchitis in the fall, but it occurs in sporadic outbreaks. Parainfluenza 2 will often alternate years of occurrence with parainfluenza type 1. Although children of the age group 8 to 36 months are at greatest risk of infection, the morbidity from parainfluenza 2 infections is substantially less than that from parainfluenza type 1.

Parainfluenza virus type 3 is associated with bronchiolitis and pneumonia in infants less than 1 year of age, with croup in children 1 to 3 years old, and with tracheobronchitis in older children. This virus is similar to respiratory syncytial virus, with its predilection for causing infection in infants during the first 6 months of life, as well as through 3 years of age. The majority of primary infections in infants and children are associated with febrile illness of approximately 4 days duration, and at least one third of these illnesses are complicated by pneumonia or bronchiolitis. Serologic studies have demonstrated that approximately one half of children have been exposed to this agent by the end of their first year of life.

Parainfluenza type 4 has been recovered much less frequently from children and adults with mild respiratory illness. The laboratory isolation of this agent is more difficult, which contributes to its less frequent association with illness. The common symptoms of infection with any of the parainfluenza agents in adults are nasal congestion, sore throat, and malaise. These viruses have been associated with exacerbations of chronic bronchitis, pharyngitis, and tonsilitis in college-age students, and asymptomatic reinfection.

Several studies have demonstrated excretion of parainfluenza virus type 3 for 2 to 5 months in a population of adult patients with chronic bronchitis and emphysema. Several of these patients had virus-specific local antibody detected in their respiratory tract prior to detection of virus excretion. This persistence of parainfluenza type 3 infection did not produce a significant increase in local respiratory antibody. This could be contrasted to those patients showing symptomatic illness, brief excretion of virus, and an associated increase in titers of serum and respiratory secretory antibody.

Pathogenesis of Infection

These viruses are excreted in respiratory secretions, and therefore virus is aerosolized in small and large droplets with breathing, coughing, and sneezing. Inhalation of infectious virus transmits infection. It is probable that hand-to-mucous membrane contact may also transmit infection, as has been shown with rhinovirus and respiratory syncytial virus. The incubation period is usually from 1 to 4 days. Virus has been isolated from the respiratory tract for as long as 6 days before onset of symptoms and is isolated from about two thirds of symptomatic patients during the first week of illness. The parainfluenza viruses are found in secretions as long as the second and third week after onset of symptoms more often than are respiratory syncytial viruses or influenza viruses.

The replication of each of these agents is normally limited to the respiratory tract. The two membrane glycoproteins, the hemagglutinin/neuraminidase (HN) and fusion protein (F) are spike-like surface projections on the virion and are anchored in the viral membrane by the hydrophobic portion of the proteins. The HN protein has receptor binding activity and requires a receptor with neuraminic acid residues for adsorption of the virus to the cell. Glycoproteins and glycolipids with neuraminic acid are ubiquitous on vertebrate cells. These viruses can therefore adsorb to many cell types, and thus virus–cell receptor interaction does not explain the tissue tropism of parainfluenza viruses. The fusion of virus and cell membranes is involved in virus penetration and, therefore, infection of the host cell. The F protein is essential for infectivity of these viruses and must be cleaved by a proteolytic enzyme provided by the host. Host-dependent proteolytic activity therefore determines tissue tropism and host range. It has even been shown that a specific amino acid sequence at the N terminus of the activated F polypeptide is essential for biologic activity and that homology for this region exists between the proteins of various members of the paramyxovirus group. Proteolytic cleavage occurs in the same site on the F protein of different parainfluenza viruses, and oligopeptides resembling the N terminus have been used experimentally to inhibit fusion/penetration.

Since adsorption occurs independently of fusion, it is possible to hypothesize different outcomes of the virus–host cell interaction. If the virus with cleaved F protein infects cells lacking an appropriate protease, virus replication may occur, but progeny virus particles will have uncleaved F protein and therefore will not be infectious. If these virus particles can adhere to cells capable of cleaving F protein during adsorption, they become infectious. If cells cannot activate F protein after adsorption, the virus is not infectious. Although details are yet to be determined, the limitation of virus replication to the human respiratory tract probably is a result of specific proteolytic cleavage of the F protein, which occurs efficiently in the respiratory tract.

In vitro, tracheal ring cultures have been utilized to describe the sequential morphologic events attendent upon parainfluenza infection. Epithelial cell cytoplasmic antigens are easily demonstrable with immunofluorescence by 24 hours after infection. Ciliary motion is lost, and the pseudostratified columnar organization of the epithelial layer disappears as some ciliated cells are lost and others fuse to form multinucleate giant cells. Such fusion is also seen in the lamina propria and cartilage, and budding virus particles from these cells are visible by electron microscopy. Virus replication can be sustained for 2 weeks in vitro before focal destruction of the epithelium occurs.

The available pathology of pulmonary tissue from infected children shows an increase in bronchial-associated lymphoid tissue, peribronchial infiltrates, and exudates in lamina of the bronchus. Interstitial pneumonia with associated atelectasis may also be present.

Host Response

A single infection does not confer immunity to infection or symptomatic illness. Reinfections occur frequently, although the presence of antibody may modify the clinical manifestations. In fact, studies with parainfluenza 2 have demonstrated that protection against clinical reinfection is best correlated with the presence of detectable local neutralizing antibody in nasal secretions. Patients show homologous IgA antibody formation in nasal secretions, usually within 7 to 10 days after onset of symptoms, which peaks in about 2 weeks. Virus neutralizing activity is also demonstrable but does not necessarily correlate with IgA. This may be because neutralization is only one measure of antibody function, and all neutralization is not due to specific IgA antibody.

Infection causes the host to produce humoral antibody, as measured by hemagglutination inhibition, neutralization, and complement fixation. The neutralizing and hemagglutination-inhibitory antibodies are directed against the HN protein. Antibody to the F protein is also critical to limitation of virus replication. Antibodies to both proteins are probably necessary to prevent clinical infection.

Reinfection stimulates an anamnestic response with heterotypic antibodies to other serotypes of the parainfluenza viruses.

Lymphocytic cellular host defenses seem to be important in the normal response to these viruses and may be essential for their eradication. Severe combined immunodeficient children have persistent respiratory excretion of these viruses for months or years and have had virus isolated from peripheral blood, liver, CSF, and pericardial fluid. Systemic infection is well documented, but whether these are mutant viruses that have evolved in a defective host or whether this is only due to the host's deficits remains to be determined.

Diagnosis

The overlapping spectrum of respiratory disease produced by a number of viral pathogens can be etiologically defined only by specific identification of the infecting virus. Rapid and accurate diagnosis by immunofluorescence of nasal secretions has been accomplished by several laboratories. Careful collection of materials and fluorescent staining of the exfoliated epithelial cells from the upper respiratory tract provide a diagnosis within 1 day of obtaining the specimen. The fluorescence is cytoplasmic and has been observed in the ciliated epithelial cells.

Isolation and identification of these agents in susceptible cells in tissue culture may require up to 2 weeks. The infected tissue culture can be examined by immunofluorescence with successful demonstration of viral antigens during the first several days of culture. More commonly, hemadsorption employing guinea pig red blood cells is utilized in 4 to 7 days to detect the presence of a hemadsorbing agent.

Tissue culture cells that are used for parainfluenza virus isolation include primary human embryonic kidney, human amnion, and primary monkey kidney cells. Unfortunately, the presence of hemadsorbing simian viruses must be taken into consideration when working with simian cell cultures.

The parainfluenza viruses do hemagglutinate guinea pig and chicken red blood cells. Thus, hemagglutination inhibition can be useful for identification of virus and for determining the titers of specific serum or secretory antibody against known virus strains. With primary infection, the response to the infecting agent tends to be type-specific. With each subsequent infection, there is an increased heterologous antibody response.

Treatment

The treatment of these respiratory infections is only by the provision of supportive therapy. Hydration, maintenance of an adequate airway, and therapy of bacterial superinfection are important in the management of these patients. The severity of the lower respiratory tract disease is greatest in the youngest age group.

Parainfluenza virus 3 infection has been documented to be a significant nosocomial infection, with increased morbidity to the patients who acquire these infections in the hospital. All of the viruses causing severe respiratory infections in children should be regarded as communicable within the hospital, and appropriate precautions should be taken to prevent spread of the infection within the hospital.

Prevention

As implied in the preceding paragraphs, immunity to parainfluenza viruses is only partial. That is, reinfection may occur naturally, although the severity of the illness may be considerably diminished.

Parainfluenza viruses grown in embryonated eggs or tissue culture have been administered as formalin-inactivated vaccines. Two to three injections of the individual parainfluenza types are necessary before seroconversion occurs in young infants. These materials have been tested as monovalent or trivalent immunogens. The vaccine can produce a 95 to 100 percent seroconversion rate in antibody-negative subjects, but no resulting significant protection against naturally occurring infection has been demonstrated. Parenteral administration of these inactivated products does not produce local secretory antibody. It has been learned that formalin destroys the F protein of measles and RSV. It seems likely that such treatment destroys the F glycoprotein of the parainfluenza viruses, too, and therefore no antibody to this protein was produced. Thus, the failure to achieve protection with inactivated antigen may be due to destruction of an antigen essential for protection. This explanation is important in view of suggestions that preexisting antibody might enhance disease and provide an explanation for severe disease in infants with maternal antibody. A Syrian hamster model of pulmonary infection with live virus has been used to show no enhancement of disease by the administration of passive antibody or by reinfection of an animal.

Significant morbidity results from infection with these agents in the youngest infants. Prevention of infection is a desirable goal, but the available immunogens have not been successful. Our better understanding of the surface glycoproteins may facilitate successful immunization.

Respiratory Syncytial Virus

Clinical Illness

Respiratory syncytial virus (RSV) was first described in 1956 and since that time has become recognized as the single most important respiratory tract pathogen of infants and young children. Severe disease caused by RSV is most often manifest as bronchiolitis or pneumonitis and occurs predominantly in children less than 6 months of age. Studies of hospitalized young children with acute respiratory disease reveal 20 to 30 percent of their illnesses are attributable to RSV. RSV is the only known virus of humans in the genus *Pneumovirus* of the Paramyxoviridae family. The virus is enveloped; it has a nonsegmented single-stranded RNA genome in a helical nucleocapsid. RSV has a fusion protein but lacks a hemagglutinin.

The virus comes in contact with the mucosal surfaces of the nasopharynx, and virus replication occurs. Immunofluorescence of nasal secretions provides evidence that ciliated epithelial cells and macrophages contain RSV antigen and are, therefore, sites of virus replication. Infection is normally limited to the respiratory tract, and virus is generally isolated only from respiratory tissues and secretions. The incubation period preceding clinical illness is ordinarily 1 to 4 days after exposure to virus.

A calculated risk for hospitalization due to RSV infection during the first year of life is 5 per 1000 live births based on studies in low income families. These very young children are severely ill, have fever, lethargy, and apnea, which is a prominent feature of their respiratory tract disease. Passively acquired maternal serum antibody levels correlate with acquisition and severity of illness. Infants born with higher titers of antibody acquire disease at a later age, and those who have moderate levels of antibody have milder illnesses. Bronchiolitis and/or pneumonia is manifest by labored, rapid respirations, with radiologic changes ranging from hyperaeration to consolidation. Involvement of the lungs may be sufficiently extensive to necessitate respiratory assistance and, in a small percentage of children, is fatal. Infection in the youngest infants is their primary encounter with the virus. In a day-care setting where longitudinal observations are possible, virtually all antibody-negative children develop infections, as documented by virus excretion and seroconversion after their first exposure to RSV. Clinically apparent illness, including fever, lower respiratory illness, and middle ear effusions, occurs significantly more often with primary infection. One infection will produce some resistance to reinfection, so about 75 percent of these exposed seropositive youngsters develop infection with the second exposure to virus, as evidenced by antibody rise and/or virus shedding.

Children between the ages of 1 and 3 years who have symptomatic illness are less likely to have bronchiolitis. The age-related occurrence of bronchiolitis suggests anatomic determinants of this manifestation of RSF infection. Middle ear effusion is a common concomitant finding after the age of 6 months. Older children and adults are more likely to have colds, with cough, nasal congestion, or asymptomatic infection evidenced only by serologic or cultural evidence of infection. The percentage of asymptomatic/mild illness increases from 2 percent to 50 percent from the first to the third or fourth infection, respectively. This reduction in the number of symptomatic infections is independent of age and correlates with previous infections. Even mild symptomatic illness can produce measurable morbidity for periods up to 8 weeks. There may be an increase in respiratory tract resistance, apparently due to altered reactivity of small airways.

Reinfection with RSV is the rule. Antigenic variation of RSV does not seem to explain reinfection of humans, since the measured antibody response to different isolates of virus does not detect any antigenic difference. As indicated above, 75 percent of infants will become infected with their second exposure to virus and 65 percent with their third. School-age children have a risk of infection of about 40 percent. Thus, immunity is reinforced by subsequent infections.

Host Response

The severity and frequency of RSV infections in infants have led to rather extensive study of the virus in an attempt to guide the development of preventive procedures. Serum antibody against RSV is largely IgG and, as such, crosses the placenta to the fetus as delineated above. Serum antibodies appear in the infant in approximately 10 days to 2 weeks after the onset of infection, persist for months, and then show an anamnestic response with natural or artificial challenge with virus. Antibody persists longer after reinfection as compared to primary infection. The presence of humoral antibody in the youngest infants correlates with protection against serious lower respiratory tract disease. The mechanism of protection is unknown, and hypotheses, such as diffusion of humoral antibody at the alveolar or bronchiolar level or mediation of antibody-dependent cell-mediated cytotoxicity (ADCC), have been suggested. A ^{51}Cr release assay showed ADCC in nasopharyngeal secretions collected from infants that was primarily mediated by IgG. It is possible that humoral antibody itself may not be the protective factor. These antibodies do not cross-react with any other known virus.

Antibody to RSV in nasopharyngeal secretions as demonstrated by immunofluorescence appears promptly during illness, usually within 3 days of onset. IgG and IgM are detectable with peak titers available for IgG and M from 8 to 15 days after onset. IgA is the predominant class of antibody, with peak titers attained from 14 to 28 days after onset and sustained for about 2 months in the face of waning IgG and IgM. Infants older than 6 months produce higher IgA titers in response to primary infection than do younger infants. Secondary infection stimulates an anamnestic response in all three classes of immunoglobulin in nasopharyngeal secretions, with a less rapid decline in antibody.

Studies demonstrate a better correlation with protection against RSV infection by secretory antibodies than by serum IgG antibodies. It has been shown in virus challenge studies in adults that there is an inverse correlation of the titer of nasal wash antibody with the quantity of virus excreted and the antibody rise. Those persons with high levels of specific IgA antibody challenged with RSV excrete less virus and may show no antibody rise in secretions or serum. Those adults with low or absent levels of specific nasal IgA show excretion of increased amounts of virus and do develop rises in antibody. Clinical illnesses were observed only in the volunteers with low nasal levels of IgA who received the larger of two inoculation dosages of virus.

More recently, RSV-specific IgE has been demonstrated more frequently and in higher titers in the nasopharyngeal secretions of infected children with wheezing. The degree of RSV-IgE response correlated with hypoxia and, thus, with severity of illness.

RSV-specific IgA has been measured in colostrum and milk, and because virus replicates only in the respiratory tract, it would seem that this is the site of antigen exposure to lymphocytes, suggesting a bronchomammary axis in the immune response. Any protective or ameliorating effect of specific antibody in breast milk is still to be determined, although epidemiologic evidence suggests that some protection may be provided.

RSV antigens are expressed on the surface of infected cells, and as expected, increased blastogenic responses of lymphocytes to RSV are seen in children with RSV infection. The combined immunodeficient children have prolonged shedding of this virus from their respiratory tracts. Cellular immunity is probably important in limiting infection with this enveloped respiratory virus.

Pathology

Infants with RSV infection show severe changes in their lungs. Pulmonary tissues from children with pneumonia show marked inflammation, with mononuclear cell infiltrates in interstitial tissues, alveoli, small bronchioles, and alveolar ducts. There may be demonstrated syncytia formation and intracytoplasmic inclusions, which are consistent with, but not pathognomonic of, RSV infection. Infants with bronchiolitis show less extensive interstitial and alveolar involvement but instead have moderate to marked changes in the bronchioles. Epithelial necrosis and plugs consisting of cell debris and fibrin are seen, as well as peribronchiolar lymphocytic infiltrates. Virus has been isolated from tissues of children with both types of illness.

Epidemiology

RSV infection is worldwide in distribution and tends to cause yearly outbreaks of illness alternating from midwinter to late spring in occurrence. Infection has been experimentally produced by introduction of virus into the upper respiratory tract of volunteers and animals (chimpanzees). Within the hospital setting, RSV transmission is readily demonstrable when persons have close contact with infected infants, suggesting transmission by touch or large droplets. Small particle aeresol transmission does not transmit infection easily in this setting. Experimental inoculation of adults shows the eye and nose to be efficient portals of entry, whereas the mouth is less sensitive. The increased frequency of severe disease in infants has been noted, and during community studies, attack rates of 30 to 60 percent are estimated for exposed infants less than 1 year old. RSV infection seems to be introduced into a family by an older (2 years or more) sibling. The secondary attack rate is then greatest for infants less than 1 year of age, but appreciable attack rates occur at all ages, with approximately 50 percent of family members acquiring infection. Investigations conducted simultaneously on different populations in the same geographical setting pointed out that patients seen in private practice had RSV infection at an older age than either urban or rural clinical patients. These older infants with less severe disease were seldom hospitalized.

A final epidemiologic consideration is that of nosocomial infections with RSV. The hospitalized infant excretes virus for days, and it is transmitted to ward personnel as well as to patients. The acquired illness also results in prolongation of hospitalization for infants and may produce fatal illness in those infants hospitalized with other underlying problems. Consideration should be given to patient isolation and careful handwashing in providing care for infected infants.

Diagnosis

Presumptive clinical diagnosis can be made in an infant with bronchiolitis or pneumonia with no demonstrable bacterial pathogens. A definite etiologic diagnosis of RSV infection can be made by detection of viral antigen or serologic tests. The virus can be isolated from nasal secretions utilizing tissue cultures of cells such as the Hep2 line. Longitudinal study of families has demonstrated that virus can be detected as long as 6 days before symptoms occur and in about 73 percent of infants during the first week but in only 6 percent in the second week (after onset of symptoms). Hospitalized children may excrete virus for longer periods. The mean titer of virus detected in secretions of hospitalized children is 5.0 $\log_{10}$ $TCID_{50}$. Children less than 2 years of age excrete virus longer than do older children or adults. Although this information may assist in management of severely ill infants, all too frequently it is not known until the patient has completed the natural course of illness.

The virus is extremely labile, and respiratory secretions, throat swab material, lung biopsy, or postmortem material must be kept at 4C and immediately processed by a knowledgeable laboratory utilizing specific techniques in order to preserve cells for immunofluorescence or infectious virus for tissue culture inoculation. Several laboratories have demonstrated RSV antigens in cells present in nasal secretions by fluorescent antibody techniques or ELISA assay. The indirect immunofluorescent method employing bovine anti-RSV serum and fluorescein-conjugated antibovine globulin has been successful in the few laboratories familiar with the procedure. The technique affords a means of identification of RSV infection within hours but is not generally available. Later in disease, it can also identify viral antigen despite the presence of antibody, which may neutralize the infective virus in secretions.

Serologic techniques allow the recognition of RSV antibodies by complement-fixation, neutralization, or plaque-reduction techniques, with the latter being the most sensitive method. Experimentally, radioimmune and enzyme-linked immunosorbent assays are presently being developed. Acute and convalescent sera are necessary to define the significance of measured antibody. As with other virus infections, a four-fold or greater antibody rise indicates recent infection, but a single value will indicate only previous experience with the virus at an undetermined time. Investigational use of a specific IgM radioimmunassay may prove helpful in defining acute illness.

Therapy

The therapy of RSV infection is entirely nonspecific and consists of support of the respiratory system, control of fever, adequate hydration and nutrition, and therapy of secondary bacterial infection.

Prevention

The prevalence of RSV infection has resulted in attempts to develop an effective vaccine. A formalin-inactivated, alum-precipitated virus vaccine was prepared and utilized in field trials. The vaccine produced a rise in serum antibodies as measured by neutralization in adults and children but no rise in secretory antibody. Although antibody to the F protein was not measured, it is probable that formalin destoryed this protein, rendering the immunogen incomplete. During naturally occurring outbreaks of RSV disease, the attack rate among infants immunized with inactivated vaccine was the same as that in the control (unimmunized) populations. This indicated that this immunization did not protect from subsequent infection. In addition, the clinical illness was more severe in vaccinees, and the age group suffering severe disease was extended to include older infants. It is probable that immunization was analogous to that with inactivated measles virus. The infants could identify RSV antigens except the fusion protein, and therefore virus replication and cell-to-cell spread occurred until antibody to the F protein was formed. The host response to other viral components resulted in destruction of some infected cells. Such unanticipated observations stopped the use of inactivated vaccine.

Attempts are being made to develop a live virus vaccine that will be protective. It is predicted that an effective vaccine will induce formation of respiratory tract IgA because of its recognized importance in protection against disease. The first RSV vaccine administered intranasally was a cold-adapted strain that was found to be attenuated in adults but produced mild disease and prolonged virus shedding in seronegative infants. Temperature-sensitive RSV mutants multiplying only at 33 to 35C have been isolated. It was hoped that such mutants would multiply only in the upper respiratory tract and thus reproduce the immunologic events of natural infection without causing illness in the infants. Administration of the temperature-sensitive mutant produced asymptomatic infection in seropositive children and infection with mild rhinitis in seronegative children. Using intranasal administration of 100 $TCID_{50}$, children with preexisting nasal antibody were not infected. Virus shedding was monitored, with recovery of a small population of genetically altered virus with partial loss of the temperature-sensitive property in a few instances. The vaccine virus was not transmissible to control children in intimate contact with vaccinees. Sequential studies have shown that subsequent natural RSV infection occurred in vaccinees. Additional trials with a genetically stable, temperature-sensitive mutant of RSV having a defect consistent with an altered fusion protein have been conducted. The virus was poorly infectious when administered intranasally in chimpanzees, adults, and children. A similar vaccine administered parenterally was not efficacious.

The natural history of RSV infection suggests that no immunogen will prevent multiple infections with this virus. If the initial infection with an attenuated virus could prevent severe illness, which is more likely to occur in the younger children, it would be worthwhile. Perhaps multiple immunizations will be necessary. To date, prevention of illness has never been demonstrated, and no candidate immunogen clearly modifies subsequent infections.

Mumps

Mumps virus infection was recognized as epidemic parotitis as early as the fifth century BC by Hippocrates. From its position as a universal infection of childhood, mumps has receded to an uncommon illness in nations employing vaccine. The most frequently recognized symptom of infection is parotitis, although the illness may have multiple manifestations, indicating the widespread multiplication of virus. The last decade has added far more substantive understanding to the molecular virology of mumps virus, and it is possible to incorporate some of these facts into our understanding of the clinical consequences of infection with this agent. Mumps virus is a member of the paramyxovirus family and, as such, is pleomorphic, with a diameter of approximately 150 nm. The lipid envelope surrounds a helical nucleocapsid containing a single-stranded, nonsegmented RNA genome. There are two surface glycoproteins on the envelope that are equivalent to the hemagglutinin/neuraminidase (HN) and fusion (F) proteins described for other paramyxoviruses.

Clinical Illness and Pathogenesis

The portal of entry is thought to be the upper respiratory tract, as the virus gains direct access to the mucous membranes of the mouth and nose. Virus is transmitted by the saliva or other secretions of infected persons. The virus replicates after entering the host, although the specific tissue in which primary multiplication of virus occurs is unknown. Sialic acid residues are ubiquitous on mammalian cells and may be the host cell receptors for this virus. Although the functions of the mumps glycoproteins have been incompletely studied, by analogy with other paramyxoviruses the HN protein probably determines the initial virus–host cell interaction. The HN protein induces antibody that inhibits hemagglutination and neuraminidase activity and neutralizes the infectivity of the virus.

Viremia occurs with uncomplicated infection, and mumps is therefore different from parainfluenza infections where virus replication is limited to the respiratory tract. Secondary infection of multiple tissues can occur. The fusion protein on the viral envelope is essential for cell-to-cell spread for this virus. Cleavage of the F protein by the host cell protease(s) is necessary for its activation, and it can be postulated that this protein has cleavage sites susceptible to different enzymes than the parainfluenza viruses because the tissue tropism is far more generalized. Such tissues as the salivary glands (predominantly the parotids), meninges, testes, pancreas, ovaries, thyroid, and heart can support virus replication. Virus is excreted in the urine, and transient abnormalities in renal function have been found in adult males with mumps infection, implying that virus replicates in renal tissue.

The temporal relationships of virus excretion and communicability of the illness with clinical symptoms and host–antibody response are shown in Figure 19-1. Salivary gland infection with pain, edema, and consequent swelling results in the characteristic parotid gland enlargement diagnosed as mumps. This infection may involve the parotids, submandibular, and, less often, the sublingual salivary glands. Salivary gland involvement usually precedes other clinical symptoms, lasts for 2 to 7 days, and may be unilateral or bilateral. Any of the other manifestations of mumps infection occasionally precede, coincide with, or occur in the absence of salivary gland involvement.

Mumps virus may involve the central nervous system. The vast majority of such recognized illness is transient meningitis with few sequelae. The incidence of this type of central nervous system infection has been estimated to be as high as 65 percent when lumbar punctures have been done on a group of hospitalized patients with clinical mumps. The central nervous system involvement was manifest in each case by a predominantly lymphocytic pleocytosis of the cerebrospinal fluid. Only one half of these individuals evidenced clinical signs of meningitis. Signs of meningeal involvement are most often manifest 2 to 10 days after the onset of parotitis, last for 3 to 4 days, and are self-limited.

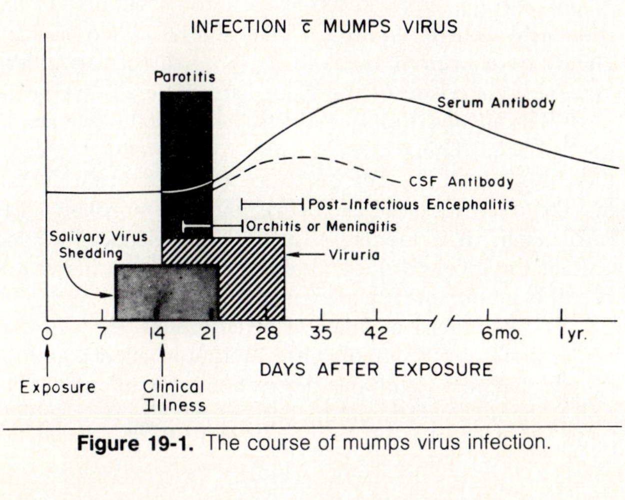

Figure 19-1. The course of mumps virus infection.

A more serious, and fortunately much less common, central nervous system manifestation of mumps is postinfectious encephalitis or encephalomeylitis. The reported ratio of mumps encephalitis to mumps cases is 2.5/1000 cases for each year from 1968 to 1972, but because of the lack of a uniform definition, meningitis cases are probably included, giving a falsely high case ratio. The time of onset is usually later than the transient meningitis and occurs 10 to 14 days after the clinical salivary gland involvement. The patient appears severely ill, is deeply obtunded, and may succumb to the illness. Although occurring less often than the postinfectious encephalitis associated with measles or varicella, it is clinically and pathologically indistinguishable from them.

Clinicians have studied the antibody response to mumps central nervous system infection and find that specific mumps IgG becomes detectable in the cerebrospinal fluid and is thought to be synthesized within the central nervous system. Titers of antibody usually reach a peak in 4 to 10 days after the onset of meningitis and decrease thereafter (Fig. 19-1). The IgG antibodies are oligoclonal, and in several patients with prolonged pleocytosis, antibodies could be detected as long as 11 to 12 months after meningitis. Similarly, interferon activity could be measured during the peak of clinical illness and tended to parallel the evidence of inflammation in the cerebrospinal fluid. Individuals with a prolonged pleocytosis had demonstrable interferon for longer periods of time.

An observation recorded in 1967 demonstrated the development of hydrocephalus in hamsters after experimental mumps infection. Suckling hamsters were inoculated intracerebrally with mumps virus isolated from the cerebrospinal fluid of a patient and passaged only once in cell cultures. Sequential studies demonstrated virus replication and associated inflammatory changes during the first week after inoculation. Virus was localized almost entirely within ependymal cells of the ventricles and choroid plexus. The animals did not show any signs of acute illness, but hydrocephalus became evident in 3 to 6 weeks after infection. These animals had aqueductal stenosis secondary to the resolving inflammation. Thus an inapparent, acute inflammation resulted in later sequelae at a time when viral antigen and infectious virus were no longer evident. The clinical application of such observations remains to be established. Although there are several case reports recording mumps infection in children who subsequently developed aqueductal stenosis, it has not been proven that the infection caused the subsequent hydrocephalus.

An occasional sequel of mumps virus infection is deafness, which may occur even in the absence of other evidence of central nervous system involvement. The loss of hearing may be preceded by tinnitus and a sense of fullness of the ear. Such deafness is relatively uncommon but occurs suddenly during the period of parotid swelling. It is usually unilateral, but an estimated 20 percent of those so affected may have bilateral disease. Once deafness has occurred, the damage is irreversible and is apparently due to virus replication, inflammation, and subsequent destruction of the organ of Corti.

The complication of mumps infection best known by nonmedical persons is the involvement of the testes. Orchitis most commonly develops during the first week of infection and occurs predominantly in postpubertal males, with 20 to 30 percent of this age group manifesting testicular involvement during the course of the mumps infection. Bilateral disease is present in approximately 2 to 6 percent of the total number of patients with orchitis. Inflammation of the testes is extremely painful, but the fear of this affliction stems from the concern that sexual impotence and sterility will follow. It is common to have some atrophy of the involved testes, but the incidence of sterility following mumps orchitis is extremely infrequent, and experience during World War I and II failed to show that either impotence or sterility was an important consequence of this infection. Once it has occurred, therapy of orchitis is symptomatic, without any clearly demonstrated benefits from either steroid therapy or immune globulin.

Pancreatitis with typical symptoms of abdominal pain, fever, and vomiting may occur in association with mumps infection. Recent in vitro work has demonstrated by fluorescence mumps infection of beta cells and non-beta cells of human pancreas in cell culture. Much less frequently, thyroiditis, mastitis, myocarditis, and oophoritis are seen.

In the normal individual, a single infection with mumps virus confers permanent immunity against clinically evident infection. It is probable that reinfection, defined as an antibody rise after exposure to the virus, may occur, but neither virus shedding nor clinical illness has been demonstrated with such reinfection. Second attacks of parotitis have been observed in the same individual but without documentation by culture or serology of two clinical attacks of mumps virus infection. Serologic cross-reactivity with other paramyxoviruses may be responsible for the rare seropositive person who develops mumps.

Special consideration should briefly be given to persons commonly thought to be at increased risk from virus infections. The pregnant woman or her fetus is frequently considered at higher risk with regard to particular infections, such as varicella and rubella. At this time, conflicting reports relating to mumps infection during pregnancy have been published. There is no confirmed evidence of the occurrence of congenital anomalies in the human fetus as a result of mumps infection sustained by the pregnant mother and transmitted to her fetus in utero. Although there have been documented cases of mumps in mothers during pregnancy and in the immediate postpartum period, neither clinical mumps nor excretion of virus has been documented in these infants. Patients who have altered immunity, either humoral (e.g., the agammaglobulinemics) or cellular (the naturally occurring lymphopenic or the immunosuppressed patient), have not been shown to be at increased risk with respect to mumps infection.

Host Response

The host initially responds to mumps virus infection with serum IgM antibodies and subsequently antibodies predominantly in the IgG class. Neutralizing antibodies are formed within the first week of symptoms and ordinarily persist for a lifetime. Hemagglutination-inhibiting and complement-fixing antibodies may appear from the first through the third week and usually reach a peak within 3 to 6 weeks after the onset of symptoms (Fig. 19-1). Complement-fixing antigens have been differentiated into two distinct types. The first is the soluble (S) or nucleoprotein antigen, and the second is the viral (V) or surface antigen, which includes the HN and F proteins. Complement-fixing antibodies against the S antigens are present within 2 to 3 days of onset, peak at about 10 days, and disappear in 8 to 9 months. Complement-fixing antibodies against the V antigen appear at about the tenth day of infection and persist for years. The transient nature of the S antibodies may sometimes assist in defining recent infection, and the presence of V antibodies may define the presence of previous experience with this virus.

Specific antibodies to the two surface glycoproteins HN and F are measurable after natural infection and are essential for protection from disease. Neutralization of infectivity, inhibition of hemagglutination, and the inhibition of neuraminidase activity are functions attributable to antibodies to the HN protein.

Mumps virus can replicate in vitro in human continuous lymphoblastoid cell lines with T cell characteristics or in human peripheral blood mononuclear cells. In the presence of pokeweed mitogen, replication is enhanced and occurs primarily in T lymphocytes, suggesting that these cells may be infected during natural infection. A T cell-mediated cytolytic response by human lymphocytes has been demonstrated after natural infection in humans.

Pathology

Examination of involved tissues is unusual because of the ordinarily benign nature of the illness. When salivary glands have been studied, there is no disruption of the general architecture of the gland after several days of illness. The involved salivary ducts demonstrate changes in the epithelial lining cells, ranging from swelling to complete desquamation. The ducts are dilated, and the lumen may be filled with cellular debris and polymorphonuclear cells. There is a moderate amount of periductal edema around the involved ducts, and the interstitial inflammatory cell is predominantly mononuclear.

The pathology of other involved tissues, e.g., the testes, is similar, with mononuclear infiltrates, edema, and no specific hallmarks allowing the diagnosis of mumps infection to be made solely on the basis of the observed pathology.

Epidemiology

In susceptible populations, mumps virus infection is predominantly a disease of childhood, with the majority of clinically evident infections being seen between the ages of 5 and 10 years. It has been estimated that in the prevaccine era 90 percent of the population were immune by the time they reached 15 years of age. Although mumps virus infection is contagious, it is less communicable than measles and varicella. The degree of communicability is estimated most accurately by serologic surveys of exposed individuals because as many as one fourth of the infections with mumps virus occur without clinical symptoms.

Isolation of the patient within the hospital setting or in homes, when it is attempted, has not effectively curtailed spread of disease. This is usually attributed to the period of virus shedding that occurs prior to the symptomatic onset of illness and thus precedes the recognition of infection. As previously mentioned, one fourth of patients have an asymptomatic infection, but they also excrete virus. Their infection is self-limited, and their immunity is comparable to those with symptomatic infection. To the best of our knowledge, there are no animal reservoirs or human carriers of mumps virus.

Diagnostic Approach

The work of Johnson and Goodpasture first established that mumps was caused by a filterable virus and demonstrated that rhesus monkeys could be experimentally infected. The description of the complement-fixation test and successful propagation of virus in chick embryo preceded the now generally employed standard tissue culture techniques. These methods employ monolayers of one of several cell types, including primary monkey kidney, human amnion, or human kidney and cell lines, such as HeLa. In vitro multinucleate giant cells are seen, and hemabsorption inhibition provides a practical means of identification of the virus. With these techniques, virus has been isolated from such varied sources as blood, cerebrospinal fluid, urine, saliva, salivary gland tissue, and human milk.

In many academic and large hospital settings, viral diagnostic laboratories are available, and virus isolation can be attempted from clinical materials. The responsible laboratory will provide directions for submitting materials for culture. Saliva and urine can be collected at the time of clinical central nervous system symptoms and submitted for culture. Mumps isolation in tissue culture is usually not necessary for either diagnosis or management of patients with parotitis, but the techniques and facilities are available for defining the unusual or complicated situation.

For practical reasons, many diagnostic laboratories can offer more extensive serologic diagnosis than cultural facilities for virus isolation. They will evaluate sera for the presence of antibodies to mumps virus. The serum for evaluation should be obtained as early as possible in the illness, and a convalescent specimen should be obtained after an interval of 2 to 3 weeks. A pair of sera can determine whether a specific illness is mumps infection by demonstrating an increase in antibody titer. A single serum can determine whether a person has ever had mumps infection but cannot define when it occurred. As indicated above, there are several types of antibody elicited by mumps infection.

Treatment

There is no specific therapy available for mumps infection. Symptomatic management of patients includes adequate hydration and analgesic and antipyretic therapy.

Prophylaxis and Immunization

The problem repeatedly occurs of what to do after exposure to mumps infection. Usually the person concerned is an adult without previous symptomatic mumps infection. Hyperimmune globulin or pooled serum IgG has been administered after exposure, with no proven efficacy. However, there has been a controlled study purporting to demonstrate that the administration of hyperimmune globulin after the appearance of parotitis can decrease the incidence and severity of orchitis. For this reason, hyperimmune globulin has been administered to postpubertal males who already have parotitis.

There has been limited experience in Scandinavia using a formalin-inactivated mumps vaccine, which affords some short-term protection from infection. No anti-F protein antibodies are demonstrable. It is probable that the F protein, which is sensitive to formalin, is not present. However, animal studies suggest that whole virus preparations can only induce anti-HN antibodies when the virus fails to replicate in the host. Purified F protein is an effective immunogen, and antibody to this protein is necessary to limit cell-to-cell spread of virus.

Live attenuated mumps virus vaccine was licensed in January 1968 and is available for prophylactic use. It is recommended for administration to children more than 1 year old and to young adults for induction of immunity parallel to that induced by natural infection. Vaccine should not be given to pregnant women because of the potential vulnerability of the fetus. Although no data exist that demonstrate transmission of attenuated virus to the fetus, placental infection has been documented after maternal immunization. For practical purposes there is only a single serologic strain of mumps virus, hence a single infection with either natural or attentuated virus confers immunity. The vaccine is a live attenuated virus produced in tissue cultures of chick embryo fibroblasts and is administered parenterally. Virus is not shed by the vaccinee, and immunization does not cause any side effects. The vaccine produces 95 to 100 percent serologic conversion from antibody-negative to antibody-positive in vaccinated susceptibles. The antibody levels, although considerably lower, parallel those produced by natural infection and persist for the 12 to 15 years that vaccine has been available for study. Immunized children in contact with naturally occurring mumps in their families, institutional settings, or the community have been protected against clinical illness.

The vaccine will not offer protection against mumps if someone has already been exposed to natural infection and is in the incubation period of illness. On the other hand, no harmful effects have been noted after administration of vaccine to an exposed susceptible.

Over 40 million doses of mumps vaccine have been administered since its licensure in 1967. The incidence of mumps has declined from 90 to 200/100,000 reported prior to 1967 to 2/100,000 in 1981. This is a decrease of 97 percent from 1968. Based on this reported occurrence of the disease, the vaccine has been effective in reducing disease morbidity, mortality, and the calculated costs of illness.

FURTHER READING

PARAINFLUENZA VIRUSES

Chanock RM, Parrott RH, Cook MK, et al.: Newly recognized myxoviruses from children with respiratory disease. N Engl J Med 258:207, 1958

Choppin PW, Scheid A: The role of viral glycoproteins in adsorption, penetration, and pathogenicity of viruses. Rev Infect Dis 2:40, 1980

Frank AL, Taber LH, Wells CR, et al.: Patterns of shedding of myxoviruses in children. J Infect Dis 144:433, 1981

Gardner PS, McQuillin J, McDuckin R, et al.: Observations on clinical and immunofluorescent diagnosis of parainfluenza virus infections. Br Med J 3:7, 1971

Glezen WP, Denny FW: Epidemiology of acute lower respiratory disease in children. N Engl J Med 288:498, 1973

Glezen WP, Fernald GW: Effective or passive antibody on parainfluenza type 3 pneumonia in hamsters. Infect Immun 14:212, 1976

Gross PA, Green RH, Curnen MG: Persistent infections with parainfluenza type 3 virus in man. Am Rev Respir Dis 108:894, 1973

Gross PA, Green RH, Lerner E, et al.: Immune response in persistent infection. Further studies on persistent respiratory infection in man with parainfluenza type 3 virus. Am Rev Respir Dis 110:676, 1974

Hall CB, Geiman JM, Breese BB, et al.: Parainfluenza viral infections in children: Correlation of shedding with clinical manifestations. J Pediatr 91:194, 1977

Kim HW, Canchola JG, Vargosko AJ, et al.: Immunogenicity of inactivated parainfluenza type 1, type 2, and type 3 vaccines in infants. JAMA 196:111, 1966

Klein JD, Collier AM: The pathogenesis of human parainfluenza type 3 virus infection in hamster tracheal organ culture. Infect Immun 10:883, 1974

Musson MA, Mocega HE, Krause HE: Acquisition of parainfluenza 3 virus infection by hospitalized children. I. Frequencies, rates, and temporal data. J Infect Dis 128:141, 1973

Workshop on broncholitis. Pediatr Res 11:209, 1979

Yanagihara R, McIntosh K: Secretory immunological response in infants and children to parainfluenza virus types 1 and 2. Infect Immun 30:23, 1980

RESPIRATORY SYNCYTIAL VIRUS

Belshe RB, Van Voris LP, Mufson MA: Parenteral administration of live respiratory syncytial virus vaccine: Results of a field trial. J Infect Dis 145:311, 1982

Chin J, Magoffin RL, Shearer LA, et al.: Field evaluation of a respiratory syncytial virus vaccine and a trivalent parainfluenza virus vaccine in a pediatric population. Am J Epidemiol 89:449, 1969

Fishaut M, Murphy D, Neifert M, et al.: Bronchomammary axis in the immune response to respiratory syncytial virus. J Pediatr 99:186, 1981

Fishaut M, Tubergen D, McIntosh K: Cellular response to respiratory viruses with particular reference to children with disorders of cell-mediated immunity. J Pediatr 96:179, 1980

Frank AL, Taber LH, Wells CR, et al.: Patterns of shedding of myxoviruses and paramyxoviruses in children. J Infect Dis 144:433, 1981

Fulginiti VA, Eller JJ, Sieber F, et al.: Respiratory virus immunization. I. A field trial of two inactivated respiratory virus vaccines; an aqueous trivalent parainfluenza virus vaccine and an alum-precipitated respiratory syncytial virus vaccine. Am J Epidemiol 89:435, 1969

Glezen WP, Paredes A, Allison JE, et al.: Risk of respiratory syncytial virus infection for infants from low-income families in relationship to age, sex, ethnic group, and maternal antibody level. J Pediatr 98:708, 1981

Hall CB, Douglas RG Jr, Geiman JM: Quantitative shedding patterns of RSV in infants. J Infect Dis 32:151, 1975

Hall WJ, Hall CB, Speers DM: Respiratory syncytial virus. Infection in adults. Clinical, virologic, and serial pulmonary function studies. Ann Intern Med 88:203, 1978

Henderson FW, Collier AM, Clyde WA Jr, et al.: Respiratory-syncytial-virus infections, reinfections and immunity. N Engl J Med 300:530, 1979

Kapikian AZ, Mitchell RH, Chanock RM, et al.: An epidemiologic study of altered clinical reactivity to respiratory syncytial (RS) virus infection in children previously vaccinated with an inactivated RS virus vaccine. Am J Epidemiol 89:405, 1969

Kaul TN, Welliver RC, Wong DT: Secretory antibody response to respiratory syncytial virus infection. Am J Dis Child 135:1013, 1981

Kim HW, Canchola JG, Brandt CD, et al.: Respiratory syncytial virus disease in infants despite prior administration of antigenic inactivated vaccine. Am J Epidemiol 89:422, 1969

Klein BS, Dollete FR, Yolken RH: The role of respiratory syncytial virus and other viral pathogens in acute otitis media. J Pediatr 101:16, 1982

Welliver RC, Wong DT, Sun M, et al.: The development of respiratory syncytial virus-specific IgE and the release of histamine in nasopharyngeal secretions after infection. N Engl J Med 305:842, 1981

Wright PF, Belshe RB, Kim HW, et al.: Administration of a highly attenuated, live respiratory syncytial virus vaccine to adults and children. Infect Immun 37:397, 1982

Wright PF, Shinozaki T, Fleet W, et al.: Evaluation of a live, attenuated, respiratory syncytial virus in infants. J Pediatr 88:931, 1976

MUMPS

Brunell PA, Brickman A, O'Hara D, et al.: Ineffectiveness of isolation of patients as a method of preventing the spread of mumps. N Engl J Med 279:1357, 1968

Fryden A, Link H, Norrby E: Cerebrospinal fluid and serum immunoglobulins and antibody titers in mumps meningitis and aseptic meningitis of other etiology. Infect Immun 21:852, 1978

Koplan JP, Preblud SR: A benefit-cost analysis of mumps vaccine. Am J Dis Child 136:362, 1982

Morishima T, Miyazu M, Ozaki T, et al.: Local immunity in mumps meningitis. Am J Dis Child 134:1060, 1980

Orvell C: Immunological properties of purified mumps virus glycoproteins. J Immunol 41:517, 1978

Orvell C: Structural polypeptides of mumps virus. J Immunol 41:527, 1978

Server AC, Merz DC, Waxham MN, et al.: Differentiation of mumps virus strains with monoclonal antibody to the HN glycoprotein. Infect Immun 35:179, 1982

Vandik B, Norrby E, Steen-Johnsen J, et al.: Mumps meningitis: Prolonged pleocytosis and occurrence of mumps virus-specific oligoclonal IgG in the cerebrospinal fluid. Eur Neurol 17:13, 1978

Weibel RE, Buynak EB, McLean AA, et al.: Persistence of antibody after administration of monovalent and combined live attenuated measles and rubella virus vaccines. Pediatrics 61:5, 1978

Yamauchi T, Wilson C, St. Geme JW Jr: Transmission of live attenuated mumps virus to the human placenta. N Engl J Med 290:710, 1974

CHAPTER 20

Measles and Subacute Sclerosing Panencephalitis

Measles (Rubeola)

Because of its distinctive clinical features, measles was recognized as a disease entity by Hebrew and Arabic physicians long before the demonstration of its viral etiology. Home, a Scottish physician, demonstrated in 1758 the transmissibility of the disease by scarification of susceptible individuals with blood taken from infected patients. Measles virus was first isolated successfully in tissue culture in 1954 by Enders and his associates. This permitted investigations of the virus, studies of immunity, and the development and selection of variants for vaccine evaluation.

The use of live attenuated vaccines began in 1963 and has extended to many parts of the world, altering dramatically the incidence and epidemiology of the disease. Where infant measles immunization is widely practiced, the illness has become uncommon. In other lands, especially among economically disadvantaged nations, measles persists in epidemic fashion responsible for the deaths of approximately 1.5 million infants and children each year.

Pathogenesis and Pathology

Measles is acquired as an infection of the respiratory tract, with principal damage to surface mucosal lining cells. Secondary bacterial infections may be enhanced by diminished function of alveolar macrophages. The virus spreads via lymphatics and through the blood to give widespread involvement, particularly in lymphoid cells. The large, inclusion-bearing, multinucleated giant cells found in tissues are quite similar to those produced by measles virus when grown in vitro. Patients excrete large amounts of virus during the catarrhal phase. Virus can be recovered from the blood, particularly from the white cell fraction, for several days before rash appears but rarely thereafter. The urine may remain positive for virus up to 4 days after the onset of rash. The pathology of acute central nervous system involvement includes edema, congestion, and scattered petechial hemorrhages, with perivascular cuffs of round cells. There may be some perivascular demyelination in the later stages.

The exact nature of the measles rash is uncertain but involves a vasculitis. Viral microtubular aggregates have been observed by electron microscopy of nuclei and cytoplasm of skin biopsies. They are also found in the oral lesions (Koplik spots). An important host mechanism for controlling the virus infection is the recognition and lysis of measles-infected cells by cytotoxic T lymphocytes. Malnourished, immunodeficient, or immunosuppressed children often undergo more severe measles, with prolonged virus replication, giant cell pneumonia, virus dissemination to many organs, and high case-fatality rates. Depressed T cell function appears to be the liability shared by these patients. Further evidence of an interaction of measles infections and cellular immune mechanisms is the loss of delayed hypersensitivity to tuberculoprotein among tuberculin-positive patients with measles. This persists for weeks to months following acute infection. A worsening of underlying tuberculosis in children or adults who acquire measles infection has been reported.

Clinical Course

Measles has an incubation period of 10 to 14 days (Fig. 20-1). A prodromal stage marked by catarrhal symptoms of cough, coryza, and conjunctivitis is accompanied by fever, which rises steadily until the appearance of rash 2 to 4 days after onset. Preceding the rash, the pathognomonic Koplik spots appear on the lateral buccal mucosa. They are pinpoint and grayish white surrounded by bright red inflammation and found over the lateral buccal mucosa and the inner lips, occasionally involving the entire inner mouth. They also may be detected in the palpebral conjunctiva. The exanthem begins on the head, behind the ears, on the forehead, and on the neck. Discrete red macular and papular lesions progress downward to involve the trunk and upper extremities. Over a period of 3 days, the entire body is involved. When the lower extremities show discrete lesions, those on the head and neck have begun to coalesce. With rash on the lower extremities, fever recedes dramatically. The bright red rash fades, to leave a brown discoloration that does not blanch with pressure.

The respiratory tract manifestations vary in severity but include laryngitis, tracheobronchitis, bronchiolitis, and interstitial pneumonitis from the primary virus infection that damages surface mucosal cells. With defervescence, there is improvement, but secondary bacterial infections of the respiratory tract may complicate the recovery phase in 5 to 10 percent of patients. These include otitis media, sinusitis, mastoiditis, and pneumonia. Encephalomyelitis occurs in approximately 0.1 percent of cases. This follows a 3 to 4 day period of recovery from the acute illness and is marked by a sudden onset, with seizures, confusion, and

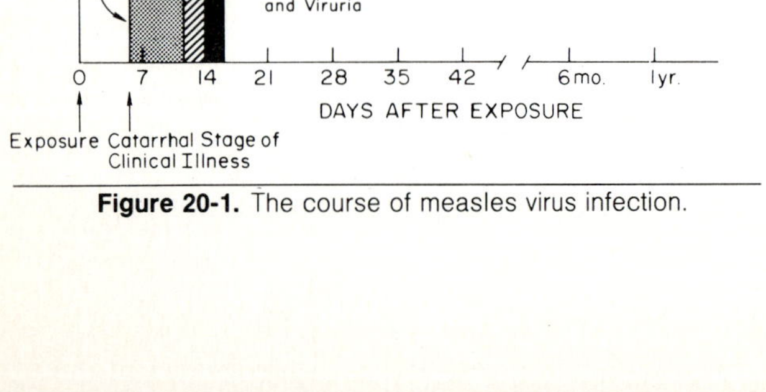

Figure 20-1. The course of measles virus infection.

coma. The mortality rate of central nervous system involvement approaches 25 percent. Nearly half of those who survive are left with some sequelae involving impaired intellectual, motor, or emotional development. The responsibility of measles virus for a late central nervous system complication, subacute sclerosing panencephalitis (SSPE), has been firmly established. This occurs in 1 or 2 per 100,000 cases and is discussed in greater detail later in this chapter.

Epidemiology

Measles is one of the most highly communicable of all virus infections, so that nearly all susceptible children acquire the infection. In rural settings or among isolated communities, it has been possible for a population to reach adult life without exposure. Under such circumstances, the introduction of measles virus produced devastating epidemics. An epidemiologic classic is Panum's description in 1846 of such an outbreak in the Faroe Islands. He showed the persistence of lifelong immunity among individuals who had acquired the infection 6 and 7 decades previously.

In the temperate zones, measles has occurred in winter–spring epidemics in 2- or 3-year cycles, apparently related to the new groups of susceptible children born since the last outbreak. Maternal antibody is transplacentally acquired by the infant, so that infection under 6 months of age is rare. As shown in Figure 20-1, the catarrhal stage of the illness is marked by extensive respiratory virus excretion, so that infected droplet nuclei provide the usual mode of transmission within families, schoolrooms, or other crowded settings. A single attack confers lifelong immunity.

Although measles is a member of the genus *Morbillivirus*, which includes the agents of canine distemper and rinderpest of cattle, there is no evidence of natural spread from one species to another. Except for minor variations, only one distinct serotype of measles virus has been identified. Infection sustained in any part of the world confers enduring, uniform geographic protection. With the striking decline of indigenous measles in the United States (Table 20-1) an increasing proportion of cases arise as a result of disease importations from other countries. Of the 1697 cases of measles reported in the United States in 1982, 36 percent were imported or the result of transmission to a family or social contact from an imported case. A second change has been an upward shift in the age-specific incidence rate, with sporadic outbreaks on college campuses among previously unimmunized students.

Diagnosis

Diagnosis is clinical, based on the characteristic history and findings. Examination of the urinary sediment or of nasal smears will show characteristic inclusion-bearing

TABLE 20-1. REPORTED MEASLES CASES IN THE UNITED STATES, 1963–1982

Year	Cases	Rate (per 10^5 Population)
1963	385,156	204.3
1964	458,083	239.7
1965	261,904	135.3
1966	204,136	104.4
1967	62,705	31.8
1968	22,231	11.1
1969	25,826	12.8
1970	47,351	23.2
1971	75,290	36.5
1972	32,275	15.5
1973	26,690	12.7
1974	22,094	10.5
1975	24,374	11.4
1976	41,126	19.2
1977	57,345	26.5
1978	26,871	12.3
1979	13,597	6.2
1980	13,506	6.0
1981	3,032	1.3
1982	1,697	0.7

syncytia, and there is peripheral leukopenia. Indirect immunofluorescent microscopy has been used to show measles antigen in nasopharyngeal cells. Although virus can be isolated from blood, respiratory tract secretions, conjunctival secretions, or urine, this is not ordinarily required or available.

A number of serologic tests are available, utilizing the antigens of the measles virion or its infectivity. These include virus neutralization, hemagglutination inhibition, complement fixation, enzyme-linked immunosorbent assay (ELISA), and immunofluorescence. Antibodies rise very rapidly after the appearance of rash and reach high titers in the next 30 to 60 days. A pair of sera obtained early in the course of illness and 7 to 14 days thereafter will show a marked rise in antibody titer by any of the methods described. Because of its ease and rapidity, the hemagglutination-inhibition test is most often utilized.

Treatment and Prevention

The primary viral disease is not amenable to any current therapy. Supportive measures may be employed to reduce fever, ameliorate cough, and maintain hydration. Secondary bacterial complications are treated with antibiotics selected by culture of appropriate specimens. The treatment of encephalomyelitis is also symptomatic, with careful attention to the maintenance of an airway, reduction of increased intracranial pressure, control of seizures, and provision of fluid, electrolyte, and caloric requirements. The administration of immune globulin early in the incubation period of measles may completely abort or modify the infection, depending on the amount employed. At a dose of 0.04 ml per kg body weight, immune globulin will reliably modify measles so that a more benign course ensues, followed by lasting immunity. Using a dose of 0.2 ml per kg body weight, it is possible to abort the infection completely, and the patient remains susceptible to future infection after catabolism of the exogenous globulin.

The prevention of measles by proper use of the available attenuated active virus vaccines offers the most reliable and enduring protection. Vaccines are recommended for all healthy children shortly after 1 year of age. The virus is propagated in chick embryo fibroblast or human diploid cell cultures. It is given parenterally, with successful infection in at least 95 percent of susceptibles. The infection is usually occult but may cause fever in 15 percent of recipients. Rarely, there is moderate, transient rash following the fever. This attenuated infection is noncommunicable and results in antibody responses somewhat lower than those that follow the natural infection. In patients studied to date, antibodies have persisted for periods up to 20 years after immunization. When exposed to natural infection, immunized children remain solidly protected. From 1963 to 1967 an inactivated measles vaccine was available. It has been abandoned because a severe unusual illness followed the exposure of children to naturally occurring measles several years after the receipt of inactivated vaccine. They developed fever, pneumonitis, and an unusual rash with petechiae. It seemed to represent a hypersensitivity reaction. The formalin or detergent treatment required to prepare the inactivated vaccine apparently degraded the F (penetration, fusion, hemolytic) protein of the measles virus so that recipients lacked specific antibody to that antigen despite the presence of antibodies to the other five virion proteins. On exposure to natural measles, virus penetration occurred, with spread of newly synthesized virus by cell-to-cell fusion. These inactivated vaccines have been withdrawn from the market.

In the initial 5 years after the onset of vaccine use in the United States, reported cases of measles were reduced by 90 percent. Table 20-1 demonstrates the striking decline in reported cases of measles in the United States since vaccine licensure in 1963 and public health immunization programs began in 1966. Studies of patients involved in current small outbreaks in the United States showed a heterogeneous population with illness. The majority had never received measles vaccine and had not previously acquired natural immunity to the infection. Some had received inactivated vaccine in the past. Others had been given active attenuated vaccine prior to their first birthday, at a time when persistent maternally transmitted antibody aborted the vaccine infection. In some instances vaccine failures were traced to improper storage of the attenuated vaccine, so that heat and/or light had reduced the infectivity of the material injected.

Recent public concerns about the hazards of immunization have prompted the collection of data, such as those displayed in Table 20-2, to permit a statistical evaluation of the comparative risks of the natural disease and the attenuated vaccine infection. The higher rates of pneumonia and deaths represent figures collected in India, Nigeria, Gambia, Bangladesh, and other nations with developing

TABLE 20-2. RATES OF COMPLICATIONS OF MEASLES AND MEASLES IMMUNIZATION

Adverse Reaction	Measles per 10^5	Vaccine per 10^5
Encephalomyelitis	50–400	0.1
SSPE	0.5–2.0	0.05–0.1
Pneumonia	3800–7300	—
Seizures	500–1000	0.02–19
Deaths	10–10,000	0.01

Adapted from reports of the Centers for Disease Control and World Health Organization.

health systems. Continued attention to immunization of all children 1 year of age or older is needed in order to attain the goal of measles eradication.

Subacute Sclerosing Panencephalitis (SSPE)

This degenerative disease of the brain was first described in 1933, but it was not attributed to measles infection until 1967. Since that time abundant laboratory data have confirmed the etiologic agent as measles virus (or a defective variant) that persists in the host after initial conventional measles in infancy or early childhood.

Clinical Features

SSPE occurs almost exclusively in children and adolescents, usually between the ages of 5 and 10 years and predominantly in males (3:1). Rarely, young infants are affected, and a few cases have been reported in adults. The usual clinical course is outlined in Table 20-3. The progress of the disease may appear to be arrested for periods of years, usually when the patient is in coma, but almost invariably the patients die, often of intercurrent infection. A very few older patients with well-documented disease have recovered.

Epidemiology

Although the incidence of SSPE varies in many countries and among population groups within nations, it is estimated that 1 case follows each 100,000 cases of measles. The majority of patients give a history of uncomplicated natural measles at a younger age than average, and all remain well during the interim of approximately 5 years until the onset of their central nervous system disease. Occasionally, no prior history of measles is elicited, or live attenuated measles vaccine is the only known exposure to measles virus. No consistent immunologic defects have been demonstrated in SSPE patients.

Data have suggested that the disease may have been more common in the Southeastern United States, that the primary measles infection occurred at a younger age in such patients, and that rural rather than urban residents were at greater risk. With the widespread use of measles vaccine and the resultant decline of measles in the United States, there has been a parallel, sharp decrease in reported cases of SSPE. Prior to measles vaccination programs, 20 to 40 cases of SSPE occurred annually, whereas only 4 or 5 new patients are now reported each year.

Diagnosis and Pathogenesis

The diagnosis should be suspected on the basis of the history and the clinical findings of progressive personality changes, myoclonus, and variable focal neurologic deficits. A characteristic spike wave discharge is seen on the EEG, and the cerebrospinal fluid is usually normal apart from a first-zone colloidal gold sol curve. The diagnosis is confirmed by the finding of measles antibodies in the cerebrospinal fluid. Brain biopsy is not necessary for diagnosis, but should tissue become available, it may show perivascular round cell infiltration, neuronal degeneration, gliosis, and type A Cowdry intranuclear inclusion bodies when stained with hematoxylin and eosin and examined with the light microscope. With the electron microscope, these inclusion bodies contain microtubular filaments, corresponding in size and configuration to the nucleocapsids of measles virus. With appropriate fluorescent antibody staining, measles antigen can be demonstrated at these sites. Finally, when brain tissue is cocultivated in the laboratory with permissive cells, complete infectious virus may be re-

TABLE 20-3. SUBACUTE SCLEROSING PANENCEPHALITIS (SSPE)

Clinical	Laboratory	
Personality change; declining school performance; intellectual deterioration often manifested by impaired memory, altered judgment, and inappropriate behavior; occasionally chorioretinitis; impaired motor activity, gait difficulty, speech difficulty; myoclonic jerks progressing to repetitive, often sound-sensitive myoclonic seizures; paralysis; gradual deterioration in consciousness; coma; death	EEG	Paroxysmal, synchronous spike discharges with interim suppression of electrical activity
	CSF	Usually acellular; normal total protein; increased gamma globulins (IgG); detectable measles antibody
	Blood	Markedly elevated measles antibody
	Brain	Specific immunofluorescence to measles antigen; microtubular filaments within nuclear inclusions on electron microscopy; SSPE virus recovered in tissue culture

EEG, electroencephalogram; CSF, cerebrospinal fluid.

covered. Analysis of serum and cerebrospinal fluid antibodies reveals that SSPE patients lack detectable response to the M (membrane) protein of measles virus, although they respond to all the other five major structural proteins of the virion. This observation coincides with the failure of maturation of the measles nucleocapsids detected in the neuronal and glial cells.

Although measles virus infects central nervous system cells, there is no incorporation of the newly replicated components into cell membranes to form complete new infectious virus. Direct analysis of measles-virus proteins in central nervous system tissue of SSPE patients shows a lack of synthesis of M protein. This host cell-dependent restriction is consistent with the findings of accumulated viral nucleocapsids intracellularly, failure to recover infectious measles virus except by cocultivation with known permissive cells, antibodies in serum and cerebrospinal fluid to the other five measles proteins, and the abortive persistent infection.

Treatment

Although numerous approaches to therapy for this condition have been attempted, all have failed. At present one can only offer general supportive care for the patient, attempt to control seizures, and try to provide early diagnosis and proper explanation.

FURTHER READING

MEASLES

Abu Beer Mohammed Ibn Zacariya Ar-Razi (Rhazes): A Treatise on the Smallpox and Measles. Translated from the original Arabic by WA Greenhill, Sydenham Society, London, 1848

Annunziato D, Kaplan MH, Hall WW, et al.: Atypical measles syndrome: Pathologic and serologic findings. Pediatrics 70:203, 1982

Centers for Disease Control: Measles Surveillance Report No. 11, 1977–1981, issued September 1982

Frank JA Jr, Hoffman RE, Mann JM, et al.: Imported measles: A potential control problem. JAMA 245:264, 1981

Hall WW, Choppin PW: Measles-virus proteins in the brain tissue of patients with subacute sclerosing panencephalitis. N Engl J Med 304:1152, 1981

Katz SL, Krugman S, Quinn TC: International symposium on measles immunization. Rev Infect Dis 5:389, 1983

Lucas CJ, Biddison WE, Nelson DL, el al.: Killing of measles virus-infected cells by human cytotoxic T cells. Infect Immun 38:226, 1982

Machamer CE, Hayes EC, Zweerink HJ: Cells infected with a cell-associated subacute sclerosing panencephalitis virus do not express M protein. Virology 108:515, 1981

terMeulen V, Stephenson JR, Kieth HW: Subacute sclerosing panencephalitis. In Fraenkel-Conrat H, Wagner RR (eds): Comprehensive Virology. New York, Plenum Press, 1983, vol 18, p 105

CHAPTER 21

Rubella (German Measles)

From the mid-19th century until 1941, rubella was regarded as a benign childhood exanthem. When the Australian ophthalmologist, Sir Norman Gregg, reported the association of intrauterine rubella infection with congenital cataracts, this attitude changed completely. Subsequently, deafness, congenital heart disease, and other malformations were found to result from maternal rubella during the first 4 months of pregnancy. The recovery in 1962 of rubella virus in cell culture systems led to the development and, in 1969, the licensure of attenuated active vaccines that have proven safe and effective. Congenital rubella has become infrequent in the United States as a result of widespread use of these vaccines.

On the basis of its biochemical and biophysical properties, rubella is classified as a togavirus, but it has no involvement with arthropod vectors. Because many different viruses may cause a similar clinical illness with rash and fever, but only rubella is teratogenic, virus isolation techniques and specific serologic tests for antibody have provided the necessary differentiation of etiologic agents.

Clinical Features and Pathogenesis

Rubella is a mild rash disease that occurs principally in children but is seen at all ages. As shown in Figure 21-1, the incubation period is approximately 2 weeks, with minimal prodromal signs or symptoms. Most often, the first awareness of illness is mild fever and respiratory signs immediately preceding the onset of rash. The exanthem is pink macules and papules, at first on the face and then on the neck, trunk, and extremities, where they remain discrete and rarely coalesce. The rash has ordinarily disappeared by the third day. Preceding and accompanying the rash there is lymphadenopathy, which may involve the postauricular, suboccipital, and cervical nodes. Rash is observed commonly among children, but infection may be occult or only a febrile pharyngitis in as many as one third of adult patients. Although major complications are rare (thrombocytopenic purpura and encephalitis), the incidence of arthralgia and arthritis is much greater than generally appreciated. The frequency of joint involvement is directly correlated with increasing age and appears also to be more common among women. In a few patients, persistence of rubella virus in synovial cells has been associated with polyarthritis and arthralgia of lengthy duration. Usually joint involvement is acute and transient without sequelae (Fig. 21-1).

The route of infection is via the respiratory tract, with spread to lymphatic tissues and then to the blood. Both viremia and respiratory tract shedding of virus may precede the rash by 1 week, and the latter may follow it for another several weeks. Because much virus excretion occurs prior to the recognition of illness, secondary infection of intimate contacts has usually transpired before the primary patient has been diagnosed. Little is known of the actual pathology of the postnatal disease because it is not a fatal one. However, the pathogenesis of congenital infection has been well studied during and since the 1964 pandemic. Maternal viremia is followed by infection of the placenta, which may lead to virus invasion of the fetus. Multiple tissues and organs support the replication of virus, which continues to multiply throughout the remainder of pregnancy and in the postnatal period. A large percentage of maternal infections that occur in the first 3 months of pregnancy result in fetal illness. There is a diminishing number in the fourth month, and it is uncertain whether any fetal infections have resulted from maternal rubella in later pregnancy. Although the exact mechanism of damage to fetal organs is not clear, rubella infection of human embryonic cells in vitro is associated with both chromosomal breakage and inhibition of normal mitosis. Infants with

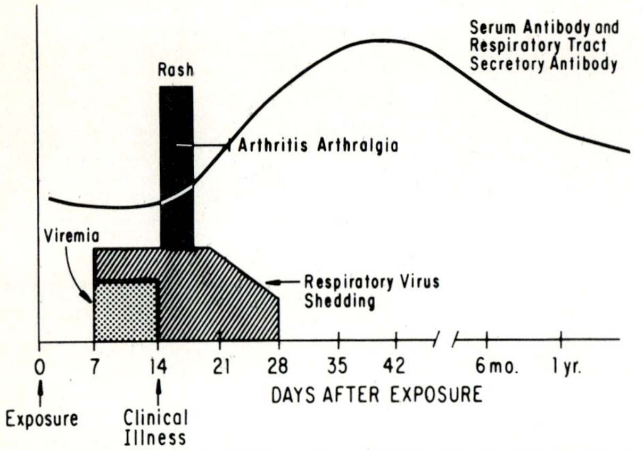

Figure 21-1. The course of postnatal rubella virus infection.

congenital rubella undergo intrauterine growth retardation and have a subnormal number of cells in some infected organs, suggesting that these same features may also occur in vivo.

Congenital rubella infection may result in a large variety of abnormalities, including deafness, congenital heart disease, eye defects (cataracts, glaucoma, retinitis, microphthalmia), growth retardation, thrombocytopenic purpura, osteitis, hepatitis, pneumonitis, encephalitis, and cerebral damage with mental retardation. In contrast to the postnatal infection, intrauterine disease is marked by a continued replication and excretion of virus, which may persist throughout the first year of life and has been demonstrated in selected tissues, such as the lens of the eye, as long as 3 or 4 years postnatally. In addition to malformations compatible with life, intrauterine rubella infection may produce fetal death, abortion, or neonatal death. Although many of the acute neonatal manifestations resolve over the first months of life, long-term sequelae result in multiple developmental handicaps. Recent studies also indicate a significant increase in diabetes mellitus, chronic pneumonitis, thyroiditis, and degenerative encephalitis among long-term survivors of intrauterine infection.

The immunity that follows naturally acquired postnatal rubella is enduring. Only one serologic type of virus has been identified, and a single attack confers lifelong immunity. The immunologic events that accompany intrauterine infection differ strikingly. The antibody response in utero is principally one of IgM rather than IgG. Although IgG specific for rubella is found in fetal circulation, it is mainly of maternal origin and transplacentally acquired. Despite the presence of specific IgM and IgG in the fetal circulation, chronic infection of cells continues. Postnatally, the infected infant synthesizes rubella-specific IgG. Virus replication diminishes gradually over ensuing months. A small number of congenitally infected infants have developed unusual forms of hypogammaglobulinemia in the first year of life. Another group have lost all their detectable rubella antibody postnatally but have nonetheless proven resistant to challenge with attenuated rubella viruses. The explanations for a number of these immunologic paradoxes are not yet known.

Epidemiology

In most urban communities, rubella infection was acquired during early childhood, principally in the school years. Because it is not as highly communicable as measles or varicella, 15 to 20 percent of women reached childbearing age without having acquired natural immunity. In the United States, large epidemics occurred at 6- to 8-year intervals, with smaller numbers of cases in the intervening years. This cycle was interrupted in 1969 by the onset of rubella vaccine programs, and no large epidemic has developed in the United States in the 19 years since the 1964–1965 pandemic. The usual transmission is by the respiratory route, but the prolonged viruria of congenitally infected infants may be of importance in spread to close contacts. In situations where adolescents and young adults have been placed in crowded living conditions, rubella outbreaks have been observed. Examples are regularly seen among Armed Forces recruits, preparatory school and college groups, and summer camps. With widespread use of rubella vaccines, childhood outbreaks have disappeared, and sporadic clusters of cases are reported now on college campuses, in Armed Forces training camps, and among other teenage groups who have escaped both immunization and natural infection.

Diagnosis

Until 1962, the diagnosis was entirely a clinical one and unreliable. Currently, virus isolation techniques are not readily available. They involve the use of cell culture systems susceptible to the virus, with direct observation for cytopathic effect, or the use of an interfering agent as an indicator of virus replication. Because these are time consuming and fastidious, serologic tests are more commonly used. The antigens of rubella virus are responsible for the induction of a number of antibody types that can be assayed in serum. These include complement-fixing (CF), virus-neutralizing, hemagglutination-inhibiting (HI), immunodiffusion, enzyme-linked immunosorbent assay (ELISA), and immunofluorescent antibodies. The HI test has been the most commonly employed. Paired serum specimens obtained early in the course of illness and 10 to 20 days thereafter will demonstrate an antibody rise. The presence in many sera of nonspecific inhibitors of hemagglutination makes the HI test susceptible to some error unless care is taken first to treat the sera to remove inhibitors. The HI test is also valuable for screening populations to determine serosusceptibility or immunity and in the consideration of the use and efficacy of vaccines. The diagnosis of intrauterine rubella is more complicated but may be accomplished on a single serum specimen if neonatal blood is assayed for IgM antibodies specific to rubella virus. If such a technique is not available, it may be necessary to test paired specimens obtained over a period of several months in order to determine whether there is active postnatal antibody synthesis by the infant or merely a decline of transplacentally acquired antibody.

Treatment and Prevention

There is no specific therapy for rubella virus infection. In the case of documented maternal infection during the first trimester of pregnancy, therapeutic abortion is commonly employed. Even though rubella is confirmed virologically and/or serologically in the mother, it is not possible to be certain that fetal infection has occurred. It is estimated that maternal rubella in the first month of gestation carries a 30 to 50 percent incidence of fetal infection, in the second month of gestation a 25 percent risk, and in the third month a 10 percent incidence. After the third month there are insufficient numbers to quantitate the minimal risk of fetal involvement. Amniocentesis has been employed in a few cases to examine cells and fluid for evidence of rubella virus infection. However, there are insufficient data to evaluate the reliability of this method.

The use of immune serum globulin to prevent fetal rubella in an exposed pregnant woman has been ineffective and misleading. In most situations, it has been difficult to ascertain for how long a mother has been exposed to the virus. As depicted in Figure 21-1, she may have had a week's exposure to respiratory shedding from a contact by the time the contact develops rash disease.

Since 1969, attenuated active rubella virus vaccines have been used. These vaccines confer lasting effective immunity. They have been prepared in cell cultures of duck embryo, canine kidney, rabbit kidney, and a human diploid line (WI-38). Their use is followed by some respiratory shedding of the vaccine virus for 7 to 28 days after vaccination. In contrast to that following natural infection, this is not transmissible. The human diploid cell vaccine (RA 27/3) is most widely available in this country. A serologically detectable HI antibody response is produced in more than 95 percent of susceptible vaccine recipients within 4 to 6 weeks of immunization. As with naturally acquired rubella, vaccination may be followed by joint complaints but in a smaller percentage of recipients. Approximately 25 percent of adult female vaccinees experience arthralgia and only 1 percent arthritis. Whether the attenuated strains of virus might also be teratogenic for the fetus or embryo is uncertain. Vaccine virus can cross the placenta to reach the products of conception. The risk of any teratogenesis is negligible in 14 years' accumulated experience but theoretically possible. Of 215 infants born to seronegative mothers who inadvertently received rubella vaccine in early pregnancy, none had a detectable congenital malformation. The use of vaccine in pregnant women remains nonetheless contraindicated. Before administering attenuated rubella vaccine to a susceptible woman of childbearing age, it is important to be certain she is not pregnant and that she will follow an acceptable method of pregnancy prevention for 2 to 3 months thereafter.

Reinfection with wild rubella virus has been demonstrated to occur following either naturally acquired or vaccine-induced immunity. This usually happens in individuals whose antibody titers have fallen to low levels. It is more likely to occur in vaccinated individuals who lack detectable rubella-specific respiratory tract secretory immunoglobulins (sIgA). The virologic events of such reinfections are markedly abbreviated and have not been accompanied by viremia. There is a rapid secondary type of antibody response with no overt illness. Such a reinfection does not threaten the fetus of a woman in early pregnancy. Continued study will be required to answer fully all the questions raised by the vaccines. In 15 years of utilization in the United States, they have produced a striking reduction in reported cases of intrauterine and postnatal rubella. Prospective surveillance will be required to determine the long-range effects of these changes in population immunity and of the reduction in circulation of rubella virus.

FURTHER READING

Chantler JK, Ford DK, Tingle AJ: Persistent rubella infection and rubella-associated arthritis. Lancet 1:1323, 1982

Crawford GE, Gremillion DH: Epidemic measles and rubella in Air Force recruits. J Infect Dis 144:403, 1981

Gregg NM: Congenital cataract following German measles in the mother. Trans Ophthal Soc Aust 3:35, 1942

Herrmann KL, Halstead SB, Wiebenga NH: Rubella antibody persistence after immunization. JAMA 247:193, 1982

Hinman AR, Bart KJ, Orenstein WA, et al.: Rational strategy for rubella vaccination. Lancet 1:39, 1983

Horstmann DM: Rubella. In Evans AS (ed): Viral Infections of Humans. New York, Plenum, 1982, chap 21, p 519

Sever JL, Cleghorn BA: Rubella diagnostic tests. Postgrad Med 71:73, 1982

CHAPTER 22

Arboviruses

Rift Valley fever really pulled a surprise act near the end of the decade (1970s) in affecting thousands of people as well as domestic animals in an invasion of Egypt.

—*RW Chamberlain: Am J Trop Med Hyg 31:434, 1982*

Arboviruses (*ar*thropod *bo*rne) are maintained in nature usually by cyclical transmission between susceptible vertebrates and bloodsucking arthropods, with the virus multiplying in both. In vertebrates, arboviruses produce, after an incubation period, a viremia of sufficient titer and duration to permit infection of arthropods. In arthropods, virus multiplication results in the capacity to transmit virus by bite to new vertebrates after a period of time known as the "extrinsic incubation period." This biologic transmission, which depends on the multiplication of virus in the arthropod, is in contrast to mechanical transmission, which occurs as the result of rapid carriage of virus by an arthropod from one host to another. The consequences of infection of the vertebrate range from total absence of disease to major illness and death. With rare exceptions, no effect on the arthropod has been detected.

Most arboviruses are members of the families Togaviridae and Bunyaviridae; some are Reoviridae and Rhabdoviridae. A small number, generally of no significance in human disease, may be found in other families. Proof of biologic transmission by arthropods has not been obtained for many arboviruses but is inferred from epidemiologic and taxonomic characteristics. The discipline of arbovirology often deals, in addition, with some viruses, such as arenaviruses, that probably are not arthropod-borne and for which other modes of transmission have been demonstrated. This is because of a historical, initial presumption of arthropod transmission based on clinical and epidemiologic similarities to known arbovirus disease.

The year 1900 marked the beginning of arbovirology, when Walter Reed demonstrated the biologic transmission of yellow fever by the mosquito *Aedes aegypti.* The facts, so convincingly elucidated by the commission of which Reed was chairman, proved the remarkable perception of Dr. Carlos Finlay and the essentials of the basic definition of arboviruses.

During ensuing decades, other viruses, many of which are human pathogens, were recognized to possess life cycles that involve arthropod–vertebrate transmission. By the end of the 1930s, there were approximately 16 arboviruses. Since World War II, hundreds more have been discovered, so that now there are in excess of 445 known arboviruses. More than 100 may infect and produce disease in humans.

Beginning in the 1920s with the yellow fever program of its International Health Division, the Rockefeller Foundation has provided one of the major physical and intellectual bases of arbovirology. Besides developing the conceptual base, much of the basic technology, and most of the facts of arbovirology, the Foundation's conquest of yellow fever by the development of the first tissue culture-attenuated, live virus vaccine stands as a major achievement.

Classification and Nomenclature

Initially, arboviruses were named for the disease that they caused, for example, dengue and yellow fever. Later, combined names were devised that comprised both geography and diseases, such as St. Louis encephalitis. Names currently derive from the place of collection of the specimen from which the first isolation was made, especially for those agents for which no disease is recognized. Most arboviruses fall into this group.

Arboviruses are classified according to morphologic and serologic relationships based on tests employing complement fixation, hemagglutination inhibition, and infectivity neutralization. At first, serogroups were designated A, B, and C; these groups have been renamed alphaviruses, flaviviruses, and bunyaviruses, respectively. More recently, groups are given the name of the first virus isolated. Fifty-seven serogroups have been identified, and 97 viruses are as yet ungrouped.

There are several other ways of grouping arboviruses that may be useful in certain circumstances. These include classification according to vector, geographic range, type of disease, or combinations of these, such as "tickborne hemorrhagic fevers." Because this text is intended primarily for medical students, it seems appropriate to use a clinically oriented classification (Tables 22-1, 22-2, and 22-3).

Technology

The epidemiologic and clinical study of arboviruses involves two basic technologies: virus isolation and measurement of antibodies. The major culture medium for isolation is the infant mouse, in which nearly all arboviruses are pathogenic when inoculated intracerebrally. Cell cultures are the next most useful medium, especially for the study of many established isolates. In the usual search for arboviruses, serum or tissue specimens from humans or other vertebrates, as well as aqueous suspensions of ground-up arthropods, are routinely inoculated intracerebrally into each infant mouse in a litter. The mice are observed for signs of illness over the next month. Brain tissue from mice that become sick during this time is used for further passage. Serial passages are made until mouse pathogenicity is constant, at which time a large pool of infected brain tissue is stored frozen for use in biologic, physical, chemical, and serologic characterization of the agent.

Serum antibody measurements are usually essential in the diagnosis of individual patients (Fig. 22-1). Antibodies also provide a record of past infection that permits detection of the involvement of specific populations of humans and other vertebrates in the transmission cycle. These seroepidemiologic investigations are of great value to the understanding of the geographic distribution of arboviruses. Geographic distribution is also delineated through the use of sentinel animals, such as caged mice or chickens placed in the forest. Presence of virus in these animals is revealed by disease or by a rise in serum antibodies.

The techniques of virus isolation and antibody measurement may be applied to captured or colonized vertebrates and arthropods to determine their potential as natural hosts for a given virus. Experts in field and labora-

TABLE 22-1. SUMMARY OF SELECTED HUMAN ARBOVIRUS DISEASES CHARACTERIZED BY FEVER WITH OR WITHOUT RASH

Virus			Maintenance Hosts		
Name*	Group	Geography	Vertebrate	Arthropod	Clinical (Other than Fever) and Epidemiologic Features
Dengue	Flavivirus	Tropics and subtropics throughout world	Humans, monkeys	Mosquito	Headache, myalgia, rash, arthralgia, endemic and epidemic
Colorado tick	Orbivirus	Western North America	Small mammals	Tick	Headache, myalgia, rash, biphasic fever, spring and summer focal endemicity
West Nile	Flavivirus	Mediterranean, Africa, Middle East, Russia, Asia	Birds	Mosquito, ? ticks	Headache, lymphadenopathy, rash, meningoencephalitis, endemic and epidemic
Sandfly	Phlebotomus fever	Mediterranean, Asia, tropical America	Humans, small mammals	Phlebotomus flies	Myalgia, headache, gastrointestinal symptoms, seasonally epidemic and sporadically endemic
Rift Valley	Phlebotomus fever	Africa	Large mammals, humans, ? forest rodents	Mosquito	Headache, myalgia, photophobia, retinal damage may occur; sporadic from mosquito or by contact with tissue from infected animals
O'nyong-nyong	Alphavirus	Africa	Humans	Mosquito	Like dengue, epidemic
Chikungunya	Alphavirus	Africa, Asia	Humans	Mosquito	Like dengue, epidemic and endemic
Mayaro	Alphavirus	South and Central America	Monkeys	Mosquito	Like dengue, forest-associated, endemic and epidemic
Ross River	Alphavirus	Australia, South Pacific	Humans, ? marsupials	Mosquito	Like dengue, arthritis, endemic and seasonal epidemic
Oropouche	Simbu	Tropical America	Humans, monkeys, birds	Culicoides gnats	Headache, fever, myalgia, epidemic

*Disease name is generally the virus name plus fever, e.g., Colorado tick fever.

TABLE 22-2. SUMMARY OF SELECTED HUMAN ARBOVIRUS DISEASES CHARACTERIZED BY ENCEPHALITIS

Virus			Maintenance Hosts		Clinical (Other than Encephalitis) and Epidemiologic Features
Name*	Group	Geography	Vertebrate	Arthropod	Case Fatality (F) and Sequelae (S)
Western equine	Alphavirus	Western and South America	Birds	Mosquito	Summer epidemics North America, equine epizootics F = high, S = severe
Eastern equine	Alphavirus	Eastern North America, Caribbean, South America	Birds	Mosquito	Summer epidemics and equine and bird epizootics F = high, S = severe
Venezuelan equine	Alphavirus	South and Central America	Rodents, birds, horses	Mosquito	Influenza-like, CNS involvement far less common, encephalitis epizootics in equines F = low, S = moderate
St. Louis	Flavivirus	Western hemisphere, especially U.S.	Birds	Mosquito	Summer epidemics in U.S. F = low, S = moderate
Rocio	Flavivirus	Brazil	Birds	Mosquito	Seasonal epidemics F = low, S = moderate
California (La-Crosse)	Bunyavirus-California	USA	Small mammals	Mosquito	Summer outbreaks and sporadic cases F = low, S = ?
Japanese	Flavivirus	Asia, Japan	Birds, pigs	Mosquito	Summer and fall epidemics in temperate areas F = high S = severe
Murray Valley	Falvivirus	Australia and New Guinea	Bird	Mosquito	Epidemic F = high
Powassan	Flavivirus	U.S. and Canada	Small mammals	Tick	Two cases of human disease recognized, one fatal
Russian spring–summer	Flavivirus	Russia	Birds, mammals	Tick†	Diphasic pattern, bulbospinal paralysis F = high, S = severe
Central European	Flavivirus	Europe	Birds, mammals	Tick†	Diphasic pattern F = low, S = mild
Kyasanur Forest disease	Flavivirus	India	Birds, mammals	Tick†	Hemorrhagic manifestations more common F = low, S = 0
Louping ill	Flavivirus	British Isles	Birds, mammals	Tick†	Diphasic pattern F = 0, S = 0

*Disease and virus name listed plus, usually encephalitis, e.g., St. Louis encephalitis.
†Transovarially transmitted.

tory zoology and entomology are therefore essential. As a result, the arbovirus laboratory is staffed by a broad-based medical zoology group.

Ecology, Epidemiology, and the Public Health

Arboviruses are distributed throughout the world. While most exist in the tropics and subtropics, some have also been isolated from arthropods and vertebrates in climatically less hospitable areas, such as Finland, Canada, Siberia, and Alaska. Their epidemic potential continues to surprise us. Outbreaks of major and often new clinical disease in the savannahs, forests, and swamps of the tropical world provide episodes of romance and high adventure as well as tragedy and misery. Here in the United States, St. Louis and LaCrosse encephalitis viruses cause epidemics of serious disease.

The conceptual and technical base of arbovirus ecology grew from the work in the late 1920s and 1930s on yellow fever. Yellow fever initially was thought to be entirely a problem of human-to-human transmission by the relatively domestic mosquito *A. aegypti.* When the entirely nonhuman jungle cycle was discovered and the study broadened zoologically, several arthropod-transmitted viruses were discovered that were not yellow fever. After World War II, an extraordinary global effort was made to study these agents. Arbovirus laboratories were established around the tropical world in such places as Jamaica, Trinidad, Egypt, India, Malaya, Taiwan, Brazil, Panama, Nigeria, and Uganda. The hundreds of arboviruses that we know today were discovered in this effort.

Arboviruses generally maintain themselves in nature by constant and fairly frequent transmission between an arthropod and a vertebrate host (Fig. 22-2). Many variables influence the likelihood and frequency of successful transmission. For example, the frequency of feeding of an

TABLE 22-3. HEMORRHAGIC FEVERS DUE TO ARBOVIRUSES, ARENAVIRUSES, AND OTHER (SIMILAR TO RHABDO) VIRUSES

Fever	Causative Agents	Vector(s)	Vertebrate Host(s)	Geographic Distribution	Epidemiologic Features of Involvement of Humans	Control	Remarks
Yellow fever (urban)	Flavivirus	*Aedes aegypti*	Humans	Human populations in tropics of Africa and South America	Person-to-person passage by *Aedes*	*A. aegypti* control: vaccination	Sylvan YF can spread to *A. aegypti* cycle
Yellow fever (sylvan)	Flavivirus	*Haemagogus* mosquitoes in New World, *Aedes* species in Africa	Monkeys	Forests and jungles of South America and West, Central, and East Africa	Humans infected by exposure in jungles (i.e., woodcutters, hunters, and so on)	Vaccination	Human cases epidemic or sporadic and unpredictable, monkey deaths signal epidemic in tropical America
Dengue homorrhagic fever	Flaviviruses	*Aedes aegypti*	Humans	Tropical and subtropical cities of Asia and Caribbean	Small children usually involved in cities where *A. aegypti* densities are high	*A. aegypti* control: mosquito repellent, screens, and so on	Disease probably due to immune enhancement following sequential infection with different dengue serotypes
Omsk hemorrhagic fever	Alphavirus	Ticks of genus *Dermacentor*	Small rodents and muskrats	Omsk region of U.S.S.R., northern Romania	People exposed in fields and wooded lands	Tick repellents and protective clothing	
Kyasanur forest disease	Flavivirus	Ticks of several species in genus *Haemaphysalis*	Monkeys (rhesus and langur) and small rodents and birds	Mysore State, India	People exposed in fields and wooded lands	Tick control: tick repellents and protective clothing	Monkey mortality signals epidemic
Argentinian hemorrhagic fever	Junin virus, an arenavirus	None recognized	Small rodents, *Akodon, Calomys*	Argentina, NW of Buenos Aires Province extending west to Province of Cordoba	Field workers at harvest time are particularly at risk	Rodent control in fields	Infected rodents contaminate environment with urine
Bolivian hemorrhagic fever	Machupo virus, an arenavirus	None recognized	Small rodent, *Calomys callosus*	Beni Province of Bolivia	Residents of small rodent-infested villages and homes, 1971 nosocomial outbreak in Cochabamba, Bolivia	Rodent control in fields	High mortality in humans
Lassa fever	Lassa virus, an arenavirus	None	Small rodent, *Mastomys natalensis*	West Africa; Nigeria, Liberia, Sierra Leone	Residents of small rodent-infested villages, dramatic nosocomial outbreaks	None known, possibly rodent control	High mortality in humans
Crimean hemorrhagic fever	CHF Congo virus, (bunyavirus)	Ticks of several genera	Larger domestic animals implicated, also African hedgehog	Southern U.S.S.R., Bulgaria, East and West Africa	Cowhands and field workers in U.S.S.R., nosocomial outbreaks reported	Tick control relating to livestock, full isolation in patient care	Human disease important in U.S.S.R., importance to humans in Africa not known

(continued)

TABLE 22-3. (cont.)

Fever	Causative Agents	Vector(s)	Vertebrate Host(s)	Geographic Distribution	Epidemiologic Features of Involvement of Humans	Control	Remarks
Korean hemorrhagic fever (hemorrhagic fever with renal syndrome)	Hantaan virus (bunyavirus)	Not known	Rodents	Korea, northern Eurasia to and including Scandinavia	Rural or sylvan exposure (military, forest occupations, farmers), outbreaks in laboratories related to white rats	None	Antibodies found in Norway rats worldwide
African hemorrhagic fever (Marburg disease)	Marburg and Ebola viruses, similar to rhabdoviruses	Not known	Unknown	Africa	Person-to-person	Clinical isolation techniques	Highly fatal

Adapted from Johnson: In Beeson and McDermott (eds): Textbook of Medicine, 14th ed, 1975, p 239. Philadelphia, W.B. Saunders Co.

arthropod on a vertebrate host depends on numerous innate and behavioral factors of each animal that may be environmentally determined. These factors may differ from time to time and from place to place. Arthropod longevity, a major determinant, depends in turn on climatic factors, such as humidity and temperature, availability of food, and the prevalence of predators, as well as on noxious physical, chemical, and biologic agents. Many other complex factors similarly influence transmission. Clearly, a systems analysis approach is needed to assess the effect of any change in any variable. Because of the large number of agents, the numerous nonhuman hosts, and the great gaps in our knowledge, this approach has not yet come into its own.

Although viremia is usually of sufficient intensity for transmission only for a matter of days, there is evidence that long-lasting infections in some hibernating vertebrates, such as rodents infected with Eastern equine encephalitis virus, may permit a virus to remain in an area during a period of unsuitable climate and to be transmitted again when arthropod feeding resumes. Transovarial transmission through generations of arthropods occurs with many viruses and provides the prospect of indefinite survival of virus without cyclical transmission. The important subject of how arboviruses survive periods when cyclical transmission cannot occur has been reviewed recently by Reeves. Other than transovarially, arthropod-to-arthropod transmission of some viruses may occur venereally. Direct transmission may occur between vertebrate hosts, as in the case of Eastern equine encephalitis virus, which is passed from pheasant to pheasant under crowded conditions of commercial pheasant farms. The importance in nature of these alternate maintenance cycles is an area of active, current research.

Humans are generally incidental hosts and a dead end for virus transmission. Notable exceptions are the human–mosquito cycles of dengue, yellow fever, Ross River, and Chikungunya viruses. As a rule, arboviruses are clinically

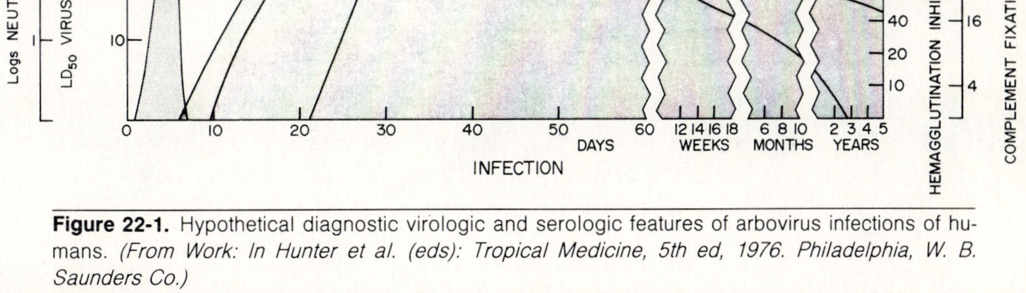

Figure 22-1. Hypothetical diagnostic virologic and serologic features of arbovirus infections of humans. *(From Work: In Hunter et al. (eds): Tropical Medicine, 5th ed, 1976. Philadelphia, W. B. Saunders Co.)*

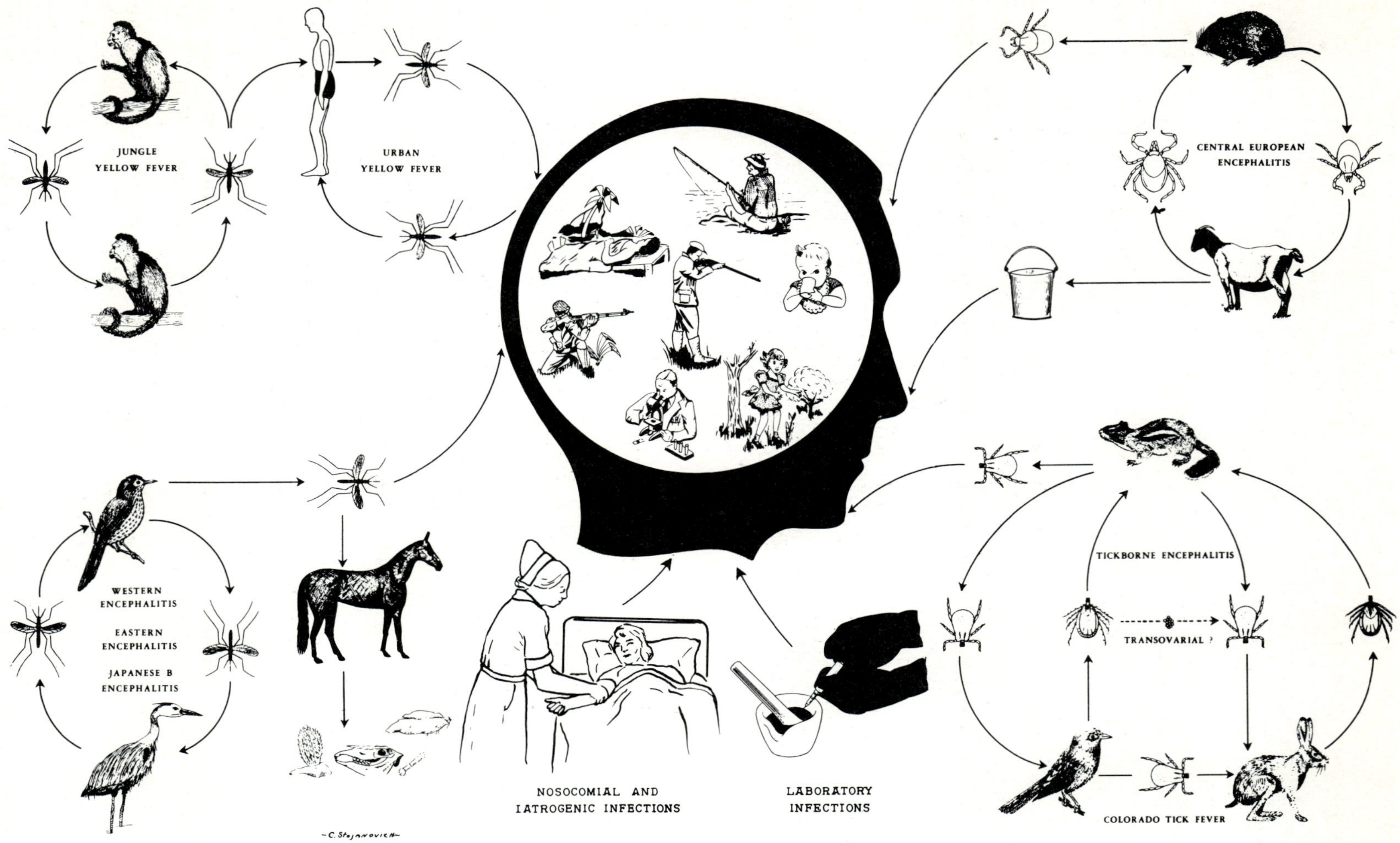

Figure 22-2. Occupational and recreational exposure of humans to arbovirus and other vertebrate virus infections. *(From Work TH et al.: In Feigin RD, Cherry JD (eds): Textbook of Pediatric Infectious Diseases, vol II, 1981. Philadelphia, Saunders.)*

silent as they cycle in nature. Disease occurs in unnatural hosts, such as humans and horses, and these hosts are of no consequence to viral transmission.

There are two basic ecologic mechanisms that ensnare humans and other animals: either humans enter the geographic area of the transmission cycle, or the cycle changes and moves closer to them. Yellow fever ecology provides examples of both. The former occurs when a person enters a forest where yellow fever virus is cycling between monkeys and the tree-top mosquitoes. Without the intrusion, these mosquitoes might never feed on humans. When the infected person returns to town, he may introduce yellow fever virus into a cycle involving humans and the peridomestic mosquito *A. aegypti*, and an urban epidemic may result. Some viruses may come in contact with humans by another mechanism, the amplification cycle. These viruses have a basic cycle away from humans that involves arthropods that feed almost exclusively on animals. With seasonal build-up of populations of different arthropods and, let us say, birds, another cycle is started that carries the virus closer to humans and arthropods that are more likely to bite humans.

From time to time an arbovirus disease appears where it has been previously unknown. Dengue hemorrhagic fever of Southeast Asia, Kyasanur Forest disease in India, Chikungunya and O'nyong-nyong fevers in East Africa, and Rift Valley Fever in Egypt are all examples of new disease situations that have been recognized within the past 2 decades. Did O'nyong-nyong fever virus become more pathogenic for humans as a result of passage in anopheline mosquitoes? This is a possibility, since all other group A arboviruses (alphaviruses) are transmitted by culicenes. Was pick-up and transmission by a certain genus of tick responsible for human pathogenicity of Kyasanur Forest disease virus? It is difficult to prove that pathogenicity for humans may be enhanced by a change in the transmission cycle, but the question is of great importance, since we persist in meddling with our environment. The possibility that the clinical consequences of infection may be affected by sensitization from prior infection by a related virus has been raised to explain the hemorrhagic fever syndromes in the Philippines and Southeast Asia caused by dengue viruses. Before the 1950s, dengue virus was known only in connection with classic dengue, a relatively benign disease characterized by fever and nonhemorrhagic rash. Thus one disease may change as a result of a change in the ecology of another infection. Whatever the reasons prove to be, we are clearly in an unstable situation, with some surprises in the future. Additional expression of some basic concepts that help to explain the behavior of arboviruses can be found in the paper by Chamberlain.

Arboviruses cause disease and death in thousands of persons each year. From year to year and decade to decade, the epidemic potential results in wide swings in incidence in a given geographic area. In the United States, the number of known and reported cases of arboviral encephalitis varies from tens to thousands each year. In the 1960s, there was an epidemic of yellow fever in remote areas of Ethiopia that is believed to have killed 10,000 persons. Dengue hemorrhagic fever in the Philippines and Southeast Asia affects thousands each year, with substantial mortality. Laboratories must not be overlooked in a discussion of epidemiology. Human curiosity about arboviruses has resulted in more than 400 reported laboratory infections, of which 18 caused the deaths of investigators.

Disease in Humans

Arboviruses cause acute febrile illnesses that range from minimal severity to highly fatal diseases with devastating sequelae for the survivors. There are three general types of disease. One type is characterized by undifferentiated fever that may or may not be accompanied by rash and arthralgia (Table 22-1). In another type, there is viral invasion of the central nervous system, productive of an often severely damaging encephalitis (Table 22-2).

In the third category are those arboviruses that cause hemorrhagic fever, as in yellow fever, hemorrhagic dengue fever, and a number of tickborne hemorrhagic fevers. Hemorrhagic fevers (Table 22-3) are also caused by a number of arenaviruses and agents similar to rhabdoviruses. Additional material on this category of diseases is found in the appropriate chapters.

The pathogenetic mechanisms of arbovirus disease are only beginning to be understood. In some diseases direct tissue destruction occurs for unknown reasons. In others, such as dengue, an immunologically modulated pathologic process seems to occur. The conditions permitting this chain of events are briefly referred to in the section below on hemorrhagic dengue.

There follow brief descriptions of representatives of each of these categories, somewhat arbitrarily selected because they occur within the United States or because of their significance to the public health elsewhere.

Arboviruses that Cause Fevers, Rash, Arthralgia

Undifferentiated arbovirus fevers with or without rash and arthralgia are generally of low mortality, and recovery is complete with rare exceptions. Classic dengue fever is the prototype, and many of the other members of the group often are described as dengue-like. Members of the group that are transmitted in the United States include Colorado tick fever and vesicular stomatitis viruses.

Dengue fever is a disease of rapid onset, with the temperature rising suddenly to high levels and persisting for several days. Accompanying the fever are headache and aching in the muscles and joints. There is an associated macular rash that blanches with pressure; later in the disease it may become papular and morbilliform, sparing only the palms and soles. Lymphadenopathy is usually present. After 5 to 10 days, the acute symptoms disappear, but generalized weakness and lassitude may delay complete recovery for weeks. In the midst of the acute disease, there may be one or several days when manifestations of illness disappear. This provides the biphasic course that characterizes many arbovirus diseases. Leukopenia is the most striking and consistent laboratory abnormality. Etiologic diagnosis is confirmed by virus isolation from the blood or by the demonstration of a rise in serum antibody titer. Death is rare, and most patients recover completely. The disease occurs throughout the tropical world. Epidemics may be widespread, affecting a very high proportion of the population. Typically, the virus cycles between humans and *Aedes* mosquitoes, especially *A. aegypti.* In some areas (Malaysia and West Africa) there may be a jungle cycle involving primates.

O'nyong-nyong, Chickungunya, Mayaro, and *Ross River* are four related, mosquitoborne alphaviruses that cause dengue-like disease in Africa, southern Asia, South and Central America, and Australia.

Colorado tick fever is characterized by fever, headache, myalgia, and lethargy. Rash and central nervous system signs and symptoms occur less commonly. The rash is maculopapular, sometimes petechial, and does not have any particular distribution. A biphasic fever pattern occurs in about half of the cases. Disease begins approximately 5 days from tick bite and lasts for about a week, although malaise may continue for several more weeks, especially in the older patient. Approximately 20 percent of patients require hospitalization. Rarely, pericarditis or orchitis occurs; very rarely, a hemorrhagic syndrome with death has been reported. Diagnosis is confirmed by laboratory methods that detect antibodies in serum, infectious virus in blood, or viral antigen in erythrocytes. Curiously, infectious virus and/or viral antigens may be detected in the blood for up to several weeks after onset of disease. There are some reports of transmission by blood transfusion.

The disease is transmitted throughout the Rocky Mountain states from March to October, with peak incidence in May and June. During 1973 and 1974, active search revealed 228 cases in Colorado alone. The arthropod host is *Dermacentor andersoni.*

Arboviruses that Cause Encephalitis

The arthropodborne viral encephalitides are a group of serious illnesses that occur sporadically or in epidemic form throughout the tropical and subtropical world, except in Africa. Infected persons are at varying risk of death or severe central nervous system damage depending on their age and on the type of virus. In the United States since 1960, there have been an average of 300 arbovirus encephalitis cases reported to the Centers for Disease Control annually, ranging from a low of 45 in 1960 to a high of 2113 cases in 1975. In recent years, California and St. Louis encephalitis viruses account for most of these cases, followed by Western, Eastern, and Venezuelan equine encephalitis viruses, with Powassan virus making its appearance in human disease for the first time in single cases in 1971 and 1972. Rociovirus encephalitis emerged as an epidemic disease in southern Brazil in 1975.

In Britain, louping ill is a tick-transmitted encephalitis of sheep and humans. Central European and Russian spring–summer encephalitides are found in Europe and Russia, while Japanese encephalitis occurs in Japan, Asia, and the Pacific. Kyasanur Forest disease in India entails signs of central nervous system involvement, as well as abnormal bleeding, and is thus classified both as an encephalitis and a hemorrhagic fever. Murray Valley encephalitis is found in Australia.

Western equine encephalitis is an acute generalized illness characterized by fever, meningeal signs, somnolence, coma, convulsions, and paralysis. In infants and young children fatality is high, and permanent brain damage is common. The virus cycles in nature between a variety of small birds and the mosquito *Culex tarsalis.* Humans and equines are dead-end hosts because viremia adequate for mosquito infection does not occur. The overwintering mechanism is unknown. Diagnosis depends on demonstration of a rise in antibodies between acute and convalescent serum specimens. Virus isolation attempts from human tissue are rarely successful. The disease is confined to western North America, and it occurs in epidemic form in early and midsummer.

Eastern equine encephalitis is an acute generalized illness characterized by fever and central nervous system signs and symptoms, including those of meningeal irritation, lethargy, coma, pareses, and convulsions. Death is frequent, and in survivors residual central nervous system damage is common and severe. A striking polymorphonuclear leukocytosis occurs in blood and in cerebrospinal fluid. Etiologic diagnosis depends on virus isolation from brain tissue or the demonstration of an increase in serum antibody. Mosquitoborne epidemics and equine epizootics occur in late summer along the eastern strip of North America from Florida to Canada and the Caribbean.

California encephalitis is an acute febrile illness of 7 to 10 days' duration, characterized by headache, vomiting, lethargy, disorientation, seizures, and focal neurologic signs. Although convalescence may be prolonged, fatality and morbidity are low. The cerebrospinal fluid contains abnormally high protein and increased numbers of white blood cells during the acute phase. Etiologic diagnosis depends on demonstration of a rise of specific antibodies. The virus has been recovered from brain tissue from two fatal cases. It is a disease of children and occurs during summer months, principally in the north central United States. Mosquitoes of the genus *Aedes* transmit the virus to humans. Overwintering of the virus occurs by transovarial transmission in vector mosquitoes; the eggs survive the winter in tree holes. Vertebrate hosts include small animals.

St. Louis encephalitis is an acute febrile illness that occurs in a small percentage of those infected. It is usually characterized by fever and headache, tremors, and abnormalities of coordination and motor cranial nerve function. The disease is most common in older persons. Signs of urinary tract inflammation may occur. Fatality may reach 25 percent, and mental and emotional sequelae are common. Cerebrospinal fluid changes are consistent with virus infections. Diagnosis depends on demonstration of a serum antibody rise; virus isolation is rarely achieved from human specimens. The virus cycles between birds and *Culex* mosquitoes. Large urban and suburban outbreaks occur in the United States.

Powassan virus encephalitis has been identified as the cause of encephalitis in an occasional patient for the past 20 years in northern United States and Canada. While human infections are very uncommon, clinical consequences can be severe, with fever, headache, seizures, coma, and paralysis. Permanent neurologic damage may follow. Powassan virus is transmitted by ticks, although history of tick bite is frequently lacking.

Venezuelan equine encephalitis is characterized by fever, severe headaches, chills, and gastrointestinal symptoms. In a few children, serious encephalitis occurs, with convulsions, coma, paralysis, and abnormal reflexes. Myalgia, conjunctivitis, and sore throat commonly appear as the disease progresses. Leukopenia is typical. Diagnosis is suspected in patients who have been in appropriate geographic areas during epidemics. Demonstration of a rise in antibodies in serum samples obtained in the acute and convalescent stages of disease is necessary.

The disease occurs as equine epizootics in South and Central America, the Caribbean, Mexico, and southern United States. Strains of the virus that are responsible for endemic cases cycle in mosquitoes, small rodents, and birds. Epidemic strains cycle in equines and a variety of mosquitoes; it is this poorly understood amplification cycle that results in humans becoming infected. A live attenuated vaccine has been shown capable of immunizing humans and horses. While it may be too dangerous for widespread use in people, this vaccine can be applied on a mass basis to horses, with prompt cessation of both equine and human cases. Insecticides can be used concurrently.

Japanese B encephalitis is an acute illness that occurs in a small percentage of those infected with the virus. The usual consequence of infection is either inapparent or mild, undifferentiated disease. The encephalitis disease is similar to St. Louis encephalitis, with more severe neurologic involvement. Fatality is high, especially in young children and older persons. Diagnosis is confirmed serologically, and virus isolation from human specimens is unusual. The virus cycles annually between *Culex* mosquitoes and birds or pigs in temperate areas, including Japan, Siberia, Korea, Taiwan, Pacific islands, and in tropical areas of southeast Asia. Japanese encephalitis also produces disease in horses, and large epizootics are reported.

The tickborne flaviviruses comprise a group of related agents that are found, each in a circumscribed domain, in North America, Britain, Europe, Russia, and Asia. The most common ones are Powassan, Russian spring–summer, central European, and louping ill encephalitides, and Omsk hemorrhagic fever and Kyasanur Forest disease. The clinical spectrum includes hemorrhagic fever or encephalitis or a combination of the two. They are listed in both Tables 22-2 and 22-3. The diseases vary greatly in fatality and in the severity of permanent neurologic damage. Diagnosis is by virus isolation from blood or brain tissue and by serologic tests.

Arboviruses that Cause Hemorrhagic Fevers

The viral hemorrhagic fevers comprise 10 distinct diseases with widely differing epidemiologies and geographic loci. They are caused by viruses representing several taxonomic groups (Table 22-3). Some are mosquitoborne, others are tickborne, and the arthropod vectors of a third group are unknown or nonexistent. In addition to humans, vertebrate hosts generally include primates or small mammals or rodents. The diseases are severe, with high fatality, but are self-limited, and survivors usually recover completely. None of these diseases is transmitted within the United States, although recently, antibodies to Hantaan virus (hemorrhagic fever with renal syndrome) have been found in Norway rats in the United States.

Yellow fever and hemorrhagic dengue are described here, and others are described in Chapters 23 and 24.

Yellow Fever. In spite of the presence of a safe, effective, attenuated vaccine that has been available since the 1930s, yellow fever remains today a real or potential public health problem for many peoples of the tropical world. Clinically, the disease is marked by the sudden onset of fever associated with severe headache, myalgia, back pain, conjunctivitis, and photophobia. As the disease progresses, prostration increases, and there are signs of involvement of the liver, kidneys, and heart with hepatomegaly, albuminuria, and a striking slowing of the heart rate. A hypovolemic shock phase associated with bleeding gums, hematemesis, oliguria, and jaundice follows. Case fatality is high; recovery is complete. Diagnosis is confirmed by the isolation of the virus from the blood or from the liver or by demonstration of a specific serologic response.

The characteristic histopathology of midzonal necrosis in the liver lobule has given rise in some areas to an epidemiologic method wherein mandatory postmortem corings of the liver are obtained from all deaths and sent in fixative to a central examining point, thus permitting an assessment of the proportion of deaths that are due to yellow fever.

Yellow fever has two distinct cycles in nature. One is an *A. aegypti*–human cycle that is operative in the large urban epidemics that are now, fortunately, history in the new world and Europe. In parts of Africa, however, large epidemics with transmission by this vector still occur. The virus also cycles in the forest, involving monkeys and different genera of mosquitoes. The virus is carried from the forest cycle to the urban cycle by infected monkeys or humans. Transmission can be effectively interrupted, in the case of the urban cycle, by *A. aegypti* control measures. Such measures, used prior to the recognition of the sylvan cycle, rid the urban centers of the Western hemisphere of dreadful epidemics that affected cities as far north as Philadelphia into the first decade of the present century. These same measures permitted completion of the Panama Canal. They are however, less useful when one is dealing with zoophilic forest mosquitoes. As if in defiance of the best human effort, yellow fever epidemics occur today in areas where lack of basic logistical underpinnings of health services prevent vector control or immunization programs.

Hemorrhagic Dengue. This acute febrile illness begins abruptly like classic dengue with fever, nausea, vomiting, and cough. However, after a day or two, hemorrhagic manifestations appear, first as petechiae, followed by purpura and signs of gastrointestinal hemorrhage. The clinical picture of shock ensues. Hypoproteinemia, rising hematocrit, and hemostatic abnormalities, including thrombocytopenia, are present. During the next days the patient either dies or begins a complete recovery. Left untreated, fatality can be as high as 50 percent, but with proper medical management, the fatality rate is less than 3 percent. Diagnosis is confirmed by the demonstration of rise in antibodies or by isolation of virus from specimens of blood.

This hemorrhagic form of dengue was first seen in the 1950s in the Philippines and Southeast Asia and subsequently in India, Indonesia, and Oceania. In 1981, the disease appeared in this hemisphere in an outbreak in Cuba. Children comprise the vast majority of those affected.

Recently, substantial progress has been made in the development of data that support the hypothesis that dengue hemorrhagic fever/dengue shock syndrome (DHF/DSS) occurs in circumstances where circulating antibody to one dengue virus type from a prior infection changes the clinical expression of a second infection to include DHF/DSS. In this sequence, called "immune enhancement," antibody and virus form immune complexes that are phagocytized by monocytes. Virus multiplies within the monocyte, which in turn interacts with sensitized T cells. Factors are then released that activate a complement pathway, increase vascular permeability, and effect blood clotting systems. The resulting hypocomplementemia, thrombocytopenia with hemorrhage, and increased vascular permeability with hypovolemia and shock are the hallmarks of DHF/DSS. An impressive array of results from in vitro laboratory experiments and field epidemiologic observations support this hypothesis. The well-documented, although far less frequent, occurrences of DHF/DSS in association with primary dengue infection remain unexplained, however.

The usual vector is *A. aegypti,* as it is for classic dengue. Accordingly, the frequency of transmission is governed by climate and numerous domestic factors (such as those relating to collections of standing water) that affect breeding and feeding of this mosquito. Control measures entail all those measures that reduce the frequency of the vector mosquito feeding on potential patients. No vaccine is available.

Treatment, Control, and Prevention

There are no therapeutic agents that are specific for arboviruses. The management of patients with disease involves measures designed to restore and maintain nutrition and reasonably normal physiology. The latter might include, for example, restoration of intravascular volume during the hypovolemic shock phase of hemorrhagic fever or measures to reduce destructive degrees of cerebral edema in patients with encephalitis.

With the exception of the highly effective, safe, attenuated, tissue culture vaccine that has been in use since the 1930s for yellow fever, there are no arbovirus vaccines in general use.

Venezuelan equine virus vaccine has a restricted use for laboratory workers and can protect humans indirectly by preventing the development of a large reservoir of infected horses. Many experimental vaccines are under trial or laboratory development.

For arboviruses with limited host range and an accessible vector, there have been instances of effective prevention based on vector control. Urban yellow fever was eradicated in the early decades of this century by measures against *A. aegypti.* The task becomes infinitely more complex when one considers arboviruses that cycle silently in a variety of natural settings in birds, mammals, and arthropods. In these situations, where no ecologically acceptable vector control is available, the possibilities may be restricted to lessening human exposure to the ecosystem in question. Such a measure may fail because of anticipated and unacceptable consequences as, for example, might beset a woodcutter denied access to the forest.

FURTHER READING

Berge TO: International Catalogue of Arboviruses, 2nd ed. Dept. HEW, Washington, D.C., US Govt Printing Office, 1975. *See also* Karabatsos N (ed): Supplement to International Catalogue of Arboviruses Including Certain Other Viruses of Vertebrates. Am J Trop Med Hyg [Suppl] 27:372, 1978

Chamberlain RW: Arbovirology—then and now. Am J Trop Med Hyg 31:430, 1982

Halstead SB: The pathogenesis of dengue molecular epidemiology in infectious disease. Am J Epidemiol 114:632, 1981

Johnson KM, Monath TP, Tesh RB, et al.: Arthropod-borne viral fevers, viral encepalitides and viral hemorrhagic fevers (arboviruses and arenaviruses). In Wyngaarden JB, Smith LH (eds): Textbook of Medicine, 16th ed. Philadelphia, Saunders, 1979

Johnson KM: Nephropathia epidemica and Korean hemorrhagic fever: The veil lifted? J Infect Dis 141:135, 1980

Monath TP (ed): St. Louis Encephalitis. Washington, D.C., American Public Health Assoc, 1980

Morens DM: Dengue fever and dengue shock syndrome. Hosp Pract 17:103, 1982

Strode GK: Yellow Fever. New York, McGraw-Hill, 1951

Theiler M, Downs WG: The Arthropod-Borne Viruses of Vertebrates. New Haven, Yale University Press, 1973. *See also review of this book*: Work TH: Science 182:273, 1973

World Health Organization. Rift Valley Fever—An Emerging Human and Animal Problem. WHO Offset Publication #63. Geneva, WHO, 1982

Work TH, Monath TP, Gear JHS, et al.: Arbovirus infections and other zoonotic virus infections and diseases. In Feigin RD, Cherry JF (eds): Textbook of Pediatric Infectious Diseases. Philadelphia, Saunders, 1981, vol II

CHAPTER 23

Rhabdoviruses and Marburg and Ebola Viruses

A rabid racoon recently cost the State of South Carolina approximately $10,000 by coming in contact with at least 25 people.

— *USPHS, Centers for Disease Control Veterinary Public Health Notes, Feb. 1980, p. 1*

On May 10, 1980, a rabid dog in Yuba County, California, bit three persons. A total of 70 persons were identified as having been exposed to the dog and were given rabies vaccine. The total cost of the episode was $105,790.

— *USPHS, Centers for Disease Control MMWR 30:527, 1981*

There are more than 60 rhabdoviruses. Of these, 10 are known to cause disease in humans (Table 23-1). Two important agents, Marburg and Ebola, although previously so classified, possess distinctive physicochemical characteristics that may lead to the formation of a new group. Rabies, Marburg, and Ebola cause serious illnesses, often with very high fatality rates. Rabies is nearly 100 percent fatal, while for Marburg and Ebola, fatality rates ranging from 20 to 90 percent have been observed. Other members of the group, such as Isfahan virus, isolated in Iran in 1975, probably infect humans, as evidenced by a high prevalence of antibodies, but no disease has been observed. Rabies was the first rhabdovirus isolated, in the early years of this century, while the newest member of the group was isolated in the 1970s.

Transmission from human to human or animal to animal is clearly by arthropod with certain viruses, while others are transmitted mainly through animal-to-animal contact. For Marburg and Ebola, in addition to person-to-person transmission, humans probably acquire infection as a result of environmental contamination by chronically infected viruric rodents.

Serologic relationships and morphology define the subgroups of the Rhabdoviridae and individual members of subgroups. Arbovirologists often have been drawn into the study of rhabdoviruses either because of definite arthropod transmission or epidemiologic features that were initially highly suggestive of arthropodborne transmission. In addition, rhabdoviruses possess complex life cycles and transmission patterns, and these aspects in themselves attract the attention of medical scientists and clinicians whose interests are broadly based zoologically. Other than support of physiologic processes in the sick individual, the only protection that humans and animals have from rhabdoviruses is natural or induced immunity and environmental manipulations based on an understanding of the zoonotic details of the life cycles.

In this chapter, attention will be paid only to those agents known to cause human disease: rabies, Marburg, Ebola, and certain members of the vesicular stomatitis group.

Rabies

Rabies has been recognized for centuries. In the late 1800s, Pasteur sorted out the confusion concerning the etiologic agent and pathogenesis of the disease. He then crowned these extraordinary achievements with the development of a method of active immunization, which, although never tested in a controlled trial in humans, is generally believed to have been effective. Today, rabies

TABLE 23-1. RHABDOVIRUSES AND SIMILAR AGENTS THAT CAUSE ILLNESS IN HUMANS

Virus				
Group	Serotype	Year of Original Isolation	Natural Geographic Distribution	Disease in Humans
Rabies	Rabies	1903	Worldwide	Meningoencephalitis
	Mokola	1968	Africa	Meningoencephalitis
	Duvenhage	1971	Africa	Meningoencephalitis
Marburg	Marburg	1967	Africa	Hemorrhagic fever
	Ebola	1976	Africa	Hemorrhagic fever
Vesicular stomatitis	Indiana	1925	Western hemisphere	Fever and vesicles
	New Jersey	1952	Western hemisphere	Fever and vesicles
	Alagoas	1964	Western hemisphere	Fever
	Piry	1960	Western hemisphere	Fever
	Chandipura	1965	Asia and Africa	Fever

continues to frighten human beings, and it poses a distinct and usually fatal hazard to them as well as to their domestic animals. In the 1960s the physical and chemical properties and the morphology of the rabies virus were established. Markedly improved vaccines were developed in the late 1970s.

Epidemiology

Rabies virus persists in nature by passage from animal to animal, usually during direct contact. Adequate contact generally requires that virus-containing saliva be inoculated through broken skin by bite or scratch into a susceptible animal. The infected animal's illness alters behavior in favor of transmission by making the animal deranged and aggressive and thus more likely to attack or bite more frequently and to less purpose than normally. The timing and duration of virus excretion in saliva of infected animals vary dramatically according to species of the infected animal, strain of virus, and dose of virus inoculated. For dogs, virus in the saliva has been documented as long as 2 weeks prior to onset of disease, although a few days appears to be a more probable period. Infected, unvaccinated dogs have been observed to excrete virus intermittently for months in the absence of disease. How frequently this occurs, however, is not known.

In some situations rabies virus may be transmitted by aerosol. Such situations occur in caves that contain large populations of insectivorous bats. At certain times of the year, when bats are being born and are developing and when their mothers are lactating, sufficient quantities of rabies virus may be present in the air of the cave to infect susceptible animals placed in such a fashion as to be exposed only to cave air. Beyond such observations as these, however, the ecology of bat cave rabies is poorly understood.

Some biologic determinants of transmission include the following. The saliva must contain an adequate titer of virus. In this connection, infected skunks have been found to develop the highest titers. The bitten animal must be of a susceptible species. In the laboratory, the route of inoculation is important, with intracerebral being among the most sensitive routes, whereas intraperitoneal injection is less likely to transmit infection. Transmission transplacentally or via the gastrointestinal tract by drinking milk of infected animals or by arthropod vector does not seem to occur to any significant degree in nature. The age of the receiving animal can be important; generally, the younger the animal, the more susceptible.

The site of the inoculation is clearly important. In humans, bites about the head and neck are likely to result in disease earlier than are bites at areas more peripheral to the central nervous system. This is thought to be because there is a greater density of nerve endings about the head and face, providing more neurologic pathways for the virus to travel to the central nervous system. In addition, the distance to the brain is shorter from the head and neck area.

Virus multiplies first in muscle tissue at the site of inoculation. Thereafter virus enters peripheral nerves and progresses, probably passively, in the axoplasm to the spinal cord and then to the brain. Virus spreads rapidly throughout the brain. Disease ensues after a variable incubation period, which is not explained solely by the time it takes the virus to migrate from peripheral inoculation site to brain.

Virus also migrates toward the periphery from the brain, reaching such sites as skin and cornea, where it may be detected by immunofluorescent techniques.

Sources of infection for humans and their economically important domestic animals vary to some extent geographically. For example, in North America, foxes, skunks, racoons, cattle, dogs, cats, and bats are the usual reservoir and vector hosts. In Latin America, bats of various species seem to be the most important, while in the Mediterranean area the wolf, in India the jackal, and in certain Caribbean areas, such as Cuba, Puerto Rico, and Granada, the mongoose is the most significant reservoir/vector animal.

Bat rabies may be transmitted in two ways. In South America, vampire bats transmit rabies to domestic cattle while taking their blood meal. This results in enormous economic and nutritional losses to people in these areas. As mentioned above, aerosol transmission can occur in some insectivorous cave-dwelling bats of North America. Presumably this mechanism, as well as transmission by bite, can be operative in vampire populations.

The epizootic and enzootic behavior of rabies in domestic and wild animals may display swings of incidence in one or another species and from one place to another that are often poorly understood. For example, in the United States during the past few years there has been a sharp increase in rabies in domestic cattle and wild racoons.

Spread of animal rabies into a geographic area typically involves but one species. Evidence that strains of wild rabies may differ in their pathogenicity for one species as compared to others may explain such epizootic behavior.

Density of susceptible and infected animal populations, the biology of the virus in the infected host, the degree to which rabies can become latent, and factors that influence aggressive behavior, other than the rabies infection itself, all require further understanding before the determinants of rabies transmission are completely elucidated.

Serologic surveys for the purpose of detecting rabies antibodies indicative of nonfatal, past infection has not been helpful in rabies because no adequately sensitive, specific, and inexpensive test is available. Accordingly, the question of whether latent or clinically silent infections are epidemiologically significant is not yet answered.

There is seasonal variation in rabies in animals as well as humans. In animals the greatest number of cases occur in the spring and early summer during the breeding season. In humans, most cases occur in the summer, possibly as a result of more outdoor contact with rabid animals.

In the 1970s two viruses, Mokola and Duvenhage, were found in Africa that are morphologically and serologically related to rabies. For each agent there is at least one reported case of fatal central nervous system disease.

Disease in Humans

Generally, disease begins within 2 to 8 weeks of exposure, with extremes of the incubation period ranging from 9 days to more than a year, and even many years in very rare instances (Fig. 23-1). Early symptoms include loss of appetite, nausea, vomiting, and fever associated with feeling poorly, pain, and paresthesias at the site of the bite. Anxiety, depression, and agitation ensue. As the disease progresses, spasms begin to occur. When they involve the muscles of deglutition, the inability to drink liquids or to swallow one's own saliva properly gives rise to the picture of hydrophobia. Soon, a wide variety of central nervous system signs appear, including hyperactivity, confusion, delirium, hallucinations, disorders of coordination, and paralyses. Finally, coma develops, and by this time secondary infection, nutritional deficiencies, and respiratory problems bring on death.

Recovery from rabies is considered to be extremely rare. There is one definite, well-documented case of recovery reported in the literature.

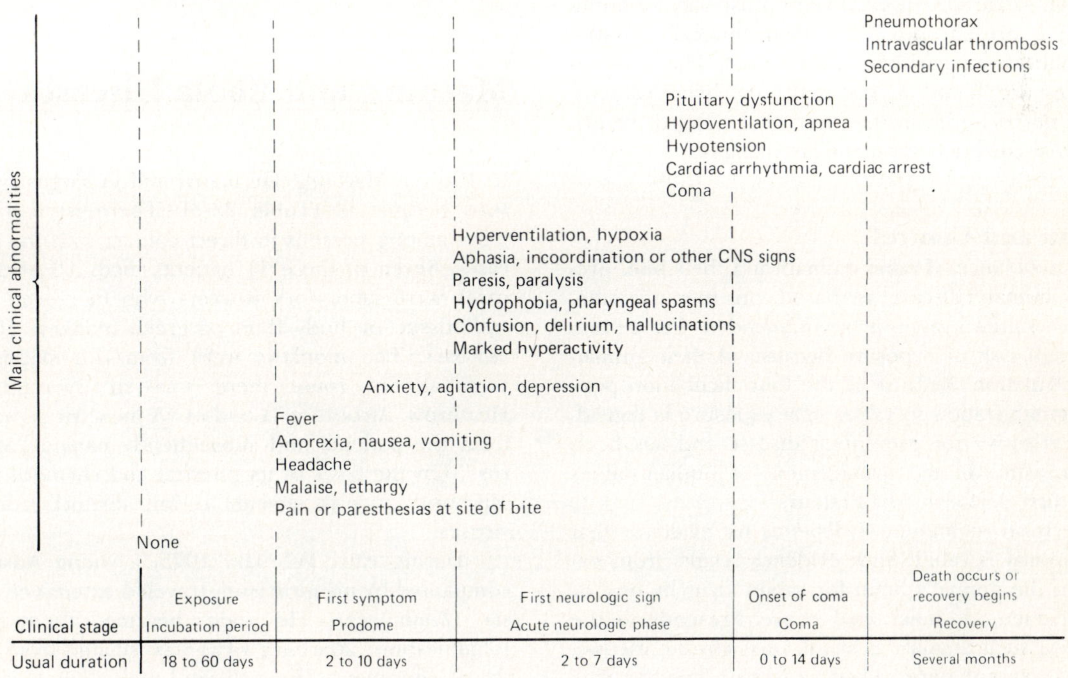

Figure 23-1. The natural history of clinical rabies in humans; hypothetical composite case. All clinical abnormalities need not be present in each case. *(From Hatwick, Gregg: In Baer (ed): The Natural History of Rabies. New York, Academic Press, 1975, vol 2, p 289.)*

Laboratory findings include an elevated white cell count of 20 to 30 thousand cells per cu mm associated with an increased percentage of polymorphonuclear leukocytes. Cerebrospinal fluid is usually normal, but a mild pleocytosis may be observed consisting of less than 100 mononuclear cells per cu mm. Protein, sugar, and hyaline casts may be seen in the urinary sediment.

The clinical features described above following a bite by a rabid animal are the major criteria for diagnosis. Virus isolation attempts from saliva, cerebrospinal fluid, tears, urine, and nasopharyngeal secretions may be successful, but they are meaningless if negative. Fluorescent antibody staining of smears of corneal epithelial cells or of sections of skin from face or neck may reveal virus antemortem after disease has begun. A rise in serum antibodies is generally not detectable by the time the patient dies. Following death, virus can be demonstrated in the central nervous system by one or more of the three methods used to detect rabies virus in animal brain specimens. One method, the most rapid, involves the detection of intracellular rabies virus antigen by the use of fluorescent antibody. A second method is the identification of typical intracytoplasmic, eosinophilic inclusions (Negri bodies, see Color Plate) in nerve cells in certain areas of the central nervous system. Third, intracerebral inoculation of mice with suspensions of brain tissue is followed by identification of rabies virus in brain tissue after a suitable period of time for virus multiplication to occur.

The principal pathologic finding in rabies is inflammatory necrosis that chiefly involves the brain. Grossly, the brain is swollen and congested. Microscopically, nerve cells are seen to be destroyed, and perivascular, mononuclear cuffing is present in addition to meningeal mononuclear cell infiltrates. Negri bodies are found. The most severe changes are found in the thalamus, hypothalamus, and cranial nerve nuclei in the floor of the fourth ventricle. The spinal cord may show similar changes.

Prevention and Control

Other than avoidance of rabid animals and their bite, prevention of human disease is based on immunization. Preexposure immunization is recommended for certain people at high risk of exposure because of their animal-handling occupation. Because of the long incubation period, active immunization to rabies *after* exposure is considered to be effective for preventing disease and has been the basic measure in the management of human rabies since it was first performed by Pasteur.

The decision to immunize depends on evidence that the biting animal is rabid. Such evidence results from examination of the animal's brain for rabies virus by one or more of the methods mentioned above. Presently in the United States, such animals as skunk, fox, coyote, racoon, or bat that carry out unprovoked attacks on humans may be presumed rabid.

Effective vaccines for human use both pre- and postexposure are available. These modern vaccines are prepared from the strain of virus originally isolated by Pasteur in 1882. Virus is grown in cell cultures derived from human embryo lung. Physical, chemical, and immunologic studies of rabies virus reveal that the glycoprotein found in the form of spikes in the viral envelope stimulates neutralizing and protective antibody. Based on this work of the 1960s and 1970s, a number of vaccines employing either whole virion or glycoprotein split product are now in use. Antiserum derived from hyperimmunized people is used concurrently with vaccine in certain clinical situations. Details of active and passive rabies immunization procedures for animals and humans are constantly changing as products exhibiting fewer undesirable side effects and better antigenicity are developed. Groups, such as the Advisory Committee on Immunization Practices of the U.S. Public Health Service, publish their recommendations periodically in the Morbidity and Mortality Weekly Report of the Centers for Disease Control.

The control of rabies is considerably more difficult in wild animals than in domestic animals and humans. Human rabies in the United States has decreased to less than 3 cases per year for the past 19 years. Dog rabies has decreased from 8000 cases in 1947 to 216 in 1981 as a result of immunization practices. On the other hand, thousands of cases of wild animal rabies continue to be recognized. Measures for control of wild animals rabies include quarantine or slaughter. More recently, some innovative work employing baited food with live virus vaccine designed to attract specific species, such as foxes, is being tried in certain parts of the world. The Morbidity and Mortality Weekly Report should be consulted for the latest status reports and recommendations for control of animal rabies.

Marburg and Ebola Diseases

In 1967 in Marburg, Germany, and in Yugoslavia, 25 persons became ill (Table 22-3). There were 6 secondary cases among persons in direct contact with the primary 25 cases. Seven of these 31 patients died. All of the primary cases were laboratory workers who had been in contact with tissue or body fluid of green monkeys (*Cercapithicus aethiops*). The monkeys were from two shipments from Uganda. On route there was an overnight stay at Heathrow Airport in London. A new virus was isolated from the patients and subsequently named "Marburg virus." On the basis of its physical and chemical properties, Marburg virus is similar to but distinct from rhabdoviruses.

During early February 1975, a young Australian, accompanied by his girlfriend, traveled extensively in Rhodesia (Zimbabwe). He then became ill and died in Johannesburg. Marburg virus was isolated from blood and throat specimens. His girlfriend and a nurse who assisted her in caring for him during his fatal illness suffered a similar illness but recovered. Intensive epidemiologic investigations have failed to reveal the source of their infections.

Between August and November 1976, in two towns

COLOR PLATE

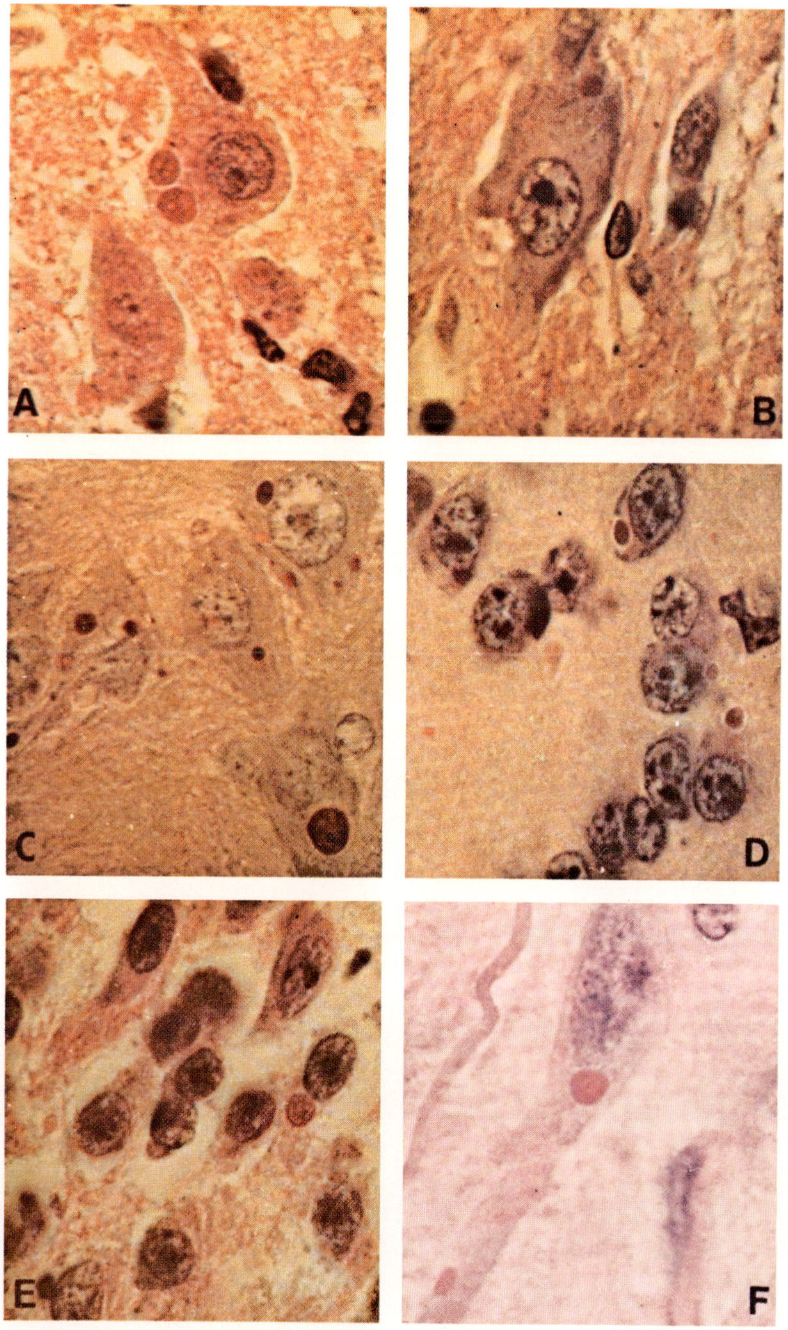

Negri bodies are shown here as the round eosinophilic cytoplasmic inclusions in brain cells from a variety of animals. **A,** Human; **B,** Cat; **C,** Dog; **D,** Mouse; **E,** Bovine; **F,** Fox. All sections are magnified approximately 1000–1400 ×. *(From Atanasiu P, Sisman J: In Baer GM (ed): The Natural History of Rabies, Vol 1. New York, Academic Press, 1975, p 374.)*

600 miles apart, one in southern Sudan and the other in northeastern Zaire, hundreds of persons became ill, and most died. From these patients a virus was isolated that was found to be antigenically distinct from but morphologically identical to Marburg virus. This agent was named "Ebola virus," for the river that runs near the location of the outbreak in Zaire. In Zaire, except for the index case, all 235 cases were linked by intimate contact or by syringes and needles used for medicinal purposes. Of these cases, 201 died, including all of those infected by syringe and needle transfer. Ebola hemorrhagic fever was again seen in Zaire in 1977–1978.

Thus, Marburg and Ebola viruses have struck at humans only occasionally but always with devastating effect. While the method of spread within a given outbreak has become evident quickly, the natural life cycle and the source of the infection for the index cases remain a mystery except in the original outbreak involving green monkeys from Uganda. But even in that instance, the epidemiologic determinants of the monkey infection are not at all clear. Investigations in Uganda failed to reveal serologic evidence in the monkeys at the time of the Marburg outbreak. Moreover, the nearly universal mortality in this species makes it unlikely that monkeys serve as reservoir hosts in a maintenance cycle. Thousands of green monkeys shipped from Uganda during the years before the Marburg incident were apparently not infected. As one prominent worker in this field has stated, "The green monkey is a red herring."

Exhaustive studies of the 1975 Rhodesian cases provide evidence suggestive of arthropod transmission of infection to the index case, but no proof could be obtained. Similarly, the sources of infection in the index cases of the two simultaneous 1976 outbreaks are unknown. Serologic surveys show that between 1 and 20 percent of persons, depending on the geographic area surveyed, may show antibodies, and it is thus likely that considerable human transmission occurs in clinical silence. Beyond that, however, routes of transmission, reservoir hosts, and all of the other facts that permit rational defense are totally lacking. Recently, Ebola antibodies were found in domesticated guinea pigs living in village huts in Zaire. The source of the infection remains a mystery.

Transmission routes within outbreaks, however, are much better understood. Close personal contact during acute illness clearly results in transmission. Handling of secretions, tissues, and body fluids from acutely ill patients is another source. In several instances, venereal transmission has occurred through infected semen long after the acute disease. In Zaire, improper use of syringes and needles spread the infection nosocomially in a uniformly fatal manner among hundreds of persons.

Clinically, Marburg/Ebola disease begins with fever, headache, nausea, vomiting, myalgia, and diarrhea. After a few days, sore throat, conjunctivitis, abdominal pain, and rash appear. The rash is fine and maculopapular and may appear initially in relation to hair follicles. It begins either on the trunk or limbs, spreading thereafter to involve both. After 5 to 7 days, severe bleeding begins, involving chiefly the gastrointestinal tract. Shock and death often follow soon thereafter.

Laboratory findings include leukopenia, thrombocytopenia, and often the findings of disseminated intravascular coagulation. Proteinuria and markedly elevated serum amylase and transaminases are also found.

The major pathologic finding is focal hepatocellular necrosis. Eosinophilic cytoplasmic inclusions are seen, and on electron microscopy numerous virus particles are seen in the liver.

Diagnosis rests on isolation of virus in Vero cell cultures or guinea pigs from blood or oropharyngeal secretions from acute-phase specimens. After approximately 2 weeks, serum antibodies may be best detected by fluorescent antibody and various other techniques.

Case fatality approaches 100 percent under some circumstances, but this has been held to 20 percent when first class intensive care facilities are available. The roles of heparin to combat intravascular coagulation, specific antibody-containing plasma, and interferon in the treatment of the acute disease are not fully defined, but all have been used.

Index cases cannot be prevented for lack of knowledge. Secondary cases resulting from person-to-person contact or the handling of patient's secretions or tissues can be controlled by rigorous isolation and protective practices. Laboratory work on Marburg viruses must be confined to maximum containment laboratories, such as the facility at the Centers for Disease Control in Atlanta.

Vesicular Stomatitis Virus

The vesicular stomatitis virus (VSV) group is generally considered to comprise seven serologically related but distinct viruses; they are the Indiana, New Jersey, Cocal, Alagoas, Piry, Chandipura, and Isfahan strains of VSV. The first of these was isolated in 1925 and the latest in 1975. All but two have been found solely in the western hemisphere, while the remainder have been found in Africa, Asia, and Iran.

As a group, the vesicular stomatitis viruses have been found in nature in a variety of animals ranging from insects to humans. Evidence for arthropod-borne transmission includes the fact that VSV has often been isolated from naturally infected insects, including sandflies, mites, blackflies, and mosquitoes. With some serotypes, insect transmission has been achieved experimentally. For other serotypes, the above information is lacking. In addition, the seasonal pattern of transmission of some of these agents strongly suggests arthropod vectors.

The disease, vesicular stomatitis, is most frequently seen in cattle, pigs, and horses, where it occurs in outbreaks of illness associated with vesicular lesions in the mouth and elsewhere on the body. Lesions may also be seen on the feet, thus mimicking foot-and-mouth disease, a much more severe condition. Although three quarters of a herd may become ill, fatality is less than 5 percent. Transmission among domestic animals seems to require contact with very sharply circumscribed pasture areas, epidemiologic conditions that are difficult to explain on the basis of arthropod transmission.

The disease in humans is an acute, self-limited, benign, febrile illness associated with general malaise, myalgia, nausea and vomiting, and headache. No deaths have been reported. In some instances, vesicles may be seen on the gums and buccal and pharyngeal mucosa. Herpes-like lesions on the lips may also be seen. Illness is generally of less than a week's duration. Many laboratory infections have occurred, and the illnesses resulting from these infections seem to be identical to those occurring as a result of natural transmission.

In the United States, small outbreaks have been detected wherein direct transmission from animal to human is the most probable route of infection. Several serologic surveys in a variety of populations throughout the world suggest that infections with these viruses may be quite widespread. No serious public health problem, however, in the form of human disease at least, has seemed to occur as a result of these widespread infections. Because of the nonspecific nature of the illness, it is possible that many cases of human disease go undetected.

No characteristic clinical laboratory or histopathologic features have been recognized. Diagnosis depends on the clinical picture and the knowledge of close contact with diseased animals. Specific, complement-fixing, and neutralizing antibodies are detectable approximately 2 weeks after the onset of illness.

Except for avoidance of contact with diseased domestic animals, no preventive measures are known. No specific treatment of the sick individual is available.

FURTHER READING

RABIES

Centers for Disease Control, U.S. Public Health Service: Morbidity and Mortality Weekly Report:
- Rabies—United States, 1980. 30:147, 1981
- Rabies prevention (ACIP). 29:265, 1980
- Supplementary statement on rabies vaccine and serologic testing (ACIP). 30:535, 1981
- Supplementary statement on pre-exposure rabies prophylaxis by the intradermal route. 31:279, 1982
- Rabies in racoons—Virginia. 30:354, 1981
- Compendium of animal rabies vaccines, 1983. 31:685, 1982

Familusi JB, Osunkoya BO, et al.: A fatal human infection with Mokola virus. Am J Trop Med Hyg 21:959, 1972

Fekadu M, Shaddock JH, Baer GM: Excretion of rabies virus in the saliva of dogs. J Infect Dis 145:715, 1982

Hattwick MAW, et al.: Recovery from rabies: A case report. Ann Intern Med 76:931, 1972

Meredith CD: An unusual case of human rabies thought to be of Chiropteran origin. South Afr Med J 45:767, 1971 (Note: This virus is known as Duvenhage.)

Mertz GJ, Nelson KE, Vithayasai V, et al.: Antibody responses to human diploid cell vaccine for rabies with and without human rabies immune globulin. J Infect Dis 145:720, 1982

Plotkin SA: Rabies vaccine prepared in human cell cultures: Progress and perspective. Rev Infect Dis 2:433, 1980

Shope RE: Rabies. In Evans AS (ed): Viral Infections of Humans, Epidemiology and Control. New York, Plenum, 1976

Shope RE, Baer G, Allen WP: Summary of workshop on the immunopathology of rabies. J Infect Dis 140:431, 1979

Sikes RK: Rabies. In Hubbert WT, et al. (eds): Diseases Transmitted from Animals to Man, 6th ed. Springfield, Ill., Thomas, 1975

Steele JH: The epidemiology and control of rabies. Scand J Infect Dis 5:299, 1973

MARBURG AND EBOLA VIRUS DISEASE

Centers for Disease Control, U.S. Public Health Service: Marburg Virus Disease, Kenya. Morbidity and Mortality Weekly Report 29:145, 1980

Conrad LT, et al.: Epidemiologic investigation of Marburg virus disease, Southern Africa, 1975. Am J Trop Med Hyg 27:1210, 1978

Editorial: After Marburg, Ebola. . . . Lancet 1:581, 1977

Editorial: Ebola virus infection. Br Med J 1:539, 1977

Esmond RTD, et al.: A case of Ebola virus infection. Br Med J 1:541, 1977

Gear JSS, et al.: Outbreak of Marburg virus disease in Johannesburg. Br Med J 4:489, 1975

Heymann DL, Weisfeld JS, Webb PA, et al.: Ebola hemorrhagic fever: Tandala Zaire, 1977–1978. J Infect Dis 142:372, 1980

Johnson KM, et al.: Isolation and partial characterization of a new virus causing acute hemorrhagic fever in Zaire. Lancet 1:569, 1977

Johnson KM, Scribner CL, McCormick JB: Etiology of Ebola virus: A first clue. J Infect Dis 143:749, 1981

Kissling RE: Marburg virus. In Hubbert WT, et al. (eds): Diseases Transmitted from Animals to Man, 6th ed. Springfield Ill., Thomas, 1975

Pattyn SR (ed): Ebola Virus Hemorrhagic Fever. Amsterdam, Elsevier, 1978

Regnery RL, Johnson KM, Kiley MP: Marburg and Ebola viruses: Possible members of a new group of negative strand viruses. In Bishop DHL, Compans RW (eds): The Replication of Negative Strand Viruses. Amsterdam, Elsevier/North Holland, 1981, p 971

VESICULAR STOMATITIS VIRUS DISEASES

Bhatt PN, Rodrigues FM: Chandipura: A new arbovirus isolated in India from patients with febrile illness. Indian J Med Res 5:1295, 1967

Fields BN, Hawkins K: Human infection with the virus of vesicular stomatitis during an epizootic. N Engl J Med 277:989, 1967

Tesh RB, Johnson KM: Vesicular stomatitis. In Hubbert WT, et al. (eds): Diseases Transmitted from Animals to Man, 6th ed. Springfield, Ill., Thomas, 1975, chap 73

Tesh RB, Saidi S, Javadian E, et al.: Isfahan virus, a new vesiculovirus infecting humans, gerbils and sandflies in Iran. Am J Trop Med Hyg 26:299, 1977

Watson WA: Vesicular diseases: Recent advances and concepts of control. Can Vet J 22:311, 1981

CHAPTER 24

Arenaviruses

Human Diseases
Lymphocytic Choriomeningitis
Hemorrhagic Fevers

Junin Virus in Argentina
Machupo Virus in Bolivia
Lassa Fever in West Africa

. . . the most spectacular outbreaks in Africa (in the 1970s) were of Lassa fever and African hemorrhagic fever.

—*RW Chamberlain: Am J Trop Med and Hyg 31:434, 1982*

Arenaviruses have in common a similar morphology, related antigens, and the capacity to cause chronic infections in rodents. Three of them—Junin, Machupo, and Lassa—can cause serious, highly fatal, hemorrhagic fever in humans; one—lymphocytic choriomeningitis (LCM)—causes a sporadic, relatively benign meningoencephalitis. The arenaviruses are listed in Tables 2-4, 22-3, and 24-1, together with some of their clinical and epidemiologic features. LCM virus is found worldwide. Other arenaviruses are found in the Americas and in Africa, as shown in Figures 24-1 and 24-2. Perhaps the most impressive feature of arenaviruses is their capacity to surprise us. Lassa fever outbreaks warned us in the 1970s, as Machupo and Junin did in the 1960s, of the dire consequences of our ignorance and of our constant meddling with the balance of nature.

Arenaviruses establish chronic infections in a variety of laboratory and wild rodent species. When the young animal is inoculated perinatally, a chronic, lifetime infection can result, with continuous viremia, as well as high titer viruria. It is this sort of rodent infection that is of great importance in the perpetuation of the virus in nature, as well as the main source of human infection. Inoculation of normal adult rodents, on the other hand, may cause severe, acute, often fatal disease. By varying such factors as dose, route of inoculation, strain, and age of animal, intermediate results may be produced with, for example, chronic immune complex disease being the result of the infection.

The virologic and immunologic events characterizing these three types of host response (acute disease, asymptomatic carrier state, and chronic immune complex disease) have been extensively studied for LCM virus with development of knowledge that, in many particulars, is applicable to an understanding of the pathogenesis of viral disease in general. The most striking result of these studies is the fact that both the acute and chronic forms of disease are the result of immunopathologic processes.

The events depicted in Figure 24-3 occur in the acute disease situation. It has been demonstrated repeatedly by a variety of techniques, that compromise of the infected animal's immune system results in less severe disease. Subsequent studies showed that the acute disease is mediated by specifically oriented cytotoxic T cells. Furthermore, the capacity of such T cells to damage infected cells requires, in addition to viral antigen at the cell surface, an appropriate histocompatibility complex. This additional requirement is known as the "H-2 restriction" phenomenon and was described first with LCM virus infection. The roles of interferon, natural killer cells, the increase in number and changes in morphology of macrophages, the B cell activation and immunoglobulin production in the outcome of acute disease are not clearly understood.

In the chronic disease situation, humoral antibody is produced but is not detectable unless one searches for it in immune complexes that are deposited in certain tissues, such as glomeruli. The chronic disease is a progressive glomerulonephritis and arteritis resulting from the deposited immunocomplexes. Antibody production also occurs in asymptomatic carrier animals. Due to complex formation, this antibody is not detectable by older, conventional methods, and it was thought formerly that such animals were immunologically tolerant to their LCM virus infection. The situation in chronic disease and in the carrier state with regard to T cell activation and function is not clear.

Transmission by arthropods has been demonstrated

TABLE 24-1. ARENAVIRUSES

Virus	Date and Source of Specimen Yielding Initial Isolate			Disease in Humans
Lymphocytic choriomeningitis	1934	United States	Humans	Meningoencephalitis
Tacaribe	1956	Trinidad	Bats	None
Junin	1958	Argentina	Humans	Hemorrhagic fever
Machupo	1963	Bolivia	Humans	Hemorrhagic fever
Amapari	1964	Brazil	Rodent	None
Latino	1965	Bolivia	Rodent	None
Parana	1965	Paraguay	Rodent	None
Pichinde	1965	Columbia	Rodent	None
Tamiami	1965	United States	Rodent	None
Lassa	1969	Nigeria	Humans	Hemorrhagic fever
Mozambique	1977	Mozambique	Rodent	None

experimentally for one of these agents (Junin), but such transmission does not seem to be of importance in nature.

Human Diseases

When a person is infected, one of a spectrum of consequences ensues. On the one hand, no clinical disease appears, with infection detectable only by a rise in titer of serum antibody. On the other hand, virulent disease with a 25 percent fatality rate may result. In many instances during the acute stages of infection, virus may be isolated readily from a variety of body fluids or tissues by the use of laboratory rodents or cell cultures.

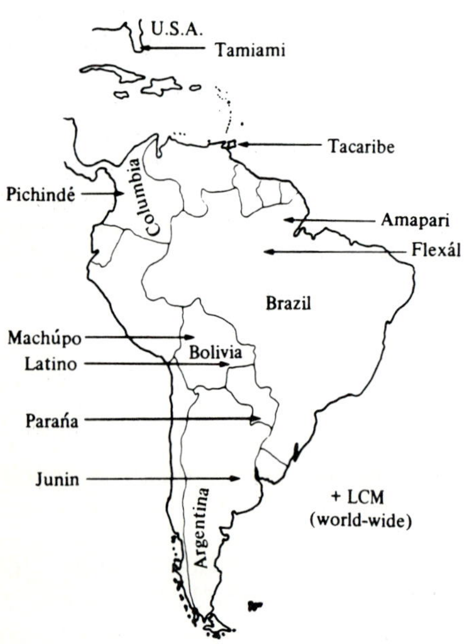

Figure 24-1. Geographic locations of arenavirus isolates in the New World. All viruses with the exception of LCM virus are serologically defined as being members of the Tacaribe complex. *(From Howard and Simpson: J Gen Virol 51:1, 1980.)*

Lymphocytic Choriomeningitis

LCM virus was isolated initially in the 1930s from patients with acute aseptic meningitis. From the very beginning, it has been recognized that LCM virus causes but a fraction of a percent of the overall number of these cases.

In nature the virus is found in house mice, where, as a result of natural perinatal inoculation, chronic infection with no clinical manifestations is established in a high proportion of animals. Contact with mice or their excreta brings the virus to humans; a dead end for the virus, as person-to-person or person-to-animal spread does not seem to occur. Captive Syrian hamsters have been found to be a source of human infection. There have been sizable outbreaks in laboratory personnel who have been in contact with infected hamsters that were being used in cancer research. In one instance, the infected hamsters were widely dispersed to many cancer laboratories from a single provider's colony.

Disease begins with fever, headache, myalgia, and malaise. Conjunctival infection and cough may be present. Within a few days the disease may subside, with rapid return of well-being. In some, however, it may worsen, with the addition of confusion and somnolence. Stiff neck, vomiting, and marked increase in the severity of the headache may become prominent. Gross disorientation may be a feature. Physical examination reveals fever and meningeal and encephalitic signs. Children tend to have less severe disease than adults.

The total and differential white blood counts are often normal, as is the urine. Cerebrospinal fluid, especially from those persons showing a meningeal or encephalitic clinical picture, is generally under abnormally high pressure, with an elevated number of lymphocytes and increased protein concentration. Low spinal fluid sugar is often found.

The disease is rarely, if ever, fatal, and it generally subsides after a few days so that the acute febrile stage of the illness is usually over within 7 to 14 days. In older and more severely affected patients, convalescence may be prolonged.

Clinically, there is often little to suggest LCM viral eti-

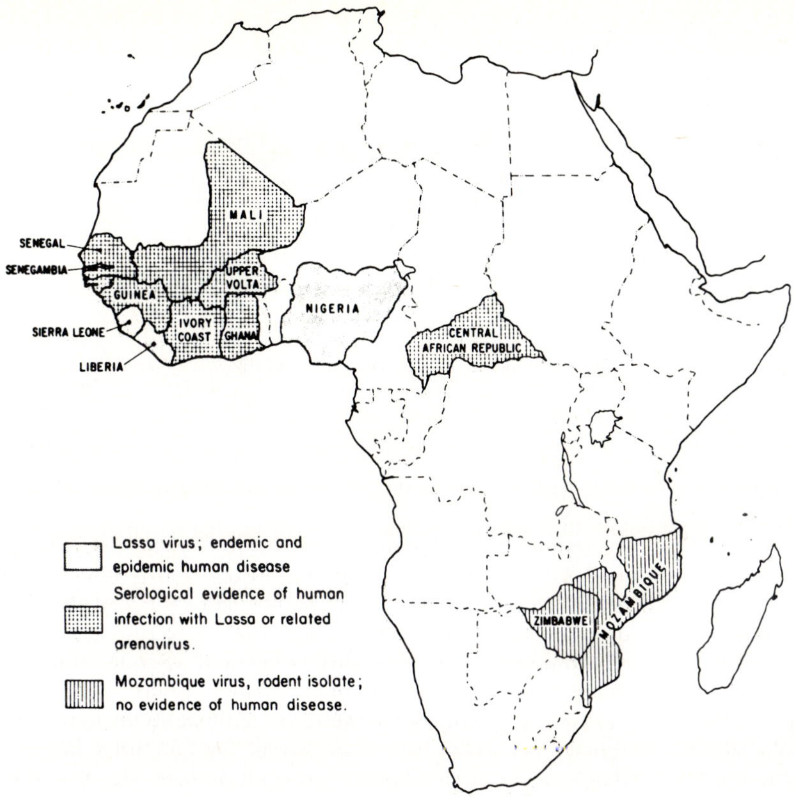

Figure 24-2. Geographic distribution of Lassa and Mozambique viruses in Africa. *(Courtesy of Dr. P. Monath.)*

ology as being any more probable than many of the far more usual causes of viral meningitis, such as enteroviruses. Diagnosis is made by isolation of virus and/or demonstration of high titer, complement-fixing antibodies

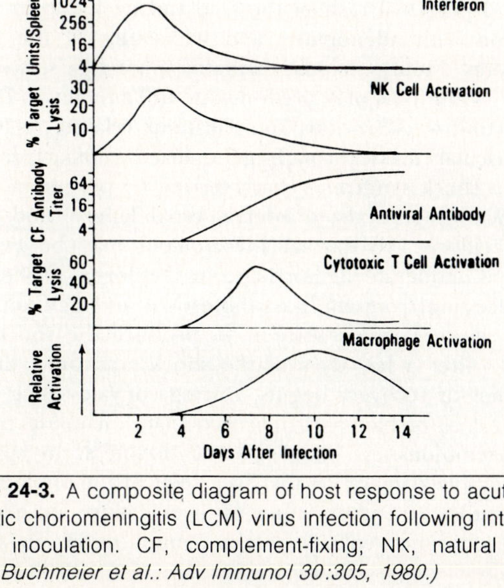

Figure 24-3. A composite diagram of host response to acute lymphocytic choriomeningitis (LCM) virus infection following intraperitoneal inoculation. CF, complement-fixing; NK, natural killer. *(From Buchmeier et al.: Adv Immunol 30:305, 1980.)*

in serum obtained during the acute disease or by a rise in titer between samples obtained early in the acute stages and again in convalescence. Adult white mice from colonies known to be free of LCM virus are the medium of choice for isolation. Following intracerebral inoculation, the mice become ill at about 10 days, at which time antigen can be detected in brain tissue by immunofluorescent techniques.

Human deaths are very rare. Consequently, the pathology of LCM infection must be inferred from that observed in experimental animals, such as mice and monkeys, where lymphocytic infiltrates of the meninges and choroid plexus are prominent features from which the name of the virus is derived.

Treatment is supportive; there are no specific measures available.

Hemorrhagic Fevers

Argentinian and Bolivian hemorrhagic fever and Lassa fever are similar diseases.

Junin Virus in Argentina

Argentinian hemorrhagic fever occurs in certain agricultural areas of northern Argentina. The disease was recognized in the 1940s, and in the 1950s definitive epidemiologic and clinical studies culminated in the identification of Junin virus as the causative agent. The disease occurs predominantly in male field workers, who in the course of their labors contact the virus, which contaminates the environment from the excreta of chronically infected wild rodents of the genus *Calomys.* During the period from February to May when agriculture, especially of maize, is intense, thousands of cases a year may occur, with a 10 to 20 percent case fatality. Concurrent transmission of LCM virus and arboviruses may confound the clinical and epidemiologic features of the annual outbreaks.

Machupo Virus in Bolivia

Bolivian hemorrhagic fever was recognized in 1959 as a disease of agricultural workers in specific areas of Bolivia. In 1962 and 1963, the disease moved into the town of San Joaquin. Intensive investigation of this outbreak revealed Machupo virus to be the etiologic agent, and the source of human infection to be the contamination of the household environment with the excreta of chronically infected rodents of the species *Calomys.* These mice, normally found in the fields, invaded the houses of the town and thereby brought the virus to family groups in the general population. The reasons for this ecologic shift are not well understood but serve to remind us of the complexity of the balances of nature. The efficacy of domestic rodent control was established in the San Joaquin outbreak. In 1971, a small, highly fatal outbreak in an area where there are no *Calomys* was due to person-to-person spread of the infection.

Lassa Fever in West Africa

Lassa fever was first encountered in 1969 in a small outbreak of serious disease among the hospital personnel from missions in the towns of Lassa and Jos in northeastern and central Nigeria (Fig. 24-2). Subsequent to the startling events surrounding this initial outbreak, a more balanced picture of this zoonosis has emerged. Additional nosocomial outbreaks occurred in the subsequent years, and considerable concern spread to Europe and America as the result of the importation of nine cases from West Africa. Fortunately, very little spread, if any, resulted from these importations, and it can be definitively stated now that careful isolation procedures are adequate to protect hospital staff and visitors. Handling of specimens and tissues in the laboratory, however, must be done with extreme care, as fatal laboratory infections have occurred. Presently, maximum security laboratory facilities, such as the one available at the Centers for Disease Control in Atlanta, are the only laboratories where work with this virus should be carried on.

The virus, as is so far known, seems to be present in several countries of West Africa, including Liberia, Nigeria, and Sierra Leone. Studies in West Africa, guided by knowledge gained from studies of LCM, Junin, and Machupo viruses, resulted in the recognition that the rodent *Mastomys natalensis* (Fig. 24-4) carries the agent in nature with the lifelong infection that characterizes arenaviruses.

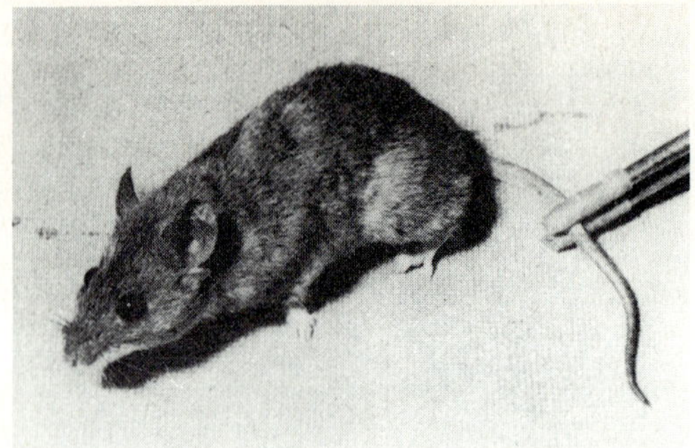

Figure 24-4. *Praomys* (*Mastomys*) *natalensis*, chronically infected reservoir host of Lassa fever virus. *(From Isaacson: Bull WHO 52: 631, 1975.)*

Humans provide the only overt indication that virus is present (indicator host) and are of little significance in the perpetuation of this agent in nature. Humans probably acquire infection from contamination by these rodents of the environment with infectious urine and excreta. Human practices that entail field burning and capture of rodents fleeing therefrom contribute to the intimate human–rodent contact necessary for transmission. For all three hemorrhagic fever arenaviruses, human-to-human transmission has been documented but is relatively unusual.

A Lassa-like virus has been isolated from the other side of Africa. This agent, named Mozambique virus, was isolated from pools of rodent (*Mastomys*) organs. So far, it is not known to cause human disease.

The clinical consequences of infection with the three viruses range from no disease and simple seroconversion to a fulminant and highly fatal condition. Following an incubation period of 1 to 2 weeks, disease begins in a nonspecific manner with fever, headache, sore throat, and myalgia. Toward the end of the first week, flushing, edema, and petechial rash of the face and neck appear in association with adenopathy and worsening of the above symptoms. Mouth lesions, exudative pharyngitis, and pulmonary symptoms may predominate in Lassa fever. During the second week, serious complications relating to loss of intravascular mass through generalized capillary leakage cause a shock syndrome characterized by peripheral vasoconstriction, generalized edema, renal failure, and metabolic acidosis. Myocardial involvement may be evident. There is moderate hemorrhage in the form of petechiae and bleeding from the gastrointestinal and genitourinary tracts, which is not sufficient to produce the shock syndrome. After a few days of the shock syndrome, the patient dies or recovery begins. During convalescence, there may be loss of hair and neurosequelae, including nystagmus, tremulousness, and episodic dizziness. In spite of considerable damage to the liver seen histopathologically, no jaundice or other signs of liver failure occur. The spleen does not enlarge. Major complications in severe

Lassa fever occur in no more than 5 percent of cases and include deafness, abortion, pleural effusion, pericarditis, orchitis, and iridocyclitis.

Laboratory findings include leukopenia, decreased platelets, increased prothrombin time, and evidence of disseminated intravascular coagulation. Protein, cells, and casts are found in the urine. The cerebrospinal fluid is normal. A chest x-ray may reveal a patchy pneumonia, and there may be electrocardiographic changes consistent with diffuse myocardial damage. During the shock syndrome, hemoconcentration may be evident.

Pathologic findings include little inflammatory response other than modest monocytic infiltrates. There is widespread edema indicative of the capillary damage that permits leakage of plasma from the intravascular space. Cellular damage may be found in many organs, including heart, muscles, lungs, liver, adrenals, kidneys, spleen, lymph nodes, and brain.

Diagnosis depends on isolation of virus from either body fluids or from tissue specimens. Mice, hamsters, or cell cultures are inoculated, depending on the virus suspected. The presence of virus in the laboratory system is detectable by a variety of means, including disease, cytopathology, and immunofluorescent techniques. Antibody response in man occurs within a few weeks of onset and is generally detected in testing for a rising titer of group-specific complement-fixing antibodies or type-specific neutralizing antibodies. Immunofluorescent antibodies appear as early as 7 days after the onset of symptoms in Lassa infections. A satisfactory neutralization test for Lassa fever has not been developed.

The general theme of clinical management of arenavirus disease calls for efforts to support basic physiologic processes long enough for the body to cure itself. There are no specific therapeutic agents except humoral antibodies derived from persons who have survived natural infection. Such immunotherapy has seemed to improve dramatically a few patients who appeared to be in imminent danger of dying. No vaccine is currently available, although experimental vaccines have been prepared and tested.

Prevention of person-to-person transmission can be achieved in any hospital by standard strict isolation techniques. Outbreaks can be controlled with measures aimed at breaking the intimate contact between the excreta of certain rodents and humans. A protocol for the management and containment of imported cases of Lassa fever has been used and is available through the Center for Disease Control of the U.S. Public Health Service.

FURTHER READING

Arenaviruses in perspective. Br Med J 1:529, 1978

Buchmeier MJ, Welch RM, Dutko FJ, et al.: The virology and immunobiology of lymphocytic choriomeningitis virus infection. Adv Immunol 30:275, 1980

Buckley SM, Casals J: Pathobiology of Lassa fever. Int Rev Exp Pathol 18:97, 1978

Cooper CB, Gransen WR, et al.: A case of Lassa fever: Experience at St. Thomas's Hospital. Br Med J 285:1003, 1982

Dowdle WR: Exotic viral diseases. Yale J Biol Med 53:109, 1980

Emond RTD, Bannister B, et al.: A case of Lassa fever: Clinical and virological findings. Br Med J 285:1001, 1982

Fuller JG: Fever! The Hunt for a New Killer Virus. New York, Readers Digest Press, 1974

Howard CR, Simpson DIH: The biology of the arenaviruses. J Gen Virol 51:1, 1980

International Symposium on Arenaviral Infections of Public Health Importance, July 14–16, 1975, Atlanta, Georgia. Bull WHO 52:381, 1975

Jahrling PB, Hesse RA, Eddy GA, et al.: Lassa virus infection of rhesus monkeys: Pathogenesis and treatment with ribavirin. J Infect Dis 141:580, 1980

Johnson KM, Monath TP, Tesh RB, et al.: Arthropod-borne viral fevers, viral encepalitides and viral hemorrhagic fevers (arboviruses and arenaviruses). In Wyngaarden JB, Smith LH (eds): Textbook of Medicine, 16th ed. Philadelphia, Saunders, 1982.

Kiley MP, Tomori O, Regnery RL, et al.: Characterization of the arenaviruses Lassa and Mozambique. In Bishop DHL, Compans RW (eds): The Replication of Negative Strand Viruses. Amsterdam, Elsevier, North Holland, 1981

CHAPTER 25

The Hepatitis Viruses

Although recognized since the fifth century BC, hepatitis is only recently becoming well understood. By the 1940s and into the 1950s, viral agents were accepted as etiologic agents of hepatitis. The most notable of these were the MS-1 and MS-2 strains of hepatitis virus reported by Krugman and later identified as hepatitis A and hepatitis B, respectively. More detailed understanding of these viruses began with the discovery of the Australia antigen in 1964 by Blumberg. This chapter summarizes current concepts in viral hepatitis, and reflects largely the data acquired by many investigators since 1964.

Characterization of the Hepatitis Viruses

By definition, viral hepatitis is an infection of the liver caused by one of four or more distinctly different viruses: hepatitis A virus (HAV), hepatitis B virus (HBV), non-A, non-B hepatitis virus or viruses (NANB), and δ-associated agent. Table 25-1 summarizes some of their known characteristics.

Noted in Table 25-2 is the terminology used for the hepatitis viral antigens and antibodies, which serve as the basis for identification. Because the sequence of development and disappearance of these viral markers is generally predictable, it serves as the basis for diagnosing the specific diseases that each virus causes. Although there is a simple interpretation for each marker, as indicated in Table 25-2, it should also be noted that observation of the course of events is as useful as the presence or absence of any single marker.

Both commercial and research methods are available to test for these markers, which each have various advantages and disadvantages. The sensitivity and the specificity of each method are noted in Tables 25-3 and 25-4. In these tests, each antigen is specific to a particular virus; that is, antigen has been detected that is common to more than one class of virus. Within each individual group, all strains are alike in terms of virulence, disease produced, complications, and cross-protection, except for NANB, which in all probability is composed of distinctly different virus types.

Pathogenesis and Pathology

Direct viral-induced cytopathogenicity is one plausible explanation for some of the pathologic features of the disease, but immune mechanisms (both humoral and cellular) may better account for some of the extrahepatic manifestations. In acute hepatitis, pathologic findings typically consist of an accumulation of inflammatory cells and parenchymal necrosis, which are variously distributed in the portal, periportal, and lobular areas of the liver. These findings usually disappear completely after clinical recovery. Among the four groups there are currently no accepted differences in the pathology of acute hepatitis. Chronic hepatitis, a disease peculiar to HBV and NANB, is described in the following section.

Clinical Disease

As well as being pathologically indistinguishable, the acute infections are also symptomatically indistinguishable. Patients are commonly anicteric, a finding present in from 30 to 70 percent of the reported cases. NANB hepatitis may

TABLE 25-1. CHARACTERISTICS OF THE HEPATITIS VIRUSES

Virus	Virus Family: Genus	Size	Nucleic Acid	Cloned	Grown in Tissue Culture	Identified by Electron Microscopy	Specific Serologic Tests	Infectious for Animals	Special Characteristics
HAV	Picornaviridae: *Enterovirus 72*	27 nm	Single-stranded RNA	No	Yes	Yes	Yes	Yes	—
HBV	Not yet classified	42-nm Dane particle 22-nm surface antigen	Primarily circular, double-stranded DNA	Yes	Yes*	Yes	Yes	Yes	—
NANB	Unknown	Unknown	Unknown	No	No	No	No	Yes	Probably two or more different viruses
δ-associated agent	Unknown	35–37 nm	RNA-associated	No	No	No	Yes	Yes	Requires HBV for replication

*Reported but unconfirmed.
HAV, hepatitis A virus; HBV, hepatitis B virus; NANB, non-A, non-B hepatitus virus or viruses.

be the one most likely to fall into this category. The typical illness, when it occurs, consists of lassitude, anorexia, weakness, nausea, vomiting, headache, chilliness, abdominal discomfort, fever, dark urine, and a variety of less frequent symptoms and signs. Laboratory findings reflect liver cell necrosis, such as aminotransferase abnormalities. Bilirubin and, less frequently, alkaline phosphatase may also be abnormal. Each type of abnormality may persist beyond the typical 2 to 4 weeks of illness, may appear to relapse after apparent resolution, or may resolve completely save for persistent hyperbilirubinemia, but these courses are unusual. These unusual courses are benign, like most cases of acute hepatitis, in that they resolve completely and spontaneously. The diagnostic laboratory tests that can identify the specific disease are noted in Table 25-2.

Despite the general similarity of symptoms and pathology, each class of virus has unique features. Figure 25-1 shows schematically the usual course of acute hepatitis for each virus, and Table 25-5 outlines the sequelae associated with each. Distinctive features are as follows:

Hepatitis A

Hepatitis A is characterized by an absence of many of the features found in other forms of hepatitis. In particular, there are no extrahepatic manifestations of the acute infection, no chronic hepatitis, no long-term carrier state, and

TABLE 25-2. NOMENCLATURE OF THE HEPATITIS VIRUS ANTIGENS AND ANTIBODIES AND THEIR GENERAL INTERPRETATION

	Antigens		Antibodies	
Virus	Name	Interpretation	Name	Interpretation
HAV	HA Ag* (Major antigen of HAV)	Acute infection	Anti-HA	
			IgG†	Immune to HAV
			IgM†	Recurrent or current acute infection
HBV	HBsAg† (Surface antigen of HBV)	Prior exposure to HBV	Anti-HBs†	Immune to HBV
	Subtypes adr, adw, ayw, ayr	Distinctive strains of HBV		
	HBcAg* (Core antigen of HBV)	Infectivity—acute or chronic	Anti-HBc†	Early or late convalescence or chronic hepatitis
	HBeAg† (A core-related antigen)	Infectivity—acute or chronic	Anti-HBe†	Late convalescence
NANB	—‡	—	—‡	—
δ-associated agent	δ antigen*	Acute δ-associated hepatitis	Anti-δ*	Immune to δ-associated hepatitis

*Research tools only.
†Tests currently clinically available.
‡Reportedly identified but not confirmed.
HAV, hepatitis A virus; HBV, hepatitis B virus; NANB, non-A, non-B hepatitis virus or viruses.

TABLE 25-3. METHODS FOR DETECTING HEPATITIS B s ANTIGEN (HBsAg)

Methods	Relative Sensitivity	Ease of Performance	Time Required for Completion (hours)
Immunodiffusion (ID, AGD)	1	Simple	24–72
Counterimmunoelectrophoresis (CIE)	2–10	Simple	2
Complement fixation (CF)		Moderate	18–24
Reversed passive latex agglutination		Simple	0.1–0.2
Passive hemagglutination inhibition (HAI)		Moderate	2
Immune adherence hemagglutination		Moderate	2
Radioimmunoassay (RIA)	100		
Solid phase		Moderate	4–24
Double antibody (DA-RIA, RIP)		Complex	24–72
Reversed passive hemagglutination (RPHA)		Simple	1–4
Enzyme-linked immunosorbent assay (ELISA)		Moderate	2–24

Adapted from Howard, Burrell: Structure and nature of hepatitis B antigen. Prog Med Virol 22:36, 1976.
AGD, agar gel diffusion; RIP, radioimmunoprecipitation.

no recognized association with either cirrhosis or primary hepatocellular carcinoma. A fulminant form of acute hepatitis occurs in 1 to 4 percent of patients, as it does in hepatitis B.

Hepatitis B

Hepatitis B differs from hepatitis A in a number of significant respects. First, there is a wide range of extrahepatic manifestations including arthralgias, particularly of the small joints, and a variety of immunologically mediated diseases such as arteritis, nephritis, and dermatitis.

Second, there are chronic forms of hepatitis B, defined as those illnesses lasting longer than 6 months. These fall into two general classifications: chronic persistent hepatitis and chronic aggressive hepatitis. In terms of ultimate outcome, chronic persistent hepatitis is a benign illness. This form of hepatitis B is ordinarily not symptomatic, but patients who are tested show abnormal findings on liver function tests and the persistence of many HBV markers, including hepatitis B s antigen (HBsAg), hepatitis B e antigen (HBeAg), and antihepatitis B c (HBc) antibody. Liver biopsy findings further reveal the transient abnormalities associated with acute hepatitis and, most importantly, the absence of the more advanced pathology found in the serious and second form of chronic hepatitis B, namely chronic aggressive hepatitis.

TABLE 25-4. METHODS FOR DETECTING ANTI-HBs

Method	Relative Sensitivity
Immunodiffusion	1
Counterimmunoelectrophoresis	1–4
Complement fixation	2–10
Passive hemagglutination	1000–10,000
Solid-phase radioimmunoassay	1000–10,000
Radioimmunoprecipitation	10,000–100,000

Adapted from Howard, Burrell: Structure and nature of hepatitis B antigen. Prog Med Virol 22:36, 1976.

In chronic aggressive hepatitis, the patient is clinically indistinguishable from the one with chronic persistent hepatitis. However, the anti-HBc antibody may be present in very high titer, and the liver biopsy shows widespread lymphocyte infiltration of portal tracts and lobules, piecemeal necrosis, and bridging necrosis. This pathologic picture is a recognized precursor to cirrhosis and possibly to primary hepatocellular carcinoma. As yet, it is not possible to predict the frequency with which this sequence of events occurs, but the cause-and-effect association seems certain. How long it takes to develop these very serious consequences is also not known. Once it has developed, however, most cases of chronic aggressive hepatitis seem to persist indefinitively. This is most unlike the expected course with chronic persistent hepatitis, which resolves spontaneously and completely, without progression to the more serious sequelae. As desirable as it might be to be able to predict which cases of acute hepatitis B will become chronic, no reliable markers have yet been identified to allow this prognostication. Once chronic hepatitis develops, HBeAg should be measured.

HBeAg was described by Magnius and Espmark in 1972. Distinct from either the 22-nm free HBsAg and the 42-nm Dane particle, this antigen is a soluble protein that correlates with HBcAg and DNA polymerase, is a marker of infectivity, and suggests continued activity of chronic hepatitis. In addition, HBeAg–IgG immune complexes are thought to be pathogenetic in the induction of membranous glomerulonephritis. On the other hand, antibody to HBeAg correlates with the absence of HBcAg and DNA polymerase; much less infectivity; a better prognosis for chronic hepatitis; and, possibly, omission of nephritis. Continued liver disease, however, may be observed independent of infectious virus, and immunopathologic mechanisms may continue to play a role in the pathogenesis.

The third way that hepatitis B differs from hepatitis A is that the patient with hepatitis B may continue for a long time to be a carrier of either the whole infectious virus or the HBsAg. About 0.1 to 1 percent of the adult population

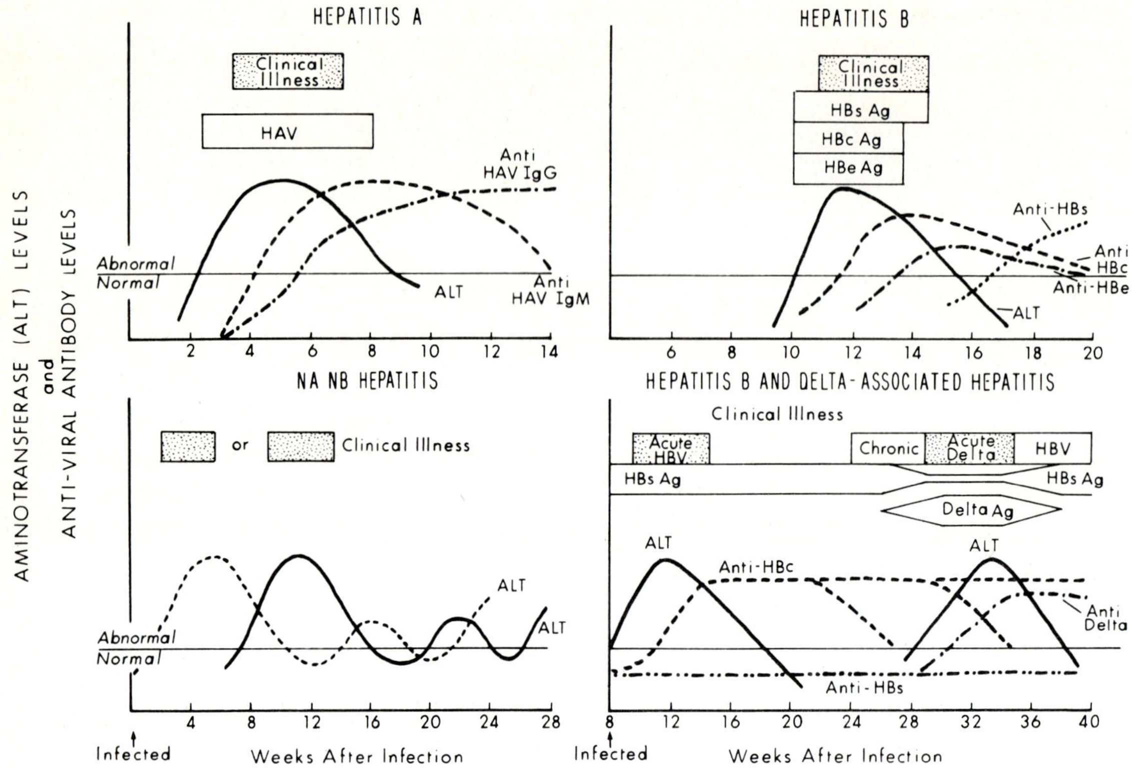

Figure 25-1. The panels illustrate the sequence of development of clinical illness, liver function abnormalities, and hepatitis antigen and antibody for each of the four currently recognized forms of viral hepatitis.

are asymptomatic carriers, and approximately 5 percent of the recognized cases of acute HBV infection become carriers of HBV. Some patients spontaneously cease to be carriers, but most persist beyond 6 months after the acute infection. Patients more likely to be long-term carriers are: (1) nonwhites; (2) males; (3) infants; and (4) those who are immunosuppressed, such as dialysis patients or patients receiving immunosuppressive drugs. The carrier may or may not be infectious. There are currently no available tests that make this distinction, but among the several types of patients more prone to being infectious carriers are: (1) those who have had a recent infection; (2) those with a high titer of anti-HBc antibody; (3) those with detectable HBeAg; and (4) those who are immunocompromised. In contrast, those with anti-HBs or anti-HBe antibodies are less likely to be infectious. From a practical point of view, all carriers should be considered potentially infectious.

The fourth difference is that cirrhosis and primary hepatocellular carcinoma are probable sequelae of hepatitis B because the HBV genome is integrated into the DNA of tumor cells. Furthermore, epidemiologic studies have confirmed a significant association of HBV infection and the incidence of hepatocellular carcinoma.

TABLE 25-5. CLINICAL CHARACTERISTICS OF VIRAL HEPATITIS

						Chronic Hepatitis			Associated with Cirrhosis
Virus	Anicteric: Icteric	Incubation Period	Acute	Extra-hepatic Manifestations	Fulminant/ Mortality	Persistent	Aggressive	Carrier	Primary Hepatocellular Carcinoma
HAV	1:2.1	25 days	+	–	+/1–4 percent	–	–	–	–/–
HBV	1:2.1	75 days	+	+	+/1–4 percent	2–4 percent	2–4 percent	5 percent	+/+
NANB	4–6:1	50 days post-tx sporadic	+	+	+/0.1–0.2 percent	15 percent	30 percent	+(? percent)	+/–
δ	Unknown	Unknown	+	Unknown	Unknown	Unknown	Unknown	Unknown	Unknown

HAV, hepatitis A virus; HBV, hepatitis B virus; NANB, non-A, non-B hepatitis virus or viruses; post-tx, post-transfusion; +, present; –, absent.

Non-A, Non-B Hepatitis

Non-A, non-B hepatitis is a diagnosis of exclusion. It can be made only after the exclusion of HAV with an IgM anti-HAV antibody; HBV with an HBsAg and an IgM anti-HBc antibody; and a variety of other infectious and noninfectious diseases, i.e., infectious mononucleosis, cytomegalovirus, syphilis, measles, varicella, rubella, mumps, leptospirosis, bacterial sepsis, cholecystitis, ischemic necrosis, and Wilson's disease. Several investigators have reported promising antigen/antibody systems for making a positive diagnosis of NANB, but none is completely satisfactory.

Evidence is substantial that more than one virus causes NANB hepatitis. For one, there is a wide range of incubation periods. A preliminary suggestion is that there are at least two broad categories—one of rather short incubation (2 to 4 weeks), and the other of rather long incubation (16 to 24 weeks). For another, there are second episodes of NANB. Other evidence is the suspected histopathologic differences and the definite cross-challenge experiments in chimpanzees. Aside from these, three general groups of NANB have been identified based on its occurrence—the epidemic form, those cases associated with parenteral exposures, and sporadic cases.

As with HBV, NANB seems to be transmitted primarily by parenteral routes and is the leading cause of posttransfusion hepatitis (PTH). In efforts to obviate this complication, it has been found that a significant reduction in the incidence of PTH can be achieved by using donor blood that has an aminotransferase activity of less than 45 IU/liter. Unfortunately, most donors have normal alanine transferase (ALT) levels, and the logistic and financial costs of routine donor testing make this a problematic solution to the unacceptable frequency of PTH.

Both a carrier state and the incidence of chronic hepatitis have been documented with NANB. The frequency of chronic hepatitis seems to be even greater with this virus than it is with HBV. Posttransfusion chronic hepatitis may occur in up to 54 percent of cases, whereas sporadic occurrence may account for only 20 percent. Although the frequency of chronic non-A, non-B hepatitis is high, the severity is usually more benign than that accompanying HBV. Also, complete resolution without sequelae is usual, especially among the sporadic. But parenterally acquired (e.g., that involving PTH, illicit drug use, or hemodialysis) chronic hepatitis may persist and progress. Symptoms and liver function tests are not necessarily infallible indicators of continuously active liver disease.

δ-Associated Agent

Rizzetto and his colleagues described the δ/anti-δ antigen–antibody system in 1977. They had detected δ antigen in the nuclei of liver cells of only HBsAg-positive patients with chronic liver disease. Antibody to δ was later found to be associated with, but distinct from, HBV (it was present in 19.1 percent of patients with chronic hepatitis; in 2.6 percent of chronic carriers of HBsAg; and in low titers transiently in 4.8 percent of patients with acute HBV infection), and it was not detected in the sera of HBsAg-negative controls. Patients who had been multiply transfused and were HBsAg-positive had a higher incidence of anti-δ antibody than nontransfused HBsAg carriers did. These data suggested that the δ-associated agent was transmitted both parenterally and nonparenterally by superinfection or coinfection of HBsAg carriers. Animal studies confirmed that it is transmittable and that it requires HBV as some sort of helper while it inhibits the replication of HBV. It has been further characterized biochemically and biophysically as being a protein that is encapsulated with low molecular weight RNA in a particle 35 to 37 nm in diameter. Recent studies suggest that it may be a very important determinant in the development of the carrier state and chronic liver disease.

Epidemiology

Consideration of the trends in occurrence, risk factors, and modes of transmission is extremely important for understanding viral hepatitis. Between 1970 and 1980 the number of new reported cases of hepatitis of all types has decreased. This decrease is accounted for by a reduction in the rate (cases per 100,000 population) of hepatitis A from 27.87 in 1970, to 12.84 in 1980. Hepatitis B increased from 4.08 to 8.35 over the same interval, and unspecified hepatitis increased from 3.95 to 5.39 from 1974 to 1980.

Viral hepatitis is transmitted by a wide variety of routes. Table 25-6 summarizes these routes and their relative frequency. HAV is present in the feces of infected patients during the 2 weeks preceding and several weeks following the onset of clinical disease. It may be present in the blood and other body fluids for a short period of time, but fecal–oral transmission of the HAV virus is by far the most prevalent route. The finding of an unexpectedly high incidence of HAV among male homosexuals suggests the possibility of sexual transmission, but more likely, this is due to fecal–oral transmission during oral–anal contact.

For HBV, NANB, and δ-associated diseases, blood is the major route, although other body fluids may possibly transmit virus as well. This has been especially well documented for HBV. In contrast with HAV, feces are not infectious or, if they are, it is at a very low level unless contaminated by blood. Therefore, not surprisingly, the usual mode of transmission is by parenteral exposure to viral-contaminated blood or blood products. This mechanism is facilitated because HBV and NANB may persist in the serum in carriers. It is especially important to recognize that blood and blood products from different sources have a different risk of possessing infectious virus. Most whole blood and its derivatives, which are not prepared by the pooling of units, have a relatively smaller risk of inducing infection with HBV. This is largely due to the infrequency of HBV carriage in the normal adult population, the exclusion of potentially infected donors, and perhaps

TABLE 25-6. MAJOR ROUTES OF HEPATITIS VIRUS TRANSMISSION

Virus	Major Infectious Body Fluid	Route of Transmission*			
		Parenteral	Fecal/Oral	Sexual	Vertical
HAV	Feces	–	4+	+/–	–
HBV	Blood and other body fluids	4+	+/–	2+	3+
NANB	Blood	4+	+/–	+/–	+/–
δ	Blood	4+	–	–	–

*Estimates of the relative frequency (from – to 4+).
HAV, hepatitis A virus; HBV, hepatitis B virus, NANB, non-A, non-B hepatitis virus or viruses; +, present; –, absent.

most importantly, the routine testing of donor blood for HBsAg. Preparations generally considered to be safe are serum albumin, thrombin, profibrinolysin, fibrinolysin, immune serum globulin (ISG), and all hyperimmune globulins. At higher risk are blood and blood products derived from commercial (as opposed to volunteer) donors, and those derived from pools of plasma and clotting factors I, II, VII, IX, and X. Washed and frozen human blood cells are not reliably virus free, and should also be considered a risk. Furthermore, as no tests are available to exclude NANB from blood or blood products, none of the above measures are known to eliminate this virus. As it might be expected, posttransfusion hepatitis is most often due to NANB. Hepatitis caused by either HBV or NANB may be acquired by other parenteral routes, such as illicit drug use or accidental needle-stick, or accidental injury such as might occur during surgery.

Nonparenteral routes of transmission have also been reported for HBV, NANB, and δ-associated disease. There is strong evidence that all these viruses, but particularly HBV, may be transmitted by close personal contact, including sexual contact.

Prevention

The mainstays of viral hepatitis prevention are the correct diagnosis and reporting of new cases, attention to standard principles of cleanliness and hygiene, and specific

TABLE 25-7. RECOMMENDATIONS FOR USE OF IMMUNE GLOBULINS

Virus Exposure	Time of Evaluation	Nature of Exposure	Recommended Immune Globulin: Immune Serum Globulin*	Recommended Immune Globulin: Hyperimmune Hepatitis B Immune Globulin†
HAV	Preexposure	Travel to endemic area	+	–
	Postexposure	Household	+	–
		School or work	–	–
		Institution	+	–
		Primate handler	+	–
		Medical and paramedical personnel	+	–
		Common source epidemic	+	–
HBV	Preexposure	Personnel or family members attending and infected patient	+	–
	Postexposure	Parenteral		
		Transfusion of HBsAg positive blood	–	+
		Accidental	–	+
		Needle-stick, surgical injury, blood on open wound, or mucous membrane		
		Nonparenteral		
		Intimate contact	+	–
		Postnatal	–	+
NANB	Postexposure	Parenteral		
		Transfusion	+	–
		Accidental	+	–
δ-associated agent‡				

*0.01–0.02 ml/kg body weight dose within 14 days of exposure, if possible.
†0.05–0.07 ml/kg body weight dose within 7 days of exposure, and repeated 1 month later.
‡No present indications for use of globulins with δ-associated agent exposure.
HAV, hepatitis A virus; HBV, hepatitis B virus; NANB, non-A, non-B hepatitis virus or viruses; +, indicated; –, not indicated.

measures to eliminate the sources of infection. These methods are only partially successful, and additional measures have, therefore, been used.

Passive immunity through the use of immune globulin is one such approach. Table 25-7 summarizes current recommendations for the use of ISG and hyperimmune hepatitis B immune globulin. It should be noted that there is general, but not complete, agreement on these recommendations among authorities.

Active immunization is now a viable option for the prevention of HBV, for a vaccine is now available. The vaccine is a preparation of purified HBsAg from HBsAg carriers who are free of infectious virus of all known types. In studies performed on over 10,000 recipients, the vaccine has been shown to induce anti-HBS antibody in over 95 percent of normal adult recipients. Because anti-HBs antibody is considered to be the immunologic defense that confers immunity, it is not surprising that it is 85 to 95 percent effective in the prevention of naturally acquired hepatitis B. In the same studies, minor self-limited side effects were observed at a rate equal to that of the placebo control. No serious long-term side effects were observed in the period up to 7 years after immunization. It appears that this vaccine will be an extremely useful preventive in the control of this disease.

Treatment

No specific effective therapy has been identified for any of the diseases associated with the hepatitis viruses. Supportive measures are still the best therapy. Although corticosteroids have been used for a variety of the sequelae of hepatitis, there are no proved indications for this form of therapy. In fact, these agents may have adverse effects.

FURTHER READING

Barker LF, Gerety RJ, Tabor E: The immunology of the hepatitis viruses. Adv Intern Med 23:327, 1978

Beasley RP, Hwang LY, Lin CC, et al.: Hepatocellular carcinoma and hepatitis B virus. A prospective study of 22,707 men in Taiwan. Lancet 2:1129, 1981

Bernstein LH, Koff RS, Siegel ER, et al.: The hepatitis knowledge base—A prototype information transfer system. Ann Intern Med 93:165, 1980

Blumberg BS: Polymorphisms of the serum proteins and the development of iso-precipitating antibodies in transfused patients. Bull NY Acad Med 40:377, 1964

Centers for Disease Control Hepatitis Surveillance. Washington, D.C., U.S. Department of Health and Human Services, Public Health Service, Report 47, 1981

Dienstag JL: Immunopathogenesis of the extrahepatic manifestations of hepatitis B virus infection. Springer Semin Immunopathol 3:461, 1981

Francis DP, Hadler SC, Thompson SE, et al.: The prevention of hepatitis B with vaccine: Report of CDC multicenter efficacy trial in homosexual men. Ann Intern Med 97:362, 1982

Gerety RJ: Non-A, non-B hepatitis. New York, Academic Press, 1981

Howard CR, Burrell CJ: Structure and nature of hepatitis B antigen. Prog Med Virol 22:36, 1976

Ishak KG: Light microscopic morphology of viral hepatitis. Am J Clin Pathol 65:787, 1976

Koff RS: Viral hepatitis. New York, Wiley, 1978

Krugman S, Giles JP, Hammond J, et al.: Infectious hepatitis—Evidence for two distinctive, epidemiological and immunological types of infection. JAMA 200:365, 1967

Krugman S, Gocke DJ: Viral hepatitis. Philadelphia, Saunders, 1978

Levy GA, Chisari FV: A proposed role for the immune system in the pathogenesis of hepatitis B virus induced liver disease. CRC Crit Rev Clin Lab Sci 15:335, 1981

Seeff LB, Hoofnagle JH: Immunoprophylaxis of viral hepatitis. Gastroenterology 77:161, 186, 1979

Szmuness W, Stevens CE, Harley EJ, et al.: Hepatitis B vaccine—Demonstration of efficacy in a controlled clinical trial in a high-risk population in the United States. N Engl J Med 303:8323, 1980

Szmuness W, Alter HJ, Maynard JE (eds): Viral Hepatitis. Philadelphia, Franklin Institute Press, 1981

Szmuness W, Stevens CE, Harley EJ, et al.: HBV vaccine in medical staff of hemodialysis units. Efficacy and subtype cross-protection. N Engl J Med 307:1481, 1982

Vyas GN, Cohen SN, Schmid R (eds): Viral Hepatitis—A Contemporary Assessment of Etiology, Epidemiology, Pathogenesis and Prevention. Proceedings of the Second Symposium on Viral Hepatitis. Philadelphia, Franklin Institute Press, 1978

CHAPTER 26

Miscellaneous Viruses: Reoviruses and Rhinoviruses

Reoviruses

Possession of a segmented genome of 10 to 12 genes of double-stranded RNA is now the criterion for classifying viruses as Reoviridae. The family name has evolved from the original designation of human isolates as respiratory enteric orphan (REO) viruses.

Human reoviruses were first isolated in the early 1950s and initially identified as echovirus type 10 until 1959, when these agents were designated as reovirus serotype 1. A macaca monkey isolate (SV59) was designated reovirus type 2 in 1960, and a human virus pathogenic for mice, first reported in 1953, was designated reovirus type 3 in 1961.

Mammalian reoviruses are inhabitants of the human gastrointestinal tract. They have been detected in healthy persons and occasionally in persons with an array of inconsequential respiratory and/or gastrointestinal illnesses. Three different serotypes have been isolated from sporadic cases of encephalitis, hepatitis, meningitis, fatal pneumonia, and other diseases. They have no clearly defined role in these associated human illnesses. In infants, reovirus infection has been associated with mild febrile illness, diarrhea, and exanthem. The most characteristic pattern of adult infection as judged by recovery of virus is that of an afebrile coryzal illness occurring in the winter. It is clear that asymptomatic infections, as documented by virus isolation, are common. The presence of neutralizing antibody in serum seems to be relatively protective against infection with the homologous serotype and may give some degree of protection against infection with heterologous types. The reoviruses have not been of major epidemiologic importance, but infection of humans is common throughout the world.

A recent clinical serologic association of reovirus type 3 with human biliary atresia is a provocative observation in view of the ability of reovirus type 3 to infect bile duct cells and produce obstructive jaundice in a weanling mouse model.

The three serotypes of mammalian reoviruses have also been obtained from many species of animals including chimpanzees, calves, pigs, cats, and sheep. Serologic evidence of infection has been shown in virtually all of the biologic species tested.

Pathogenesis of Infection

The reoviruses have been studied in great detail in mouse models of infection. The segmented genome has facilitated their study because gene assortment occurs easily and is readily detected in recombinant progeny. Thus, the molecular virology of these viruses has been utilized to gain insight into clinical problems. It has been possible to dissect several virulence factors of these viruses for mice, thus illustrating the complexity of interaction of the host and the virus. The direct relevance of these observations to the pathogenesis of human infection is not yet established.

A summary of the interaction of the virus with the murine host follows. The virus gains entry to the host through the gastrointestinal tract. Reovirus type 1, but not type 3, successfully establishes infection in the mouse gut. Through the use of recombinant viruses, it has been demonstrated that an outer capsid protein, μlC (a cleavage product of protein μ1), coded for by gene M1, varies in its sensitivity to proteases. The μ1C protein of reovirus type 1 confers resistance to proteolysis in the gastrointestinal tract, and enables pinocytosis of the virus by M epithelial cells, subsequent access to Peyers patches, replication in lymphoid tissue, and dissemination of virus. Thus, one facet of virulence is the ability to resist nonspecific degradation of infectious virus to noninfectious cores by the action of host proteases within the gastrointestinal tract. Specific antibody directed against μ1C does not neutralize infectivity or prevent hemagglutination, but will bind and precipitate virus particles.

Of great importance in virulence is the σ1 protein encoded by the S1 gene. Only 24 molecules of this protein are present per virion in contrast with an estimated 900 of another outer capsid protein, σ3. Protein σ1 specifies cell tropism, as it is the attachment protein of the virus that interacts with specific receptors on the cell surface. The specificity of the σ1 protein of reovirus type 1 is for ependymal cells, whereas that of reovirus type 3 is for neurons. Thus, intracerebral inoculation of reovirus type 1 produces infection of ependymal cells, an inflammatory response, and scarring of the aqueduct with resulting hydrocephalus at a later time. In contrast, intracerebral inoculation of reovirus type 3 produces infection of neurons and rapidly fatal encephalitis. Thus, a single gene, S1, encodes a protein that determines specific cell interactions and tissue tropism in the host.

The σ1 protein is also the hemagglutinin, and the first of three proteins stimulating the formation of neutralizing antibody. These functions are on separate domains of the σ1 protein. This protein is also responsible for the association of reovirus particles with microtubules in cells. Sensitized T lymphocytes, both cytolytic and suppressor cells, identify this protein, which is also expressed on the surface of infected cells.

The outer capsid shell of reovirus is largely (about 99 percent) composed of the μ1C and σ3 proteins. They have a strong affinity for each other and probably exist as complexes in the capsomers. Proteins σ1 and σ3 are removed after virus gains entry into cells. The loss of part of the outer capsid shell results in activation of enzymes essential for mRNA synthesis. Antibody to protein σ3 also neutralizes infectivity and inhibits hemagglutination. Thus, a second protein is capable of stimulating a host antibody response, which may contribute to protection of the animal.

The third protein inducing neutralizing antibodies is λ2, a core protein, present in about 60 copies per virus particle. It is the major component of the 12 core projections or spikes through which single-stranded transcripts of reovirus genes can be liberated. The fact that antibodies to this protein neutralize infectivity of virus and inhibit hemagglutination indicates that these spikes project through the outer capsid shell. It has been shown that antibody to λ2 prevents antibody to σ1 from binding to this protein. Thus, σ1 must be near λ2, and the λ2 antibody may neutralize infectivity by blocking the σ1 protein from access to specific host cell receptors. Finally, antibody to λ2 of any of the three serotypes of reovirus interacts with the λ2 protein of all three serotypes. Therefore, by definition, this protein is group reactive, which suggests common determinants are present on the λ2 protein of all three serotypes of reovirus.

As would be predicted from the above information, creating a recombinant virus with a serotype 1 M1 gene and a serotype 3 S1 gene produces a virus capable of infecting the mouse by the oral route, of disseminating infection, and of establishing a fatal encephalitis. Reovirus has two proteins defined thus far that are essential to their virulence in animals. Proteins located on the surface of the virus are involved in adsorption to host cells, stimulation of neutralizing antibodies and sensitization of lymphocytes.

Diagnosis

The mammalian reoviruses replicate and produce visible cytopathic effects in a wide variety of cell cultures. Primary rhesus cell cultures are satisfactory for routine isolation, but primary human kidney cells have been used when it was essential to exclude the possibility of endogenous infection of monkey kidney cells. The cytopathic effect consists of a granular change in the cytoplasm and the cells do not slough off the glass quickly. Often they remain attached to the surface by a single cytoplasmic process and may appear to be undergoing nonspecific degeneration. Stained preparations show intracytoplasmic eosinophilic inclusions. Isolates have been obtained primarily from fecal specimens and, less often, from the respiratory tract. They have also been seen on occasion from other sources such as urine, cerebrospinal fluid, and various tissues obtained at autopsy.

The serotypes of reoviruses have been identified by the hemagglutination inhibition technique. Human infection is associated with a demonstrable antibody rise to the homotypic serotype. The antibody rise is measured by type-specific hemagglutination inhibition or neutralization. The heterologous rise in antibodies to other serotypes is explained by the antibody to group reactive λ2 protein. The high prevalence of reovirus antibodies makes it mandatory that an antibody titer rise be demonstrated to document the presence of acute infection. The detailed studies of the antigens associated with reoviruses have made it possible to measure an antibody response to individual proteins and to use measurements other than neutralization or inhibition of hemagglutination. These methods include radioimmunoprecipitation, immunodiffusion, and immunofluorescence. For example, studies that have examined the potential role of reovirus type 3 in biliary atresia have utilized patient sera for indirect immunofluorescence of infected cells. This has demonstrated that these sera have reovirus antibodies despite the absence of neutralizing antibodies. Although the antigens (and the induced antibody) responsible for the immunofluorescence remain to be defined, it seems probable that the $\sigma 1$ protein will not be one of these antigens. Thus, if this is reovirus infection, the absence of neutralizing antibodies suggests an unusual virus–host interaction.

Rhinoviruses

Over 100 serotypes constitute the genus Rhinovirus of the Picornaviridae family. These 25- to 30-nm particles have a naked icosahadral nucleocapsid containing a single-stranded RNA genome. The first isolate in 1956 was initially classified as echovirus 28, but subsequently it has been appreciated that, in contrast to other picornaviruses, the rhinoviruses are acid labile and are destroyed at a pH of less than 3. This property explains their failure to survive passage through the gastrointestinal tract. The rhinoviruses have a buoyant density of 1.38 to 1.41 g/cm^2 in cesium chloride, which is higher than that of enteroviruses. The picornaviruses all share the property of capsid assembly in the cytoplasm of infected cells, and mature virus particles contain four capsid proteins as a result of cleavage of a common precursor. Rhinoviruses (nose viruses) are important causes of acute respiratory infections, with predominant illness occurring in the airway above the larynx.

Clinical Illness

The usual symptoms of a rhinovirus common cold are nasal obstruction and discharge, sneezing, scratchy throat, mild cough, and malaise. Virus replication is limited to the respiratory tract. Human epithelial cells containing rhinovirus antigens have been demonstrated in the nasal mucus of infected individuals, but the amount of damage to the nasal epithelium appears to be minimal. Severe tracheobronchitis and even atypical pneumonia may occur rarely in adults, and rhinovirus infection has been associated in a few studies with acute exacerbation of chronic obstructive pulmonary disease. As with influenza and respiratory syncytial virus (RSV) infections, hyperreactive small airways have been demonstrated in adult volunteers with rhinovirus-caused illness. Fever and significant lower respiratory tract involvement in the form of bronchiolitis or pneumonia are more common with rhinovirus infection of children, and symptomatic infections have been temporally associated with the precipitation of asthma attacks. There is need to clarify the role of rhinoviruses in these illnesses and, although they are infectious agents contributing to the overall occurrence of respiratory disease, they are not of the importance of respiratory syncytial virus and the parainfluenza viruses.

Detectable serum antibody correlates positively with resistance to infection. Repeated infections with these agents occurs throughout life and, therefore, antibody positivity increases with age. Nasal antibody is often detected in individuals with naturally occurring serum antibody. Experimental work suggests that the quantity of serum antibody is a good indicator of type-specific resistance to rhinovirus infection, and that nasal antibody is an important component of immunity to rhinoviruses. Volunteer study has shown initial appearance of IgA and IgG in nasal secretions after infection and specific antibodies become detectable within the first several days after experimental infection. If this is the first experience with the virus, the serotype specific antibody is present after approximately 1 week of infection. Similarly, serum antibody—usually IgG, but occasionally IgM—also begins to be detectable at about 1 week into the infection, with peak levels occurring at approximately 1 month. If the person has experienced rhinovirus infection previously, an anamnestic response is observed.

Epidemiology

Rhinovirus infections have been documented in all populations studied. They occur throughout the year, but in a temperate climate there is some tendency for an increased incidence from April through October. Children frequently serve to introduce rhinoviruses into the family unit, with subsequent illnesses occurring usually after a 2- to 3-day incubation period. Occasional epidemics with a single serotype have been described, but more often multiple serotypes appear to be circulating at the same time. Rhinoviruses seldom repeat within a population from year to year. Human rhinoviruses are limited in their host range, and only the chimpanzee and gibbon have been shown to be experimentally susceptible.

Shedding of rhinoviruses in respiratory tract secretions has been amply documented. Experimental studies of transmission of these viruses have shown that transmission may occur by way of aerosols under intimate circumstances, but, surprisingly enough, a more efficient means of transmission of virus is by hand contact and self-inoculation of the mucous membranes of the eye or nasal mucosa. Comparative studies have indicated that this route of infection is more efficient than that of either large or small particle aerosols. The importance of hand contact and self-inoculation observed in experimental circumstances where the variables are well controlled raises questions as to the main mode of transmission of infection in naturally occurring infection. Viral contamination of objects in the environment frequently occurs. Experimental studies tend to support the concept that rhinoviruses will not ordinarily be transmitted in public gathering places or with relatively short exposure to friends or relatives with colds. Rather, transmission is far more likely where hand contact with viral-containing secretions occurs. The observed unpredictability of intrafamilial transmission of these viruses tends to support the concept that virus is not easily transmitted by aerosol. Finally, recent studies have successfully interrupted experimental rhinovirus transmission by the use of local application of aqueous iodine solution to the hands. Effectiveness of iodine in interrupting viral transmission in volunteers suggests that hand contamination and self-inoculation of the virus may be the most important route by which these agents are transmitted.

Diagnosis

Acute upper respiratory symptoms can be caused by multiple viruses. A tentative assignment of probable rhinovirus etiology can be made to illnesses occurring in the characteristic seasonal pattern and producing typical mild symptoms. To specifically distinguish rhinovirus infection from other etiologic agents requires virus isolation and demonstration of a rise in antibody titer between acute and convalescent sera. The assays for antibody must be done with neutralization tests against the specific rhinovirus causing the infection. This specific serologic identification of the agent requires multiple cross-neutralization tests and is impractical for general use.

Rhinoviruses are best recovered by inoculating a nasal specimen into human fibroblast cells or human embryonic kidney cell cultures. To obtain an optimal yield of these viruses, the culture should be incubated at 33C to 35C and at a neutral pH. The cytopathic effects usually become visible within the first week after inoculation and infected cells are visible as a focus of oval or refractile cells. Cell lysis and diminution in cell number occurs. At the present time, detection of antigen by immunofluorescence of respiratory secretions is impractical because the large number of rhinovirus serotypes requires multiple antisera. No commerically available sources of hyperimmune sera exist. An isolate can be identified as a rhinovirus by its physicochemical properties, especially acid lability, which will distinguish rhinoviruses from enteroviruses.

Treatment

Treatment of rhinovirus infection is generally aimed at relief of symptoms. Hydration and preventing obstruction of the airways, paranasal sinuses, and eustachian tubes are the mainstays of therapy. Aspirin has been commonly prescribed and although some diminution in symptoms may occur, increased virus shedding has been documented in persons receiving aspirin therapy. Interferon has been tested for effectiveness against the rhinoviruses. The total number of infections was unaltered, although some diminution in the frequency of symptomatic illness could be attributed to the administration of low doses of prophylactic human leukocyte interferon applied topically to the nasal mucosa. The quantity of interferon appears to be of critical importance, and thus far there is no practical or inexpensive way in which this material can be used. Finally, in apparently well-designed studies, vitamin C has not significantly decreased the number of colds.

Prevention

Resistance to reinfection with the same rhinovirus serotype can be shown following an initial infection. The major obstacle to the formation of any proposed vaccine is the existence of the more than 100 antigenically distinct serotypes of rhinoviruses. Trials have suggested that production of materials of appropriate potency is difficult, and there are questions concerning whether a parenterally administered rhinovirus vaccine is protective because of the need for stimulation of nasal antibody. At the present time, vaccination appears unlikely to be a successful method of prophylaxis against rhinovirus colds.

Probably of greater importance is the possibility of diminishing the spread of infection. Recognition that contaminated hands play a role provides the opportunity to interrupt transmission with such basic measures as hand disinfection. One study has shown that iodinated paper, which is virucidal for rhinoviruses, successfully diminished the incidence of respiratory illness.

FURTHER READING

REOVIRUSES

Epstein RL, Powers ML, Weiner HL: Interaction of reovirus with cell surface receptors. III. Reovirus type 3 induces capping of viral receptors on murine lymphocytes. J Immunol 125:1800, 1981

Fontana A, Weiner HL: Interaction of reovirus with cell surface receptors. II. Generation of suppressor T cells by the hemagglutinin of reovirus type 3. J Immunol 125:2660, 1980

Morecki R, Glaser JH, Cho S, et al.: Biliary atresia and reovirus type 3 infection. N Engl J Med 307:481, 1982

Rubin DH, Fields BN: Molecular basis of reovirus virulence. Role of the M2 gene. J Exp Med 152:853, 1980

Sabin AB: Reovirus: A new group of respiratory and enteric viruses formerly classified as ECHO type 10 is described. Science 130:1387, 1959

Weiner HL, Drayna D, Averill DR, et al.: Molecular basis of reovirus virulence. Role of the S1 gene. Proc Natl Acad Sci USA 74:5744, 1977

Weiner HL, Powers ML, Fields BN: Absolute linkage of virulence and central nervous system cell tropism of reovirus to viral hemagglutinin. J Infect Dis 141:609, 1980

RHINOVIRUSES

Butler WT, Waldmann TA, Rossen RD, et al.: Changes in IgA and IgG concentrations in nasal secretions prior to the appearance of antibody during viral respiratory infection in man. J Immunol 105:584, 1970

Cate TR, Roberts JJ, Russ MA, et al.: Effects of common colds on pulmonary function. Am Rev Resp Dis 108:858, 1973

Greenberg SB, Harmon MW, Couch RB, et al.: Prophylactic effect of low doses of human leukocyte interferon against infection with rhinovirus. J Infect Dis 145:542, 1982

Gwaltney JM, Moskalski PB, Hendley JO: Hand-to-hand transmission of rhinovirus colds. Ann Intern Med 88:463, 1978

Gwaltney JM, Moskalski PB, Hendley JO: Interruption of experimental rhinovirus transmission. J Infect Dis 142:811, 1980

Stanley ED, Jackson GG, Panusarn C, et al.: Increased virus shedding with aspirin treatment of rhinovirus infection. JAMA 231:1248, 1975

Turner RB, Hendley JO, Gwaltney JM Jr: Shedding of infected ciliated epithelial cells in rhinovirus colds. J Infect Dis 145:849, 1982

CHAPTER 27

Subacute Spongiform Encephalopathies/Unconventional Viruses

The agents considered in this chapter are those causing progressive degenerative central nervous system diseases with very similar histopathologies. It is from this histologic appearance that the term subacute spongiform encephalopathy is derived. The four known naturally occurring diseases of the central nervous system caused by unconventional viruses include two in humans, kuru and Creutzfeldt–Jakob disease (CJD), and two in animals, scrapie and transmissible mink encephalopathy. The agents causing the subacute spongiform encephalopathies have been more difficult to characterize than the conventional viruses. Examination of their chemical and physical properties suggests that they are simpler and smaller than conventional viruses. Recognizable virus particles have not been visualized by electron microscopy of infected cells or in preparations concentrated by density gradient banding that have subsequently been shown to have a high infectivity. Perhaps the best working hypothesis for a model of these agents is one similar to a membrane protein, featuring a small nucleic acid capable of coding for a single polypeptide.

The illnesses caused by these agents are transmissible conditions characterized by slow evolution of the clinically evident symptomatology, which invariably involves the central nervous system. Each of these diseases has an incubation period of months to years, and a protracted, relentlessly progressive illness that is almost invariably fatal. All of these diseases have been transmissible to animals by injection of infected tissues. One of the unique features of this group of illnesses is the lack of inflammatory reaction of involved tissues (central nervous system), and the normal cerebrospinal fluid in the face of devastating illness. In accord with these findings, there has been no measurable host cellular or humoral immunity to these agents, although infected hosts have no impairment of the overall function of their immune system.

The technical difficulties of working with these agents are immense. Quantitation of virus is dependent upon infection of animals. The prolonged incubation period, as well as the species specificities (Table 27-1), make quantitation tedious, expensive, and time-consuming.

It is yet to be determined if a single "unit" causes infection or if successful infection requires many "units." Similarly, the basic question of whether these agents are truly self-replicating or whether they liberate an undefined infectious product whose properties are specified by cellular genes is not yet known. It is clear that infectivity of tissue is associated with cellular membranes.

Primary cell lines maintaining the infectious viruses of kuru, CJD, and scrapie have been derived from the brains

TABLE 27-1. HOST RANGES OF THE UNCONVENTIONAL VIRUSES

	Nonprimate	Primate
Scrapie, kuru, and Creutzfeldt–Jakob disease		Capuchin, squirrel, cynomologous macaque, rhesus, spider
Kuru and Creutzfeldt–Jakob disease	Ferret	Chimpanzee; marmoset; wooly monkey, African green monkey, mangabey, pig-tailed macaque
Kuru	Mink	Gibbon, bonnet
Creutzfeldt–Jakob disease	Cat, goat, guinea pig, hamster, mouse	Stump-tailed macaque, patas
Scrapie	Gerbil, goat, hamster, mink, mouse, rat, sheep, vole	Not susceptible: cat, chimpanzee

of patients and animals with spongiform encephalopathies. The cultures do not differ morphologically from those of uninfected tissues, and infectivity is ultimately lost after several months. The infected cultures contain amounts of virus much smaller than those from the original tissues and, thus, investigations must continue primarily to use animals as sources of virus.

Infections of Humans

Kuru

The Fore people of Papua, New Guinea's eastern highlands, used the word *kuru* to describe trembling from fear or cold. This came to be the name of a disease characterized by tremors, which was confined to this Melanesian tribe of 35,000 persons in isolated mesolithic villages. At the time of the first description of this illness by Gajdusek and Zigas in 1957, the disease was the most common cause of death among these people, and the death rate was as high as 2 to 3 percent annually.

Kuru is a distinctive neurologic syndrome, and there is an extraordinary uniformity of the clinical signs, symptoms, and course of the disease. Clinical disease is initially recognized by clumsiness in walking or inability to maintain balance. There may be associated minor changes in mood and personality. The relatively minor changes in coordination may be present for 12 to 18 months before generalized disease becomes readily apparent. After definite neurologic symptoms are recognized, the course of the disease is ordinarily fatal over the next 12 to 18 months. The initial clumsiness progresses so that the patient becomes unable to balance and finally unable to sit, stand, or perform any voluntary movement. At this stage, excessive contraction of synergistic muscles and associated movements in other limbs create exhausting ineffective muscular activity. Speech is slurred and becomes unintelligible, and chewing and swallowing are affected. Clinical examination reveals signs of cerebellar dysfunction. Changes in mood, emotional lability, depression, and episodes of confusion are common. Disability of memory and language functions are apparent. Unable to eat, aspirating secretions, and developing pneumonia and decubitus ulcers, the patients die.

Epidemiology

The incubation periods of kuru range from 4.5 years to more than 30 years. Pregnant women have been infected, but the agent was not transmitted transplacentally. Found commonly in children of both sexes and women, kuru is uncommon in adult males. The ritualistic cannibalism of the immediate family members ordinarily involved women and small children, and it is likely that the handling of the infected tissues allowed access of the agent to breaks in the skin or mucous membranes, with the consumption of infected tissue less important in transmission of disease. No one born after cannibalism ceased has acquired kuru, and no outsider in contact with patients has ever acquired the disease. Human-to-human transmission has been limited exclusively to the ritual of cannibalism.

Pathology

The pathology of this disease is as uniform as the clinical illness. Macroscopically the cerebral hemispheres appear normal, whereas the cerebellum is atrophied. Microscopically the most severe degeneration occurs in the cerebellum, where there is a loss of Purkinje and granule cells. The spongiform changes of gray matter of the cerebral cortex and cord seem to be vacuolar enlargements of neuronal processes, and are apparently of intradendritic origin. Accumulations of membranous material in these swellings are apparent. Microglial cells are seen in all stages of phagocytic activity, and there is a proliferation of astrocytes with a dense gliosis throughout the cerebellar cortex. Amyloid plaques are also apparent. There has never been any evidence of inflammatory reaction or demyelination of white matter.

Kuru has been transmitted to experimental animals and the pathology of nonhuman primates resembles that of humans. Infectivity is as high as 10^9 infectious units per gram of brain tissue, and animal inoculation studies have shown lower titers sometimes present in spleen, liver, or nodes. Infectivity has not been found in blood, cerebrospinal fluid, urine, white blood cells, milk, amniotic fluid, or placenta. Intracerebral, intravenous, intramuscular, subcutaneous, or intraperitoneal injections regularly transmit infection, but incubation periods range from 1 to 8.5 years. A single experiment successfully transmitted infection orally to a squirrel monkey, whereas many other experiments have failed. Thus, experiments suggest penetration of skin or mucosal membrane is a far more likely avenue of infection.

Creutzfeldt–Jakob Disease

Clinical and Epidemiologic Features

Creutzfeldt–Jakob disease, a progressive fatal disease of the central nervous system, occurs in middle life and affects both sexes. It was originally described as a rare form of presenile dementia in approximately 1920. Vague prodromal symptoms are followed by dementia, with subsequent rapid progression to coma and death, usually within 2 years after recognition of symptoms. The dementia can be accompanied by other neurologic disturbances, which may include focal cortical degeneration, both upper and lower motor neuron signs, extrapyramidal signs, cerebellar ataxia, and seizures. Associated myoclonus is characteristic, and there is often a typical electroencephalogram. There is great variability in the clinical syndrome.

This disease occurs throughout the world, with the rate thought to be 1 or 2 per 1 million population. Libyan Jews have a rate of over 30 times higher, and there may be a familial form of the disease in approximately 10 percent of patients, involving several generations of a family. It is not highly transmissible, as evidenced by the fact (1) that there are only two reports of conjugal cases of disease and (2) that none of the people in closest contact with CJD patients, including wives, friends, and health care professionals, appear to be at any higher risk of contracting infection than the general population. Thus far, neuropathologists, research scientists, and laboratory personnel do not appear to be at excessive risk.

The only definitive evidence of transmission has occurred with the recognition of several patients who presumably acquired infection from contaminated stereotactic electroencephalographic electrodes or from a corneal transplantation. The incubation period is estimated to be at least 15 to 20 months in these situations, where direct inoculation has occurred. The natural latency period must be much longer because of the absence of disease in children or young adults.

There can be no doubt about the transmissibility of this disease, as Gadjusek and associates have reported that 111 inoculations of 373 specimens resulted in successful transmission of disease to nonhuman primates. The results of additional inoculations are still pending. The agent has been found less regularly and in lower concentrations in lymph nodes, liver, kidney, spleen, lung, cornea, and cerebrospinal fluid than in the brain and spinal cord. The brain has been shown to contain at least 10^8 infectious units per gram. This agent has not yet been isolated from body surfaces, secretions, or excretions. It therefore seems that acquisition of diseases occurs by tissue penetration.

Pathology

The diverse clinical manifestations are matched by the spectrum of the distribution and severity of the pathologic lesions. Brains may look normal or they may be small and atrophic. The microscopic changes always include neuronal loss, status spongiosus (less marked than in kuru), and proliferation of hypertrophic astrocytes. Brains of inoculated animals also show status spongiosus as one of the major pathologic findings, together with neuronal loss, proliferation of astrocytes, and absence of inflammation.

Disinfection for Creutzfeldt–Jakob Disease Agent

No special ward isolation procedures are warranted. In fact, such procedures may be an inconvenience to patient and personnel alike, and, if specified, may prevent optimal care of the patient or admission to a long-term facility. Exposure to breath, saliva, nasopharyngeal secretions, or urine of CJD patients should not cause special concern. Washing of hands or other exposed areas of the skin with appropriate detergent is recommended, as in contact with any other patient with potentially transmissible agents. Although a patient's blood or cerebrospinal fluid could be potentially infectious, simple washing should be sufficient to protect exposed persons. Caution must be taken to avoid accidental percutaneous exposure to blood, cerebrospinal fluid, or brain tissue. If a puncture occurs, careful washing in iodine solution, phenolic antiseptic, or 0.5 percent sodium hypochlorite is appropriate. Some of the physical and chemical properties of these agents are listed in Table 27-2. The preferred method of disinfection of equipment is either a 1-hour exposure to 5 percent sodium hypochlorite or autoclaving at 121C. Choice of method depends upon the material being treated. Surgical instruments, tonometers used on demented patients, and all instruments used in eye operations should be considered contaminated.

TABLE 27-2. SOME PHYSICAL AND CHEMICAL PROPERTIES OF UNCONVENTIONAL AGENTS

1. Sensitive (loss of infectivity) to: autoclaving (121C, 15 ψ, 60 min), phenol, sodium hypochlorite (5 percent), ether, acetone (moderate)
2. Resistant to: formaldehyde, glutaraldehyde, B-propriolactone, EDTA, 80C (partial inactivation at 100C), proteases (trypsin, pepsin, pronase, proteinase K), nucleases (DNase, RNase, micrococcal nuclease), phospholipases, nonionic or mildly ionic detergents (triton, NP-40, deoxycholate, sarkosyl)

Subacute Spongiform Encephalopathies in Animals

Scrapie

Scrapie has been known for some 200 years as a clinical entity in sheep in Europe, and for over a 100 years a chronic disease affecting the central nervous system of sheep was prevalent in a region of northern Iceland. The name of the disease in Icelandic, *rida,* means either ataxia or tremor. This is a progressive disease of adult sheep, which is inevitably fatal. The sheep fail to thrive, become frightened and excitable, and then the tremor and uncoordinated movements of the head appear. The animal becomes clumsy, with initial involvement of hind limbs. Finally, the animal is unable to walk, and despite remaining alert, is totally immobilized by tremors and spastic movements. This disease is scrapie, but without the characteristic pruritus seen in other geographic locations. Vertical transmission of infection to offspring is usual and, in nature, lateral transmission is also quite common. Hadlow first suggested that the neuropathology was similar to that of kuru, and Gajdusek then pursued the possibility that kuru was caused by an infectious agent.

Scrapie can be transmitted by inoculation to a number of animals (Table 27-1), and sheep, goats, and mice have been infected with scrapie by the oral route. The pathogenesis of scrapie has been studied in mice and, although the route of infection influences the incubation period and ultimate outcome, several general features emerge. Inoculated virus can be almost completely recovered from spleen in the first week after infection. Infectivity is no longer detectable for the subsequent several weeks. About 1 month after inoculation, replication becomes apparent, with initial reappearance of the agent in the spleen and nodes, then spreading through the lymphoid system. Replication in lymphoid tissue does not alter immune function or produce any apparent pathology. About 3 months after inoculation, infectivity is detectable in the central nervous system. It also is detectable in salivary glands, lung, intestine, and other tissues. The animals remain asymptomatic for a total of 4 to 5 months.

Transmissible Mink Encephalopathy

Transmissible mink encephalopathy is a rare sporadic disease occurring only in ranch mink. It was first noted in 1947 in Wisconsin, with additional outbreaks from 1961 through 1963. It, too, is a chronic progressive neurologic disease characterized by early behavioral changes, ataxia, and somnolence. The incubation period is approximately 8 to 9 months after oral inoculation, and 5 to 6 months following parenteral inoculation. Experimentally, the disease is transmitted to mink by various routes of inoculation using suspensions of infected brain or other tissues. The similarity to scrapie was noted in 1965. Like the other diseases discussed above, pathologic lesions are restricted to the central nervous system and the pathology is similar. Differences from the other illnesses consist only of variation in the topographic distribution of the lesions.

Experimental studies demonstrate detectable virus 16 weeks after inoculation, visible pathologic lesions 24 weeks after inoculation, and recognizable clinical disease approximately 30 weeks after inoculation. It is now thought that transmissible mink encephalopathy most likely originates from mink having been fed scrapie-infected sheep or goat tissues. Experimentally, mink are susceptible to United States sources of scrapie, but not those from the United Kingdom. It has also been suggested that the natural route of infection in mink is from bite wounds inflicted by litter mates. These observations have led to questions concerning the identities of these agents relative to each other. Is there only one such agent, i.e., scrapie that has been transmitted to mink and humans? Is kuru a result of CJD spreading in the Fore by inoculation through cannibalism? At the present time there is no evidence for epidemic spread of any of the spongiform encephalopathies.

FURTHER READING

Books and Reviews

Prusiner SB, Hadlow WJ (eds): Slow Transmissible Diseases of the Nervous System. Vol I. Clinical, Epidemiological, Genetic and Pathological Aspects of the Spongiform Encephalopathies. Vol II. Pathogenesis, Immunology, Virology, and Molecular Biology of the Spongiform Encephalopathies. New York, Academic Press, 1979

Selected Papers

Brown P, Gibbs CJ Jr, Amyx HL, et al.: Chemical disfunction of Creutzfeldt–Jakob disease virus. N Engl J Med 306:1279, 1982

Gajdusek CD, Gibbs CJ Jr, Asher DM, et al.: Precautions in medical care of, and in handling materials from patients with transmissible virus dementia (Creutzfeldt–Jakob disease). N Engl J Med 297:1253, 1977

Gibbs CJ Jr, Amyx HL, Bacote A, et al.: Oral transmission of Kuru, Creutzfeldt–Jakob disease and scrapie to non-human primates. J Infect Dis 142:205, 1980

Klatzd I, Gajdusek DC, Zigas V: Pathology of Kuru. Lab Invest 8:799, 1959

Manuelidis EE, Angelo JN, Gorgacz EJ, et al.: Experimental Creutzfeldt–Jakob disease transmitted via the eye with infected cornea. N Engl J Med 296:1334, 1977

Sigierdsson B: Observations on three slow infections of sheep. Br Vet J 110:255, 307, 341, 1954

Zigas V, Gajdusek DC: Kuru: Clinical study of a new syndrome resembling paralysis agitans in natives of the Eastern Highland of New Guinea. Med J Aust 2:765, 1957

Index